THE PSYCHOLOGY OF THINKING
ABOUT THE FUTURE

THE PSYCHOLOGY OF
THINKING ABOUT THE FUTURE

EDITED BY

Gabriele Oettingen
A. Timur Sevincer
Peter M. Gollwitzer

THE GUILFORD PRESS
New York   London

Printed in the United States of America

This book is printed on acid-free paper.

Last digit is print number: 9   8   7   6   5   4   3   2   1

Library of Congress Cataloging-in-Publication Data is available from the publisher.

ISBN 978-1-4625-3441-8 (hardcover)

About the Editors

Gabriele Oettingen, PhD, is Professor of Psychology at New York University and the University of Hamburg, Germany. Dr. Oettingen's research differentiates among various types of thinking about the future and examines their developmental and situational origins, as well as their effects on the control of cognition, emotion, and behavior. She has pointed out the perils of positive thinking and discovered mental contrasting, an imagery-based self-regulation technique that, by drawing on nonconscious processes, is effective for mastering one's everyday life and long-term development. Dr. Oettingen has published in journals of social, personality, developmental, educational, health, clinical, organizational, and consumer psychology, as well as in neuropsychological and medical journals. Her work led to the creation of effective and easy-to-apply behavior change interventions, and she is the author or coauthor of several books in the area of behavior change.

A. Timur Sevincer, PhD, is Assistant Professor in the Institute of Psychology at the University of Hamburg, Germany. Dr. Sevincer's primary research interest is motivation and self-regulation, including, for instance, the spontaneous use of self-regulation strategies, their effect on physiological energization, the effect of alcohol on motivation and self-regulation, and motivational underpinnings of migration toward cosmopolitan cities. Dr. Sevincer is the author or coauthor of more than 25 scholarly publications in such journals as *Psychological Science*, the *Journal of Personality and Social Psychology*, the *Journal of Abnormal Psychology*, *Personality and Social Psychology Bulletin*, and *Motivation and Emotion*.

Peter M. Gollwitzer, PhD, is Professor of Psychology at New York University and the University of Konstanz, Germany. Dr. Gollwitzer's research examines how goals and plans affect people's cognition, affect, and behavior. He has developed various models of action control: the theory of symbolic self-completion (with Robert A.

Wicklund), the Rubicon model of action phases (with Heinz Heckhausen), the auto-motive model of automatic goal striving (with John A. Bargh), the mindset model of action phases, and the theory of implementation intentions. In these theories, the underlying mechanisms of effective action control are delineated, and respective moderators are distilled. Dr. Gollwitzer's recent research focuses on developing easy-to-conduct but powerful behavior change interventions. He has published many influential journal articles, book chapters, and books.

Contributors

Francis T. Anderson, BA, BS, Department of Psychological and Brain Sciences, Washington University in St. Louis, St. Louis, Missouri

Cristina M. Atance, PhD, Department of Psychology, University of Ottawa, Ottawa, Ontario, Canada

Daniel M. Bartels, PhD, The University of Chicago Booth School of Business, The University of Chicago, Chicago, Illinois

Roger Buehler, PhD, Department of Psychology, Wilfred Laurier University, Waterloo, Ontario, Canada

Adam Bulley, BA, School of Psychology, The University of Queensland, St. Lucia, Queensland, Australia

Charles S. Carver, PhD, Department of Psychology, University of Miami, Coral Gables, Florida

Marina Chernikova, MS, Department of Psychology, University of Maryland, College Park, College Park, Maryland

James F. M. Cornwell, PhD, Department of Behavioral Sciences and Leadership, United States Military Academy, West Point, New York

Christina Crosby, BA, Department of Psychology, New York University, New York, New York

Franziska Damm, MSc, Institute of Psychogerontology, Friedrich-Alexander University Erlangen–Nuremberg, Nuremberg, Germany

Maria K. DiBenedetto, PhD, Science Department, Bishop McGuinness High School, Kernersville, North Carolina

Carol S. Dweck, PhD, Department of Psychology, Stanford University, Stanford, California

Gilles O. Einstein, PhD, Department of Psychology, Furman University, Greenville, South Carolina

Andrew J. Elliot, PhD, Department of Psychology, University of Rochester, Rochester, New York

Kai Epstude, PhD, Department of Psychology, University of Groningen, Groningen, The Netherlands

Angelica Falkenstein, MA, Department of Psychology, University of California, Riverside, Riverside, California

Ayelet Fishbach, PhD, The University of Chicago Booth School of Business, The University of Chicago, Chicago, Illinois

Michael Gilead, PhD, Department of Psychology, Ben-Gurion University of the Negev, Beer-Sheva, Israel

Paul W. Glimcher, PhD, Center for Neural Science, New York University, New York, New York

Peter M. Gollwitzer, PhD, Department of Psychology, New York University, New York, New York, and Department of Psychology, University of Konstanz, Konstanz, Germany

Dale Griffin, PhD, UBC Sauder School of Business, The University of British Columbia, Vancouver, British Columbia, Canada

Hal E. Hershfield, PhD, UCLA Anderson School of Management, University of California, Los Angeles, Los Angeles, California

E. Tory Higgins, PhD, Department of Psychology, Columbia University, New York, New York

Lucian Hölscher, PhD, Department of Modern History, Ruhr University Bochum, Bochum, Germany

Jeremy P. Jamieson, PhD, Department of Psychology, University of Rochester, Rochester, New York

Katarzyna Jasko, PhD, Institute of Psychology, Jagiellonian University, Krakow, Poland

Evan M. Kleiman, PhD, Department of Psychology, Harvard University, Cambridge, Massachusetts

Anna B. Konova, PhD, Center for Neural Science, New York University, New York, New York

Arie W. Kruglanski, PhD, Department of Psychology, University of Maryland, College Park, College Park, Maryland

Frieder R. Lang, PhD, Institute of Psychogerontology, Friedrich-Alexander University Erlangen–Nuremberg, Nuremberg, Germany

Gary P. Latham, PhD, Rotman School of Management, University of Toronto, Toronto, Ontario, Canada

Nira Liberman, PhD, Department of Psychology, Tel Aviv University, Tel Aviv, Israel

Edwin A. Locke, PhD, Department of Management and Organization, Robert H. Smith School of Business, University of Maryland, College Park, College Park, Maryland

Andrew K. MacLeod, PhD, Department of Psychology, Royal Holloway, University of London, Egham, United Kingdom

James E. Maddux, PhD, Department of Psychology, George Mason University, Fairfax, Virginia

Mark A. McDaniel, PhD, Department of Psychological and Brain Sciences, Washington University in St. Louis, St. Louis, Missouri

Rory C. O'Connor, PhD, Institute of Health and Wellbeing, University of Glasgow, Glasgow, United Kingdom

Gabriele Oettingen, PhD, Department of Psychology, New York University, New York, New York

Jonathan Redshaw, PhD, School of Psychology, The University of Queensland, St. Lucia, Queensland, Australia

Daniel L. Schacter, PhD, Department of Psychology, Harvard University, Cambridge, Massachusetts

Michael F. Scheier, PhD, Department of Psychology, Carnegie Mellon University, Pittsburgh, Pennsylvania

Dale H. Schunk, PhD, School of Education, University of North Carolina at Greensboro, Greensboro, North Carolina

A. Timur Sevincer, PhD, Institute of Psychology, University of Hamburg, Hamburg, Germany

Paschal Sheeran, PhD, Department of Psychology and Neuroscience, University of North Carolina at Chapel Hill, Chapel Hill, North Carolina

Oliver J. Sheldon, PhD, Rutgers Business School, Rutgers, The State University of New Jersey, Newark, New Jersey

James A. Shepperd, PhD, Department of Psychology, University of Florida, Gainesville, Florida

Sushmita Shrikanth, BA, BS, Department of Psychology, University of Illinois at Chicago, Chicago, Illinois

Kate Sweeny, PhD, Department of Psychology, University of California, Riverside, Riverside, California

Karl K. Szpunar, PhD, Department of Psychology, University of Illinois at Chicago, Chicago, Illinois

Yaacov Trope, PhD, Department of Psychology, New York University, New York, New York

Thomas L. Webb, PhD, Department of Psychology, University of Sheffield, Sheffield, United Kingdom

David S. Yeager, PhD, Department of Psychology, The University of Texas at Austin, Austin, Texas

Marcel Zeelenberg, PhD, Department of Social Psychology, Tilburg University, Tilburg, The Netherlands

Contents

PART III. GOALS AND PLANS

Introduction

Gabriele Oettingen
A. Timur Sevincer
Peter M. Gollwitzer

Thinking about the future means thinking about experiences that one may or may not have, about a world that may or may not develop, and about actions one may or may not perform. Though we all mentally experience future events and scenarios in our minds, the imagined future almost always looks different from what will actually happen in real life. The future is uncertain, and thinking about the future evokes feelings of uncertainty. Much of what we wish for the future will never materialize. Is thinking about the future, then, a waste? All idle daydreams and fantasies, hopes that will never be fulfilled, and threats feared in vain? But if so, why would we still spend so much time in daily thinking about the future, planning scenarios that will never occur, daydreaming about satisfactions that will never happen, and making predictions that eventually turn out wrong? How much of our time do we "waste" thinking about the future during our lives? People report thinking about the future approximately once every 15 minutes, on average, when asked to record all their future-oriented thoughts during a day (D'Argembeau, Renaud, & van der Linden, 2011). Compared with the past, people think about the future about two to three times more often (Baumeister, Vohs, & Hofmann, 2015; Gardner & Ascoli, 2015).

In this volume, we hope to show that thinking about the future is not necessarily a waste of time. Quite the opposite, in fact: The ability to think about the future is a gift to humankind. Given that the future is still yet to come, it is open to change and malleable and therefore particularly relevant for behavior. This book is about the psychology of thinking about the future. To that effect, it examines the question of how thinking about the future influences our behavior, and thus ourselves, our surroundings, and the world at large. In relation to behavior, thinking about the future has three separate functions, each with its own mechanisms: (1) It allows us to mentally explore the future, visualizing its endless possibilities; (2) it helps us predict the future based on extrapolations from the past; and (3) it helps us to focus on specific objectives in the future, paving the way to reaching our goals.

Past research has largely focused on the second and third functions of thinking about the future: that is, making predictions, as manifested in our beliefs and judgments about the future, and maintaining focus, as manifested in our goals and plans. In comparison, the exploratory function of thinking about the future, how we imagine and conceptualize the many possible futures yet to emerge in our minds, has attracted less research attention.

Using these three functions of thinking about the future as a guide, we decided to group the chapters into a setting-the-stage section and three subsequent parts corresponding with each functional aspect. The first part refers to imagery and the exploratory aspects of thinking about the future; the second part refers to beliefs and judgments and the predictive aspects of thinking about the future; and the third part refers to goals and plans and the focusing aspects of thinking about the future. Dividing the book in this way has thus resulted in an unequal number of chapters in each section. Part II, on beliefs and judgments, and Part III, on goals and plans, have 9 and 11 chapters, respectively, both more than double Part I, on imagery, which has 4. We interpret this inequality as a signal of the large opportunity and space for future research in studying the psychology of thinking about the future, particularly its imagery and how it is conceptualized.

Next to providing an overview of research regarding the three functional aspects of thinking about the future, another aim of this volume is to bring together scientists from different disciplines who study future-thinking. To that end, we asked scholars from different subdisciplines within psychology, including clinical, cognitive, comparative, developmental, educational, health, organizational, and social psychology, as well as neuroscientists, for contributions. We also invited scholars from the fields of history and economics for their perspectives.

Scrutinizing the terminology used across the research literature on the psychology of thinking about the future, we find a wide variety of seemingly unrelated terms. Researchers investigate predictions, expectations, the sense of self-efficacy, beliefs of control, optimism–pessimism, current concerns, goals, intentions, plans, possible selves, future selves, mental time travel, episodic future thinking, mental simulations, mind wandering, future fantasies, and many more. We hope to show with this volume that although unconnected at first sight, these different and varying terms frequently overlap in their operationalizations and are used in ways that often serve similar descriptive functions.

We seek to bridge research investigating similar phenomena, albeit using different terms and theoretical approaches. Communicating across the different lines of research might open up new questions that would eventually lead to a reduction of terms and to a deepening of our understanding of why, how, and with what consequences people spend so much time "living" in the future. We hope this interdisciplinary approach will facilitate connecting phenomena that scientists have previously investigated in isolation and that it will link together innovative basic and applied research that, ultimately, will help people to more effectively pursue and fulfill their desired futures.

Readers will learn how the way people think about the future affects such important variables as well-being, physical health, academic performance, job performance, ethical behavior, financial spending, prosocial behavior, and many more everyday concerns and behaviors. They will also learn how thinking about the future changes in childhood and across the lifespan. Finally, throughout the volume, readers will learn about the most effective self-regulation strategies that help people to effectively pursue and realize their desired futures in many domains (e.g., achievement, interpersonal, health).

This volume should be of interest to undergraduate and graduate students in psychology, as the topic of future-thinking touches many of the most influential psychological concepts (e.g., self-efficacy, mindsets, approach–avoidance motivation). With its interdisciplinary approach, it should attract not only students and scholars in psychology but also those in neighboring disciplines, such as neuroscience, sociology, economics, medicine, and educational science. Finally, with its translational perspective on how to use future-thinking to foster effective self-regulation, it should be of help to lay people who wish to learn how to effectively pursue their goals, make better decisions, and regulate their thoughts, emotions, and behavior.

OVERVIEW OF THE CHAPTERS

Setting the Stage

We start the book by setting the stage. Three chapters elucidate how thinking about the future can be approached from the perspectives of different fields. The first contribution examines the topic from a historical perspective, showing that across history people had different conceptions of the future. The second comes from the perspective of comparative psychology, exploring future-oriented cognition and behavior in nonhuman species. Finally, the third contribution comes from a neurocognitive perspective, providing a broad psychological classification of different forms of thinking about the future derived from what we know about thinking about the past.

In the first of the three opening chapters (Chapter 1), Lucian Hölscher gives a historical account of how people conceived of the future throughout different historical time periods. These "past futures" (i.e., the visions people of the past had regarding what their futures would look like) shaped their subsequent decisions and actions, regardless of whether these visions became true or not (and, indeed, most did not). Hölscher argues that the concept of the future itself and the degree to which people were oriented toward the future has changed over time. The future as a temporal "space of time" is a relatively new invention, arising around the time of the European Enlightenment. Many societies' thinking about the future has continually cycled through phases of optimism and pessimism, but the current technological changes may be giving way to a new way of thinking, in which people become less future-oriented and more attuned to the present.

In Chapter 2, Jonathan Redshaw and Adam Bulley explore future-oriented cognition and behavior in nonhuman species. They propose that members of nonhuman species are capable of considerably more sophisticated future-oriented behavior than was once thought. For example, in the domain of navigation and route planning, they are capable of delaying gratification, preparing for future threats, acquiring and constructing tools to solve future problems, and acquiring, saving, and exchanging tokens for future rewards. Redshaw and Bulley suggest that animals have mental representations that go beyond the here and now, even though they may not conceive of them as representations of the future. Accordingly, simultaneously preparing for multiple, mutually exclusive versions of the future and setting reminder cues for successfully acting in prospective memory tasks is difficult for members of nonhuman species. Thus the metacognitive ability to conceive of future representations as future representations seems to be unique to humans, allowing humans to reflect on their future-thinking limitations and to compensate for them.

In the final chapter of the stage-setting section (Chapter 3), Karl K. Szpunar, Sushmita Shrikanth, and Daniel L. Schacter offer a neurocognitive perspective on thinking about the future akin to thinking about the past (i.e., episodic vs. semantic memory). They distinguish four modes of future thought—simulation, prediction, intention, and plans—and suggest that each of these modes can vary in the degree to which the contents focus on autobiographical experiences or abstract states of the world. The authors describe the methods that are typically employed in studying the different forms of future thought and discuss neuropsychological underpinnings of some of these differentiated forms.

Part I: Imagery

After setting the stage, Part I of the book examines the first form of thinking about the future outlined in this preface: imagery. We define future-oriented imagery as thoughts and images involving possible futures that occur in the stream of consciousness and that are distinct from beliefs and judgments, especially in their relations to decision making and behavior (Oettingen & Mayer, 2002; Oettingen, 2012). Related concepts are fantasies about the future, mental simulations, and mental time travel into the future. We also consider thoughts about possible pasts—both realized and unrealized—that influence future-thinking and subsequent action.

The opening chapter of Part I (Chapter 4) discusses the development of future thinking during childhood. Focusing on episodic future thinking, Cristina M. Atance suggests that the capacity to mentally project into the future develops between 3 and 5 years of age. Atance discusses different ways to assess future-thinking in children, such as asking children to select an object for future use and analyzing children's future-event narratives. She then points out similarities and differences between thinking about past episodes (mentally reexperiencing events) and thinking about future episodes. Atance also reports research exploring how future-thinking is affected by younger and older children's executive functions as assessed by the discounting of delayed rewards and prospective memory performance (i.e., forgetting to act on one's behavioral intentions). In closing, she suggests various ways to improve children's future-oriented reasoning, such as letting them experience the consequences of acting versus not acting while keeping the future in mind or encouraging them to take the perspective of another person.

In Chapter 5, Hal E. Hershfield and Daniel M. Bartels explore how thoughts about one's future self can affect present decision making, as many decisions involve making tradeoffs between the present and the future (i.e., intertemporal tradeoffs). In doing so, Hershfield and Bartels describe three theoretical perspectives on the future self: the future self as another person, continuity between selves, and failure to imagine the future consequences of one's actions. They then discuss the implications of these perspectives for decisions on behalf of the future self in various life domains such as finances, health, and ethical decision making. In closing, Hershfield and Bartels discuss possible interventions that might help people change their thinking about their future selves, connecting them more to their present incarnations, and thus foster more careful decision making involving the future.

In Chapter 6, Kai Epstude outlines the consequences of counterfactual thinking for both thinking about the future and future actions. Counterfactual thoughts are reflections about how events in the past could have turned out differently. Epstude presents a dual-pathway model that differentiates two mechanisms by which counterfactuals affect behavior: the content-specific pathway and the content-neutral pathway. Whereas the content-specific pathway refers to focusing on the specific problem at hand, the content-neutral pathway refers to broader consequences for information processing and general motivation. He argues that counterfactual thoughts represent a bridge between past possibilities and future opportunities. By simulating alternative ways in which past situations could have developed differently, counterfactuals help people to prepare for similar situations in the future. Epstude also discusses how counterfactuals relate to different forms of future-oriented cognition (e.g., prefactual thoughts, fantasizing).

In Chapter 7, Gabriele Oettingen and A. Timur Sevincer argue that positive fantasies about desired future events facilitate the mental exploration of future possibilities but are a clear hindrance when it comes to reaching that desired future and fulfilling our wishes. Experimental evidence shows that such positive thoughts and images make people feel accomplished but sap their energy. Because positive future fantasies reflect people's needs, it is important to enrich people with the energy required to fulfill those fantasies. Oettingen and Sevincer describe Fantasy Realization Theory (FRT) and the principles and mechanisms behind mental contrasting, a research-backed self-regulation strategy based on FRT. Mental contrasting which asks people to juxtapose their future fantasies with potential obstacles of reality has proven to foster behavior change and constructive action. The chapter ends with a description of the research and interventions involving mental contrasting, as well as efforts to disseminate mental contrasting as an easy-to-use and effective everyday self-regulation tool.

Part II: Beliefs and Judgments

Part II of the book focuses on the second form of future thought differentiated in this preface: beliefs and judgments. Future-oriented beliefs and judgments are subjective estimates of the likelihood with which certain future events will occur or not (Bandura, 1977; Mischel, 1973). Examples of such beliefs and judgments are expectations about the occurrence of certain future outcomes, self-efficacy expectations, general optimism and pessimism, estimates of the expected value of future outcomes, and emotions one expects to feel in the future.

The first two chapters in Part II focus on various types of expectations. In Chapter 8, Dale H. Schunk and Maria K. DiBenedetto discuss the role of expectations in the academic domain. They differentiate various types of expectations relevant in academic settings (self-efficacy expectations, outcome expectations, and expectations of success) and review research suggesting that high expectations of learning and accomplishment consistently benefit learning, motivation, self-regulation, and academic achievement. They also describe interventions that successfully raise students' expectations and in this way foster academic performance. In sum, this chapter highlights the important role that students' expectations of learning and accomplishment play in their academic development.

In Chapter 9, James E. Maddux and Evan M. Kleiman focus on self-efficacy expectations and their role in physical and psychological health. Self-efficacy expectations are people's beliefs about whether they can do what is necessary to achieve desired future outcomes and prevent undesirable ones. Maddux and Kleiman explain how self-efficacy expectations differ from related constructs, how they are assessed, and how they develop and change over life. The authors also outline the research establishing how high self-efficacy expectations help people achieve desired outcomes in the domains of physical health and mental well-being via increased exercising, dieting, managing stress, and smoking cessation.

The importance of future-thinking for mental health is the subject of Chapter 10. Andrew K. MacLeod and Rory C. O'Connor distinguish between positive and negative expectations about the future. They show that people with depression, and especially those who are suicidal, hold fewer positive expectations but not necessarily more negative expectations about their future than people without depression. MacLeod and O'Connor also suggest that people with depression and those who are suicidal have difficulties disengaging from unattainable goals and engaging with new goals. This chapter underlines how important it is for well-being to let go from overly aspirational goals and commit to goals that are more feasible.

The topic of the next two chapters is optimism and pessimism. Optimism has been defined as the expectation that things will work out well, and pessimism as the expectation that things will work out badly. Charles S. Carver and Michael F. Scheier take a closer look at generalized optimism as a personal attribute or trait (Chapter 11). They argue that dispositional optimism has both genetic and environmental origins and that it is relatively stable over time. They further suggest that optimism is a social resource because optimists are good social partners. Optimists also have more positive emotional lives because they effectively cope with adversity. Finally, optimism is related to better physical health because optimists exert more effort to maintain their health and because they show better emotional well-being. Finally, Carver and Scheier discuss the question of whether optimism may also have some drawbacks (e.g., when it comes to disengaging from a failing course of action).

Chapter 12 follows up on optimism from a different angle. James A. Shepperd, Angelica Falkenstein, and Kate Sweeny investigate unrealistic optimism, defined as people's tendency to expect that their futures will be better than those of similar others and better than the future suggested by objective indicators. The authors propose that unrealistic optimism originates from desires and motivations but also from biases in information processing. Unrealistic optimism is not observed when subjective feelings of control over undesirable outcomes are low and when people have prior experience with these undesirable outcomes. People also abandon their unrealistic optimism in favor of more realistic or even pessimistic predictions when the future moves closer. This shifting away from optimism arises when people acquire new information or are motivated to avoid disappointment in case of failure and when the predicted outcomes are rare, serious, and personally relevant.

The next three chapters deal with decision making. Chapter 13 examines intertemporal decision making (i.e., decisions that involve tradeoffs between present and future outcomes) from a neuroeconomic perspective. Anna B. Konova and Paul W. Glimcher first provide a historical account of economic theories in decision making and discuss experimental methods commonly used in neuroeconomics. They then elaborate on delay discounting, the observation that people value positive outcomes less the longer they have to wait for them. The authors present research on neurobiological correlates of delay discounting and discuss whether the phenomenon stems from a lack of self-control and whether a unified-system or a dual-system approach is best at explaining the phenomenon of delay discounting. Finally, the authors address the relevance of delay discounting in understanding psychopathologies of choice (e.g., drug addiction).

In Chapter 14, Marcel Zeelenberg explores how people's anticipated emotional responses to selected and rejected choice options influence their decision making. He focuses on anticipated regret, the emotion that decision makers feel when they think about how their choices could go awry. Zeelenberg reviews economic and psychological theories on anticipated regret, and he reports research showing that anticipated regret fosters strong intentions and intention–behavior relationships. He also discusses whether anticipated regret is an emotion or simply a belief about a future emotion, and he argues that the experience of anticipated regret is qualitatively distinct from retrospective regret. Zeelenberg closes by offering various empirically tested mental strategies that people can use to regulate anticipated regret when making decisions.

In Chapter 15, Michael Gilead, Yaacov Trope, and Nira Liberman argue that the human capacity to imagine future scenarios goes hand in hand with the capacity for abstract thought. They discuss the cognitive and neural underpinnings of mental time travel and abstract thought based on construal level theory and point to similar processes involved in mental time travel and abstract thought. In addition, they discuss research demonstrating that the more temporally distant events are, the more abstract they are construed mentally. In closing, the authors outline the consequences of increased temporal distance for judgment and decision making in the domains of financial investments, altruistic behavior, and negotiations.

In the closing chapter of Part II (Chapter 16), Frieder R. Lang and Franziska Damm examine how people's future-thinking and their perspectives on time change during adulthood. Lang and Damm review research showing that, as adults age and their experience of the future becomes more limited, their perception of the passage of time accelerates, and they anticipate more negative outcomes in their expectations of the future (losses rather than gains). Lang and Damm propose that the age-related changes in future-time perspective may promote selection, optimization, and compensation processes that facilitate adaptive ways of dealing with the undesirable and burdening aspects of the perceived future time. Adults may thus flexibly and differentially respond to perceived challenges and risks of future time, as well as to the threats associated with the finitude of life.

Part III: Goals and Plans

Part III of the book addresses the third form of future thought: goals and plans. Goals are mental representations of desired future outcomes that imply a commitment to realizing these outcomes. Plans, on the other hand, are mental representations of the steps conducive to attaining a goal; they imply a commitment to strive for the respective goal in a certain, prespecified way (Gollwitzer & Moskowitz, 1996; Oettingen & Gollwitzer, 2001).

In the first chapter of Part III (Chapter 17), Peter M. Gollwitzer and Christina Crosby present research on planning out in advance how one wants to act, feel, and think in a critical future situation (opportunity, hindrance) so that one's goals can be attained. Specifically, the chapter scrutinizes if–then plans (also referred to as implementation intentions). These types of plans specify a critical situation in the *if* part and the intended response in the *then* part. The chapter begins by examining the question of why such simple plans are so effective in triggering future behavioral, affective, and cognitive responses. It then turns to highlighting studies demonstrating that if–then planning is effective in guiding all kinds of future actions, feelings, and cognitions in people. Finally, Gollwitzer and Crosby discuss potential moderators of if–then planning effects, as well as potential costs of using if–then plans in guiding one's future behavior, feelings, and cognition.

In Chapter 18, Carol S. Dweck and David S. Yeager highlight the importance of different mindsets for tackling future challenges. People with a growth mindset view their abilities as malleable and tend to set learning goals aimed at improving their abilities. People with a fixed mindset, in contrast, view their abilities as stable and tend to set performance goals aimed at getting a positive evaluation of their abilities. People with a fixed mindset tend to see negative feedback as due to their lack of relevant ability rather than lack of effort. They therefore exhibit less effort and persistence in pursuing intellectual and social goals than people with a growth mindset. Dweck and Yeager present various interventions geared toward promoting a growth mindset. It is suggested that creating growth mindsets with respect to intelligence, personality, and interpersonal relations allows people to see beyond a problematic present and begin to work toward a more promising future.

In Chapter 19, Edwin A. Locke examines why it can be difficult for people to think long range about the future even though doing so is important for many aspects of living a meaningful daily life. First, he gives a brief overview of goal-setting theory and the expansive research it has spawned since it was first introduced by Edwin A. Locke and Gary P. Latham in 1990. He then identifies a multitude of techniques that can help promote engagement in long-range thinking, illustrating each with case examples. Strategies include tying short-term goals to long-term goals, obtaining support and guidance from others, writing about one's goals, seeking feedback and tracking progress, identifying role models, evaluating one's pleasures in terms of long-term benefits, and introspecting about one's emotions, priorities, and moral values.

From the domain of organizational and industrial psychology, Gary P. Latham, in Chapter 20, begins by describing goal-setting theory, which he developed with Edwin A. Locke, before moving on to discuss the possibility of activating goals outside of people's awareness (i.e., goal priming) in organizational and industrial contexts. He describes research showing that primed goals can produce reliable effects on organizationally relevant outcome variables similar to those of consciously set goals. He also reports findings that primed learning goals produced the same differential behavioral consequences as consciously set learning goals when each are evaluated against respective performance goals. Moreover, conscious and primed goals geared for fairness have been found to have additive effects on counteracting self-serving tendencies that typically arise during negotiations. Latham closes by underlining the practical and theoretical significance of goal-priming research in organizational and industrial contexts.

In Chapter 21, Arie W. Kruglanski, Marina Chernikova, and Katarzyna Jasko discuss regulatory mode theory. Locomotion regulatory mode is the aspect of self-regulation concerned with motion and progress from state to state, whereas assessment regulatory mode is the aspect of self-regulation linked to a critical evaluation of goals and means. Given that locomotion is generally a forward-oriented movement, it is proposed that locomotors' preoccupation with movement leads to a greater future focus. A review of the literature indeed suggests that high locomotors plan more for the future, focus less on the past, and more readily initiate and maintain commitments toward desired futures. The authors further highlight that a locomotion focus can be situationally induced and discuss benefits (e.g., faster goal completion), as well as drawbacks, of a high locomotion focus (e.g., reduced readiness to learn from the past).

James F. M. Cornwell and E. Tory Higgins, in Chapter 22, start out by presenting regulatory focus theory, which distinguishes between two motivational orientations referred to as promotion and prevention focus. Applying the insights from this theory to thinking about the future, the authors reason that people with a strong promotion focus should be concerned with improving their future prospects relative to their status quo, whereas those with a strong prevention focus should be concerned with preventing the future from deteriorating relative to status quo. Cornwell and Higgins also discuss how a strong promotion focus versus a strong prevention focus, in conjunction with one's current relation to a given status quo, can lead people to prefer different options (e.g., risky vs. less risky options) in their prospective decision making. They explicate how promotion and prevention focus and the perception of one's current standing in relation to the status quo may affect risky financial investments and even the selection of presidential candidates as real-world case examples.

Chapter 23 focuses on how people appraise future performance situations. Jeremy P. Jamieson and Andrew J. Elliot describe recent research on the biopsychosocial (BPS) model of challenge and threat. According to the model, people appraise performance situations as either challenging or threatening, depending on whether their coping resources exceed situational demands or the situational demands exceed their coping resources. Jamieson and Elliot integrate the BPS model with three other approaches: the extended process model of emotion regulation, implicit theories of personality, and the analysis of achievement goals. By integrating these approaches, the authors aim to generate more accurate and process-focused predictions of a person's future cognition, affect, and action.

How people anticipate unethical temptations and how they plan to resist them is evaluated in Chapter 24. Oliver J. Sheldon and Ayelet Fishbach propose that people first identify an upcoming situation as an ethical dilemma that poses a self-control conflict and, second, plan to exercise self-control to counteract that temptation. Sheldon and Fishbach review situational factors involved in identifying upcoming ethical dilemmas, including breadth of decision frame, either a narrow or broad frame (i.e., the critical situation is seen as singular or as one of many similar upcoming situations), psychological connectedness to the decision at hand (i.e., the decision having more or less impact on other decisions to be made), and the degree of self-diagnosticity of the critical decision (i.e., indicating what kind of person one is). They argue that advanced warning of temptations, coupled with employing self-regulation strategies, facilitates resisting an experienced temptation and the urge to behave in an unethical manner. People who anticipate a future temptation have a better chance of resisting it than people who confront a temptation in the present without preparation.

In Chapter 25, Paschal Sheeran and Thomas L. Webb review research on the intention–behavior gap. Research suggests that people translate their intentions to carry out future behavior into actual behavior only to a small degree. This effect is demonstrated in a range of studies including correlational studies, statistical simulations, and experiments. Sheeran and Webb suggest moderators of the intention–behavior gap: actual and perceived control, habits and experience with the behavior, the basis of the intention (e.g., feelings of moral obligation), and properties of the respective intention (e.g., intention stability). The authors discuss what makes it so hard for people to realize their intentions and address what kind of interventions could potentially aid in the realization of intentions.

Prospective memory refers to remembering to perform future actions. In Chapter 26, Gilles O. Einstein, Mark A. McDaniel, and Francis T. Anderson suggest that people rely on multiple processes for prospective memory retrieval. Behavioral and neuroscience research supports that prospective memory retrieval can be accomplished through sustained monitoring processes, as well as through transient spontaneous retrieval processes initiated by the processing of cues that have been associated with the intention. Which process people rely on likely depends on the circumstances. For example, people rely on spontaneous retrieval when remembering to give a message to a friend and on monitoring processes when multiple intentions have to be kept in mind in a demanding air traffic control setting. In their chapter, Einstein, McDaniel, and Anderson focus on spontaneous retrieval and suggest that it occurs without the intention to retrieve at the moment that a relevant cue is processed.

The planning fallacy, the topic of Chapter 27, refers to people's tendency to underestimate the time it will take to complete a certain task, despite knowing that similar tasks have taken longer than planned. Roger Buehler and Dale Griffin write about the widely documented phenomenon of people underestimating completion times. This underestimation can happen for reasons pertaining to focusing too narrowly on plans for task completion and to the neglect of other information, such as previous experience, competing priorities, and potential barriers. Buehler and Griffin suggest that the planning fallacy extends to other domains beyond completion time predictions, including people's predictions of how much money they will spend in the future. In closing, they present interventions for reducing the planning fallacy: consideration of potential obstacles; task decomposition; consulting observers, as well as switching to an observer perspective; and engaging in backward planning.

ACKNOWLEDGMENTS

We thank Seymour Weingarten, Editor-in-Chief, and Carolyn Graham, Editorial and Contracts Administrator, at The Guilford Press for their excellent guidance from the outset of the book project to its completion. Doris Mayer deserves special thanks for her support in preparing the volume. We hope that *The Psychology of Thinking about the Future* will inspire many future research collaborations between scientists from different fields and that a better understanding of thinking about the future will help people lead constructive and meaningful lives.

REFERENCES

Bandura, A. (1977). Self-efficacy: Toward a unifying theory of behavioral change. *Psychological Review, 84,* 191–215.

Baumeister, R. F., Vohs, K. D., & Hofmann, W. (2015, February). What were you thinking?: Past, present, and future in a random sample of everyday thoughts. In G. Oettingen & A. T. Sevincer (Chairs), *Spontaneous thoughts and images.* Symposium conducted at the 16th annual meeting of the Society for Personality and Social Psychology, Long Beach, CA.

D'Argembeau, A., Renaud, O., & Van der Linden, M. (2011). Frequency, characteristics, and functions of future-oriented thoughts in daily life. *Applied Cognitive Psychology, 25,* 96–103.

Gardner, R. S., & Ascoli, G. A. (2015). The natural frequency of human prospective memory increases with age. *Psychology and Aging, 30,* 209–219.

Gollwitzer, P. M., & Moskowitz, G. B. (1996). Goal effects on action and cognition. In E. T. Higgins & A. W. Kruglanski (Eds.), *Social psychology: Handbook of basic principles.* (pp. 361–399) New York: Guilford Press.

Mischel, W. (1973). Toward a cognitive social learning reconceptualization of personality. *Psychological Review, 80,* 252–283.

Oettingen, G. (2012). Future thought and behaviour change. *European Review of Social Psychology, 23,* 1–63.

Oettingen, G., & Gollwitzer, P. M. (2001). Goal setting and goal striving. In A. Tesser & N. Schwarz (Eds.), *The Blackwell handbook of social psychology* (pp. 329–347). Oxford, UK: Blackwell.

Oettingen, G., & Mayer, D. (2002). The motivating function of thinking about the future: Expectations versus fantasies. *Journal of Personality and Social Psychology, 83,* 1198–1212.

SETTING THE STAGE

CHAPTER 1

Future-Thinking
A Historical Perspective

Lucian Hölscher

At first it may seem odd to discuss the future in terms of history. History is, after all, by definition a study of humanity's recorded past. Attempts to learn about the future are left to biblical prophets and mystical oracles, or, lately, pollsters and statisticians. But an undercurrent of the future runs through historical narratives; it is manifested in people's thoughts, motivations, plans, and aspirations, which in turn guide their actions and behavior. It is impossible to truly understand the events of the past without examining the major players' roles and the ambitions, hopes, and dreams for the future that fueled them.

The future, like the past, is not a static event. Both are continually moving targets, relative to where we stand in the present. One's perspective changes with the passage of time, as the present catches up with the future and eventually becomes the past. Take the assassination of Julius Caesar as an example: In the 2,000 years following it, the event was continuously interpreted and reinterpreted—Caesar's killers saw the assassination of the increasingly dictator-like leader as a necessary action to preserve the Roman Republic. Instead, it touched off a series of civil wars and ushered in a new age of Roman emperors. A thousand years later, it was interpreted as a template for the Holy Roman Empire, before being reinterpreted yet again in 19th-century France, when Caesar was hailed as the prototype for Napoleon and the new political regime of Bonapartism.

Seen from the perspective of various observers in the past, the same person and event carry different significance for the future, largely dependent on the time in which the story is told. Reinhart Koselleck coined the term *past futures* in the early 1960s to refer to past societies' visions of time beyond their own (Koselleck, 1985). In addition to changing perspectives over time, past futures encompass the many different and sometimes conflicting visions of the future held by contemporaries at a single point in history. Unsurprisingly, most bygone visions of the future did not come true. Despite not being borne out in reality, they nonetheless had important effects on people's actions and mentalities, and in that and other respects they are as much a part of history as the futures that do come true.

Unrealized past futures call to mind an often mocked genre of historical fiction, the alternate history (Ferguson, 2011). These narratives take on a science fiction flavor and often begin from a speculative premise: What would have happened if, instead of the Allies, Hitler had won the Second World War? Although much satirized, alternate histories, in fact, raise important questions: How settled are the events of the past? Was Germany doomed to lose the Second World War from the beginning, or only after committing a series of missteps?

Looking at these past futures portrayed in alternate histories reveals more than looking at the events of history alone. Alternative histories break up and bring to light the different competing views of the future that guided the various past actors, which often get lost when looking at the big picture. In identifying those actors' motivations in any given moment, they help us pinpoint just how determined the events of the past were; what, if any, were the pivotal turning points; and how close history was to taking another shape entirely. Finally, even those visions of the future that fail to become reality continue to influence ideas about the future into today— in guiding our expectations of it and how we see our own place in time.

DISCOVERING THE FUTURE

The concept of the future has changed significantly over time. In fact, people did not think about the future much at all, at least not in long terms, until relatively recently. Our modern understanding of the future as a discrete unit, or temporal "space of time," only took shape by the 17th and 18th centuries, around the European Enlightenment (Grimm & Grimm, 1954, vol. 31, p. 569, s. v. zeitraum)—a development that has led me to speak of a "discovery of the future" in Western history (Hölscher, 2016).

At the beginning of the modern age, there was a shift in how people thought about time. People began to view events that occurred close together in time and influenced each other as thematically linked and grouped them into discrete periods or eras, which marched along in an unbroken line (Hölscher, 2014). Only when the past began to be viewed in this way, as taking up discrete space in a timeline, did the future begin to be seen this way as well, as a distinct period that would follow the present. Unlike the past, however, which was filled with significant events in history, the future was seen as open and largely undetermined.

This temporal conception of the future stands in stark contrast to the Middle Ages. Up until around 1700 C.E., the vast majority of people had a firm conviction that the end of the world was near. The long-term future, at least in this world, did not exist. Rather, people lived in something of an extended present. Another perspective on time also existed in the ancient world, in Greece and Rome, as well as in non-European civilizations, such as the Maya in South America, which believed in a circular structure of time, that events would be repeated again and again.

We can see the shift in thinking about the future around 1700 in Western Europe by looking at how people wrote about things to come. Surprisingly few languages originally featured a future tense. Greek and Latin are among the few that did. Many European languages that did not—including English, French, and German—borrowed the future tense and also the word *futurum* itself from Latin in the late Middle Ages, when the modern conception of the future was first emerging (Bloch & von Wartburg, 1968; Grimm & Grimm, 1954, vol. 32, p. 479; *Oxford English Dictionary*, 1933, pp. 626 ff.). In Latin texts of classical and medieval times, *futurum* never indicated a discrete chunk of time like we think of today, however. Instead of a noun, *futurum* was always used as an adjective, a signifier marking events to come. Still today, in languages that adopted the word and idea of the future from Latin, the future is expressed as an add-on, as in English, in which auxiliary verbs such as *will* or *to come* or *to be on the way to* are inserted before the action, and adjectives and adverbs such as *once* and *tomorrow* are placed around it (Hölscher, 2016, pp. 40–42).

The language that sprang up to describe the future, and time in general, frequently derived from spatial relations. The word *progress* evolved out of a word that originally meant the action of moving the feet step by step, for example, and the word *development* from rolling a ball of wool. The etymologies of the words for *future* are themselves convenient metaphors for how man saw his position on earth and how that perspective changed over time: the German *Zukunft*, literally meaning "time to come," for example, is derived from *zukommen*, "to come to me"—similar to the French *avenir*, stemming from *advenire* (to come, to arrive). This transformation of the individual from a stationary, passive observer of history—viewing events as emerging from the future and passing before one's eyes before receding into the past—to an active agent, moving through time oneself, represents one of the defining changes from the premodern to the modern age in Western history.

We tend to take for granted the idea of the future as inherently uncertain and mysterious—that the events have not happened yet and largely depend on how things shake out today. In premodern societies, however, it was common understanding to think of objects of the future and past as being existent at any time. The past and future had the same metaphysical status in people's imaginations. Although the specific course and character of events was not known, it was not because they were uncertain, however. Rather, only God was said to be aware of them. Instead of shaping the course of history, humanity was continually flogged by the events of the past as they emerged whole from some unknown realm. This mindset is seen in Augustine's famous Chapter 11 of *The Confessions*, when the early Christian theologian asked: "Do future and past things exist, and if, from which 'hidden place' (*occultum*) do future things (*futura*) come when they become present, and to which 'hidden place' do they disappear when they become past?"[1] (p. 216).

As man's role in time morphed from passive to active, from observer to agent, people began to attempt to explore the future, not only in the material sense of trying to predict what will happen but also in the abstract: They began to reflect on the human condition and the extent of their ability to predict, to produce, and to arrange the future.

---

[1] "An et ipsa sunt, sed ex aliquo procedit occulto, cum ex futuro fit praesens, et in aliquod recedit occultum, cum ex praesenti fit praeteritum?" Translation by L. Hölscher.

IDEAS ABOUT THE FUTURE IN PREMODERN EUROPE

The extent to which premodern people in Europe were aware of the distant future is debated (Brakensiek & Scheller, 2011). The primary source of thought about cosmology and time in the Middle Ages was Christian mythology. Early Christian theologians heavily adopted the idea of the near end of the world developed in antiquity and modified it to fit the emerging religious tradition (Koselleck & Widmer, 1980). In the first few hundred centuries C.E., early Roman Christian scholars, including Symmachus, Claudian, Prudentius, Augustine, and Ambrosius, believed the world was grown old and had reached its *senectus,* the last stage of its vital circle before it would be reborn to the "golden age" of childhood again.

Later in the millennium, Christian mythology held on to the idea of the world grown old but turned away from the idea of returning to the beginning and instead predicted its permanent end. It was widely accepted that the world would last 6,000 years, as foretold in the *Vaticinium Eliae,* a Talmudic prophecy originating in late antiquity that was adopted by many Christian scholars in medieval times. Medieval scholars became fascinated with trying to date the creation of the world and, following from there, its destruction. According to their calculations, made by adding up the ages of the biblical forefathers of Jesus taken from different holy books, the world was created somewhere between 5,000 and 4,000 years before Jesus was born, leading many to predict that the Last Judgment would come by the year 1000, or 2000 C.E. at the absolute latest if God did not in His mercy destroy the Earth sooner.

These feverish calculations occurred despite an explicit prohibition on searching for the exact date of the end of the world. The Bible clearly condemned attempts to estimate the age of the world as folly, hubristic attempts to learn what only God can know (Froom, 1946–1954). Christian scholars justified their actions by arguing that the knowledge that the Second Coming was imminent would promote increased moral vigilance and willingness to repent sins and to return to the path of salvation on the part of humanity (Krüger, 1972).

Whether this rather optimistic prediction had the intended effect is debatable and contravened by the many horrific acts committed by humanity in the Middle Ages, but church dogma did have a tangible impact on how regular people considered the future. Like today, people had short- and even long-term goals, as evidenced by investment in long-term projects, and therefore must have considered the future in a limited sense. Peasants planted for the harvest, and merchants sent ships that would not return for several months or even years. Expectations for the future even extended beyond individual lifetimes, manifested, for instance, in the construction of Gothic cathedrals expected to survive not just for the next 10 or 50 years but long into the future. But, unlike today, this vision of the future did not involve the expectation of anything new or change the image of a distant period of time. The cathedral would still be standing at the end of the world, but the scenery surrounding it would look essentially the same.

There are very few sources from before the 17th century that contain long-term predictions for the future, other than to say that the world would end. In medieval times, most human affairs had the form of an endless repetition: sowing and harvesting, disease and health, war and peace, the rise and fall of kingdoms—there was little reason to believe in long-term change or even improvement in human affairs. Hence, if we take the future as a dimension of fundamental change, a time different from the past and present—as we are used to in modern times, in which we view time as a progressive march—a far distant future was not meaningful or relevant for premodern people. With the circular expectations of life and the experience of little fundamental change, it is fair to say that in the Middle Ages the future—a time of events and conditions of life different from the past and present—did not exist. Another reason for such a static concept of time came from the Bible, then considered the primary source and authority documenting the beginning and first periods of human life. Although it supposedly contained all of human history, the Bible did not report much about the changing conditions of human life—people seemed to live under different political regimes, but more or less in the same way as ever.

This future myopia started to lift only by the early modern period, from the 17th century onward. When adventurers such as Columbus in the West and the Portuguese Jesuits in the Far East discovered nations that the Bible had no knowledge of, scholars began to ask where these peoples were represented in the Bible. In order to come to terms with the discrepancy and reconcile how people outside the Christian world could be included into the history of salvation, historians such as the French librarian Isaak de La Peyrère in 1655 began to postulate a "pre-Adamite" mankind, of people living before Adam and Eve, first challenging the biblical timeline (Klempt, 1960, pp. 89–96).

The credibility of the Bible as a primary source of history, and thus the postulated 6,000-year age of the world, was also thrown into question by the emerging scholarship of natural sciences. Some decades after La Peyrère's concept of a "pre-Adamite" mankind, geologists such as the Englishman John Ray concluded from mussels found on top of mountains that these animals had once lived under the sea. From that, it followed that surface of the Earth had moved, with mountains rising from under the ocean—impossible within the short period of human life on earth (Toulmin & Goodfield, 1982). Gradually, and with much resistance from the Church, it became clear that the Earth was much older than the 5,000 years put forth by prominent theologians. Once the date of creation was questioned, it was only a short step to question the date of the end of the world. In the words of a mid-18th-century encyclopedia: "There is no convenient argument, why God should have created the world 5,000 instead of a hundred thousand years ago." Nevertheless, it still seemed to be a "bad speculation" to deduce that the world "would last forever" (Zedler, 1747, pp. 1674, 1678).

Only in 1755, Immanuel Kant declared: "There will be millions and millions of centuries, in which new worlds and world orders will be generated. . . . Creation is never finished. It once had its beginning, but it will never end" (Kant, 1755/1960a, p. 335). At the time this was a sacrilege. Even in the second half of the 19th century, most ordinary people in the West, as well as the Church and many secular scholars, still believed in the 6,000-year history of mankind (*Meyers neues Konversationslexikon*, 1871). Nevertheless, the advanced age of the world became harder to deny. Already in the mid-18th century in Europe, the modern calendar, beginning with the year of Jesus' birth and counting the years back and forth in endless succession, began to replace the old calendar of counting the years from world creation in 4000 B.C.E. onward (Klempt, 1960).

The Early Modern Era: From Theological Speculation to Rational Prognostics

This reevaluation of the Bible as a historical authority, and consequently of time itself, beginning around the 17th century led to what I have deemed a "discovery of the future," in early modern Europe. The process of such a discovery and the construction of modern ideas of the future as a dimension of time were long and complex and continue to evolve today.

As Europe emerged from the Dark Ages and entered the early modern age, theology was still the leading discipline concerned with the science of the cosmos. Theologians naturally resisted questions about the accuracy of the biblical account of time and near end of the world—for one thing, the threat of imminent destruction was crucial for their argument that sinners should repent post haste. For another, in its descriptions of the end of days, the Bible explicitly warned that, along with catastrophic events portending the Second Coming, false prophets would appear and seduce many people with their ideas, according to the Gospel of Matthew (Ch. 24). The German Pietist theologian Johan Jacob Spener was one of the first who argued that if the end of the world was farther away than traditionally contended, instead of freeing mankind to debauchery, the extra time on Earth would allow humanity to improve its condition step by step (Spener, 1694).

Although Spener's call for earthly transformation rankled traditional theologians, none could deny his point about man's inherent imperfection and need for change. Because God was not able to create something imperfect, man's clear state to the contrary created a paradox, raising the question, at what point would man's transformation occur? In the 1730s the English bishop of Durham Samuel Butler argued that the paradox proved human life after death, with this postmortal life lasting perhaps 10,000 years, which time man would spend improving his moral condition (Butler, 1736).

Swedish scholar Emmanuel Swedenborg argued similarly in his main work *Arcana coelestia* (1749–1756), in which he described a celestial society in which the dead lived in distinct communities, communicated and traveled by their thoughts alone, learned at schools in order to approach step by step to a state of perfection, and even gave birth to spiritual children. Swedenborg's fantastical account stimulated Kant to discuss the possibility of the future life of "spirits" and prompted intense consideration about the possibility of communication with dead people (Kant, 1766/1960a). Kant was only one among many intellectuals in the second half of the 18th century who were interested in the constitution of and communication with "spirits" (Sawicki, 2000).

By the late 18th century, speculation on the future of man was a commonplace and well-established theological discussion (cf., Mulsow, 2007; Sparn, 2007). The "future of man" became a synonym for his destiny after death, the "future world," an expression for a transcendent sphere that man would enter after death. What this future world—where souls lived after death but before the Last Judgment, when Jesus would send them to either Heaven or Hell—looked like was a hotly debated question. Protestants rejected the Catholic concept of a Purgatory, established in the 12th century (LeGoff, 1986), but they also argued about the details of what life after death would entail in the "realm between" (*Zwischenreich*; Lang & McDannell, 1990).

Although some skeptics challenged the belief in life after death, the idea of a future celestial world—in Germany called the *Jenseits* (the Beyond)—greatly influenced the 19th-century religious imagination (Hölscher, 2007). A handful of theologians, such as Ludwig Feuerbach, argued for the end of man's existence when he died, but Christian preachers and theologians doubled down in asserting the reality of future life after death. An extensive practice of requiems, sermons, and religious images from the time testify to how widespread and popular such concepts were.

By the end of the 18th century, however, as humanity entered the late modern period, the religious concept of the "future" began to recede and a more secular concept of the future emerged, focusing on the time to come in this world, rather than after death. This new secular idea of the future had a touch of the religious about it, expressed in people's longing for a better life, but without waiting for it in another world beyond the grave. The philosopher Immanuel Kant and the French mathematician Condorcet were among the first who elaborated on the concept of a future world history (Condorcet, 1793/94; Kant, 1784/1960b; Lessing, 1780). Their descriptions of the future envisioned a world at the end of time, but rather than borrowing from the prophetic tradition of the Bible, they drew from popular utopian novels of the time to construct the perfect state of man, following the example of Thomas More's *Utopia,* published in 1516.

Gradually, secular visions of the future moved away from an ideal utopian state to more realistic—sometimes even pessimistic—ideas. For example Adam Smith in his *Wealth of Nations* (1776), Lessing in his *Die Erziehung des Menschengeschlechts* (1780), and Kant in his essay *"Idee zu einer allgemeinen Geschichte in weltbürgerlicher Absicht"* (1784) stopped defining the future by its outcome—the Last Judgment in religious tradition and the state of perfect humanity in the secular. They began trying to deduce the future development of mankind from what had happened in the past, under the presumption that "nature" itself would lead mankind to the intended improvement and final perfection. As Johann Gottfried Herder wrote in 1797, following Gottfried Wilhelm Leibniz's already famous phrase: "The future is a daughter of the present, as this is of the time before. Two sentences are before us to conclude the third. Who has understood the first correctly and concludes from them in the right way, has made no bad usage of his reason, which is the faculty to see the connexion among things . . ." (Herder, 1830, p. 53).

Prognostics based on science and systematic observation began to displace the prophecy of the past. Secular historians and philosophers did not entirely abandon the idea of a perfect future, to be strived for through political, social, and scientific programs. But they viewed such programs as "immanent," not "transcendent." They did not proclaim final destinations of mankind, but rather the next steps on the way of human development (de Jouvenel, 1964). The future was reconceived as an almost endless process that would cover hundreds and even thousands of years. In the late 1770s, Lessing described this long-term development of human "education" by pointing out that "eternal providence" proceeds in "imperceptible steps": Nature would take "thousands of years" to accomplish its goals (Lessing, 1780, §85 ff.). Kant, too, reckoned that arriving at a perfect future would take "perhaps an incalculable series of procreations, one passing its enlightenment to the next," in order "to develop the sprout in the human species to that stage of development that is adequate to its destiny" (Kant, 1784/1960b, p. 35).

The French Revolution swung like a wrecking ball, destroying people's dreams of a future utopia and plans for a perfect society. Faced with the gruesome reality of the Revolution and its aftermath, people began to question whether the future was indeed a series of incremental steps toward perfection. The mental climate in Europe changed from optimism about the future to pessimism. As the utopian projects of the French Revolution turned out to be unworkable, sometimes even producing disastrous effects, European intellectuals became more hesitant about making long-term predictions for the future. In the romantic literature of German poets such as Friedrich von Hardenberg (known under the name of Novalis), Friedrich Schlegel, and Ludwig Tieck, the future was even suspended and replaced by images of the medieval past, which, they argued, was connected to the future in a secret dimension. "The new world is falling down beclouding the brightest sunshine; out of mossy ruins one sees a wondrous future gleaming," Novalis lamented in an unpublished fragment of his novel *Heinrich von Ofterdingen,* continuing, "Would the times be not as antisocial, future would combine with the past, spring with autumn, summer with winter" (von Hardenberg, 1815, Part 1, p. 256).

Humanity experienced something of a regression, diverging from the enlightened progressivism that had until so recently taken hold of Europe. Instead of the linear vision of time from the past through the present into the future, people again began to conceive of time as circular. After passing through the present period of alienation, historians argued that in the future human affairs would return to the past. Many concepts of history in the 19th century, from Marxism to fascism and national socialism, reflected this trend, producing images of a future society near to where history had started: Marxism in the concept of a primordial communist society, fascism in the idea of resurrecting the primordial order of Germanic tribes and morality (cf., Esposito & Reichardt, 2015).

THE LATE MODERN ERA

As the world shifted from the early to the late modern period, lasting from the 19th through the 20th century, there was another significant change in how people thought about the future. In the decades before and into the early years of the French Revolution, in many ways marking the middle of the Modern Age, writers of the time generally approached the future optimistically, with extensive, far-reaching predictions of what would come. After the war, descriptions of the future in writing became more circumspect; people scaled back their predictions, becoming more interested in near-term next steps for improving their lot.

Although the temporal conception of the future was established by the early modern era, how people thought about the future continued to change in a more limited way through the late modern period, cycling through periods split between optimism and pessimism about the future. At the beginning of each of these cycles, people were engaged and enthusiastic about building new visions of a better world, only to be disappointed when their hopes and endeavors were thwarted (Hölscher, 2016). To be sure, different people writing at the same point in history had various visions and predictions for the future, but behind all these different expectations were trends generally linked to traditional cycles of boom and of depression.

Dichotomous periods characterized by hope for the future in the first half and then pessimism in the second followed each other in waves of about two generations, or 60 years, before recovering again into optimism.

The first cycle in the modern era had its apex in the 1770s to 1790s, with philosophers such as Lessing and Kant, Adam Smith, and Condorcet. The second cycle, starting around 1830, with the beginning of the late modern period, was chiefly characterized by concerns for democracy. In the following two decades many programs of social reform, such as those of the "utopian socialists," including Saint-Simon, Fourier, Owen, and at some occasions even Marx in his early writings of the 1840s, spread all over Europe and the United States, with the goal of improving the lives of urban populations of many countries. Democracy was seen as the only form of government that would survive in the long run—in 1834 Francois-René de Chateaubriand observed, "L'Europe court a la démocratie" (*Revue de deux mondes*)—and collective labor was held as the organizational form of future societies. But after 1848, a new period of disappointment began, lasting until the 1890s, when utopian hopes again began to agitate industrial societies.

Starting in the late 1890s, a vision of the future by far the strongest and most influential of all modern booms set off, which penetrated and revolutionized all parts of society in ways that are still felt today (Briggs, 1996). Future projects began to crop up everywhere, in technology, politics, and social reform, in newspapers, in scientific programs, in economic organizations, and even in the arts. To give but two examples: By the 1890s big industrial enterprises such as the Allgemeine Elektrizitätsgesellschaft (AEG) in Germany began to build up departments for long-term technological projects, which could only be realized in the long-term future, within 50 or even 100 years (cf., Bechtel, 1967). Technological progress became the standard rather than a by-product of accidental inventions. Military planning adopted the character of technological planning, with new generations of weapons horrifically realized in the First World War.

Around 1900 the future was omnipresent in modern society. People heavily anticipated technological miracles right around the corner; it seemed to be only a question of how to get rid of all the old traditions and make way for the new. The Italian poet Tommaso Marinetti articulated the overweening optimism of the time in describing his art movement *futurism*, promising that even war would not lead only to death and destruction but to something new that would come after and could only be achieved by having cleared the world from the past. This perspective was seen in art, as with the abstract paintings of Picasso, as well as in technology, in the streamlined design for motorcars, aeroplanes, rockets, and other modes of transportation (Hölscher, 2010). The sleek lines promised faster and superior objects compared with anything before, and the look took on a symbolism indicating a product of the future. To be "new" was a value in itself. It was not associated with dangerous alteration (as in the Middle Ages), but with progress, advantage in the competition of daily survival (Koselleck, 1979). It became common wisdom that natural order dictated that man had to change in order to be fit for the future. By the turn of the century, the "new man", the "new woman", and the "new society" were synonyms for their ideal forms.

This willingness to destroy the past to make room for a new future is acutely articulated in the plans of Swiss-French architect Le Corbusier for Paris after the

First World War. In his *"plan voisin"* of 1922 he proposed to raze the whole city, from the Place de la Concorde in the west up to the Place de la Bastille in the east, and erect a dozen monotone skyscrapers on the old center of Paris. In the following decades, similar plans were proposed for Moscow, Rome, New York, Chicago, and the new German metropolis Germania that was supposed to replace Berlin after the Second World War.

Le Corbusier clung to his proposal into the late 1950s, long after many people in postwar Europe had turned away from the idea of the wholesale destruction of the past. He wasn't alone: Modernists across Europe for decades indulged in visions of the future as a phoenix rising from the ashes. The longer into the future they attempted to look, the more willing they were to turn the existing world upside down. After the end of the First World War, utopias such as the Bolshevist and National Socialist dreams of a better future were accepted as mainstream in many European countries, with oftentimes horrific consequences.

The dark side of this appetite for destruction in the service of an ideal future is especially apparent when applied to medicine and biology. In the name of achieving a superior human race, scholars and politicians in Germany destroyed the lives of millions of Jews, Roma, people with mental illnesses, and others who were classified as having inferior constitutions. Attempting to create the so-called ideal man, totalitarian societies encouraged both eugenics and forced reproduction. Only after the terror of the Second World War was exposed to the world did these cruel dreams of a better future begin to dissipate.

The so-called thousand-year realm of the Third Reich was a popular expression of the future in Germany, but rather than a perversion of thought, the idea was perfectly in line with the historical perspective of the time. As early as 1895, the hero in Henry George Wells's novel *The Time Machine* traveled to the year 802701, farther than all writers of modern science fiction have envisioned before or since. Many cultural prophets in the early 20th century spoke in such extreme cosmological dimensions. In a 1905 sermon that embodied many popular rhetorical strategies of the time, the German pastor of Nürnberg, Friedrich Rittelmeyer, asked his congregation:

> Sure, our nation will play its role for a while, yet. But then? Then other people will follow, Americans, Russians. And then? After another hundreds and thousands of years, the black peoples of Africa may awake and lead world history for a time. And then? Then again thousands of years will pass, in which life on earth will become more and more comfortable because of new discoveries and inventions. And then? Then the earth will begin to cool down, mankind will become tired and weak, and step by step life will come to an end . . . . (Geyer & Rittelmeyer, 1912, p. 562)

It was common practice in speech and writing at the time to demonstrate the relativity of human and national ambitions by laying out a long series of nations and races that had dominated world history in the past and would rule in the future, portraying the present generation as nothing but an elusive moment in the endless course of history. The description of world civilizations following one another was often bound together with the astronomical horizon of time and the rise and decline of life on the planet, underlining the limits of human civilization itself. The sermon was meant to inspire humility, but it also in many ways portended the coming backlash against the wildly optimistic visions of the future that dominated the era up till then. The list of nations that would come to rule the world in the future referred to civilizations—such as in Africa and Asia—widely seen as "other" by Rittelmeyer's white, European audience. For the contemporary listener such visions were frightening, and sermons and political speeches commonly used the device to inspire postponing this future destiny as far as possible.

The newly extended perspective of historical time, compounded by emerging scientific theories about the rapid expansion of the age and size of the universe in the second half of the 19th century, had a toxic effect on man's view of his position in the cosmos. It made human life feel small and insignificant—a jarring departure from the inflated sense of humanity as God's special creation. Ernst Haeckel encapsulated this new eye on humanity's relative insignificance in the popular analogy: If the period of organic life on Earth would be pressed into 24 hours, the 200,000 years in which humans walked the earth wouldn't make more than the last 2 minutes of the day (Haeckel, 1992). This awareness could inspire humble self-reflection, such as in Bruno Bürgel's bestseller of 1937, *Das Weltbild des modernen Menschen:* "Sometimes, when I am in the thick of great cities. . . . I close my eyes for a moment thinking: a small ball flying around the sun, for eons" (Bürgel, 1937, p. 309). More often, however, it led to a kind of mass depression that enveloped humanity and darkened ideas about its future.

By the 1940s in the United States, however, as the economy recovered from the Great Depression and even boomed in the wake of the Second World War, thinking about the future again turned optimistic, but with an even more highly scientific and technological bent than before. New technologies, such as nuclear power and computer technology, promised to change the entire outer makeup of the future, compared with earlier times when new technologies were seen more as perfections on existing society.

The new technologies and visions of the future of the 1960s continue to provide the template for many projects today: artificial intelligence, laser technology and submarine agrotechnology were all created or pushed forward in the 1960s (Schmidt-Gernig, 2002). The wave of enthusiasm broke in the 1970s, and another period of future-depression began, as the technologies imagined in the 1960s were not immediately forthcoming and gave way to apocalyptic visions of despair and fear about the destruction and material exhaustion of the environment as people began to feel the negative repercussions of human inventions and interventions (Doering-Manteuffel & Raphael, 2008).

In the 1980s, popular authors such as Ulrich Beck, François Hartog, and Francis Fukuyama declared the future-looking orientation of modern societies finished and dismissed any expectations of future progress (Beck, 1992; Fukuyama, 1989; Hartog, 2002). This pessimism about the future was partly related to economic factors, such as the oil crisis of the early 1970s; partly to a new ecological sensibility, as people became increasingly aware of damages and risks to the environment, such as growing holes in the ozone layer; and finally partly belated reckoning with the psychic damages of the world wars earlier in the century. Philosophers declared that humanity had entered into a postmodern era and announced the conclusion of the modern age, which had spanned the past 250 years.

Somewhat paradoxically, the negative vision of the future that prompted post-modernists to declare the end of the modern era was itself a product of futuristic technologies. In the desire to prevent the worst from happening, humans have developed sophisticated prognostic methods and statistical models for predicting the future, which themselves in turn alter the course of history by simply being there. Attempts at forecasting the future have produced all kinds of mechanisms, institutions, and structures of communication that have fundamentally changed the world: Sophisticating polling methods used by political organizations, technologies facilitating international cooperation efforts against terrorism, economic crises and other threats to humanity, the complete reorganization of daily life by the Internet and new media, and civil rights and other social movements are all the products of our attempts to look into the future.

This proliferation of prognostic tools has altered daily life so much so that we can be said to be living in a new period in history—the contemporary age, in which the future is no longer seen as a "fate" that cannot be changed but, rather, under human control, determined by actions that happen today. Different scenarios are mapped out and calculated in terms of probability. Once again we begin to speak in terms of plural "futures" (Hartog, 2002; Seefried, 2015), indicating a new understanding of the future as no longer something unconquerable barreling through our present but as the product of human choice and subject to human molding.

When the modern era began, the newly conceived temporal future was also seen as open and subject to human intervention. But unlike then, with more than 200 years of hindsight, we can see now that the future is not always a time of progress, as it was when first imagined. There are many possible futures, some good, some bad. What actually transpires depends on our actions and choices today.

ENTERING THE NOW

As the 21st century wears on, there is some hint that our conception of the future is changing yet again. When humanity is no longer shaped by history but is the shaper of it, lines between past and present and the future blur. French philosopher François Hartog has proposed that we have entered a new era in history, as humanity's position related to its past and future has again undergone a major shift in time (Gumbrecht, 2014; Hartog, 2002). Leaving the modern age of future orientation, which has dominated society from the 17th century onward, behind us, we have entered the age of "presentism," a time that is oriented only to its own present. One of the main architects and symptoms of this age is the Internet. The Internet has made everything, all knowledge, all data seem to be present at once, regardless of its actual age.

At the same time as the voices of the past have become present on the Internet, all of the voices of the present are amplified, too. We have traditionally learned about history from the information provided by the select privileged few that had the fortune to write about it—usually educated, upper-class, white males. In the 19th century, historians debated the weight of these recollections as a necessary but deficient source of historiography,[2] offering a decidedly limited perspective on the past. But the Internet has democratized the chorus of history, enabling a more diverse array of perspectives to be expressed than ever before. Even with the limits of individual bias and memory, the collective perspective that has emerged provides arguably the most accurate image of history ever produced. The same is true of forgetting. What and how societies forget is an interesting feature of their character. Until relatively recently, it was an important aspect of peace treaties that the crimes and atrocities of both sides should be forgotten. Now, however, the duty not to forget seems to be one of the most important human duties in societies that have lived through civil wars and genocides, including the Holocaust (Hölscher, 2009). Indeed, we could not forget if we wanted to—it becomes impossible to escape one's past on the Internet, where everything lasts forever.

The Internet has also facilitated another major aspect of the current age of the present: globalization. People all over the world can communicate instantly, nation's economies and futures are entwined in trade deals and treaties. At the same time, there is a growing nationalist streak in countries in reaction to unprecedented globalization and income stratification. People from different strata of society in singular nations do not have the same outlook on the future. The split in national votes resulting in Great Britain exiting the European Union in June 2016 may be an expression of this split vision of the present reality and the future. At the moment of writing this chapter, when Donald Trump is the American President, it seems that the political elites in many countries have lost contact with the needs and aspirations of people who have no confidence in the visions of the future articulated by politicians.

The future is the product of our present projections. But we also know that as time goes on our present will be seen as the backward projection of people living in the future. In politics, we assess current actions by attempting to predict how they will look to future generations. The current refugee crisis in Europe is but one example of this strategy: Will Germany be praised for wisely welcoming hundreds of thousands of immigrants? Or will it be condemned by future generations, which will see 2016 as a turning point of new ethnic tensions? Nobody knows how future generations will judge our time; we sit in anticipation of their judgment and speculate about it in an attempt to legitimize the decisions we are convinced to be necessary today.

The present future and the future past are linked to one another. This maxim becomes more and more relevant in many fields of social activity: in technology, when the future effects of present inventions are discussed; in cultural politics, when we define the world heritage of future generations; in social policy, when we discuss what justice among different generations may be, and so on (Rohbeck, 2012). Historical times, past, present and future, are not separated from one another. In defining our present time, we include definitions of the past and of the future. Historical future research is on the way to extend history and historiography beyond the lines of the past.

---

[2]The boom of memory literature started in the 1980s after the trailblazing studies of the French historian Pierre Nora (esp. Nora, 1984–1992).

REFERENCES

Augustine of Hippo (around 400 BC). Confessions. Available at *www.gutenberg.org/files/3296/3296-h/3296-h.htm#link2H_4_0011*

Bechtel, H. (1967). *Wirtschafts- und Sozialgeschichte Deutschlands* [Economic and Social History of Germany]. München, Germany: Callwey.

Beck, U. (1992). *Risk society: Towards a new modernity.* Los Angeles: SAGE.

Bloch, O., & von Wartburg, W. (Eds.). (1968). *Dictionnaire étymologique de la langue classique.* Paris: Presses Universitaires de France.

Brakensiek, S., & Scheller, B. (Eds.). (2011). *Vorsorge, Voraussicht und Vorhersage: Kontingenzbewätigung durch Zukunftshandeln* [Precaution, Foresight and Prediction: And Accomplishment to Contingency by Future-Oriented Actions]. Essen, Germany: Universität Duisburg–Essen.

Briggs, A. (1996). Past, present and future in headlines. In A. Briggs & D. Snowman (Eds.), *Fins de Siècle: How Centuries End 1400–2000* (pp. 157–197). New Haven, CT: Yale University Press.

Bürgel, B. H. (1937). *Das Weltbild des modernen Menschen* [The World View of Modern Man]. Berlin, Germany: Ullstein.

Butler, J. (1736). *The analogy of religion, natural and revealed to the constitution and course of nature.* London: James, John, & Paul Knapton.

Condorcet, N. de. (1793/94). *Esquisse d'un tableau historique des progrès de l'esprit humain.* Available at *http://classiques.uqac.ca/classiques/condorcet/esquisse_tableau_progres_hum/esquisse_tableau_hist.pdf.*

de Jouvenel, B. (1964). *L'Art de la Conjecture* [The Art of Conjecture]. New York: Basic Books.

Doering-Manteuffel, A., & Raphael, L. (2008). *Nach dem Boom: Perspektiven auf die Zeitgeschichte seit 1970* [After the Boom: Perspectives on Contemporary History after 1970]. Göttingen, Germany: Vandenhoeck & Ruprecht.

Esposito, F., & Reichardt, S. (2015). Fascist temporalities. *Journal of Modern European History, 13*(1).

Ferguson, N. (2011). *Virtual history: Alternatives and counterfactuals.* London: Penguin. (Original work published 1997)

Froom, L. E. (1946–1954). *The prophetic faith of our fathers: The historical development of prophetic interpretation.* Washington, DC: Review and Herald.

Fukuyama, F. (1989). The end of history? *The National Interest.* Available at *www.wesjones.com/eoh.htm.*

Geyer, C., & Rittelmeyer, F. (1912). *Gott und die Seele* [God and the Soul]. Ulm, Germany: Heinrich Kerler.

Grimm, J., & Grimm, W. (1954). *Deutsches Wörterbuch* [German Dictionary] (pp. 479). Leipzig, Germany: S. Hirzel Verlag.

Gumbrecht, H. U. (2014). *Our broad present: Time and contemporary culture.* New York: Columbia University Press.

Haeckel, E. (1992). *Die Welträtsel: Gemeinverständliche Studien über monistische Philosophie* [The Riddle of the Universe]. Amherst, NY: Prometheus Books. (Original work published 1899)

Hartog, F. (2002). *Regimes of historicity: Presentism and experiences of time* (S. Brown, Trans.). New York: Columbia Unversity Press.

Herder, J. G. (1830). Vom Wissen und Nichtwissen der Zukunft [Of Knowledge and Ignorance of the Future]. In J. v. Müller (Ed.), *Johann Gottfried Herder: Sämtliche Werke* (Vol. 3, pp. 53–70). Stuttgart, Germany: Cotta. (Original work published 1797)

Hölscher, L. (Ed.). (2007). *Das Jenseits: Facetten eines religiösen Begriffs in der Neuzeit* [The Beyond: Facets of a religious concept in modern times]. Göttingen, Germany: Wallstein.

Hölscher, L. (2009). Geschichte und Vergessen: Eine Funktionsanalyse im Anschluss an den "Historikerstreit" um die Einmaligkeit der nationalsozialistischen Verbrechen [History and Forgetting: A Functional Analysis on the Uniqueness of the Crimes of National Socialism Following the so-called "Historikerstreit."] In L. Hölscher (Ed.), *Semantik der Leere: Aufsätze zur Theorie der Geschichte* [Semantics of the Void: Essays on the Theory of History] (pp. 100–115). Göttingen, Germany: Wallstein-Verlag. (Original work published 1989)

Hölscher, L. (2010). Der Aufbruch der Kunst in die Zukunft [The Departure of Art into the Future]. In Museum Folkwang Essen (Ed.), *"Das schönste Museum der Welt": Museum Folkwang bis 1933: Essays* (Vol. 2, pp. 13–25). Essen, Germany: Steidl.

Hölscher, L. (2014). Time gardens: Historical concepts in modern historiography. *History and Theory, 53*, 577–591.

Hölscher, L. (2016). *Die Entdeckung der Zukunft* [The Discovery of the Future]. Göttingen, Germany: Wallstein.

Kant, I. (1960a). Träume eines Geistersehers, erläutert durch Träume der Metaphysik [Dreams of a Visionary, Explained by Dreams of Metaphysics.] In W. Weischedel (Ed.), *Immanuel Kant: Werke* (Vol. 1, pp. 923–992). Frankfurt, Germany: Insel. (Original work published 1766)

Kant, I. (1960b). Idee zu einer allgemeinen Geschichte in weltbürgerlicher Absicht [Idea of a General History in Cosmopolitan Perspective.] In W. Weischedel (Ed.), *Immanuel Kant: Werke* (Vol. 6). Frankfurt, Germany: Insel. (Original work published 1784)

Klempt, A. (1960). *Die Säkularisierung der universalhistorischen Auffassung: Zum Wandel des Geschichtsdenkens im 16. und 17. Jahrhundert* [The Secularisation of the Concept of Universal History]. Göttingen, Germany: Musterschmidt.

Koselleck, R. (1979). "Neuzeit." Zur Semantik moderner Bewegungsbegriffe. In R. Koselleck (Ed.), *Vergangene Zukunft: Zur Semantik geschichtlicher Zeiten* (pp. 300–348). Frankfurt, Germany: Suhrkamp.

Koselleck, R. (1985). *Futures past: On the semantics of historical time*. New York: Columbia University Press.

Koselleck, R., & Widmer, P. (Eds.). (1980). *Niedergang: Studien zu einem geschichtlichen Thema*. Stuttgart, Germany: Klett-Cotta.

Krüger, S. (1972). Krise der Zeit als Ursache der Pest?: Der Traktat De mortalitate in Alamannia des Konrad von Megenberg. In Max Planck Institut für Geschichte (Ed.), *Festschrift Hermann Heimpel* (Vol. 2, pp. 839–883). Göttingen, Germany: Vandenhoeck & Ruprecht.

Lang, B., & McDannell, C. (1990). *Der Himmel: Eine Kulturgeschichte des ewigen Lebens*. Frankfurt, Germany: Suhrkamp.

LeGoff, J. (1986). *The birth of Purgatory*. Chicago: University of Chicago Press.

Lessing, G. E. (1780). *Die Erziehung des Menschengeschlechts*. Berlin, Germany: Hanser. Available at *http://gutenberg.spiegel.de/buch/die-erziehung-des-menschengeschlechts-1175/2*.

Meyers neues Konversationslexikon. (1871). Hildburghausen, Germany: Bibliographisches Institut.

Mulsow, M. (2007). Das Planetensystem als Civitas Dei. In L. Hölscher (Ed.), *Das Jenseits: Facetten eines religiösen Begriffs in der Neuzeit* (pp. 40–62). Göttingen, Germany: Wallstein Verlag.

Nora, P. (1984–1992). *Les lieux de mémoire*. Paris: Gallimard.

Oxford English Dictionary. (1933). Oxford, UK: Oxford University Press.

Rohbeck, J. (2012). *Zukunft der Geschichte: Geschichtsphilosophie und Zukunftsethik*. Berlin, Germany: Akademie-Verlag.

Sawicki, D. (2000). *Leben mit den Toten: Geisterglauben und die Entstehung des Spiritismus in Deutschland 1770–1900*. Paderborn, Germany: Ferdinand Schöningh.

Schmidt-Gernig, A. (2002). The cybernetic society: Western future studies of the 1960s and 1970s and their predictions for the year 2000. In R. N. Cooper & R. Layard (Eds.), *What the future holds: Insights from social science* (pp. 233–260). Cambridge, MA: MIT Press.

Seefried, E. (2015). *Zukünfte: Aufstieg und Krise der Zukunftsforschung 1945–1980*. Berlin, Germany: de Gruyter.

Sparn, W. (2007). Jenseitskonzeptionen in der protestantischen Aufklärungstheologie. In L. Hölscher (Ed.), *Das Jenseits: Facetten eines religiösen Begriffs in der Neuzeit* (pp. 12–13). Göttingen, Germany: Wallstein Verlag.

Spener, P. J. (1694). *Behauptung der Hoffnung künfftiger besserer Zeiten*. Frankfurt, Germany: Johann David Zunners.

Toulmin, S., & Goodfield, J. (1982). *The discovery of time*. Chicago: University of Chicago Press. (Original work published 1965)

von Hardenberg, F. (1815). Heinrich von Ofterdingen: Part 2. In L. Tieck & F. Schlegel (Eds.), *Novalis Schriften* (Vol. 1). Berlin, Germany: Reimers.

Zedler, J. H. (1732–1750). *Welt Großes vollständiges Universal-Lexicon aller Wissenschaften und Künste* (Vol. 64). Leipzig, Germany: Johann Heinrich Zedler.

CHAPTER 2

Future-Thinking in Animals
Capacities and Limits

Jonathan Redshaw
Adam Bulley

> The brute is an embodiment of present impulses, and hence what elements of fear and hope exist in its nature—and they do not go very far—arise only in relation to objects that lie before it and within reach of those impulses; whereas a man's range of vision embraces the whole of his life, and extends far into the past and future.
> —ARTHUR SCHOPENHAUER, *Studies in Pessimism* (1851/1890)

Nonhuman animals (hereafter "animals") do not harness the future to dominate their environments in the immediately obvious way that humans do (Suddendorf, 2006). It is therefore unsurprising that early thinkers such as Schopenhauer and others (e.g., Bergson, 1896/2004; Köhler, 1917/1927; Nietzsche, 1876/1998) regarded animals as being largely mentally bound to the present (but see James, 1890). Contemporary scientific theorists have also made cases for strong limits on nonhuman future-thinking (Roberts, 2002; Suddendorf & Corballis, 1997), and, driven by these claims, comparative psychologists have begun to document animal behaviors that appear in some way oriented toward the future (for previous reviews, see Cheke & Clayton, 2010; Roberts, 2012; Suddendorf & Corballis, 2007, 2010). Conflicting interpretations of the results has led to the formation of two camps within the literature: one that tends to emphasize the possible continuities between human and animal future-thinking (e.g., Clayton, Bussey, & Dickinson, 2003; Corballis, 2013; Osvath & Martin-Ordas, 2014; Roberts, 2012; Scarf, Smith, & Stuart, 2014; Zentall, 2005) and one that tends to emphasize the possible discontinuities (e.g., Cheng, Werning, & Suddendorf, 2016; Hoerl, 2008; Redshaw, 2014; Suddendorf, 2013a; Tulving, 2005).

Despite much heated debate, however, the dichotomy between the continuity and discontinuity camps is, in many respects, a false one. Both sides would agree, for instance, that animals often act in ways that increase their future survival and/

or reproductive chances without mentally representing the future at all. Future-oriented behaviors need not necessarily require sophisticated planning, but instead can exist as purely innate processes (e.g., fixed action patterns) and/or arise via associative learning (Suddendorf & Corballis, 2007, 2010). Both sides would also agree that future-thinking is not an all-or-none process, an encapsulated cognitive module that an organism is either equipped with or not. Among humans, the various components involved in future-thinking come online at different ages during childhood (Suddendorf & Redshaw, 2013), and individual differences in the capacity persist into adulthood (e.g., Lebreton et al., 2013). Finally, both sides of the debate would agree that: (1) at least some animals can represent more than just perceptual information tied to the present, and (2) there are at least some differences between human and animal future-thinking (whether these differences be quantitative or qualitative in nature).

In defining future-thinking, various theoretical positions have placed differential emphasis on the subjective nature of the phenomenon and its behavioral consequences. Tulving (1985), for instance, initially put forward the notion of *autonoetic*, or "self-knowing," consciousness to refer to the first-person awareness often implicated in mental access to past and future autobiographical events. Suddendorf and Corballis (1997) later coined the term *mental time travel* to refer to these declarative mental trips into past and future and also indicated that important differences may exist between the capacities of humans and animals. Specifically, they proposed the seminal Bischof–Köhler hypothesis (cf. Bischof–Köhler, 1985; Bischof, 1985; Köhler, 1917/1927), suggesting that animals may not be able to imagine and prepare for future desire states that conflict with their current states (see the section "Acting with future desires in mind," later in this chapter). Subsequently, however, Suddendorf and Corballis (2007, 2010) emphasized how the behavioral consequences of this future-thinking might be discerned, reasoning that evolution can work only on the behavioral "output" or actions of an animal, and not on mental events per se. A number of researchers have since proposed that certain behavioral capacities (Raby & Clayton, 2009) or underlying mechanisms (Osvath, 2016; Osvath & Martin-Ordas, 2014) should be key to understanding the future-thinking of animals. The empirical goal of comparative psychologists, then, should perhaps not be to determine whether animals can mentally represent events that have not yet happened but, rather, to establish their capacities and limits in various future-oriented behavioral domains (Osvath, 2016; Raby & Clayton, 2009; Suddendorf & Corballis, 2007).

In the bulk of this chapter, we review and critique the evidence for future-oriented animal behavior from several lines of research. Future-thinking itself, of course, cannot be directly observed in nonverbal subjects, yet with careful controls simpler alternative explanations for their behavior can be ruled out with increasing confidence (Suddendorf & Corballis, 2010). Throughout our analysis, we highlight not only the achievements of animals on certain tasks, but also their failures, and suggest where their cognitive limits may lie. We then synthesize these findings and make the case for at least one overarching limit—namely, that animals (unlike humans) may not be able to reflect on their own natural future-thinking limitations and act to compensate for them to acquire additional benefits. Given that the vast majority of research has focused on primates, rodents, or corvids, we largely restrict our analysis to studies of these taxa. We do, however, point toward other branches of the phylogenetic tree that may be worth investigating.

ANIMAL FUTURE-THINKING ACROSS DOMAINS

In the following sections, we survey the behavioral evidence for animal future-thinking across six domains: (1) navigation and route planning, (2) intertemporal choice and delayed gratification, (3) preparing for future threats, (4) acquiring and constructing tools to solve future problems, (5) acquiring, saving, and exchanging tokens for future rewards, and (6) acting with future desires in mind. We then summarize animals' capacities and potential limits in each domain in Table 2.1.

Navigation and Route Planning

It is not surprising that many animals should possess mental representations of their environments in order to navigate through them safely and efficiently. Indeed, classic behavioral research demonstrates that rodents (O'Keefe & Nadel, 1978; Tolman, 1948), chimpanzees (Boesch & Boesch, 1984; Menzel, 1973) and perhaps even bees (Gould, 1986) rely on "cognitive maps" to pursue both familiar and novel paths through known environments in order to attain rewards and avoid threats. Interestingly, recent research suggests that rodents may mentally preexperience such routes before they pursue them, both inside and outside of the simulated spatial context. This inference is based on recordings from hippocampal place cells, which show similar patterns of firing before the rodents take a path and then when they actually take the path (see, e.g., Dragoi & Tonegawa, 2013; Ólafsdóttir, Barry, Saleem, Hassabis, & Spiers, 2015; Pfeiffer & Foster, 2013).

If we grant the validity of hippocampal place cell recordings as evidence of phenomenological experience (cf. Suddendorf, 2013a), then the data do indeed suggest that rodents mentally represent specific navigational sequences before they take them (Corballis, 2013). Nevertheless, even if there is a correlation between mental representations and future behavior, it need not necessarily follow that rodents (or other animals) preemptively embed these representations within a specific future context (i.e., represent them *as* future representations). Among humans, representations of potential future events are often spontaneous and detached from awareness of the temporal location of these events (e.g., during mind wandering), even though such representations may influence actual future behavior (Baird, Smallwood, & Schooler, 2011; Stawarczyk, Cassol, & D'Argembeau, 2013). If similar cognitive processes occur in rodents, then it remains plausible that they experience navigational representations as an adaptive form of temporally detached mental imagery, rather than actively planning future routes as humans can (see Redshaw, 2014). Recent computational modeling suggests that offline sequential firing in rodent hippocampal place cells may even be generated randomly by neural network activity (Azizi, Wiskott, & Cheng, 2013).

Regardless of the underlying cognitive processes, neurological studies of rodent route planning have thus far focused only on navigation through very simple spatial fields. Ecological studies with great apes, on the other hand, have claimed to provide evidence of route planning through complex natural environments. Female chimpanzees in the Tai forest, for example, have been found to prefer sleeping in nests that are closer to breakfast sites containing ephemeral, high-calorie fruits than breakfast sites containing other fruits (Janmaat, Polansky, Ban, & Boesch, 2014). They also leave their nests earlier when they breakfast on ephemeral fruits, especially when these fruits are further away. These findings led the authors to conclude that the chimpanzees were flexibly planning their sleeping and nest-leaving behaviors with breakfast in mind (for similar route-planning claims in male orangutans, see van Schaik, Damerius, & Isler, 2013).

Ecological studies are extremely valuable for documenting the natural future-oriented behaviors of great apes and other species. The problem with drawing strong conclusions about future-thinking from such research, however, is that we cannot rule out whether the behaviors observed are the product of innate predispositions, learning processes, or a combination thereof (Thom & Clayton, 2015a). Future-oriented behavior is pervasive throughout the animal kingdom and need not necessarily require sophisticated temporal representations (Suddendorf & Corballis, 2007). It seems plausible, for instance, that natural selection would favor chimpanzees with an innate preference for sleeping closer to ephemeral, high-calorie fruits, even if these individuals were not specifically considering the next day's breakfast when doing so. Natural selection would also favor chimpanzees with a predisposition toward leaving earlier in their circadian cycle when traveling to breakfast sites that were farther away (according to their cognitive map). If chimpanzees are truly able to *flexibly* plan breakfast, then they should be able to do so in an experimental setting in which the natural contingency between proximity and ease of access to the next day's food is reversed (such that they must choose to sleep further away from a breakfasting area in order to more easily access it tomorrow).

Intertemporal Choice and Delayed Gratification

Animals often forgo immediate opportunities or incur immediate costs in favor of longer term benefits (Fawcett, McNamara, & Houston, 2012; Stevens & Stephens, 2008). When a spider builds a web that may later catch prey, for instance, energy must be expended to produce the silk and to spin the threads, and other opportunities (e.g., to mate) must be forfeited. Thus building a web, along with many other activities in the animal kingdom—from hibernating to caching food to searching for a mate—can be construed as intertemporal trade-offs between immediate and delayed outcomes (Stevens, 2010). Although these behaviors are typically referred to as "choices," however, at least some of them likely involve no thinking about the future reward at all (Stevens, 2011). Few would attribute the spider in the above example with any mental representation of the rewards it stands to receive from its patience, for instance. On the other hand, larger-brained animals such as birds, rodents, and primates are also faced with intertemporal trade-offs, the underlying cognitive mechanisms of which are more contentious (Thom & Clayton, 2015b). Foraging is a classical case: An animal encountering an unripe fruit must decide whether to eat it now or wait for it to ripen in order to reap the benefits of improved taste and nutrition (Dasgupta & Maskin, 2005).

In standard laboratory intertemporal choice tasks, an animal is presented with two options: one that will trigger an immediate reward, and one that will incur a delay until reward onset. Although rats and pigeons generally exhibit a global preference for immediate reinforcement, they will sometimes choose to delay their gratification for a few seconds for a larger reward than an immediately available one in these tasks (Tobin & Logue, 1994). Both new-world and old-world monkeys tend to wait less than a minute for the larger reward (Santos & Rosati, 2015), whereas chimpanzees may wait up to 2 minutes (Rosati, Stevens, Hare, & Hauser, 2007). Other paradigms assess the related construct of delay maintenance—or how well an animal can hold out for a larger, later reward in the face of immediate temptation. In "accumulation" tasks, a small reward will gradually build up until the animal chooses to retrieve it, and chimpanzees have been shown to wait for up to 3 minutes for chocolate pieces to accumulate before consuming them (Addessi et al., 2013; Beran, 2002). In "exchange" tasks, on the other hand, a small reward must be kept in possession for a period of time before being traded back to the experimenter for a larger one. Chimpanzees may delay gratification for up to 8 minutes when the delayed reward is 40 times larger than the one initially provided (Dufour, Pelé, Sterck, & Thierry, 2007).

Although some authors have suggested that animals' intertemporal choice behavior may rely on some form of future-thinking (Roberts, 2012; Santos & Rosati, 2015), there are a number of reasons to be skeptical. Standard dichotomous choice scenarios are usually presented in highly artificial environments in which many trials are used to teach the time lag associated with the delayed options (Mazur, 1987). For instance, it generally starts with the two rewards (large and small) both being delivered immediately, with a slight delay added to the larger reward every time it is chosen. Furthermore, because these studies often present both the delayed and immediate options simultaneously, with the only difference being the inferred wait that the animal has learned previously, it is possible for the subject to simply associate each of the options with the outcome it engenders if chosen (including the negative emotion associated with waiting for the larger reward), without necessitating a mental representation of the delay itself. In the accumulation task, this problem is somewhat abated, though the animal can still see the rewards building up and is therefore reinforced in its waiting behavior with every food item that is added. Successful performance on exchange tasks probably signifies the most convincing evidence of some degree of future reward representation, though such tasks typically still involve a long period of training to teach the trade behavior, and it is difficult to rule out the possibility that the subjects simply lose interest in the small reward and subsequently exchange it when it returns to their attention.

Sometimes it is more adaptive to select an immediate reward instead of a larger but delayed one, for example, when the environment is particularly harsh or uncertain (Fantino, 1995; Fawcett et al., 2012; Frankenhuis, Panchanathan, & Nettle, 2016). A capacity to *flexibly adjust* intertemporal preferences as a function of anticipated outcomes might therefore be a particularly informative avenue for exploring future-oriented thinking in the context of intertemporal choice (Bulley, Henry, & Suddendorf, 2016; Cheke, Thom, & Clayton, 2011). Bonobos have been found to adjust the amount of time they are willing to spend waiting for future rewards when the administering experimenter has proven to be unreliable, perhaps because they are "expecting" delayed rewards to be less likely to materialize (Stevens, Rosati, Heilbronner, & Mühlhoff, 2011). Similarly, squirrel monkeys have been found to gradually change their choice preferences to a smaller reward when they learn that this choice will eventually lead to a larger reward amount (McKenzie, Cherman, Bird, Naqshbandi, & Roberts, 2004). The animals in these studies, however, were taught that their food amounts would change as a function of their choices over a number of trials, so it is plausible that they learned to associate the two options with different outcomes. To test whether an animal could flexibly adjust intertemporal choices as a function of anticipated (rather than learned) outcomes, an experiment could be devised in which the reward options varied in perishability. For instance, if a chimpanzee first learned that 1 piece of food from Tray A would always be given immediately upon selection, whereas 10 pieces of the same food from Tray B would not be given until after a delay, then would it subsequently be less likely to select Tray B if the trays contained a quickly perishing food (e.g., flavored ice)?

Avoiding Future Threats

The future holds the potential for abundant opportunities and rewards, but it also contains myriad potential threats. Whereas manifest threats tend to be responded to with a complex suite of processes collectively labelled as a "fear" or "defensive" response (LeDoux, 2014), many animals are also capable of responding to threats with a more advanced preparatory window. Such preparation for threats before they materialize is associated with a different set of physiological and cognitive reactions that together constitute an "anxiety" response (Bateson, Brilot, & Nettle, 2011; Damasio, 1995). This response entails the secretion of stress hormones and a change in heart rate, but also hypervigilance and precautionary behaviors oriented toward sampling more information and discerning the optimal reaction to the implied danger. In essence, the anxiety response can be thought of as extending the amount of time an animal has at its disposal to deal with potential threats before they eventuate. This response can be evoked both by specific cues of a possible threat, such as the smell of a predator, but also via an appraisal of "general vulnerability"; for instance, based on interoceptive signals that indicate the current healthiness of the body (Bateson et al., 2011).

The threat reaction is thereby highly flexible, and its expression varies as a function of a number of variables pertaining to, among others, the state of the organism, its recent experiences, and ecological conditions (Bateson et al., 2011; Nettle & Bateson, 2012). Many prey animals, for example, exhibit vigilant "checking" behavior in open areas where they are susceptible to predation, and nocturnal animals show anxiety in bright light (Bednekoff & Lima, 1998; Burman, Parker, Paul, & Mendl, 2009; Underwood, 1982). Despite being impressively future-oriented and often flexible, however, such a preparatory anxiety response does not necessarily demonstrate mental representations of the future. Rather, this response may be largely dependent upon perceptible cues of specific or general threat in the immediate environment, alongside physiological signals about current vulnerability (Apfelbach, Blanchard, Blanchard, Hayes, & McGregor, 2005). It is possible that animals may also employ memory traces of aversive past events associated with such cues in modifying their responses. However, to the best of our knowledge, a capacity to think about and act against specific potential future threats without relying on external or vulnerability cues has thus far been demonstrated only in humans (Miloyan, Bulley, & Suddendorf, 2016).

Thus far, nearly all experimental research into animal future-thinking capacities has focused on preparation for future opportunities and rewards, rather than for future threats. In the previous section, however, we outlined how animals tend to be largely impatient and prefer immediately available rewards relative to larger, later ones; therefore, it may be somewhat unsurprising that animals fail certain future-thinking tasks in which they must pursue delayed rewards. Still, it remains possible that they could pass structurally similar tasks requiring them to plan for upcoming dangers. Indeed, threats to fitness are a potent source of selective pressure and likely played a critical role in the evolution of future-oriented cognition (Miloyan et al., 2016; Mobbs, Hagan, Dalgleish, Silston, & Prévost, 2015). Nevertheless, given the ethical concerns with experimental manipulations that have the potential to induce strong negative emotion, future research in this area may be largely confined to observational studies.

Acquiring and Constructing Tools to Solve Future Problems

Some of the most commonly cited evidence of animal future-thinking comes from studies of great apes' capacity to select tools and use them after a delay to solve a problem and obtain a reward. In the earliest of these studies (Mulcahy & Call, 2006), bonobos and orangutans were first trained to use a tool to retrieve a food reward and were then presented with a free choice of tools (including the trained tool) to transport out of the room while the reward was unavailable. The apes transported the appropriate tool more often than inappropriate tools, and a few of them were more likely to bring the appropriate tool back to the room and use it when the reward became available again (either 1 or 14 hours later). A second study replicated these findings with chimpanzees and orangutans in a forced-choice paradigm (in which they could choose only one tool), while also showing that the subjects sometimes preferred the appropriate tool over an immediate small food reward (Osvath & Osvath, 2008). Impressively, the final experiment in this follow-up study found that the apes were more likely to choose *novel* tools that could solve the future problem than novel tools that could not.

Concerns exist over whether the apes' success in these paradigms could be explained by associative learning, given that the appropriate tools (or similar ones) had been previously reinforced during the training phases (Suddendorf, 2006; Suddendorf, Corballis, & Collier-Baker, 2009). Even setting aside this particular low-level explanation, however, such experiments can only go so far in demonstrating apes' future-thinking. It seems plausible, for instance, that seeing an appropriate tool would trigger an immediate representation of the reward it can retrieve (such representations are easily cued in humans; Tulving & Thomson, 1973); and so the apes could make their choice based on this immediate representation rather than any expectation of a specific future event in which the reward becomes available again. Then, when the reward does become available, they simply retrieve the tool to which they have convenient access. In this manner their initial representations would indeed be "future-oriented," but only from an objective perspective rather than from the apes' own perspective (Redshaw, 2014). Such explanations could potentially be ruled out by visibly destroying the reward apparatus (and then removing it from view) before testing whether the apes continued to choose the now useless tool. If they did not, it might suggest that they made their initial choices based on flexible representations of the future, rather than on rigid representations triggered by seeing the tool.

One recent study gave great apes the opportunity to construct tools that could be used to solve a future problem and obtain a reward (Bräuer & Call, 2015). Chimpanzees, bonobos, and orangutans were introduced to an apparatus that required them to bite off and insert pieces of wood into tubes in order to retrieve grapes. Once a piece of wood had been inserted into a tube, it could no longer be retrieved, such that the apes had to bite off multiple pieces of wood in order to retrieve grapes from multiple tubes. After learning how to do this, the apes' access to the apparatus was temporarily blocked by a transparent Plexiglas panel, and either zero, one, or eight of the tubes were baited with grapes. While waiting for the apparatus to become accessible again, the apes were more likely to prepare useful pieces of wood when grapes would be available in the future (for a limited time) than when they would not. They also prepared significantly more tools in the eight-grapes condition than the one-grape condition, but not excessively so (on average, they produced less than two tools in the eight grapes condition).

These results do indeed show that great apes can prepare tools that will enable them to obtain a currently unavailable reward in the near future, but they also point to important limitations. First, it remains to be seen whether apes could succeed at the task if visual access to the apparatus were blocked and the future availability of grapes (or lack thereof) had to be represented in working memory. Moreover, the pattern of responses suggests that the apes were not particularly sensitive to the specific contingencies of the problem. They showed no evidence of producing even close to the optimal number of tools in the eight-grapes condition, which suggests that they may have been producing them based on a rough rule (e.g., "more visible grapes = make more tools") rather than the precise requirements of the task (i.e., "make one tool per visible grape"). The apes' difficulty with the eight-grapes condition and the more general capacity to produce multiple tools to solve multiple future problems may be related to limitations in number representation (Matsuzawa, 2009).

Acquiring, Saving, and Exchanging Tokens for Future Rewards

Money is a powerful reinforcer for humans primarily because we recognize that it can be exchanged for desirable items and experiences in the future. Researchers have investigated whether nonhuman primates, too, can acquire, save, and eventually exchange tokens for future rewards. In one of the earliest of these studies (Dufour & Sterck, 2008), chimpanzees were first trained to return a colorful straw to an experimenter in order to receive peanuts. In the subsequent test phase, they were given the opportunity to collect straws and two types of distractor objects, transport them to another room when ushered away, and then come back to the first room an hour later and exchange the straws for peanuts. The distractor objects were also associated with rewards (a branch that could be used to retrieve honey and a stick that could be used to retrieve fruit pieces), but not in an exchange context, in order to rule out the possibility that the subjects simply preferred the straws because of their previous positive reinforcement. The results showed that the chimpanzees often transported the straws and distractor objects out of the room when ushered away but that they rarely returned and exchanged the straws for peanuts (the best performer exchanged straws on 2 of 10 trials). Critically, the subjects showed no significant preference for returning to the testing room with straws compared with the distractor objects, suggesting that they were not specifically considering the future exchange task when returning to the room.

A similar study produced contrasting results, although there was one important methodological difference. Osvath and Persson (2013) showed that chimpanzees and orangutans preferred to transport, return with, and exchange the previously reinforced token instead of distractor objects, and they also preferred to the select the token over distractors in a forced-choice paradigm. Unlike in the earlier study, however, the distractor items were novel and not positively associated with rewards in any context. Prior to training, the subjects showed no inherent preference for selecting the correct token instead of the distractors, but it seems likely that the apes would have quickly acquired a preference for the token after they had been taught to return it for food. It therefore cannot be ruled out that the subjects preferred to select and transport the correct token instead of the distractors simply because of the token's unique association with rewards. Note that this critique also applies to a recent study suggesting that ravens may be capable of exchanging tokens and selecting tools to obtain future rewards (Kabadayi & Osvath, 2017). A final study showed that bonobos and orangutans also acquired, transported, and later exchanged items for rewards (Bourjade, Call, Pelé, Maumy, & Dufour, 2014), but these results are also equivocal, as there were no distractor objects for the apes to select.

The differential pattern of responding across these studies illuminates where apes' limitations in exchange tasks may lie. Specifically, it appears that they may select and transport tokens based on their *past utility*, rather than representing and reasoning about the specific future exchange context in which they will become useful. In Dufour and Sterck's (2008) study, the distractor items also had past utility (albeit in a nonexchange context), and so they were preferred equally to the tokens. In the later studies, however, the tokens were preferred based on their unique past utility, regardless of the fact that they would become useful in the future. The preference for past utility could be based on simple associative valence (Suddendorf, 2006; Suddendorf et al., 2009), or it could be based on cued mental representations (i.e., episodic memory traces) of previous occasions when the token was useful (Cheng et al., 2016; Redshaw, 2014).

Acting with Future Desires in Mind

For nearly two decades, animal future-thinking researchers have been trying to falsify the Bischof–Köhler hypothesis (Suddendorf & Corballis, 1997), which proposes that animals cannot imagine and prepare for a future motivational state that conflicts with their current motivational state (e.g., they cannot imagine and prepare for future hunger when sated). As Suddendorf and Corballis (2007) point out, animals incapable of anticipating future drive or need states would "have little reason to concern themselves with a remote future" (p. 306), on account of the fact that only present needs would matter to such animals. Early observations suggested that animals had great difficulty imagining future desires (e.g., Roberts, 2002), but more recent studies have produced some provocative findings.

In the earliest study that claimed to falsify the Bischof–Köhler hypothesis, Naqshbandi and Roberts (2006) gave two squirrel monkeys a choice between selecting one piece of date with water available after 30 minutes, or four pieces of date with water available after 180 minutes. The monkeys eventually began to prefer the former option, with the authors arguing that they made their selection in order to reduce future thirst levels (as dates induce thirst). Nevertheless, the fact that the monkeys gradually began to prefer the one date over many trials suggests the involvement of associative learning; and, moreover, if they were truly acting for future desires, then they should have selected the four pieces of date and simply waited until water became available before eating them (Suddendorf & Corballis, 2010). The result could not be replicated in a sample of six rhesus monkeys (Paxton & Hampton, 2009).

One of the most interesting lines of evidence in this area comes from a pair of observational studies with a male chimpanzee, Santino. Zookeepers and researchers witnessed him storing piles of stones on some mornings before hurling them at zoo visitors later (Osvath, 2009; Osvath & Karvonen, 2012). These observations were met with claims that Santino may have been preparing for future occasions when he would desire to display his dominance toward the zoo visitors (the stone-collecting behavior appeared to occur in a calm state, whereas the hurling behavior typically occurred in an aroused state). Nevertheless, it remains unclear just how oriented toward specific future events his stone-storing activities were, rather than being driven by more general mental representations (i.e., episodic memory traces) of zoo visitors appearing (Redshaw, 2014). These observational findings must be replicated in an experimental setting before they can begin to seriously question the Bischof–Köhler hypothesis.

Perhaps the strongest challenge to the Bischof–Köhler hypothesis comes from a clever line of research with birds from the *Corvidae* family, which have a natural proclivity for caching and retrieving food (e.g., Correia, Dickinson, & Clayton, 2007; Raby, Alexis, Dickinson, & Clayton, 2007). The most convincing of these studies (Shettleworth, 2012) exploited the fact that corvids and other animals prefer not to eat a specific food (in comparison with other foods) once they have become sated on that food. Eurasian jays were first fed a particular food (e.g., peanuts) to the point of satiation, and they subsequently preferred to store that food in a specific cache that would be available to retrieve from only vwhen they would prefer the food again in the future (Cheke & Clayton, 2012). Thus it appeared the birds were ignoring their current distaste for the food in order to act for their future preference. Nevertheless, the authors conceded that the jays could have simply learned to associate an emotional preference for the food with the appropriate storage location during the training phase, with this preference becoming reactivated when the birds were given the opportunity to cache. In other words, the birds might have not been acting based on a "future" desire state but rather a cued current desire state that just happened to match the future desire (Redshaw, 2014).

Emotional states seem particularly susceptible to such reactivation in that they can be cued by environmental factors and experienced in the present to motivate behaviors with incidental future benefits (see Boyer, 2008; Damasio, 1989; Osvath & Martin-Ordas, 2014). So-called interoceptive states (e.g., general hunger, thirst, temperature sensitivity), on the other hand, arise more directly from the peripheral nervous system (Craig, 2002) and may be less susceptible to reactivation. Tests of the Bischof–Köhler hypothesis should perhaps therefore focus on whether animals can act for future interoceptive states if they wish to rule out associative reactivation as an explanation. Nonetheless, acting for such states may be genuinely beyond the capacity of animals. Among humans, children struggle to act for future thirst levels until at least age 7 and possibly beyond (Atance & Meltzoff, 2006; Kramer, Goldfarb, Tashjian, & Lagattuta, 2017; Mahy, Grass, Wagner, & Kliegel, 2014). Indeed, even adults struggle to preexperience future interoceptive states (try to "experience" hunger the next time you finish a very large meal, for example), and so our capacity to act for such states may be largely based on an abstract understanding of temporal shifts in motivation rather than any analogue representation of the states themselves. If there is truth to the Bischof–Köhler hypothesis, then, it may be that animals cannot represent desire states in a propositional fashion in the way that humans can.

SYNTHESIS

The previous sections have described evidence for animals' future-oriented behavior in a number of domains (see Table 2.1 for summary). In each section we have presented examples of animals acting in ways that make future events more pleasurable and/or less painful. It is not surprising that such behaviors would be apparent in the animal kingdom, given that natural selection can clearly act on how a behavior affects an animal's future survival or reproductive chances (Klein, 2013; Schacter & Addis, 2007; Suddendorf & Corballis, 2007). It is also not surprising that some of these behaviors would be underpinned by cognitive processes, in that certain animals can represent states of reality that correlate with actual future events and subsequently behave in a manner that provides tangible fitness benefits. Indeed, some of the most influential unified theories of neuroscience propose that brains are essentially "prediction machines" that, through a continuous, potentially Bayesian-like process of comparing expected and actual outcomes, become ever more optimal at anticipating events in the immediate environment (Bar, 2007; Clark, 2013; Friston, 2010). And at least some of the predictions generated by the brain may be based on episodic memory traces triggered by the presence of relevant external cues (Cheng et al., 2016; Redshaw, 2014). In this particular sense, animal future-thinking may be basically continuous with the human capacity.

In each domain, however, we have also encountered important potential limitations. Some of these potential limitations may eventually require reconsideration; future research may well demonstrate that animals are capable of more complex

TABLE 2.1. Animal Future-Thinking Capacities and Potential Limits across Domains

Future-thinking domain	Capacities	Potential limits
Navigation and route planning	• Neural simulation of familiar and novel routes through known environments and subsequent pursuit of the same routes[r]	• May involve temporally detached mental imagery, rather than active planning
	• Strategic nesting and calling behaviors that increase future foraging and reproductive success in distant locations[p]	• Ecological evidence only; behavior may be based on innate predispositions and/or associative learning
Delayed gratification and temporal discounting	• Selecting a larger, delayed reward over a smaller but immediate one[g]; waiting for food to accumulate before eating[p]; retaining a small food reward without eating before exchanging it for a larger reward[p]	• May be limited to very short periods of time and may be based on learned associations between options and outcomes
Preparing for future threats	• Anxious affect produces hypervigilance and other physiological responses to prepare for potential threats[g]	• May be limited to instances in which immediately perceptible cues of threat are available and may require learned associations between the cue and negative outcomes (and/or innate predispositions to fear the cue)
Selecting and constructing tools to solve future problems	• Selecting an appropriate tool that can solve a nonvisible future problem and using it when the opportunity arises[c, p]	• May require past experience using an identical or similar tool successfully on the same problem, and thus tool selection may be based on rigid memory traces of past tool use rather than flexible future representations
	• Making an appropriate tool to solve a future problem and using it when the opportunity arises[p]	• May require the future problem to be visible and may struggle to make multiple tools when multiple future problems can be solved
Collecting tokens and exchanging them for future rewards	• Selecting a token and returning it for a reward after a delay[c, p]	• May be based on the past utility of the token rather than its ability to be used in a specific future exchange context, given that no preference is observed when distractor items also have past utility
Acting for future desire states (Bischof–Köhler hypothesis)	• Acting in a manner consistent with a future desire state[c, p]	• May require the future desire state to be triggered (i.e., experienced in the present) by prelearned associations with the behavioral context and may not apply to interoceptive desire states that arise more directly from the peripheral nervous system

Note. Each point in the "Capacities" column corresponds to one point in the "Potential limits" column. Superscripts indicate the taxa that the evidence applies to: p, primates; r, rodents; c, corvids; g, animals in general.

future-thinking and behavior than is currently known. On the other hand, in comparison with human future-thinking at least, it seems almost certain that some genuine limits exist. Moreover, some of these limits may be overarching, in that they restrict future-oriented behavior across several domains. A recurring theme throughout our analysis, for example, has been the lack of any evidence that animals represent future representations *as* future representations—a form of "metarepresentation" that may be critically important in various flexible human future-oriented behaviors (Redshaw, 2014; Suddendorf, 1999). In fact, Schopenhauer (1818/1909) first proposed this fundamental discontinuity between humans and animals 200 years ago, when he claimed that the principal component missing from animal minds was "distinct consciousness of the past and of the eventual future, *as such,* and in connection with the present" (p. 229, emphasis in original).

Metarepresentation is important for future-thinking not necessarily in that it enables more vivid future imagery but, rather, because it allows agents to represent the *properties* of future imagery, such that potential future events can be explicitly contrasted with both current reality (Kappes & Oettingen, 2014; Oettingen, 2012; Redshaw, 2014) and with other potential future events (Gollwitzer, 2014). A predictive brain may indeed be ideally suited to representing likely outcomes of an event, but some future events cannot be anticipated with any certainty by even an optimal predictive brain (consider, e.g., the often erratic behavior of predators and prey). An agent with an additional capacity for forming metarepresentations, on the other hand, can reflect on the natural representational limits of his or her own mind and flexibly compensate for these limits. The human ability to develop and enact contingency plans, for instance, relies on an understanding that future events do not always unfold as expected or desired, and so it pays to also prepare for mutually exclusive alternatives. A traveler may imagine and prepare for a dream overseas holiday, but he or she may also purchase insurance in case something goes wrong and his or her original plan must be abandoned. On a broader scale, governments and other institutions are tasked with guiding human societies toward prosperous versions of the future, but they must also plan for potential large-scale emergencies and disasters.

One recent study examined the capacity to simultaneously prepare for two mutually exclusive outcomes of a very basic, immediate future event in 2- to 4-year-old children and a sample of eight great apes (Redshaw & Suddendorf, 2016). Subjects were given the opportunity to catch a desirable item that was dropped into a forked tube with one opening at the top and two possible exits at the bottom. The apes (like 2-year-olds) typically covered only one exit when preparing to catch the item, whereas most of the 4-year-olds consistently covered both exits from the first trial onward. The apes thus failed to provide evidence for an insightful capacity to consider and prepare for multiple, mutually exclusive future event outcomes (see also Suddendorf, Crimston, & Redshaw, 2017). Nevertheless, it remains possible that future studies with other subjects, species, and/or paradigms will discover some competence.

Another domain in which humans often reflect on and compensate for their future-thinking limitations is prospective memory, which involves remembering to perform an action at some particular future occasion. Because we recognize the chance that we will forget to perform the action, many of us use calendars, alarms, lists, and other external reminders as aids (Gilbert, 2015; Risko & Gilbert, 2016). Indeed, many human institutions would collapse entirely if it were not for future-oriented record-keeping procedures that preclude the need for perfect memories (e.g., consider legal and financial systems). There have been some claims for prospective memory in great apes (Beran, Perdue, Bramlett, Menzel, & Evans, 2012; Perdue, Evans, Williamson, Gonsiorowski, & Beran, 2014), with experiments showing that they remember to request or exchange a token for food after completing another irrelevant task (for similar claims in rats; see Crystal, 2013). Nevertheless, it remains possible that no future-thinking was involved in these studies but, instead, that the apes were simply cued into action after completing the irrelevant task. There is nothing to indicate that great apes or other animals spontaneously set their own reminders in order to improve their likelihood of remembering to perform future actions.

Certain species naturally act on their environments to store information that will be useful in the future. Consider, for example, ants that leave a pheromone trail between their nest and a food source (Sterelny, 2003). The question here, however, is whether any animals can do so in various novel contexts, as humans can. This would indicate a domain-general, flexible capacity for strategic reminder setting rather than an instinctual fixed action pattern confined to a narrow domain (for more general arguments along these lines, see Premack, 2007; Suddendorf & Corballis, 2010). One could examine this ability, for instance, in a delayed object permanence paradigm, in which an animal has to wait a specified period of time before it can select (from some options) the location where an experimenter has hidden food. Would the animal spontaneously and consistently mark the correct location with a body part (or scent) or other object during the waiting period in order to increase its chances of remembering the place?

To summarize, there remains no evidence that animals metarepresent future representations *as* future representations, as mere possibilities that could be otherwise because of the mind's inherent inability to predict some aspects of future events with certainty. Humans, on the other hand, reflect on and flexibly compensate for their future-thinking limitations to acquire enormous benefits. Nevertheless, it is important to remember that an absence of evidence is not the same as evidence of absence, and thus future studies should give animals more opportunities to demonstrate such a capacity. Here we have given two possible lines of evidence to pursue: (1) the ability to spontaneously and simultaneously prepare for multiple, mutually exclusive versions of the future and (2) the ability to spontaneously set reminder cues in prospective memory tasks. Any results suggesting that animals did or did not possess these abilities would likely inspire debate and alternative interpretations, but with increasing refinement of experimental manipulations, it is certainly possible to make progress on such important questions.

The Phylogeny of Future-Thinking

Absence of evidence is not only a specific problem for certain domains of animal future-thinking but also more a general problem when considering the relatively minuscule number of species that have been tested in controlled settings. The performance of great apes and other primates is of particular interest, of course, given the potential for shedding light on the evolution of human-like future-oriented mechanisms by studying closely related species. Nevertheless, by examining patterns of capacities and limits across vastly different taxa, one could potentially reason about the biological and environmental factors responsible for the emergence of future-thinking in general (whether that be "mere" predictive cognition or higher order capacities). For example, does future-thinking tend to arise as a by-product of domain-general cognitive specialization? Or does it tend to emerge in response to critical environmental pressures, such as highly uncertain future rewards or threats that precipitate a need for advanced preparation? And what roles do overall brain size, neocortex ratio, or other neurological factors play? These questions will remain moot, however, until more studies are carried out with nonprimate taxa other than corvids and rodents. Prime research candidates include taxa that have demonstrated impressive cognitive skills in other domains, such as elephants (e.g., Foerder et al., 2011), cetaceans (e.g., Marino et al., 2007), domestic dogs (e.g., Range, Viranyi, & Huber, 2007), and parrots (e.g., Pepperberg, Willner, & Gravitz, 1997). Even certain invertebrates, such as coleoid cephalopods (i.e., octopuses, squid, and cuttlefish), are worthy of investigation, given their notable problem-solving and tool use capacities (Vitti, 2013).

Importantly, although discussions of "animal" future-thinking are traditionally confined to extant species other than modern humans, we must also consider that the *Homo sapiens* species is only the last survivor of a rich hominin lineage. Indeed, archaeological evidence suggests that hominin future-thinking has undergone radical changes in the last few million years. Over one million years ago in east Africa, for example, our *Homo erectus* predecessors were making many more Acheulean tools than were necessary for everyday use (Kohn & Mithen, 1999). Given that such tools are notoriously difficult to craft, it is possible that these early humans were deliberately practicing tool manufacture with future expertise in mind (Rossano, 2003)—a behavior that may be out of reach for extant animals (Suddendorf, Brinums, & Imuta, 2016). Other novel future-thinking capacities are likely to have emerged in our more recent ancestors, such as *Homo heidelbergensis,* as the ability to harness the future continued to be a prime mover in human evolution (Suddendorf & Corballis, 1997). If any of our recently extinct cousins were still walking the earth—such as *Homo neanderthalensis* or the Denisova hominin—then the potential limits column in Table 2.1 would likely be considerably bare (see Suddendorf, 2013b).

CONCLUSION

Contemporary comparative psychologists have shown animals to be capable of far more complex future-oriented behaviors than was once thought possible. Here we have reviewed the available evidence and suggested that at least some of these behaviors are based on mental representations that go beyond the here-and-now. Such representations probably function to motivate present action that provides tangible future benefits across various domains. Nevertheless, there remain important questions regarding just how much insight animals have into their own future-thinking processes. There is no current evidence to suggest that animals metarepresent and behaviorally compensate for their natural future-thinking limits—an overarching capacity that enables humans to acquire additional and substantial benefits. Much further research is needed to shed light on the continuities and potential discontinuities between human and animal future-thinking capacities and on the evolutionary circumstances that give rise to these capacities.

REFERENCES

Addessi, E., Paglieri, F., Beran, M. J., Evans, T. A., Macchitella, L., De Petrillo, F., . . . Focaroli, V. (2013). Delay choice versus delay maintenance: Different measures of delayed gratification in capuchin monkeys (Cebus apella). *Journal of Comparative Psychology, 127,* 392–398.

Apfelbach, R., Blanchard, C. D., Blanchard, R. J., Hayes, R. A., & McGregor, I. S. (2005). The effects of predator odors in mammalian prey species: A review of field and laboratory studies. *Neuroscience and Biobehavioral Reviews, 29,* 1123–1144.

Atance, C. M., & Meltzoff, A. N. (2006). Preschoolers' current desires warp their choices for the future. *Psychological Science, 17,* 583–587.

Azizi, A. H., Wiskott, L., & Cheng, S. (2013). A computational model for preplay in the hippocampus. *Frontiers in Computational Neuroscience, 7,* 161. Available at *www.ncbi.nlm.nih.gov/pmc/articles/PMC3824291.*

Baird, B., Smallwood, J., & Schooler, J. W. (2011). Back to the future: Autobiographical planning and the functionality of mind-wandering. *Consciousness and Cognition, 20,* 1604–1611.

Bar, M. (2007). The proactive brain: Using analogies and associations to generate predictions. *Trends in Cognitive Sciences, 11,* 280–289.

Bateson, M., Brilot, B., & Nettle, D. (2011). Anxiety: An evolutionary approach. *Canadian Journal of Psychiatry, 56,* 707–715.

Bednekoff, P. A., & Lima, S. L. (1998). Randomness, chaos and confusion in the study of antipredator vigilance. *Trends in Ecology and Evolution, 13,* 284–287.

Beran, M. J. (2002). Maintenance of self-imposed delay of gratification by four chimpanzees (Pan troglodytes) and an orangutan (Pongo pygmaeus). *Journal of General Psychology, 129,* 49–66.

Beran, M. J., Perdue, B. M., Bramlett, J. L., Menzel, C. R., & Evans, T. A. (2012). Prospective memory in a language-trained chimpanzee (Pan troglodytes). *Learning and Motivation, 43,* 192–199.

Bergson, H. L. (2004). *Matter and memory* (N. M. Paul & W. S. Palmer, Trans.). North Chelmsford, MA: Courier Corporation. (Original work published 1896)

Bischof, N. (1985). *Das Rätsel Ödipus [The Oedipus riddle].* Munich, Germany: Piper.

Bischof-Köhler, D. (1985). Zur Phylogenese menschlicher Motivation [On the phylogeny of human motivation]. In L. Eckensberger & E. Lantermann (Eds.), *Emotion and Reflexivität* (pp. 3–47). Vienna, Austria: Urban & Schwarzenberg.

Boesch, C., & Boesch, H. (1984). Mental map in wild chimpanzees: An analysis of hammer transports for nut cracking. *Primates, 25,* 160–170.

Bourjade, M., Call, J., Pelé, M., Maumy, M., & Dufour, V. (2014). Bonobos and orangutans, but not chimpanzees, flexibly plan for the future in a token-exchange task. *Animal Cognition, 17,* 1329–1340.

Boyer, P. (2008). Evolutionary economics of mental time travel? *Trends in Cognitive Sciences, 12,* 219–224.

Bräuer, J., & Call, J. (2015). Apes produce tools for future use. *American Journal of Primatology, 77,* 254–263.

Bulley, A., Henry, J. D., & Suddendorf, T. (2016). Prospection and the present moment: The role of episodic foresight in intertemporal choices between immediate and delayed rewards. *Review of General Psychology, 20,* 29–47.

Burman, O. H., Parker, R. M., Paul, E. S., & Mendl, M. T. (2009). Anxiety-induced cognitive bias in non-human animals. *Physiology and Behavior, 98,* 345–350.

Cheke, L. G., & Clayton, N. S. (2010). Mental time travel in animals. *Wiley Interdisciplinary Reviews: Cognitive Science, 1,* 915–930.

Cheke, L. G., & Clayton, N. S. (2012). Eurasian jays (Garrulus glandarius) overcome their current desires to anticipate two distinct future needs and plan for them appropriately. *Biology Letters, 8.* Available at *http://rsbl.royalsocietypublishing.org/content/8/2/171.*

Cheke, L. G., Thom, J. M., & Clayton, N. S. (2011). Prospective decision making in animals: A potential role for intertemporal choice in the study of prospective cognition. In M. Bar (Ed.), *Predictions in the brain: Using our past to generate a future* (pp. 325–343). London, UK: Oxford University Press.

Cheng, S., Werning, M., & Suddendorf, T. (2016). Dissociating memory traces and scenario construction in mental time travel. *Neuroscience and Biobehavioral Reviews, 60,* 82–89.

Clark, A. (2013). Whatever next?: Predictive brains, situated agents, and the future of cognitive science. *Behavioral and Brain Sciences, 36,* 181–204.

Clayton, N. S., Bussey, T. J., & Dickinson, A. (2003). Can animals recall the past and plan for the future? *Nature Reviews Neuroscience, 4,* 685–691.

Corballis, M. C. (2013). Mental time travel: A case for evolutionary continuity. *Trends in Cognitive Sciences, 17,* 5–6.

Correia, S. P., Dickinson, A., & Clayton, N. S. (2007). Western scrub-jays anticipate future needs independently of their current motivational state. *Current Biology, 17,* 856–861.

Craig, A. D. (2002). How do you feel? Interoception: The sense of the physiological condition of the body. *Nature Reviews Neuroscience, 3,* 655–666.

Crystal, J. D. (2013). Remembering the past and planning for the future in rats. *Behavioural Processes, 93,* 39–49.

Damasio, A. R. (1989). Time-locked multiregional retroactivation: A systems-level proposal for the neural substrates of recall and recognition. *Cognition, 33,* 25–62.

Damasio, A. R. (1995). Toward a neurobiology of emotion and feeling: Operational concepts and hypotheses. *Neuroscientist, 1,* 19–25.

Dasgupta, P., & Maskin, E. (2005). Uncertainty and hyperbolic discounting. *American Economic Review, 95,* 1290–1299.

Dragoi, G., & Tonegawa, S. (2013). Distinct preplay of multiple novel spatial experiences in the rat. *Proceedings of the National Academy of Sciences of the USA, 110,* 9100–9105.

Dufour, V., Pelé, M., Sterck, E., & Thierry, B. (2007). Chimpanzee (Pan troglodytes) anticipation of food return: Coping with waiting time in an exchange task. *Journal of Comparative Psychology, 121,* 145–155.

Dufour, V., & Sterck, E. (2008). Chimpanzees fail to plan in an exchange task but succeed in a tool-using procedure. *Behavioural Processes, 79,* 19–27.

Fantino, E. (1995). The future is uncertain: Eat dessert first. *Behavioral and Brain Sciences, 18,* 125–126.

Fawcett, T. W., McNamara, J. M., & Houston, A. I. (2012). When is it adaptive to be patient?: A general framework for evaluating delayed rewards. *Behavioural Processes, 89,* 128–136.

Foerder, P., Galloway, M., Barthel, T., Moore, D. E., III, Reiss, D., & Samuel, A. (2011). Insightful problem solving in an Asian elephant. *PLOS ONE, 6,* e23251.

Frankenhuis, W. E., Panchanathan, K., & Nettle, D. (2016). Cognition in harsh and unpredictable environments. *Current Opinion in Psychology, 7,* 76–80.

Friston, K. (2010). The free-energy principle: A unified brain theory? *Nature Reviews Neuroscience, 11,* 127–138.

Gilbert, S. (2015). Strategic offloading of delayed intentions into the external environment. *Quarterly Journal of Experimental Psychology, 68,* 971–992.

Gollwitzer, P. M. (2014). Weakness of the will: Is a quick fix possible? *Motivation and Emotion, 38,* 305–322.

Gould, J. L. (1986). The locale map of honey bees: Do insects have cognitive maps? *Science, 232,* 861–863.

Hoerl, C. (2008). On being stuck in time. *Phenomenology and the Cognitive Sciences, 7,* 485–500.

James, W. (1890). *The principles of psychology.* New York: Holt.

Janmaat, K. R., Polansky, L., Ban, S. D., & Boesch, C. (2014). Wild chimpanzees plan their breakfast time, type, and location. *Proceedings of the National Academy of Sciences of the USA, 111,* 16343–16348.

Kabadayi, C., & Osvath, M. (2017). Ravens parallel great apes in flexible planning for tool-use and bartering. *Science, 357,* 202–204.

Kappes, A., & Oettingen, G. (2014). The emergence of goal pursuit: Mental contrasting connects future and reality. *Journal of Experimental Social Psychology, 54,* 25–39.

Klein, S. B. (2013). The temporal orientation of memory: It's time for a change of direction. *Journal of Applied Research in Memory and Cognition, 2,* 222–234.

Köhler, W. (1927). *The mentality of apes* (E. Winter, Trans.). London: Routledge & Kegan Paul. (Original work published 1917)

Kohn, M., & Mithen, S. (1999). Handaxes: Products of sexual selection? *Antiquity, 73,* 518–526.

Kramer, H. J., Goldfarb, D., Tashjian, S. M., & Lagattuta, K. H. (2017). "These pretzels are making me thirsty": Older children and adults struggle with induced-state episodic foresight. *Child Development, 88,* 1554–1562.

Lebreton, M., Bertoux, M., Boutet, C., Lehericy, S., Dubois, B., Fossati, P., . . . Pessiglione, M. (2013). A critical role for the hippocampus in the valuation of imagined outcomes. *PLOS Biology, 11,* e1001684.

LeDoux, J. E. (2014). Coming to terms with fear. *Proceedings of the National Academy of Sciences of the USA, 111,* 2871–2878.

Mahy, C. E., Grass, J., Wagner, S., & Kliegel, M. (2014). These pretzels are going to make me thirsty tomorrow: Differential development of hot and cool episodic foresight in early childhood? *British Journal of Developmental Psychology, 32,* 65–77.

Marino, L., Connor, R. C., Fordyce, R. E., Herman, L. M., Hof, P. R., Lefebvre, L., . . . Whitehead, H. (2007). Cetaceans have complex brains for complex cognition. *PLOS Biology, 5,* e139.

Matsuzawa, T. (2009). Symbolic representation of number in chimpanzees. *Current Opinion in Neurobiology, 19,* 92–98.

Mazur, J. E. (1987). An adjusting procedure for studying delayed reinforcement. *Quantitative Analyses of Behavior, 5,* 55–73.

McKenzie, T., Cherman, T., Bird, L. R., Naqshbandi, M., & Roberts, W. A. (2004). Can squirrel monkeys (Saimiri sciureus) plan for the future?: Studies of temporal myopia in food choice. *Animal Learning and Behavior, 32,* 377–390.

Menzel, E. W. (1973). Chimpanzee spatial memory organization. *Science, 182,* 943–945.

Miloyan, B., Bulley, A., & Suddendorf, T. (2016). Episodic foresight and anxiety: Proximate and ultimate perspectives. *British Journal of Clinical Psychology, 55,* 4–22.

Mobbs, D., Hagan, C. C., Dalgleish, T., Silston, B., & Prévost, C. (2015). The ecology of human fear: Survival optimization and the nervous system. *Frontiers in Neuroscience, 9,* 55. Available at *http://journal.frontiersin.org/article/10.3389/fnins.2015.00055/full.*

Mulcahy, N. J., & Call, J. (2006). Apes save tools for future use. *Science, 312,* 1038–1040.

Naqshbandi, M., & Roberts, W. A. (2006). Anticipation of future events in squirrel monkeys

(Saimiri sciureus) and rats (Rattus norvegicus): Tests of the Bischof–Kohler hypothesis. *Journal of Comparative Psychology, 120*, 345–357.

Nettle, D., & Bateson, M. (2012). The evolutionary origins of mood and its disorders. *Current Biology, 22*, R712–R721.

Nietzsche, F. (1998). *Untimely meditations* (D. Breazeale, Trans.). Cambridge, UK: Cambridge University Press. (Original work published 1876)

Oettingen, G. (2012). Future thought and behaviour change. *European Review of Social Psychology, 23*, 1–63.

O'Keefe, J., & Nadel, L. (1978). *The hippocampus as a cognitive map*. Oxford, UK: Clarendon Press.

Ólafsdóttir, H. F., Barry, C., Saleem, A. B., Hassabis, D., & Spiers, H. J. (2015). Hippocampal place cells construct reward related sequences through unexplored space. *eLife, 4*, e06063.

Osvath, M. (2009). Spontaneous planning for future stone throwing by a male chimpanzee. *Current Biology, 19*, R190–R191.

Osvath, M. (2016). Putting flexible animal prospection into context: Escaping the theoretical box. *Wiley Interdisciplinary Reviews: Cognitive Science, 7*, 5–18.

Osvath, M., & Karvonen, E. (2012). Spontaneous innovation for future deception in a male chimpanzee. *PLOS ONE, 7*, e36782.

Osvath, M., & Martin-Ordas, G. (2014). The future of future-oriented cognition in non-humans: Theory and the empirical case of the great apes. *Philosophical Transactions of the Royal Society B: Biological Sciences, 369*, 20130486. Available at *http://rstb.royalsociety-publishing.org/content/369/1655/20130486*.

Osvath, M., & Osvath, H. (2008). Chimpanzee (Pan troglodytes) and orangutan (Pongo abelii) forethought: Self-control and pre-experience in the face of future tool use. *Animal Cognition, 11*, 661–674.

Osvath, M., & Persson, T. (2013). Great apes can defer exchange: A replication with different results suggesting future oriented behavior. *Frontiers in Psychology, 4*, 698. Available at *http://journal.frontiersin.org/article/10.3389/fpsyg.2013.00698/full*.

Paxton, R., & Hampton, R. R. (2009). Tests of planning and the Bischof–Köhler hypothesis in rhesus monkeys (Macaca mulatta). *Behavioural Processes, 80*, 238–246.

Pepperberg, I. M., Willner, M. R., & Gravitz, L. B. (1997). Development of Piagetian object permanence in grey parrot (Psittacus erithacus). *Journal of Comparative Psychology, 111*, 63–75.

Perdue, B. M., Evans, T. A., Williamson, R. A., Gonsiorowski, A., & Beran, M. J. (2014). Prospective memory in children and chimpanzees. *Animal Cognition, 17*, 287–295.

Pfeiffer, B. E., & Foster, D. J. (2013). Hippocampal place-cell sequences depict future paths to remembered goals. *Nature, 497*, 74–79.

Premack, D. (2007). Human and animal cognition: Continuity and discontinuity. *Proceedings of the National Academy of Sciences of the USA, 104*, 13861–13867.

Raby, C. R., Alexis, D. M., Dickinson, A., & Clayton, N. S. (2007). Planning for the future by western scrub-jays. *Nature, 445*, 919–921.

Raby, C. R., & Clayton, N. S. (2009). Prospective cognition in animals. *Behavioural Processes, 80*, 314–324.

Range, F., Viranyi, Z., & Huber, L. (2007). Selective imitation in domestic dogs. *Current Biology, 17*, 868–872.

Redshaw, J. (2014). Does metarepresentation make human mental time travel unique? *Wiley Interdisciplinary Reviews: Cognitive Science, 5*, 519–531.

Redshaw, J., & Suddendorf, T. (2016). Children's and apes' preparatory responses to two mutually exclusive possibilities. *Current Biology, 26*, 1758–1762.

Risko, E. F., & Gilbert, S. J. (2016). Cognitive offloading. *Trends in Cognitive Sciences, 20,* 676–688.

Roberts, W. A. (2002). Are animals stuck in time? *Psychological Bulletin, 128,* 473–489.

Roberts, W. A. (2012). Evidence for future cognition in animals. *Learning and Motivation, 43,* 169–180.

Rosati, A. G., Stevens, J. R., Hare, B., & Hauser, M. D. (2007). The evolutionary origins of human patience: Temporal preferences in chimpanzees, bonobos, and human adults. *Current Biology, 17,* 1663–1668.

Rossano, M. J. (2003). Expertise and the evolution of consciousness. *Cognition, 89,* 207–236.

Santos, L. R., & Rosati, A. G. (2015). The evolutionary roots of human decision making. *Annual Review of Psychology, 66,* 321–347.

Scarf, D., Smith, C., & Stuart, M. (2014). A spoon full of studies helps the comparison go down: A comparative analysis of Tulving's spoon test. *Frontiers in Psychology, 5,* 893. Available at *http://journal.frontiersin.org/article/10.3389/fpsyg.2014.00893/full.*

Schacter, D. L., & Addis, D. R. (2007). Constructive memory: The ghosts of past and future. *Nature, 445,* 27.

Schopenhauer, A. (1890). *Studies in pessimism* (T. B. Saunders, Trans.). London: Allen & Unwin. (Original work published 1851)

Schopenhauer, A. (1909). *The world as will and representation* (R. B. Haldane & J. Kemp, Trans.; Vol. 2). London: Kegan Paul, Trench, Trübner. (Original work published 1818)

Shettleworth, S. J. (2012). Modularity, comparative cognition and human uniqueness. *Philosophical Transactions of the Royal Society B: Biological Sciences, 367,* 2794–2802.

Stawarczyk, D., Cassol, H., & D'Argembeau, A. (2013). Phenomenology of future-oriented mind-wandering episodes. *Frontiers in Psychology, 4,* 425.

Sterelny, K. (2003). *Thought in a hostile world: The evolution of human cognition.* Hoboken, NJ: Wiley-Blackwell.

Stevens, J. R. (2010). Intertemporal choice. In M. Breed & J. Moore (Eds.), *Encyclopedia of animal behavior* (pp. 203–208). Oxford, UK: Academic Press.

Stevens, J. R. (2011). Mechanisms for decisions about the future. In R. Menzel & J. Fischer (Eds.), *Animal thinking: Contemporary issues in comparative cognition* (pp. 93–104). Cambridge, MA: MIT Press.

Stevens, J. R., Rosati, A. G., Heilbronner, S. R., & Mühlhoff, N. (2011). Waiting for grapes: Expectancy and delayed gratification in bonobos. *International Journal of Comparative Psychology, 24,* 99–111.

Stevens, J. R., & Stephens, D. W. (2008). Patience. *Current Biology, 18,* R11–R12.

Suddendorf, T. (1999). The rise of the metamind. In M. C. Corballis & S. Lea (Eds.), *The descent of mind: Psychological perspectives on hominid evolution* (pp. 218–260). London: Oxford University Press.

Suddendorf, T. (2006). Foresight and evolution of the human mind. *Science, 312,* 1006–1007.

Suddendorf, T. (2013a). Mental time travel: continuities and discontinuities. *Trends in Cognitive Sciences, 17,* 151–152.

Suddendorf, T. (2013b). *The gap: The science of what separates us from other animals.* New York: Basic Books.

Suddendorf, T., Brinums, M., & Imuta, K. (2016). Shaping one's future self: The development of deliberate practice. In K. Michaelian, S. Klein, & K. Szpunar (Eds.), *Seeing the future: Theoretical perspectives on future-oriented mental time travel* (pp. 343–366). London: Oxford University Press.

Suddendorf, T., & Corballis, M. C. (1997). Mental time travel and the evolution of the human mind. *Genetic, Social, and General Psychology Monographs, 123,* 133–167.

Suddendorf, T., & Corballis, M. C. (2007). The evolution of foresight: What is mental time travel, and is it unique to humans? *Behavioral and Brain Sciences, 30,* 299–313.

Suddendorf, T., & Corballis, M. C. (2010). Behavioural evidence for mental time travel in nonhuman animals. *Behavioural Brain Research, 215,* 292–298.

Suddendorf, T., Corballis, M. C., & Collier-Baker, E. (2009). How great is great ape foresight? *Animal Cognition, 12,* 751–754.

Suddendorf, T., Crimston, J., & Redshaw, J. (2017). Preparatory responses to socially determined, mutually exclusive possibilities in chimpanzees and children. *Biology Letters, 13,* 6.

Suddendorf, T., & Redshaw, J. (2013). The development of mental scenario building and episodic foresight. *Annals of the New York Academy of Sciences, 1296,* 135–153.

Thom, J. M., & Clayton, N. S. (2015a). Route-planning and the comparative study of future-thinking. *Frontiers in Psychology, 6,* 144. Available at *http://journal.frontiersin.org/article/10.3389/fpsyg.2015.00144/full.*

Thom, J. M., & Clayton, N. S. (2015b). Translational research into intertemporal choice: The Western scrub-jay as an animal model for future-thinking. *Behavioural Processes, 112,* 43–48.

Tobin, H., & Logue, A. W. (1994). Self-control across species (Columba livia, Homo sapiens, and Rattus norvegicus). *Journal of Comparative Psychology, 108,* 126.

Tolman, E. C. (1948). Cognitive maps in rats and men. *Psychological Review, 55,* 189–208.

Tulving, E. (1985). Memory and consciousness. *Canadian Psychology/Psychologie Canadienne, 26,* 1–12.

Tulving, E. (2005). Episodic memory and autonoesis: Uniquely human? In H. Terrace & J. Metcalfe (Eds.), *The missing link in cognition* (pp. 4–56). New York: Oxford University Press.

Tulving, E., & Thomson, D. M. (1973). Encoding specificity and retrieval processes in episodic memory. *Psychological Review, 80,* 352–373.

Underwood, R. (1982). Vigilance behaviour in grazing African antelopes. *Behaviour, 79,* 81–107.

van Schaik, C. P., Damerius, L., & Isler, K. (2013). Wild orangutan males plan and communicate their travel direction one day in advance. *PLOS ONE, 8,* e74896.

Vitti, J. J. (2013). Cephalopod cognition in an evolutionary context: Implications for ethology. *Biosemiotics, 6,* 393–401.

Zentall, T. R. (2005). Animals may not be stuck in time. *Learning and Motivation, 36,* 208–225.

CHAPTER 3

>>>>>>>>>>>>>>>>>>

Varieties of Future-Thinking

Karl K. Szpunar
Sushmita Shrikanth
Daniel L. Schacter

The contents of the present volume demonstrate that the topic of future-thinking, often referred to as prospection (Gilbert & Wilson, 2007), has made a significant impact in the fields of psychology and neuroscience. However, there are many ways in which people are able to think about the future. On a daily basis, people think about and evaluate possible encounters with colleagues, family members, romantic partners, and even their future selves; form intentions to deliver messages, take prescribed medications, and pick up miscellaneous items at the convenience store; and plan daily routines, vacations, and savings strategies for retirement (see D'Argembeau, Renaud, & Van Der Linden, 2011). Despite the vast diversity in ways in which people think about the future, we recently proposed that prospective cognition can be organized into four basic modes of future-thinking (Szpunar, Spreng, & Schacter, 2014): *simulation* (construction of a detailed mental representation of the future), *prediction* (estimation of the likelihood of, and/or one's reaction to, a particular future outcome), *intention* (the mental act of setting a goal), and *planning* (the identification and organization of steps toward achieving a goal state).

In addition to proposing that prospection can be parsed into four distinct categories, our framework also holds that these modes of future-thinking can vary in terms of their representational contents. Specifically, the framework relates simulation, prediction, intention, and planning to two well-characterized types of memory or knowledge: episodic and semantic (Tulving, 2002). In this context, the term *episodic* is meant to refer to simulations, predictions, intentions, or plans in relation to specific autobiographical events that may take place in the future (e.g., thinking about an upcoming experience that will take place next week). The term *semantic* is meant to refer to simulations, predictions, intentions, and plans that relate to more general or abstract states of the world that may arise in the future (e.g., thinking about what the environmental state of the world will be like 50 years from now; for a review, see Abraham & Bubic, 2015).

It is important to highlight that even semantic variants of prospection may sometimes be infused with episodic content (e.g., simulating aspects of one's own life in the context of an abstract vision of the future world). Nonetheless, distinctions between episodic and semantic forms of prospection have led to the demonstration of striking dissociations in the literature, particularly in relation to the concept of simulation (see the subsection on semantic simulation later in this chapter), underscoring the importance of this distinction for research on prospection. Finally, in addition to the possibility that episodic and semantic prospection may at times overlap with one another, we note that not all instances of future-thinking can be strictly classified as either episodic or semantic. Specifically, some instances of future-thinking represent autobiographical states—general states of the world that are autobiographical in nature; for example, imagining that one will attain his or her career aspirations in the future. Indeed, considerable research related to goal pursuit has focused on future autobiographical states (e.g., attaining a desired job, dating a desired romantic partner; e.g., Oettingen & Mayer, 2002). To accommodate such hybrid forms of future-thinking, our framework conceptualizes the episodic–semantic distinction as a continuous variable. Thus the result of our approach to delineating prospection is a set of four basic modes of future-oriented cognition that may vary in the extent to which they draw on episodic and semantic knowledge structures (see Figure 3.1; see also Szpunar, Spreng, & Schacter, 2014).

In this chapter, we elaborate on the various modes of future-thinking that fall within the purview of our classification scheme. In order to facilitate cross-fertilization of ideas across disparate areas of research, we frame our discussion around specific methods that are used to study these different ways of thinking about the future. We focus primarily on methods used to study episodic forms of simulation, prediction, intention, and planning, because a complete survey of the methods to study future-oriented cognition would be well beyond the scope of this chapter, and many of the methods used in the study of episodic forms of future-thinking have turned out to be useful for the study of semantic and hybrid forms of future-thinking. Finally, we consider how various modes of future-thinking may interact with one another to support adaptive behavior.

Notably, psychologists have previously considered relations among various modes of future-oriented cognition as they pertain to goal pursuit and behavioral outcomes. For instance, those interested in the impact of mental simulation on behavior have shown that the specific focus of simulation (e.g., positive or negative) can interact with expected (or predicted) performance to determine behavioral outcomes (e.g., Oettingen & Wadden, 1991). Expectancy-value theorists have considered the role of expectations (or predictions) in commitment to intentions (e.g., Wigfield & Eccles, 2000). More recent work on mental contrasting—the act of juxtaposing a positive future outcome with present circumstances—has highlighted interrelations between simulation, prediction, intention, and planning (for a recent review, see Oettingen, 2012). Nonetheless, other literatures relevant to future-oriented cognition have been carried out in relative isolation from one another. For instance, recent work on the cognitive and neural mechanisms that support the

	SIMULATION	PREDICTION	INTENTION	PLANNING
EPISODIC				
↑	Construction of a mental representation of a specific autobiographical future event.	Estimation of the likelihood of and/or one's reaction to a specific autobiographical future event.	Setting a goal in relation to a specific autobiographical future event.	Organization of steps needed to arrive at a specific autobiographical future outcome.
	Construction of a mental representation of a nonspecific autobiographical state.	Estimation of the likelihood of and/or one's reaction to a nonspecific future autobiographical state.	Setting a nonspecific autobiographical future goal.	Organization of steps needed for some nonspecific autobiographical state to arise in the future.
↓ **SEMANTIC**	Construction of a mental representation of a general or abstract state of the world.	Estimation of the likelihood of and/or one's reaction to a general or abstract future state of the world.	Setting a general or abstract goal, such as the goal of an organization.	Organization of steps needed for some general or abstract state of the world to arise in the future.

FIGURE 3.1. A taxonomy of prospective cognition. From Szpunar, K. K., Spreng, R. N., & Schacter, D. L. (2014). A taxonomy of prospection: Introducing an organizational framework for future-oriented cognition. *Proceedings of the National Academy of Sciences of the USA, 111,* 18414–18421. Copyright © 2014 National Academy of Sciences. Reprinted by permission.

ability to construct detailed simulations of the future (Schacter, Addis, & Buckner, 2008), on limitations in the ability to predict future outcomes (Gilbert & Wilson, 2007), on the ability to remember to carry out intentions in the future (Kliegel, McDaniel, & Einstein, 2008), and on the ability to generate complex organizational plans for behavior (Ward & Morris, 2005) have engaged in relatively little cross-talk. Importantly, more recent work has begun to highlight possible connections between these more disparate lines of research. We use our proposed framework as a means of highlighting these exciting developments in the field.

SIMULATION

The construct of simulation has been used to define the ability to cognitively represent various aspects of personal experience, including real or imagined events (Taylor & Schneider, 1989), the minds of others (Goldman, 2006), and person–environment interactions (Barsalou, 2003). Here, we take simulation to refer to the construction of hypothetical events, both specific and general (for further discussion, see Schacter et al., 2008).

Research studies on simulation typically assess the ability to generate detailed mental representations of hypothetical events or states of the world. In most cases, participants are provided with generic cues (e.g., "Imagine a future event that might take place in your or the world's future in the next 5 years") and given a few seconds to a few minutes to simulate events/states of the world. Simulations are typically evaluated on the basis of the levels of phenomenological detail (e.g., how vivid/coherent was the mental representation?) and/or more objective measures of event detail, such as scoring participant-generated narratives for the presence or absence of internal/episodic (e.g., details about specific people, places, and so on) and external/semantic (e.g., general/background information) detail using guidelines set forth by the Autobiographical Interview (Levine, Svoboda, Hay, Winocur, & Moscovitch, 2002). Although much of the extant research of this sort has focused on episodic simulation, these methods are easily applicable to other forms of simulation, as discussed below.

Episodic Simulation

Episodic simulation is the construction of a detailed mental representation of a specific autobiographical future event (Schacter et al., 2008). Considerable work has focused on delineating the relation of episodic simulation to episodic memory and on identifying their common neural correlates. In most such studies, participants are required to provide details about past and future experiences in response to generic cues (e.g., "Tell me about your past/future"; "Remember/imagine an event in response to the time period *last/next year* or the cue word *car*"; the technique that requires participants to generate events in response to cue words is better known as the Galton–Crovitz cuing paradigm; Crovitz & Schiffman, 1974). Notably, much of the evidence demonstrating a close relation between the personal past and future has been based on neuropsychological studies of brain-damaged patients and neuroimaging studies of healthy adults.

In a seminal case study, Tulving (1985) asked an amnesic patient (K. C.) to talk about the personal past and future and found that K. C. was unable to provide details when thinking about either temporal orientation. One limitation of this observation was that K. C. had sustained diffuse brain damage following a motorcycle accident and it was impossible to know what aspect(s) of the brain damage were related to his episodic memory and simulation deficits. More recently, Hassabis, Kumaran, Vann, and Maguire (2007) tested a set of patients with brain damage largely limited to the hippocampus, a region of the brain known to play an important role in memory for specific past events, and found that those patients had deficits in constructing coherent mental images when cued to think about specific hypothetical experiences (e.g., "Imagine you're lying on a white sandy beach in a beautiful tropical bay"). Although not all patients with hippocampal amnesia demonstrate such patterns of results (e.g., Squire et al., 2010), there is good reason to believe that the hippocampus plays a pivotal role in memory for and simulation of specific autobiographical events (for reviews, see Addis & Schacter, 2012; Schacter, Addis, & Szpunar, 2017).

Taking a broader approach, functional neuroimaging studies of episodic simulation and episodic memory provide insights into the neural underpinnings of these related abilities across the entire brain. For instance, using positron emission topography, a neuroimaging technique that requires researchers to inject a nonradioactive tracer into the bloodstream and track the uptake of the tracer by blood vessels in the brain, Okuda et al. (2003) showed that extended periods of unconstrained thinking about the personal past and future were characterized by similar patterns of brain activity in various frontal and temporal regions of the brain. One important limitation of this early work is that it was not clear whether these patterns of brain activity were related to specific memories and future events. However, the subsequent development of event-related functional magnetic resonance imagining (fMRI) did enable researchers to associate estimates of neural activity to specific memories and simulated events (e.g., by cuing memories and future events using the Galton–Crovitz cuing paradigm on a trial-by-trial basis in the scanner). Importantly, studies using event-related fMRI have similarly demonstrated a striking overlap in medial and lateral regions of frontal, parietal, and temporal cortex, including the hippocampus, as participants remember and imagine events from their past and future (for a review, see Schacter et al., 2012).

More recently, researchers have been able to parse the contributions of these regions to episodic simulation. Repetition suppression (also called neural adaptation) refers to a phenomenon whereby regions of the brain responsible for processing specific stimuli will show reduced patterns of responding following repeated presentations of those stimuli (Grill-Spector, Henson, & Martin, 2006). Capitalizing on this phenomenon, Szpunar, St. Jacques, Robbins, Wig, and Schacter (2014) asked participants to repeatedly simulate various aspects of some future events (e.g., people and locations; cued by person–location dyads that were based on personal information collected from participants before scanning) but not others. By comparing repeated and nonrepeated event features across trials, the authors were able to pinpoint the contributions of stimulus-specific regions of the brain to simulation (e.g., parahippocampal cortex and retrosplenial cortex, regions known to be involved in spatial processing, were particularly sensitive to repeated simulations of simulated locations).

The collection of neuropsychological and neuroimaging findings relating episodic simulation to episodic memory have sparked various theoretical considerations. Schacter and Addis (2007) proposed the *constructive episodic simulation hypothesis,* which postulates that a constructive memory system that is prone to errors may nonetheless be adaptive in that it enables the individual to draw flexibly upon elements of past experiences in the service of simulating novel future events (for recent relevant evidence on the link between flexible retrieval and memory errors, see Carpenter & Schacter, 2017). Others have focused on more broadly relating episodic memory and simulation to other constructs. For instance, Buckner and Carroll (2007) identified episodic simulation and episodic memory as forms of self-projection, which, along with theory of mind (i.e., the ability to take the mental perspective of another person; Goldman, 2006) and spatial navigation (i.e., the ability to imagine moving through a familiar spatial location; Ekstrom et al., 2003), allow the individual to experience mental states that are removed from the immediate environment. Still others have focused on illuminating specific cognitive mechanisms involved in episodic memory, simulation, and related constructs such as spatial navigation. For instance, Hassabis and Maguire (2007) argue that scene construction—the process of mentally generating and maintaining a complex and coherent scene or event—is a key cognitive mechanism that involves retrieving and integrating disparate details stored in modality-specific regions, a process believed to be mediated by the hippocampus.

Semantic Simulation

Semantic simulation is the construction of a detailed mental representation of a general or abstract state of the world. Although semantic simulation has not received as much research attention as episodic simulation, evidence suggests that the two may be, at least to some extent, dissociable from one another. For instance, Klein, Loftus, and Kihlstrom (2002) asked a patient with episodic amnesia (D. B.) to talk about events that he or the world might experience in the future. Although D. B. was unable to reliably express what he might do in his personal future, he was nonetheless able to think about problems that might face the world in the future (e.g., global warming). Race, Keane, and Verfaellie (2013) similarly showed that patients with medial temporal lobe damage were able to generate possible issues that the world would face in the future but were impaired in their ability to elaborate on those issues, as indicated by lack of external/semantic detail that patients produced as scored by the Autobiographical Interview. This latter finding suggests that patients with episodic amnesia may possess fine-grained deficits in semantic simulation. Notably, Manning, Denkova, and Unterberger (2013) reported preserved episodic simulation but impaired semantic simulation in a patient with epilepsy whose left anteromedial temporal lobe was resected; this is a region known to play an important role in representing general or semantic knowledge (e.g., De Renzi, Liotti, & Nichelli, 1987). Hence, the available data suggest that damage to the hippocampus and more anterior portions of the temporal lobe may, respectively, lead to dissociable deficits of episodic and semantic simulation. At the same time, it is important to note that episodic and semantic knowledge may interact in the context of simulation. For instance, Irish and colleagues (e.g., Irish & Piguet, 2013) have demonstrated that episodic simulation is also impaired with damage to the anterior temporal lobes, a finding that has led to the proposal that semantic knowledge may serve as a scaffold for episodic simulation.

Some forms of simulation cannot be neatly classified as either episodic or semantic, but rather represent hybrids of episodic and semantic simulation. These hybrid forms of simulation may take the form of personal semantic knowledge (e.g., one may have an interest in business; Renoult, Davidson, Palombo, Moscovitch, & Levine, 2012) that is projected into the future (e.g., one may envision playing an important role in business in the future). Such simulations are autobiographical but not related to specific future episodes. Nonetheless, it is possible that specific or abstract simulations could accompany simulations of autobiographical states (e.g., seeing oneself in a fancy office, contemplating the stability of the future marketplace). The relations among episodic, semantic, and hybrid forms of simulation remain to be worked out in the literature.

PREDICTION

Prediction is a fundamental task of the brain (Bar, 2009; Friston & Kiebel, 2009). Predictions about the future include short-term predictions about what object may appear next in a scene (Bar, 2007) and prediction errors concerning expected rewards that are crucial to learning (Schultz, Dayan, & Montague, 1997). Our focus is on longer term predictions about specific events and general or abstract states of the world that may arise in the future and the manner in which such predictions may interact with other modes of future-thinking (e.g., Oettingen, 2012). Long-term predictions are typically assessed in the context of studies that measure participants' affective and/or behavioral reactions to some hypothetical future scenario(s) (e.g., "On a scale of 1–9, how happy do you think you will be at your child's first soccer match/if a particular political candidate is elected/if you do or do not achieve tenure?"; see Gilbert & Wilson, 2007). Note that many studies use more than one isolated psychometric measure and/or assess whether participant behaviors change in accordance with their predictions. Importantly, simulations of future events typically accompany predictions and so play an important role in this context. We elaborate on this relation below.

Episodic Prediction

Episodic prediction is the estimation of the likelihood of, and/or one's reaction to, a specific autobiographical future event. Here, we focus specifically on predictions about reactions to events (for further detail regarding predictions of event likelihood, see the following section on semantic prediction; see also Oettingen & Gollwitzer, 2010; Szpunar, Spreng, & Schacter, 2014). Perhaps the most clear-cut example of episodic prediction of reactions to events comes from work on affective forecasting, wherein social psychologists have attempted to highlight the shortcomings of the ability to predict our reactions to the outcomes of future events (Wilson & Gilbert, 2003, 2005). Gilbert and Wilson (2007) argued that people base their predictions on episodic simulations of the future and succinctly summarized three common limitations of simulations that lead to errors in prediction. Specifically, the authors highlighted that: (1) simulations are often based on easily accessible but unrepresentative memories of similar experiences (e.g., remembering a particularly negative experience of having interacted with a particular individual when predicting one's emotional reaction to having to interact with that person in the future); (2) simulations often focus on essential details (e.g., the joys of parenthood) while omitting inessential details that can influence future happiness (e.g., how it will feel to change diapers or go into work not having slept the previous night); and (3) simulations are often abbreviated and tend to focus on the initial aspects of future experience while omitting consideration of how circumstances may change over time (e.g., imagining the positive feeling associated with getting a promotion but failing to consider the extra work that would come with it).

Given the limits that simulations tend to impose on predictions, it would be of interest to determine whether improving the ability to simulate events in detail could also improve prediction accuracy. Recent studies using specificity inductions have shown that people are able to generate more detailed episodic simulations of the future when they have been trained previously to report on episodic details in the context of a cognitive interview about a recently experienced event (Madore, Gaesser, & Schacter, 2014), and fMRI evidence indicates that brain regions implicated in retrieval of episodic detail, including the hippocampus, are preferentially engaged when people imagine a future event following an episodic specificity induction compared with a control induction (Madore, Szpunar, Addis, & Schacter, 2016; for review and discussion of specificity induction studies, see Schacter & Madore, 2016). Whether such specificity inductions could help to bring to mind additional details for simulations that might otherwise be omitted and that could serve to enhance predictive accuracy remains to be tested in the literature.

Semantic Prediction

Semantic prediction is the estimation of the likelihood of, and/or one's reaction to, a general or abstract state of the world. Semantic prediction represents an important type of future-thinking that is highly valued in disciplines such as politics and economics. Research within the domain of affective forecasting has considered not only the manner in which people believe they will react to future events but also how they may react to future states of the world, such as those brought about in the aftermath of elections. In these contexts, the shortcomings that hamper episodic simulations appear to similarly limit semantic predictions. For instance, Gilbert, Pinel, Wilson, Blumberg, and Wheatley (1998) showed that people overestimated the duration of their emotional reactions to the end of personal relationships and outcomes of elections.

Nonetheless, it is possible that predictions associated with general states of the world rely to some extent upon episodic processes, because such predictions are typically made in relation to one's own predicted emotional reactions (e.g., "How will the results of an election make me feel?"). As such, more work is needed that assesses predictions related to more objectively semantic phenomena. Research on predictions about the emergence of hybrid and/or semantic states of the world should help to fill this void in the literature. For instance, Oettingen and her colleagues have demonstrated that contrasting a future vision or simulation of achieving a general state (e.g., losing weight) with present circumstances gives rise to predictions about whether that future state is achievable and whether intentions and plans should be set (for review, see Oettingen, 2012). It remains to be tested whether or not similar mental contrasting processes may determine the formulation of predictions and the intentions and plans that follow in the context of more general or abstract future states (e.g., predicting the success of a small business).

INTENTION

Understanding the conscious determinants of human action has represented a central fixture in psychological research since the cognitive revolution (Ryan, 1970). Considerable research has been devoted to illuminating the nature of the underlying intentions that guide behavior of the individual (Ajzen, 1991) and also the more general goal setting that is the driving force behind the growth and development of organizations (Locke & Latham, 2002). Within the social psychological literature, intentions are often considered in terms of attitudes, societal norms, and perceived behavioral control (e.g., to what extent do people follow through with the intention to stop smoking). In these cases, as with most cases of research on intention, observable behaviors are the key independent variable (for a review, see Ajzen, 1991). Notably, classic work on intentions focuses on what we would classify as hybrid intentions that relate to personal future states (e.g., losing weight; Schifter & Ajzen, 1985) as opposed to any one particular personal event (episodic) or state of the world (semantic). Next, we provide a brief overview of research on specific and more general or abstract intentions and identify possible links to other modes of future-oriented cognition.

Episodic Intention

Episodic intention is the mental act of setting a goal in relation to a specific autobiographical future event. Once goals are contemplated and set, whether or not those goals are actualized represents an important obstacle to adaptive behavior (for discussion about effective intention formation, see Oettingen & Gollwitzer, 2010). Although various aspects of adherence to intentions have been considered in the literature (e.g., perceived control of behavior; see earlier discussion), we focus here on a specific aspect of intentions that has received considerable attention in the context of episodic cognition—namely, remembering that intentions have been set in the first place. Consider the role of setting and actualizing goals in the context of *prospective memory* (e.g., "I need to remember to pick up bread on my way home from work"; for a review, see Kliegel et al., 2008). Studies of prospective memory have long investigated the extent to which the quality of encoding of episodic intentions predicts the success with which those intentions are carried out in the future. Early research on implementation intentions found that explicitly stating when and where an intention will be carried out (e.g., "when X occurs, I will perform Y") causes the desired intention to become more accessible and come to mind in an automatic fashion when encountered with the specific stimulus, thus enhancing prospective memory performance (for a review, see Gollwitzer, 1999, 2014; see also Gollwitzer & Sheeran, 2006). Many studies employing implementation intention instructions require participants to generate episodic simulations that revolve around themselves carrying out the future task at hand (Chen et al., 2015), and more recent studies that explicitly relate episodic simulation to prospective memory performance have reported similar benefits (e.g., Neroni, Gamboz, & Brandimonte, 2014). It is important to note that implementation intentions may be effective in part because they involve formulating a plan of action. Indeed, Gollwitzer and colleagues operationalize implementation intentions as plans of action (e.g., Gollwitzer, 1999, 2014). However, as we highlight below, most conceptualizations of planning ability extend beyond if–then contingency statements characteristic of implementation intentions and include the organization of complex action sequences (e.g., planning a shopping trip or vacation) that move beyond carrying out or not carrying out an intended action given a specific stimulus (e.g., avoiding an invitation to a party in order to study for an exam). Before we elaborate on more complex forms of planning and their relation to other modes of future-thinking, we turn to semantic intentions.

Semantic Intention

Semantic intention is the mental act of setting a general or abstract goal, such as the goal of an organization. To our knowledge, no research has been conducted in the future-thinking literature to identify the cognitive determinants that underlie the formation of a general or abstract intention for a particular organization (e.g., setting a target of 10% industry growth). The development of research programs aimed at identifying the possible overlapping and nonoverlapping cognitive and neural mechanisms that give rise to episodic and semantic intentions should have considerable implications for various fields of study, including psychology, business, and economics. As with simulation and prediction, not all instances of intention can be classified as episodic or semantic. For instance, one may possess an inherent interest in business (personal semantics; Renoult et al., 2012) and project that information forward by forming the intention to pursue a relevant career path. Note that, although both episodic and hybrid intentions reflect personal goals, episodic intentions revolve around outcomes of circumscribed events (e.g., picking up bread from the grocery store), whereas hybrid intentions focus on desired states (e.g., being a lawyer). The extent to which such hybrid intentions rely on similar or different mechanisms compared with more clear-cut examples of episodic and semantic intention awaits future work. For instance, to what extent might similar mechanisms underlie the act of forming an intention to pursue a particular career path as compared with picking up bread from the grocery store or setting a goal for a company sales team? Research on mental contrasting, as discussed earlier in the context of prediction, suggests that episodic (e.g., getting an A on an exam) and hybrid (e.g., being in a meaningful relationship) intentions are particularly likely to be realized if those intentions are based on predictions derived from comparing positive simulations of future outcomes and current circumstances (for reviews, see Oettingen, 2012, 2014; Oettingen & Gollwitzer, 2010). Whether similar cognitive operations predict the realization of semantic intentions remains to be worked out in the literature.

PLANNING

For intended behaviors to be carried out in an effective manner, plans are often necessary. Although various scholars have defined the concept of planning (Hayes-Roth & Hayes-Roth, 1979; Mumford, Schultz, & Van Doorn, 2001; Ward & Morris, 2005), most definitions commonly conform to the notion of a plan as a "predetermination of a course of action aimed at achieving some goal" (Hayes-Roth & Hayes-Roth, 1979). Here, we focus on the nature of plans that are aimed at achieving goals in relation to specific autobiographical and more general contexts and the extent to which other modes of future-oriented cognition may factor into the planning process as revealed by the tasks that are commonly used to assess planning ability.

Episodic Planning

Episodic planning is the identification and organization of steps needed to arrive at a specific autobiographical future event or goal state. One notable aspect of research on episodic planning is that tasks that are used to gauge planning ability can vary considerably in terms of how well they approximate real-life planning. For instance, in the Tower of London test, participants are typically presented with two arrays of beads organized on two separate sets of pegs, with the goal of reorganizing the beads presented in the first array to match the arrangement of the second, or goal, array. The measure of interest is the number of steps taken to achieve the goal state (Shallice, 1982). Other tests strive to more closely mimic real-world planning. For instance, the Six Elements Test (SET; Shallice & Burgess, 1991) requires participants to carry out a series of laboratory tasks in a specified time frame and order. The Multiple Errands Test is similar to the SET but involves completing daily tasks in a real-world setting (see Shallice & Burgess, 1991). Much of the research on planning has been conducted in the context of testing patients with frontal lobe damage. The fact that patients with frontal lobe damage have trouble with each of the above-noted tasks highlights the fact that processes subserved by the frontal lobes (e.g., executive control) play an important role in planning and future-thinking more generally.

More recent neuroimaging studies (e.g., Spreng, Gerlach, Turner, & Schacter, 2015; Spreng, Stevens, Chamberlain, Gilmore, & Schacter, 2010) have examined the neural underpinnings of episodic or autobiographical planning, using a task in which participants mentally construct personal plans containing specific steps in order to achieve particular personal goals (e.g., academic success, getting out of debt). Results indicate that episodic planning is associated with activity in regions of the brain traditionally associated with executive control (i.e., the frontoparietal control network; Niendam et al., 2012) and activity in the same core network of brain regions that has been linked previously to episodic simulation (the default network; Buckner, Andrews-Hanna, & Schacter, 2008), suggesting that simulation may play an important role in the context of planning. Indeed, other real-world episodic planning tasks have also highlighted the fact that episodic simulation and other modes of future-thinking feature in the context of episodic planning. For instance, one study showed that participant descriptions of strategies for completing a pseudo–shopping planning task included simulation (e.g., images of performing tasks), prediction (e.g., estimates of probability of completing tasks), and intention formation (e.g., setting specific goals based on products of simulation and prediction; Burgess, Simons, Coates, & Channon, 2005).

Semantic Planning

Semantic planning is the identification and organization of steps needed for some general or abstract goal state in the world to arise in the future. Semantic planning is perhaps best represented in the context of strategic (Blatstein, 2012) and urban (Rydin et al., 2012) planning, tasks during which steps required to achieve a particular goal state for an organization or community are explicitly mapped out. Indeed, considerable work has focused on the concept of *corporate foresight,* which is defined as a practice that permits an organization to lay the foundation for a future competitive advantage (Rohrbeck, Battistella, & Huizingh, 2015).

Although there exists a paucity of research related to the cognitive determinants of semantic planning, research with patients with frontal lobe damage has provided some initial data. For instance, patients with frontal lobe damage exhibit difficulty in formulating both episodic plans (see earlier discussion) and financial plans for others (Goel, Grafman, Tajik, Gana, & Danto, 1997). It is important to point out that financial planning, and possibly other forms of semantic planning, may incorporate episodic knowledge (e.g., people may use their own experiences to formulate plans for others; see Goel et al., 1997, p. 1882). Nonetheless, the results of this study suggest that cognitive functions subserved by the frontal lobes may be important for episodic and semantic planning.

To our knowledge, no study has directly compared episodic and semantic planning deficits in patients with frontal lobe damage, and so more work is needed to understand the extent to which these forms of planning are supported by similar and different mechanisms. Along these lines, episodic specificity inductions may play an important role in delineating underlying differences between episodic and semantic planning. For instance, Madore and Schacter (2014) recently showed that a specificity induction could be used to boost the ability of younger and older adults to generate relevant steps toward resolving personal and impersonal means–ends problems (e.g., generate steps that would enable oneself or a hypothetical person to achieve exercising more). Assuming that semantic planning does not rely on episodic processes, we would hypothesize that similar episodic specificity inductions should not provide a benefit for constructing detailed semantic plans for the future.

CONCLUSION AND FUTURE DIRECTIONS

In this chapter, we have summarized a framework for organizing key cognitions involved in thinking about the future. We suggest that decomposing prospective cognition in terms of episodic, semantic, and hybrid forms of simulation, prediction, intention, and planning provides a useful framework for discriminating between, and developing connections among, various forms of future-thinking. Nonetheless, additional cognitive, emotional, and motor processes may contribute to and support future-oriented behavior (see Szpunar, St. Jacques, et al., 2014), which will likely lead to an expanded and refined taxonomy of prospective cognition. For now, we believe that our organizational framework can encourage cross-fertilization of research and theory across various domains of cognitive, clinical, developmental, and comparative psychology and thereby broaden and deepen our understanding of the processes that support future-oriented cognition.

Although we have focused considerable attention on episodic forms of future-thinking and their methods, it will be just as important to carry out research that will allow the evaluation of cognitive factors that underlie semantic and hybrid forms of future-thinking. We suggest that one fruitful approach could be the use of talk-aloud procedures that require participants to generate narratives associated with their simulations, predictions, intentions, and plans in order to gain a more in-depth understanding of the manner in which such conceptions of the future are represented by the individual. Indeed, prior research using narrative evaluations has already demonstrated that episodic planning involves elements of episodic simulation, prediction, and intention (Burgess et al., 2005) and that semantic planning can draw upon elements of episodic planning (Goel et al., 1997). Further delineation of the manner in which various modes of future-thinking interact with one another in the context of episodic, semantic, and hybrid future-thinking would cultivate a more thorough understanding of the workings of the human mind/ brain in relation to the future.

Finally, we conclude by suggesting that our organizational framework could serve as a useful benchmark against which clinical populations with deficits in future-thinking can be assessed in order to develop a profile of their future-thinking abilities. For instance, studies of mood and anxiety-related disorders have historically focused on the fluency with which individuals with depression and anxiety think about positive and negative events that may occur in the future (MacLeod, Tate, Kentish, & Jacobsen, 1997). Although this work has provided important insights into future-thinking in these populations, relatively little is known about the extent to which these individuals are able to engage in episodic and semantic forms of simulation, prediction, intention, and planning. Development of research programs that consider the role of these various modes of future-thinking could enhance our understanding of the ability of individuals afflicted with various mood and anxiety disorders to engage in adaptive behavior.

REFERENCES

Abraham, A., & Bubic, A. (2015). Semantic memory as the root of imagination. *Frontiers in Psychology, 6*. Available at *http://journal.frontiersin.org/article/10.3389/fpsyg.2015.00325/ full.*

Addis, D. R., & Schacter, D. L. (2012). The hippocampus and imagining the future: Where do we stand? *Frontiers in Human Neuroscience, 5*, 173.

Ajzen, I. (1991). The theory of planned behavior. *Organizational Behavior and Human Decision Processes, 50*, 179–211.

Bar, M. (2007). The proactive brain: Using analogies and associations to generate predictions. *Trends in Cognitive Sciences, 11*, 280–289.

Bar, M. (2009). The proactive brain: Memory for predictions. *Philosophical Transactions of the Royal Society B: Biological Sciences, 364*, 1235–1243.

Barsalou, L. W. (2003). Situated simulation in the human conceptual system. *Language and Cognitive Processes, 18*, 513–562.

Blatstein, I. M. (2012). Strategic planning: Predicting or shaping the future? *Organization Development Journal, 30*, 31–38.

Buckner, R. L., Andrews-Hanna, J. R., & Schacter, D. L. (2008). The brain's default network: Anatomy, function, and relevance to disease. *Annals of the New York Academy of Sciences, 1124*, 1–38.

Buckner, R. L., & Carroll, D. C. (2007). Self-projection and the brain. *Trends in Cognitive Sciences, 11*, 49–57.

Burgess, P., Simons, J. S., Coates, L. M. A., & Channon, S. (2005). The search for specific planning processes. In R. Morris & G. Ward (Eds.), *The cognitive psychology of planning* (pp. 199–227). New York: Psychology Press.

Carpenter, A. C., & Schacter, D. L. (2017). Flexible retrieval: When true inferences produce false memories. *Journal of Experimental Psychology: Learning, Memory, and Cognition, 43*, 335–349.

Chen, X., Wang, Y., Liu, L., Cui, J., Gan, M., Shum, D. H. K., . . . Chan, R. C. K. (2015). The effect of implementation intention on prospective memory: A systematic and meta-analytic review. *Psychiatry Research, 226*, 14–22.

Crovitz, H. F., & Schiffman, H. (1974). Frequency of episodic memories as a function of their age. *Bulletin of the Psychonomic Society, 4*, 517–518.

D'Argembeau, A., Renaud, O., & Van der Linden, M. (2011). Frequency, characteristics, and functions of future-oriented thoughts in daily life. *Applied Cognitive Psychology, 35,* 96–103.

De Renzi, E., Liotti, M., & Nichelli, P. (1987). Semantic amnesia with preservation of autobiographical memory: A case report. *Cortex, 23,* 575–597.

Ekstrom, A. D., Kahana, M. J., Caplan, J. B., Fields, T. A., Isham, E. A., Newman, E. L., . . . Fried, I. (2003). Cellular networks underlying human spatial navigation. *Nature, 425,* 184–188.

Friston, K., & Kiebel, S. (2009). Predictive coding under the free-energy principle. *Philosophical Transactions of the Royal Society B: Biological Sciences, 364,* 1211–1221.

Gilbert, D. T., Pinel, E. C., Wilson, T. D., Blumberg, S. J., & Wheatley, T. P. (1998). Immune neglect: A source of durability bias in affective forecasting. *Journal of Personality and Social Psychology, 75,* 617–638.

Gilbert, D. T., & Wilson, T. D. (2007). Prospection: Experiencing the future. *Science, 317,* 1351–1354.

Goel, V., Grafman, J., Tajik, J., Gana, S., & Danto, D. (1997). A study of the performance of patients with frontal lobe lesions in a financial planning task. *Brain, 120,* 1805–1822.

Goldman, A. I. (2006). *Simulating minds: The philosophy, psychology, and neuroscience of mindreading.* New York: Oxford University Press.

Gollwitzer, P. M. (1999). Implementation intentions: Strong effects of simple plans. *American Psychologist, 54,* 493–503.

Gollwitzer, P. M. (2014). Weakness of the will: Is a quick fix possible? *Motivation and Emotion, 38,* 305–322.

Gollwitzer, P. M., & Sheeran, P. (2006). Implementation intentions and goal achievement: A meta-analysis of effects and processes. *Advances in Experimental Social Psychology, 38,* 69–119.

Grill-Spector, K., Henson, R., & Martin, A. (2006). Repetition and the brain: Neural models of stimulus-specific effects. *Trends in Cognitive Sciences, 10,* 14–23.

Hassabis, D., Kumaran, D., Vann, S. D., & Maguire, E. A. (2007). Patients with hippocampal amnesia cannot imagine new experiences. *Proceedings of the National Academy of Sciences of the USA, 104,* 1726–1731.

Hassabis, D., & Maguire, E. A. (2007). Deconstructing episodic memory with construction. *Trends in Cognitive Sciences, 11,* 299–306.

Hayes-Roth, B., & Hayes-Roth, F. (1979). A cognitive model of planning. *Cognitive Science, 3,* 275–310.

Irish, M., & Piguet, O. (2013). The pivotal role of semantic memory in remembering the past and imagining the future. *Frontiers in Behavioral Neuroscience, 7,* 27.

Klein, S. B., Loftus, J., & Kihlstrom, J. F. (2002). Memory and temporal experience: The effects of episodic memory loss on an amnesic patient's ability to remember the past and imagine the future. *Social Cognition, 20,* 353–379.

Kliegel, M., McDaniel, M. A., & Einstein, G. O. (2008). *Prospective memory: Cognitive, neuroscience, developmental, and applied perspectives.* Mahwah, NJ: Erlbaum.

Levine, B., Svoboda, E., Hay, J. F., Winocur, G., & Moscovitch, M. (2002). Aging and autobiographical memory: Dissociating episodic from semantic retrieval. *Psychology and Aging, 17,* 677–689.

Locke, E. A., & Latham, G. P. (2002). Building a practically useful theory of goal setting and task motivation: A 35-year odyssey. *American Psychologist, 57,* 705–717.

MacLeod, A. K., Tata, P., Kentish, J., & Jacobsen, H. (1997). Retrospective and prospective cognitions in anxiety and depression. *Cognition and Emotion, 11,* 467–479.

Madore, K. P., Gaesser, B., & Schacter, D. L. (2014). Constructive episodic simulation: Dissociable effects of a specificity induction on remembering, imagining, and describing in young and older adults. *Journal of Experimental Psychology: Learning, Memory, and Cognition, 40,* 609–622.

Madore, K. P., & Schacter, D. L. (2014). An episodic specificity induction enhances means–end problem solving in young and older adults. *Psychology and Aging, 29,* 913–924.

Madore, K. P., Szpunar, K. K., Addis, D. R., & Schacter, D. L. (2016). Episodic specificity induction impacts activity in a core brain network during construction of imagined future experiences. *Proceedings of the National Academy of Sciences of the USA, 113,* 10696–10701.

Manning, L., Denkova, E., & Unterberger, L. (2013). Autobiographical significance in past and future public semantic memory: A case study. *Cortex, 49,* 2007–2020.

Mumford, M. D., Schultz, R. A., & Van Doorn, J. R. (2001). Performance in planning: Processes, requirements, and errors. *Review of General Psychology, 5,* 213–240.

Neroni, M. A., Gamboz, N., & Brandimonte, M. A. (2014). Does episodic future thinking improve prospective remembering? *Consciousness and Cognition, 23,* 53–62.

Niendam, T. A., Laird, A. R., Ray, K. L., Dean, Y. M., Glahn, D. C., & Carter, C. S. (2012). Meta-analytic evidence for a superordinate cognitive control network subserving diverse executive functions. *Cognitive, Affective and Behavioral Neuroscience, 12,* 241–268.

Oettingen, G. (2012). Future thought and behaviour change. *European Review of Social Psychology, 23,* 1–63.

Oettingen, G. (2014). *Rethinking positive thinking: Inside the new science of motivation.* New York: Penguin Random House.

Oettingen, G., & Gollwitzer, P. M. (2010). Strategies of setting and implementing goals: Mental contrasting and implementation intentions. In J. E. Maddux & J. P. Tangney (Eds.), *Social psychological foundations of clinical psychology* (pp. 114–135). New York: Guilford Press.

Oettingen, G., & Mayer, D. (2002). The motivating function of thinking about the future: Expectations versus fantasies. *Journal of Personality and Social Psychology, 83,* 1198–1212.

Oettingen, G., & Wadden, T. A. (1991). Expectation, fantasy, and weight loss: Is the impact of positive thinking always positive? *Cognitive Therapy and Research, 15,* 167–175.

Okuda, J., Fujii, T., Ohtake, H., Tsukiura, T., Tanji, K., Suzuki, K., . . . Yamadori, A. (2003). Thinking of the future and past: The roles of the frontal pole and the medial temporal lobes. *NeuroImage, 19,* 1369–1380.

Race, E., Keane, M. M., & Verfaellie, M. (2013). Losing sight of the future: Impaired semantic prospection following medial temporal lobe lesions. *Hippocampus, 23,* 268–277.

Renoult, L., Davidson, P. S. R., Palombo, D. J., Moscovitch, M., & Levine, B. (2012). Personal semantics: At the crossroads of semantic and episodic memory. *Trends in Cognitive Sciences, 16,* 550–558.

Rohrbeck, R., Battistella, C., & Huizingh, E. (2015). Corporate foresight: An emerging field with a rich tradition. *Technological Forecasting and Social Change, 101,* 1–9.

Ryan, T. A. (1970). *Intentional behavior.* New York: Ronald Press.

Rydin, Y., Bleahu, A., Davies, M., Davila, J. D., Friel, S., De Grandis, G., . . . Wilson, J. (2012). Shaping cities for health: Complexity and the planning of urban environments in the 21st century. *Lancet, 379,* 2079–2108.

Schacter, D. L., & Addis, D. R. (2007). The cognitive neuroscience of constructive memory: Remembering the past and imagining the future. *Philosophical Transactions of the Royal Society B: Biological Sciences, 362,* 773–786.

Schacter, D. L., Addis, D. R., & Buckner, R. L. (2008). Episodic simulation of future events: Concepts, data, and applications. *Annals of the New York Academy of Sciences, 1124,* 39–60.

Schacter, D. L., Addis, D. R., Hassabis, D., Martin, V. C., Spreng, R. N., & Szpunar, K. K. (2012). The future of memory: Remembering, imagining, and the brain. *Neuron, 76,* 677–694.

Schacter, D. L., Addis, D. R., & Szpunar, K. K. (2017). Escaping the past: Contributions of the hippocampus to future thinking and imagination. In D. E. Hannula & M. C. Duff (Eds.), *The hippocampus from cells to systems: Structure, connectivity, and functional contributions to memory and flexible cognition* (pp. 439–465). New York: Springer.

Schacter, D. L., & Madore, K. P. (2016). Remembering the past and imagining the future: Identifying and enhancing the contribution of episodic memory. *Memory Studies, 9,* 245–255.

Schifter, D. B., & Ajzen, I. (1985). Intention, perceived control, and weight loss: An application of the theory of planned behavior. *Journal of Personality and Social Psychology, 49,* 843–851.

Schultz, W., Dayan, P., & Montague, P. R. (1997). A neural substrate of prediction and reward. *Science, 275,* 1593–1599.

Shallice, T. (1982). Specific impairments of planning. *Philosophical Transactions of the Royal Society B: Biological Sciences, 298,* 199–209.

Shallice, T., & Burgess, P. (1991). Deficits in strategy application following frontal lobe damage in man. *Brain, 114,* 727–741.

Spreng, R. N., Gerlach, K. D., Turner, G. R., & Schacter, D. L. (2015). Autobiographical planning and the brain: Activation and its modulation by qualitative features. *Journal of Cognitive Neuroscience, 27,* 2147–2157.

Spreng, R. N., Stevens, W. D., Chamberlain, J. P., Gilmore, A. W., & Schacter, D. L. (2010). Default network activity, coupled with the frontoparietal control network, supports goal-directed cognition. *NeuroImage, 31,* 303–317.

Squire, L. R., van der Horst, A. S., McDuff, S. G. R., Frascino, J. C., Hopkins, R. O., & Mauldin, K. N. (2010). Role of the hippocampus in remembering the past and imagining the future. *Proceedings of the National Academy of Sciences of the USA, 107,* 19044–19048.

Szpunar, K. K., Spreng, R. N., & Schacter, D. L. (2014). A taxonomy of prospection: Introducing an organizational framework for future-oriented cognition. *Proceedings of the National Academy of Sciences of the USA, 111,* 18414–18421.

Szpunar, K. K., St. Jacques, P. L., Robbins, C. A., Wig, G. S., & Schacter, D. L. (2014). Repetition-related reductions in neural activity reveal component processes of mental simulation. *Social Cognitive and Affective Neuroscience, 9,* 712–722.

Taylor, S. E., & Schneider, S. K. (1989). Coping and the simulation of events. *Social Cognition, 7,* 174–194.

Tulving, E. (1985). Memory and consciousness. *Canadian Psychology, 26,* 1–12.

Tulving, E. (2002). Episodic memory: From mind to brain. *Annual Review of Psychology, 53,* 1–25.

Ward, R., & Morris, G. (2005). *The cognitive psychology of planning.* New York: Psychology Press.

Wigfield, A., & Eccles, J. S. (2000). Expectancy-value theory of achievement motivation. *Contemporary Educational Psychology, 25,* 68–81.

Wilson, T. D., & Gilbert, D. T. (2003). Affective forecasting. *Advances in Experimental Social Psychology, 35,* 345–411.

Wilson, T. D., & Gilbert, D. T. (2005). Affective forecasting: Knowing what to want. *Current Directions in Psychological Science, 14,* 131–134.

PART I

IMAGERY

CHAPTER 4

Future-Thinking in Young Children
How Do We Measure It and How Can We Optimize It?

Cristina M. Atance

Many areas of study in psychology pertain to thought and behavior that are future oriented, including planning, prospective memory, delaying gratification/delay discounting, and goal setting. Yet it is only relatively recently that the capacity to mentally project the self into the future and its underlying mechanisms have become topics of study in their own right. All healthy adults think about the future—and do so often (e.g., D'Argembeau, Renaud, & Van der Linden, 2011)—with these thoughts ranging from routine events, such as what to have for dinner tonight, to more novel events and occurrences, such as planning a career change. Research in the last decade has shown that adults' thought about the future is related in important ways to their memory for the past (e.g., Addis, Wong, & Schacter, 2007; Okuda et al., 2003; Schacter & Addis, 2007; Szpunar, 2010) and that individuals who are impaired in remembering past events are similarly impaired in constructing future events (e.g., Klein, Loftus, & Kihlstrom, 2002; Tulving, 1985). Research about future thinking has not solely targeted adults, however, but also young children and nonhuman animals. Here, unlike the research with adults, it is not taken as a given that these two populations have the capacity to think about the future. As such, the research in these areas has focused less on identifying the mechanisms underlying this capacity and more on developing the means to test this capacity itself. In other words, the primary question is "Can young children and nonhuman animals think about the future?"

In this chapter, I focus on the development of future-thinking and planning in young children. Most of the research about this topic has centered on developments occurring during the preschool years (i.e., between ages 3 and 5), and, accordingly, most of the methodological approaches and data I discuss do, also. There are undoubtedly instances of future-directed behavior in children younger than age

3 (e.g., an infant raising her arms in anticipation of being picked up), yet because the capacities theorized to underlie and relate to future-thinking ability (e.g., perspective taking, executive functioning, understanding of self) develop substantially between ages 3 and 5, researchers often use age 3 as a starting point. In addition, because, initially, most methodological approaches in this area have required participants to have substantial expressive language ability (as I discuss shortly), these approaches were simply not suitable for children younger than 3 years of age. There is also little debate that the capacity to think about the future undergoes development after ages 5 or 6, but, to date, the bulk of the tasks used to assess this capacity are often easily passed by children of this age. However, more recent research using verbal methodologies similar to those used with adults has shown that the characteristics of children's narratives and talk about the future develop in important ways from childhood to adolescence, and I touch on this research below.

This chapter is divided into three main sections. In the first section, I discuss the various approaches that have been used to measure future-thinking and planning in young children. Throughout this section, I also highlight the research that has explored links between future-thinking and memory. In the second section, I discuss work that has addressed whether future-thinking is related to other cognitive capacities, such as executive functioning and theory of mind. I also describe findings from a growing body of research with children and adolescents that shows that the capacity to mentally project into the future may facilitate such skills as delay discounting and prospective memory. In the third and final section of this chapter, I discuss data that pertain to ways in which it may be possible to "optimize" or improve the accuracy and adaptiveness of children's future-oriented reasoning.

MEASURING FUTURE-THINKING IN CHILDREN

Although research on future-thinking, per se, in children only began in earnest in the last decade or so, developmental psychologists have nevertheless been interested in this capacity, as evidenced by prior work on planning (e.g., Haith, 1997), delaying gratification (e.g., Mischel, Shoda, & Rodriguez, 1989; Thompson, Barresi, & Moore, 1997), and temporal reasoning (e.g., Friedman, 2000). Indeed, it seems unlikely that an individual who cannot contemplate the future is the same individual who can plan or delay gratification.

What Is Being Measured?

By "contemplating the future," I am referring to the capacity to mentally project the self into the future to preexperience events, including co-occurring mental, emotional, and physiological states. In the developmental work, this capacity has most often been referred to as "episodic future-thinking/thought" (e.g., Atance & O'Neill, 2001; Russell, Alexis, & Clayton, 2010), or "episodic foresight" (e.g., Suddendorf & Moore, 2011; Suddendorf, Nielsen, & von Gehlen, 2011). Whereas Atance and O'Neill (2001) broadly define this capacity as a "projection of the self into the future to pre-experience an event" (p. 533; see also Suddendorf & Moore, 2011), others argue that certain criteria must be met for a specific behavior to be considered reflective of foresight (e.g., Suddendorf et al., 2011), including that it be in response to a novel event (thus precluding "learning" over time). By this definition, a child who brings a bucket and shovel to the beach because she has done so numerous times in the past may not be showing foresight, per se, but, rather, has learned over time that these items "belong" at the beach. Foresight may be better exemplified by a child who brings these same items to a new location (e.g., a pond) in anticipation of a novel event such as catching tadpoles. This logic underlies the kinds of tasks that I review in the section on behavioral methods later in this chapter.

Arguably, the "tadpole" example also captures two important components of the taxonomy of prospection recently introduced by Szpunar, Spreng, and Schacter (2014): simulation and planning. "Simulation" is the construction of a detailed future event involving oneself (e.g., imagining catching tadpoles at the pond), whereas "planning" involves the organization of steps (e.g., bringing the bucket and shovel) to arrive at this particular event. The other two components of Szpunar et al.'s (2014) taxonomy—prediction (e.g., affective forecasting) and intention (e.g., goal setting and implementation intentions)—are not ones that have been tackled in the developmental literature on episodic future-thinking, but I briefly return to how implementation intentions, in particular, could be used to optimize children's future-oriented decision making later in this chapter. In what follows, I describe the methods—both *verbal* and *behavioral*—used to measure episodic future-thinking in young children.

VERBAL METHODS

Perhaps reflective of the earlier (and broader) definition of episodic future-thinking as the capacity to mentally preexperience the future (e.g., Atance & O'Neill, 2001), early developmental work mostly used verbal methods to determine the extent to which children's language could be said to reflect this capacity. One of the most straightforward approaches was simply to ask children to talk about what they would be doing at a future point in time. For example, Busby and Suddendorf (2005) asked 3-, 4-, and 5-year-olds to report something that they would do tomorrow. Whereas most children were able to report a specific event (69%, 88%, and 100% of 3-, 4-, and 5-year-olds, respectively), the percentage of events judged by parents to be "accurate/correct" dropped to 31%, 69%, and 63% for the three age groups, respectively, suggesting important developments in future-oriented talk between age 3 and ages 4 and 5.

Similar age-related improvements have also been found in studies in which children were asked about more specific future events (e.g., "What are you going to eat for breakfast tomorrow?"; Quon & Atance, 2010) and to explain why a particular item might be needed in the future (e.g., Atance & Meltzoff, 2005). Although there are some exceptions to this general pattern of age-related improvement (e.g., Hayne, Gross, McNamee, Fitzgibbon, & Tustin, 2011), overall, the findings just discussed have led researchers to conclude that children's talk about the future—and hence their conception of the future—develops substantially during the preschool years. Returning to Szpunar et al.'s (2014) taxonomy of prospection, the studies just described best reflect children's growing capacity to *simulate* future events involving the self.

Links between "Past" and "Future"

Another key question has been the extent to which children's talk about the future is related to their talk about the past. In a number of studies (including some just described), children's talk about the future has been directly compared with their talk about the past. For example, Busby and Suddendorf (2005, Experiment 1) showed that 3- and 4-year-olds' capacity to produce an accurate response to the "tomorrow" question was significantly related to their capacity to produce an accurate response to a question asking them to report something that they had done "yesterday." Moreover, children's accuracy levels did not differ between these two questions, suggesting that mental time travel into the past and future emerge in tandem (see also Quon & Atance, 2010, for similar results).

Further highlighting the role of memory processes in episodic future thought, Richmond and Pan (2013) showed that performance on a relational memory task predicted preschoolers' ability to describe possible future events. In the relational memory task, children were given a series of animal names (e.g., *sheep, giraffe*), along with information about the animal's favorite place (e.g., sheep → playground; giraffe → beach). They were then given a second set of new animal names (e.g., *pig, squirrel*) paired with the same locations as in the first set (e.g., pig → playground; squirrel → beach). Children needed to reach a training criterion of 7 out of 10 on both sets (i.e., remembering at least 7 of 10 animal-location pairings) to proceed to the test trials that tapped both recognition memory (e.g., "Which place did the sheep like best? The playground? Or the beach?") and inference (e.g., "Which animal liked the same place as the sheep? The pig? Or the squirrel?"). The inference trials were of most interest to the researchers because they required children to flexibly manipulate and combine past knowledge. Results indicated that, even when controlling for age, performance on the inference trials significantly predicted the proportion of episodic details in children's future event descriptions. Importantly, this same predictive relation did not hold for the proportion of episodic details that children used when describing past events. Thus, although remembering the past and thinking about the future may indeed be related, it also appears that certain processes (e.g., manipulating and recombining information) are uniquely required for preexperiencing the future.

Children's talk about the future and its similarities to (and differences from) their talk about the past has also been explored in older children and adolescents (e.g., Coughlin, Lyons, & Ghetti, 2014; Wang, Capous, Koh, & Hou, 2014). For example, Coughlin et al. (2014) examined the development of episodic memory and episodic future-thinking in 5-, 7-, and 9-year-olds by presenting them with cue words (e.g., *family*) and asking them to generate past ("last week" and "last year") and future ("next week" and "next year") event narratives related to those words (e.g., "Think of a time *next week* that *family* makes you think of"). Narratives were scored for "episodicity" (e.g., spatial and temporal detail, imagery, emotion, and thoughts) and were also assessed by parents for their veracity/plausibility. Episodicity scores increased with age, and past event narratives contained higher levels of episodicity than future event narratives. Interestingly, however, episodicity scores did not vary as a function of temporal distance (e.g., "last week" vs. "last year"; though see Wang et al., 2014, who did find an effect of temporal distance when asking about more distant past and future events). Importantly, children's past event episodicity scores significantly predicted their future event episodicity scores, suggesting a functional relation between these two forms of thought in middle childhood. Nonetheless, results from the episodicity analyses also revealed a more protracted developmental trajectory for episodic future-thinking as compared with episodic memory. For example, whereas 9-year-olds' episodicity scores for past event narratives did not differ from those of adults, corresponding scores for future event narratives did. According to the authors, this may be because episodic future-thinking has the added challenge of retrieving relevant information from memory and flexibly recombining and manipulating this information to construct a future event scenario—a process that may tax young children's working memory abilities.

To examine similarities and differences between episodic memory and episodic future-thinking from childhood into adolescence, Gott and Lah (2014) studied a sample of 8- to 10-year-old children and 14- to 16-year-old adolescents. Participants were asked to describe two past and two future events. Along the lines of the two previous studies I discussed, reports were scored as a function of the amount of "episodic" versus "nonepisodic" details they contained. Results indicated that adolescents provided significantly more episodic details than children and also that both age groups provided significantly more episodic details for past, compared with future, events. Nonetheless, the number of episodic details provided for past and future events were significantly correlated.

Using the Past to Inform the Future

The studies that I have just described highlight the fact that those children who provide relatively more "episodic content" for past events, for example, also tend to provide relatively more episodic content for future events. Although this suggests important functional links between these two capacities, even stronger evidence of such links comes from showing that children draw on specific information from the past to inform their decisions about the future. This kind of "past–future" linkage has been explored by Lagattuta and her colleagues (for a review, see Lagattuta, 2014), along with, more specifically, children's sensitivity and understanding that their past experiences play an important role in influencing their future (and present) thoughts, emotions, and decisions.

For example, in one study (Lagattuta, 2007), children as young as 4 years of age showed an appreciation that a character (e.g., David) who had experienced a negative event in the past (e.g., having his teddy bear stolen by a red-haired boy) would worry that the event might happen again and/or take preventative action (e.g., hide his toys) when being confronted by the same (e.g., "*the* red-haired boy") or a similar (e.g., "*a* red-haired boy") stimulus. Subsequently, Lagattuta and Sayfan (2013) also showed that children are sensitive to the order in which a character experiences positive and negative events caused by another person. For example, in one condition, children were told about a focal character who experiences a positive, then a negative, event at the hands of another individual (e.g., other individual shares with focal character, then steals from focal character). In another condition, children were told about a character who experiences the reverse order of events (i.e., negative first, then positive). Children were then told that many days later the focal character reencounters the same individual, and children were then asked how the focal character would feel and whether the focal character thinks something "good" or "bad" would happen. In the study, 4- to 10-year-olds alike made more negative forecasts when the individual's behavior in the most recent event (i.e., the second event of the two-event sequence) had been negative (as opposed to positive) toward the focal character. This finding suggests that children place more weight on the most recent past event when making their forecasts.

In sum, findings using verbal methods from preschool to adolescence show that remembering the past and thinking about the future are related processes. However, all studies also show that thinking about the future requires additional cognitive capacities, such as recombining past event information into a plausible future event scenario, and is more protracted in its development. Finally, the work by Lagattuta and her colleagues highlights the importance of children's memory for the past in informing their thoughts and decisions about the future.

BEHAVIORAL METHODS

Although verbal methods remain a popular approach to determining the content and characteristics of children's concepts of the future, a more recent approach has been to devise methods that focus less on how children talk about the future and more on whether their behavior reflects the capacity to anticipate future needs and states. A number of such paradigms have been inspired by Tulving's (2005) "spoon test" (see also Suddendorf & Busby, 2005), based on an Estonian children's story: A little girl dreams about being at a party where there is a delicious chocolate pudding but, unfortunately, having not brought a spoon, she is unable to eat any. The story ends with the little girl getting a spoon before bed the next night, in anticipation of eating the pudding and avoiding future disappointment. Tulving argues that the girl's act of getting the spoon reflects her ability to mentally travel both into the past and the future. Tulving also argues that the little girl is at least 4 years of age—the age at which, he argues, the episodic system undergoes important development (e.g., Wheeler, Stuss, & Tulving, 1997).

Implementing Spoon Tests in the Lab

Developmental researchers have now designed several versions of the spoon test appropriate for children between ages 3 and 5, with the gist of these tests quite similar to what was broadly proposed by Tulving (2005). For example, children encounter a novel problem (e.g., a locked box) in one location, and then, after a brief delay, in another location are presented with the correct item (in this case, a key), along with several distractor items. Children are then asked to select one item to take back to the original location. Most researchers (e.g., Suddendorf et al., 2011) argue that if children select the item that will be useful in the future (e.g., key), they are demonstrating that they remember the past problem and can plan to address it. Arguably, then, to solve this task, children are engaging in processes of simulation (to remember the past and envision the future), as well as planning—though "planning" is used loosely here given that children need not organize a multistep sequence to obtain their desired goal.

Interestingly, whereas some versions of the spoon test are passed only at around age 4 (e.g., Atance & Sommerville, 2014; Suddendorf & Busby, 2005; Suddendorf et al., 2011)—as Tulving (2005) had predicted—others are passed by children as young as age 3 (e.g., Payne, Taylor, Hayne, & Scarf, 2014; Scarf, Gross, Colombo, & Hayne, 2013). Some of this variation may be due to the nature of the items used, as well as the information that is given to children when the problem is first encountered. For example, in the studies by Scarf and his colleagues, children were presented with relatively distinct items (e.g., ball, wind-up toy, key), whereas in Suddendorf et al.'s (2011) study, children were presented with three keys that varied only in their shape. In this last example, children needed to select the key with the correct shape (e.g., a triangular key to open a triangular lock) to open the box. In addition, the information that children were given at the time the problem was encountered differed across studies. Whereas Suddendorf et al. (2011) did not appear to mention the need for a key of a particular shape, Scarf et al. (2013) explicitly asked the children whether they had a key to open the box's padlock. When the children said "no," the experimenter stated that she did not, either. Explicitly mentioning the need for a key, in combination with presenting children with three distinct items in the test phase, may have boosted the performance of 3-year-olds in Scarf et al. (2013) to above chance levels. It is possible that this boost in performance was due to a deeper encoding of the problem, which in turn facilitated the correct future-oriented choice, "key." It is also possible that linking "key" and "box" at the time of encoding resulted in these two items having a higher associative value than "ball" and "box," for example. If so, then one concern is that correctly choosing the key may be more reflective of associative processes and/or cuing than foresight per se. Nonetheless, systematically varying these factors of interest (e.g., type and number of items, information provided at encoding) is an important direction for future research, because it would help to determine those aspects of the task that either help or hinder children's level of success, thus providing a more graded account of children's understanding.

Another important aspect to consider in spoon tests is that children cannot solve such tests without remembering the information that pertains to the past problem. This is most marked in studies such as Suddendorf et al.'s (2011), in which the difference between the correct item (e.g., triangular key) and the distractor items (e.g., square or circular key) is quite subtle. When children are later presented with differently shaped keys, a failure to remember that the box's keyhole was triangular—and not square, for example—necessarily precludes them from selecting the item needed to address the future problem. I point this out because Tulving's (2005) spoon test—though meant to test the broader construct of mental time travel—is also specifically described as a test of foresight. Yet, if children cannot remember the critical past information, they cannot possibly show evidence of foresight—at least in this particular test. Indeed, studies that have directly manipulated the delay between the time that children encounter the problem and the time that they are allowed to act on it (Scarf et al., 2013) or that have controlled for preschoolers' memory for the problem they encountered (Atance & Sommerville, 2014) strongly suggest that memory (e.g., failure to remember the original problem), not foresight (e.g., failure to select the correct item), is the rate-limiting factor for 3-year-olds. Such findings highlight the need to design tasks that better isolate the specific roles of memory and foresight. Systematically assessing children's memory for the problem or past event is one means (e.g., Atance, Louw, & Clayton, 2015; Atance & Sommerville, 2014), as is varying the delay between the time that children encounter a given problem or event and the time that they are given the opportunity to act on it (Scarf et al., 2013).

One final point about the spoon tests used with young children is that, unlike in Tulving's original description, children are not required to spontaneously seek out the required item (e.g., "spoon" or "key") but, rather, are given a forced-choice question about which item among a set to select. Doing so may remove much of the foresight (and planning) requirement of this task and also lead to strategies that rely more heavily on recognition and association (e.g., seeing the key and recognizing that this is the correct item) rather than episodic recall (e.g., spontaneously calling to mind the past problem). How one would go about designing a version of this task that relies on children spontaneously seeking out a particular item, however, is a challenge. Alternatively, one possibility is to query parents about the extent to which they observe their children engaging in these types of more "spontaneous" behaviors in naturalistic, non-laboratory-based contexts.

EPISODIC FUTURE-THINKING AND RELATED COGNITIVE CAPACITIES

To date, most of the work on episodic future-thinking (both in adults and in children) has either implicitly or explicitly highlighted its important links to memory. Irrespective of how this issue has been addressed, most data are consistent with the claim that both forms of thought are related. Other than memory, or related capacities such as relational inference (i.e., Richmond & Pan, 2013), is there evidence for links between future-thinking ability and other simultaneously developing cognitive abilities? Two strong candidates in this respect are theory of mind and executive functioning. Indeed, in a comprehensive account of the cognitive components required for mental time travel ability, Suddendorf and Corballis (2007) convincingly argue that theory of mind in the form of metarepresentational understanding (e.g., false-belief reasoning, or the understanding that someone has a mistaken belief about the world) is needed to identify with a future self whose goals and mental states may differ from those of one's present self. Similarly, inhibitory control—a critical aspect of executive functioning—may also allow individuals to override current drives to secure future outcomes.

RESEARCH WITH YOUNGER CHILDREN

So far, however, these hypothesized links have not been detected in preschoolers. Specifically, Hanson, Atance, and Paluck (2014) gave 3-, 4-, and 5-year-olds a battery of episodic future-thinking tasks, which included asking children to talk about tomorrow, plan for future events (e.g., going to the beach), select items for a future need (e.g., Band-Aids in case one gets hurt), and sequence events according to temporal information. They correlated children's performances on these tasks with their performances on a battery of theory-of-mind tasks—including those assessing false-belief reasoning and desire reasoning (e.g., children's ability to identify that another character has a desire that differs from their own)—and a battery of executive functioning (e.g., inhibition, working memory, planning, cognitive flexibility, and generativity) tasks. Despite finding age-related improvement across most of the tasks, as well as numerous first-order intertask correlations, once age and language were controlled, only one of the individual episodic future-thinking tasks (selecting an item for a future need) remained correlated with an executive functioning composite score. These null results could, however, be explained by the fact that links between episodic future-thinking and theory of mind/executive functioning become more apparent or stronger with age and, indeed, work with older children is somewhat more promising.

RESEARCH WITH OLDER CHILDREN

In the earlier study described by Gott and Lah (2014), there was some evidence that working memory (an important aspect of executive functioning), as measured by a digit-span test, was associated with the episodic details that children and adolescents provided in their future event narratives. The authors argue that working memory may be especially important in allowing children to recall past event details and recombining these to construct possible future events. Similar findings were also reported in a separate study by Abram, Picard, Navarro, and Piolino (2014). More specifically, these authors found links both between executive functioning (as measured by planning, inhibition and flexibility, and verbal fluency tasks) and working memory (as measured by visual span tasks) and the capacity to imagine specific future events in participants ages 6 through 21. Interestingly, their results also showed that the age effects (i.e., older individuals producing more episodic details and information in their future event narratives than younger participants) were no longer significant once the contribution of the cognitive variables was controlled. This finding suggests that more developed executive functioning and working memory processes, rather than age per se, are driving improvements in the capacity to imagine specific future events. In sum, the few studies conducted with older children suggest that, if anything, the contribution of cognitive factors to episodic future-thinking—executive functioning in particular—may become more marked with development.

The little work that exists on links between episodic future-thinking and cognitive factors such as executive function and theory of mind in children has approached this issue from the perspective that these factors may be necessary to allow an individual to conceive of the future (e.g., Suddendorf & Corballis, 2007). However, another potentially fruitful approach is to explore the extent to which the capacity to think about the future may contribute to the development of related capacities that would seem to hinge on the ability to mentally project oneself into the future. Recent work along these lines with children and adolescents has shown that episodic future-thinking ability is related to (and in some cases predicts) prospective memory (remembering to perform a future intention) and delay discounting—considered a measure of impulsivity that reflects people's tendency to "devalue future rewards as a function of the time to their delivery" (Bromberg, Wiehler, & Peters, 2015).

EPISODIC FUTURE-THINKING AND DELAY DISCOUNTING

A growing body of work with adults shows that engaging in episodic future-thinking can reduce delay discounting (e.g., Benoit, Gilbert, & Burgess, 2011), and several studies have now explored this link developmentally. Most notably, Bromberg et al. (2015) tested whether individual differences in episodic future-thinking were related to individual differences in levels of delay discounting in 12- to 16-year-olds. Participants were asked to provide a series of personal past and future events from varying time points (e.g., "Please tell me the details of one event that is related to your family and which you can imagine to take place within the next 6 months"). Events were scored for their episodic "richness" as assessed by the provision of internal/episodic details or details that pertained directly to the event described (e.g., "I went to school early in the morning"). Participants were also given a delay discounting task involving larger hypothetical rewards available at varying distances in the future versus smaller hypothetical rewards available immediately. Adolescents whose future event descriptions were rich and vivid showed less delay discounting, with this relation holding after controlling for a number of variables, including the richness and vividness of participants' past event reports. This is notable, as it suggests that the relation between episodic future-thinking and delay discounting is specific to temporal direction (i.e., future vs. past) rather than mental imagery or the vividness and richness with which one describes personal events, more broadly.

Daniel, Said, Stanton, and Epstein (2015) have also recently shown that episodic future-thinking reduces delay discounting and food intake in overweight/obese children and adolescents. Their 9- to 14-year-old participants engaged in a delay discounting task that required choosing between larger hypothetical rewards available at varying delays (e.g., 2 days, 1 week, 1 month) versus immediate, smaller hypothetical rewards. Importantly, prior to this task, participants in an "episodic future-thinking" (EFT) condition had been asked to generate positive personal future events that corresponded to the time periods in the delay discounting task. In contrast, participants in a control condition were asked to generate personal events that had occurred in the last 24 hours. Prior to each trial in the delay discounting task, participants in the EFT condition were asked to think about vivid future events that corresponded to the delayed time period, whereas participants in the control condition were asked to think about vivid recent events. Results showed that participants in the EFT condition showed significantly less temporal discounting than participants in the control condition. Moreover, children in the EFT condition who were categorized as having high (vs. low) dietary restraint (a measure that reflects motivation to restrict calorie intake for health reasons) consumed fewer calories than children in the control condition on an ad libitum eating task during which future and past events were cued by playing audio recordings of the participants' earlier event reports. The authors explain these findings by arguing that imagining oneself in the future leads to a stronger consideration of or sensitivity to the actual value of the delayed rewards during the decision-making process.

EPISODIC FUTURE-THINKING AND PROSPECTIVE MEMORY

There has also been research on the link between prospective memory and episodic future-thinking in children. Although a study by Atance and Jackson (2009) with preschoolers found little evidence of significant links between event-based prospective memory and episodic future-thinking in 3-, 4-, and 5-year-olds, more recent work with older children suggests that these skills may indeed be related. Nigro, Brandimonte, Cicogna, and Cosenza (2014) gave 4- to 7-year-olds both an episodic future-thinking task that entailed selecting items that another child would need on a future trip and a prospective memory task that entailed reminding the experimenter to return a cell phone to another adult who had forgotten it. Although both tasks involved another person's future, the authors justified the use of these tasks by arguing that many instances of future-oriented thoughts and behaviors are in fact prosocial—meant to benefit others—and are likely subserved by overlapping neural and cognitive mechanisms as thoughts that pertain directly to oneself (e.g., Buckner & Carroll, 2007). Results indicated that after controlling for retrospective memory abilities, age and episodic future-thinking significantly predicted 7-year-olds' performance on the prospective memory task (with the data of the 6-year-olds trending in this direction).

In sum, there is now a small body of work to suggest that children's (especially older ones') capacity to mentally project into the future relates to the extent to which they discount the value of future rewards (Bromberg et al., 2015; Daniel et al., 2015) and succeed on tasks of prospective memory (Nigro et al., 2014). These kinds of studies are promising because they suggest that interventions aimed at improving the vividness and richness with which children envision the future, as well as merely encouraging children to think about the future in contexts in which there may be conflict between current and future rewards, may serve to improve the quality of their decision making. The ultimate goal of improving future-oriented reasoning and decision making is important, given that adults and children alike have difficulties thinking about the future accurately and adaptively. Accordingly, in the final section, I outline research that has implications for this issue; specifically, that certain kinds of past experiences and modes of thought may affect the way in which children make adaptive choices for the future.

IMPROVING CHILDREN'S FUTURE-ORIENTED REASONING

Factors that lead to variation in how children think about the future can be found both in tasks that require them to talk about and construct narratives about the future and in tasks in which children's behavior is used as a marker of whether they are thinking ahead.

Directing Children's "Prospection" to a Specific Event

Recall that Busby and Suddendorf (2005) showed that 3-year-olds—as compared with 4- and 5-year-olds—had difficulty generating plausible events that would happen "tomorrow" (with about 30% of these events being rated as "accurate" by parents). However, more recent work has shown that when 3-year-olds are asked about more specific events (e.g., "What are you going to eat for breakfast tomorrow?"), their level of accuracy (again, as rated by parents) is around 60% (though 5-year-olds' accuracy level of roughly 80% is still significantly higher). Children's performance also appears to be markedly superior when the future event in question is generated by their parents. Hayne et al. (2011) asked 3- and 5-year-olds, for example, "Tomorrow your mum said that you're going to the farmer's market. What can you tell me about this?" Both 3- and 5-year-olds alike provided at least one clause of accurate information that pertained to future events that would either happen "later today" or "tomorrow." Overall, children's reports were very accurate (90%) and, importantly, this aspect did not vary as a function of age; 5-year-olds did, however, provide more information in their accounts than did 3-year-olds.

Experiencing the Consequences of Not Acting with the Future in Mind

One "behavioral" methodology that I have not yet discussed that is relevant to the issue of improving children's future-oriented behavior is a saving paradigm developed by Metcalf and Atance (2011). In this study, we defined saving as "reserving resources for future enjoyment," and we were interested in its development between ages 3 and 5. In our paradigm, children were introduced to two rooms. The first room contained a small marble run, whereas the second room contained a larger, more attractive marble run. Children were also shown that once they put a marble down the run, they could no longer retrieve it. We then told them that they would spend 3 minutes in the first room and 3 minutes in the second room. Once children understood the instructions, they were given three marbles and entered the first room. The measure of interest was the number of marbles that children saved for the second room with the larger marble run. Overall, children saved very little, and, surprisingly, the amount that they saved did not differ as a function of age, with the mean number of marbles saved for each age group hovering at or below one (though see Atance, Metcalf, & Thiessen, 2017, in which we did find age-related changes). However, to examine the extent to which children might learn from a past experience of "not having saved," immediately after children completed this first trial, the experimenter unexpectedly revealed that she had three additional marbles and then proceeded to repeat the instructions from Trial 1 (telling children they would spend 3 minutes in each room, that they would not be able to retrieve marbles once they had been put down the run, etc.). The mean number of marbles that children saved on this second trial was significantly greater than on Trial 1; moreover, whereas only 39% of children saved one or more marbles on Trial 1, 72% did so on Trial 2. The results of this second trial suggest that, regardless of age (there was no age-by-trial interaction), children tended to save more marbles—perhaps to reduce anticipated boredom/disappointment—when they could draw on a recent past experience (i.e., memory) of not having saved or "acted with the future in mind."

Adopting the Perspective of Another Person

The accuracy of children's future-oriented reasoning is also affected by whether they are asked to reason from their own perspective or from the perspective of another person. For example, my students and I (Bélanger, Atance, Varghese, Nguyen, & Vendetti, 2014) sought to determine the extent to which 3-, 4-, and 5-year-olds understand that their current and future preferences might differ. Because predicting changes in attributes such as preferences, personality, and values is difficult even for adults (e.g., Quoidbach, Gilbert, & Wilson, 2013), we gave children a task that required making judgments in which differences in preferences would be quite salient—in this case, that one's "preschool" preferences (e.g., Kool-Aid, sticker books) will differ from one's "grown-up" preferences (e.g., coffee, magazines). Accordingly, children were given a series of trials in which they had to predict which item (e.g., "coffee" vs. "Kool-Aid") they would like best when they were grown up. Interestingly, 3-year-olds were significantly *below* chance at making these predictions (suggesting that they were predicting no change in their preferences), whereas 4-year-olds were at chance. Only the 5-year-olds were above chance at predicting that their current and future preferences would differ. Importantly, however, in a second experiment, children were more accurate at judging the future grown-up preferences of a hypothetical child than they were at making these same judgments for themselves. This finding suggests that children do not lack the knowledge that preferences change over time, but, rather, that the challenge is applying this knowledge to themselves. This "other-over-self" advantage has also been reported in the context of delaying gratification (e.g., Prencipe & Zelazo, 2005).

Though not all studies that have asked children comparable questions about their own versus another person's future have detected an other-over-self advantage (e.g., Payne et al., 2014; Prabhakar & Hudson, 2014), one factor that may differentiate the ones that have from the ones that have not is the level of conflict between children's current and future states. For example, Bélanger et al.'s (2014) "preferences" task requires that children acknowledge that although an item such as Kool-Aid is preferable "right now," coffee will be preferable in the future. Overcoming this kind of conflict may require "distancing" from one's current perspective—as is arguably accomplished by reasoning for another person—thus allowing more objective and accurate reasoning about the future (Mahy, Atance, Moses, & Kopp, 2017). As noted earlier, these kinds of findings are important because they suggest ways to improve the accuracy and quality of children's future-oriented reasoning. For example, leveraging the other-over-self advantage may be possible by setting up scenarios in which children first make predictions for another person and, only then, make the comparable predictions for themselves.

Forming Implementation Intentions

One final way in which it appears possible to improve the adaptiveness of children's future-oriented thinking is by having them form what Gollwitzer and his colleagues (e.g., Gollwitzer & Sheeran, 2006) call "implementation intentions" or "if–then" plans. In the context of goal striving (e.g., losing weight), much evidence suggests that specifying relevant cues (e.g., "If I have the urge to eat chocolate") and linking these to corresponding goal-directed responses (e.g., "then I will eat a piece of fruit") benefits goal achievement (e.g., Gollwitzer, 2014; Gollwitzer & Sheeran, 2006). One can imagine this strategy being particularly effective for young children in the context of such future-oriented tasks as delaying gratification. Indeed, Gawrilow, Gollwitzer, and Oettingen (2011) showed that 10- and 11-year-olds, both with and without attention-deficit/hyperactivity disorder (ADHD), performed better on a computerized delay-of-gratification task when they had been taught relevant implementation intentions. Furthermore, a study by Wieber, von Suchodoletz, Heikamp, Trommsdorff, and Gollwitzer (2011) showed that children as young as 6 profited from using implementation intentions created by the experimenter (e.g., "If there is a distraction, then I will ignore it!") to complete a categorization task while avoiding distractions (e.g., watching cartoons). Thus a logical extension of this work is to determine whether even preschoolers might benefit from the use of implementation intentions. For example, prior to a delay-of-gratification task in which children have to wait for an experimenter to return to receive a large (vs. a small) pile of marshmallows, distraction strategies such as "When I want to take the small pile, I will put my hands on my lap and sing" could be taught.

Having children engage in the imagery exercise of "mental contrasting" (Oettingen, 2012, 2014), in which a desired future (e.g., obtaining the large pile of marshmallows) is contrasted with the reality that stands in its way (e.g., being tempted by the immediately available marshmallow), would also be a potentially fruitful path to goal achievement in young children. Second-grade children who were taught to engage in mental contrasting became more effective in learning vocabulary (Gollwitzer, Oettingen, Kirby, Duckworth, & Mayer, 2011), and adolescents enhanced their math performance (Oettingen, Pak, & Schnetter, 2001). More broadly, the extent to which children spontaneously create implementation intentions and engage in mental contrasting (and/or can be directed to do so by an adult; see Sevincer & Oettingen, 2013) would provide an important window into the development of more sophisticated forms of episodic foresight.

CONCLUSIONS

Although episodic future-thinking is a relatively new area of study in developmental psychology, important headway has been made in the last decade. Using a combination of verbal and behavioral methods, we have learned that the capacity to mentally project into the future develops in important ways between ages 3 and 5. Moreover, beyond these ages, we now know that the vividness and richness with which children envision the future continues to improve. Most of the work that has been conducted with preschoolers, children, and adolescents alike also points to important links between mentally preexperiencing the future and reexperiencing the past. As I suggested earlier in this chapter, an important direction for preschool research is to develop methods that can tease apart the extent to which children's failure on any given task is rooted in difficulties remembering the past versus preexperiencing the future.

Work in the past 10 years has also been critical in shedding light on the extent to which episodic future-thinking is related to other cognitive abilities, such as theory of mind and executive function. Much more work on this topic is needed, but the research conducted thus far suggests that the strength of these relations is weak in early childhood but appears to strengthen with age—especially between episodic future-thinking and executive functioning. There is now also work showing that episodic future-thinking in older children and adolescents may play an important role in their discounting behavior. I predict that this area of research will continue to grow, because it has very real consequences for improving future-oriented decision making. Indeed, given that we now have good measures in place to assess the development of episodic future-thinking, the time is ripe to gain a better handle on whether improvements in this capacity play a critical role in development more broadly.

REFERENCES

Abram, M., Picard, L., Navarro, B., & Piolino, P. (2014). Mechanisms of remembering the past and imagining the future: New data from autobiographical memory tasks in a lifespan approach. *Consciousness and Cognition, 29,* 76–89.

Addis, D. R., Wong, A. T., & Schacter, D. L. (2007). Remembering the past and imagining the future: Common and distinct neural substrates during event construction and elaboration. *Neuropsychologia, 45,* 1363–1377.

Atance, C. M., & Jackson, L. K. (2009). The development and coherence of future-oriented behaviors during the preschool years. *Journal of Experimental Child Psychology, 102,* 379–391.

Atance, C. M., Louw, A., & Clayton, N. S. (2015). Thinking ahead about where something is needed: New insights about episodic foresight in preschoolers. *Journal of Experimental Child Psychology, 129,* 98–109.

Atance, C. M., & Meltzoff, A. N. (2005). My future self: Young children's ability to anticipate and explain future states. *Cognitive Development, 20,* 341–361.

Atance, C. M., Metcalf, J. L., & Thiessen, A. J. (2017). How can we help children save?: Tell them they can (if they want to). *Cognitive Development, 43,* 67–79.

Atance, C. M., & O'Neill, D. K. (2001). Episodic future thinking. *Trends in Cognitive Sciences, 5,* 533–539.

Atance, C. M., & Sommerville, J. A. (2014). Assessing the role of memory in preschoolers' performance on episodic foresight tasks. *Memory, 22,* 118–128.

Bélanger, M. J., Atance, C. M., Varghese, A. L., Nguyen, V., & Vendetti, C. (2014). What will I like best when I'm all grown up?: Preschoolers' understanding of future preferences. *Child Development, 85,* 2419–2431.

Benoit, R. G., Gilbert, S. J., & Burgess, P. W. (2011). A neural mechanism mediating the impact of episodic prospection on farsighted decisions. *Journal of Neuroscience, 31,* 6771–6779.

Bromberg, U., Wiehler, A., & Peters, J. (2015). Episodic future thinking is related to impulsive decision making in healthy adolescents. *Child Development, 86,* 1458–1468.

Buckner, R. L., & Carroll, D. C. (2007). Self-projection and the brain. *Trends in Cognitive Sciences, 11,* 49–57.

Busby, J., & Suddendorf, T. (2005). Recalling yesterday and predicting tomorrow. *Cognitive Development, 20,* 362–372.

Coughlin, C., Lyons, K. E., & Ghetti, S. (2014). Remembering the past to envision the future in middle childhood: Developmental linkages between prospection and episodic memory. *Cognitive Development, 30,* 96–110.

Daniel, T. O., Said, M., Stanton, C. M., & Epstein, L. H. (2015). Episodic future thinking reduces delay discounting and energy intake in children. *Eating Behaviors, 18,* 20–24.

D'Argembeau, A., Renaud, O., & Van der Linden, M. (2011). Frequency, characteristics and functions of future-oriented thoughts in daily life. *Applied Cognitive Psychology, 25,* 96–103.

Friedman, W. J. (2000). The development of children's knowledge of the times of future events. *Child Development, 71,* 913–932.

Gawrilow, C., Gollwitzer, P. M., & Oettingen, G. (2011). If–then plans benefit delay of gratification performance in children with and without ADHD. *Cognitive Therapy Research, 35,* 442–455.

Gollwitzer, A., Oettingen, G., Kirby, T., Duckworth, A. L., & Mayer, D. (2011). Mental contrasting facilitates academic performance in school children. *Motivation and Emotion, 35,* 403–412.

Gollwitzer, P. M. (2014). Weakness of the will: Is a quick fix possible? *Motivation and Emotion, 38,* 305–322.

Gollwitzer, P. M., & Sheeran, P. (2006). Implementation intentions and goal achievement: A meta-analysis of effects and processes. *Advances in Experimental Psychology, 38,* 69–119.

Gott, C., & Lah, S. (2014). Episodic future thinking in children compared to adolescents. *Child Neuropsychology, 20,* 625–640.

Haith, M. (1997). The development of future thinking as essential for the emergence of skill in planning. In S. L. Friedman & E. Kofsky-Scholnick (Eds.), *The developmental psychology of planning: Why, how, and when do we plan* (pp. 25–42). Mahwah, NJ: Erlbaum.

Hanson, L. K., Atance, C. M., & Paluck, S. W. (2014). Is thinking about the future related to theory of mind and executive function?: Not in preschoolers. *Journal of Experimental Child Psychology, 128,* 120–137.

Hayne, H., Gross, J., McNamee, S., Fitzgibbon, O., & Tustin, K. (2011). Episodic memory and episodic foresight in 3- and 5-year-old children. *Cognitive Development, 26,* 343–355.

Klein, S. B., Loftus, J., & Kihlstrom, J. F. (2002). Memory and temporal experience: The effects of episodic memory loss on an amnesic patient's ability to remember the past and imagine the future. *Social Cognition, 20,* 353–379.

Lagattuta, K. H. (2007). Thinking about the future because of the past: Young children's knowledge about the causes of worry and preventative decisions. *Child Development, 78,* 1492–1509.

Lagattuta, K. H. (2014). Linking past, present, and future: Children's ability to connect mental states and emotions across time. *Child Development Perspectives, 8,* 90–95.

Lagattuta, K. H., & Sayfan, L. (2013). Not all past events are equal: Biased attention and emerging heuristics in children's past-to-future forecasting. *Child Development, 84,* 2094–2111.

Mahy, C. E. V., Atance, C. M., Moses, L. J., & Kopp, L. (2017). *Do children delay gratification differently for self versus other?: It depends on their age.* Manuscript submitted for publication.

Metcalf, J. L., & Atance, C. M. (2011). Do preschoolers save to benefit their future selves? *Cognitive Development, 26,* 371–382.

Mischel, W., Shoda, Y., & Rodriguez, M. (1989). Delay of gratification in children. *Science, 244,* 933–938.

Nigro, G., Brandimonte, M. A., Cicogna, P., & Cosenza, M. (2014). Episodic future thinking as a predictor of children's prospective memory. *Journal of Experimental Child Psychology, 127,* 82–94.

Oettingen, G. (2012). Future thought and behavior change. *European Review of Social Psychology, 23,* 1–63.

Oettingen, G. (2014). *Rethinking positive thinking: Inside the new science of motivation*. New York: Penguin Random House.

Oettingen, G., Pak, H., & Schnetter, K. (2001). Self-regulation of goal setting: Turning free fantasies about the future into binding goals. *Journal of Personality and Social Psychology, 80,* 736–753.

Okuda, J., Fujii, T., Ohtake, H., Tsukiura, T., Tanji, K., Suzuki, K., . . . Yamadori, A. (2003). Thinking of the future and past: The roles of the frontal pole and the medial temporal lobes. *NeuroImage, 19,* 1369–1380.

Payne, G., Taylor, R., Hayne, H., & Scarf, D. (2014). Mental time travel for self and other in three- and four-year-old children. *Memory, 23,* 675–682.

Prabhakar, J., & Hudson, J. A. (2014). The development of future thinking: Young children's ability to construct event sequences to achieve future goals. *Journal of Experimental Child Psychology, 127,* 95–109.

Prencipe, A., & Zelazo, P. D. (2005). Development of affective decision making for self and other: Evidence for the integration of first- and third-person perspectives. *Psychological Science, 16,* 501–505.

Quoidbach, J., Gilbert, D. T., & Wilson, T. D. (2013). The end of history illusion. *Science, 339,* 96–98.

Quon, E., & Atance, C. M. (2010). A comparison of preschoolers' memory, knowledge, and anticipation of events. *Journal of Cognition and Development, 11,* 37–60.

Richmond, J. L., & Pan, R. (2013). Thinking about the future early in life: The role of relational memory. *Journal of Experimental Child Psychology, 114,* 510–521.

Russell, J., Alexis, D., & Clayton, N. (2010). Episodic future thinking in 3- to 5-year-old children: The ability to think of what will be needed from a different point of view. *Cognition, 114,* 56–71.

Scarf, D., Gross, J., Colombo, M., & Hayne, H. (2013). To have and to hold: Episodic memory in 3- and 4-year-old children. *Developmental Psychobiology, 55,* 125–132.

Schacter, D. L., & Addis, D. R. (2007). The cognitive neuroscience of constructive memory: Remembering the past and imagining the future. *Philosophical Transactions of the Royal Society B: Biological Sciences, 362,* 773–786.

Sevincer, A. T., & Oettingen, G. (2013). Spontaneous mental contrasting and selective goal pursuit. *Personality and Social Psychology Bulletin, 39,* 1240–1254.

Suddendorf, T., & Busby, J. (2005). Making decisions with the future in mind: Developmental and comparative identification of mental time travel. *Learning and Motivation, 36,* 110–125.

Suddendorf, T., & Corballis, M. C. (2007). The evolution of foresight: What is mental time travel, and is it unique to humans? *Behavioral and Brain Sciences, 30,* 299–351.

Suddendorf, T., & Moore, C. (2011). Introduction to the special issue: The development of episodic foresight. *Cognitive Development, 26,* 295–298.

Suddendorf, T., Nielsen, M., & von Gehlen, R. (2011). Children's capacity to remember a novel problem and to secure its future solution. *Developmental Science, 14,* 26–33.

Szpunar, K. K. (2010). Episodic future thought: An emerging concept. *Perspectives on Psychological Science, 5,* 142–162.

Szpunar, K. K., Spreng, R. N., & Schacter, D. L. (2014). A taxonomy of prospection: Introducing an organizational framework for future-oriented cognition. *Proceedings of the National Academy of Sciences of the USA, 111,* 18414–18421.

Thompson, C., Barresi, J., & Moore, C. (1997). The development of future-oriented prudence and altruism in preschoolers. *Cognitive Development, 12,* 199–212.

Tulving, E. (1985). Memory and consciousness. *Canadian Psychology/Psychologie Canadienne, 26,* 1–12.

Tulving, E. (2005). Episodic memory and autonoesis: Uniquely human? In H. S. Terrace & J. Metcalfe (Eds.), *The missing link in cognition: Origins of self-reflective consciousness* (pp. 3–56). New York: Oxford University Press.

Wang, Q., Capous, D., Koh, J. B. K., & Hou, Y. (2014). Past and future episodic thinking in middle childhood. *Journal of Cognition and Development, 15,* 625–643.

Wheeler, M. A., Stuss, D. T., & Tulving, E. (1997). Toward a theory of episodic memory: The frontal lobes and autonoetic consciousness. *Psychological Bulletin, 121,* 331–354.

Wieber, F., von Suchodoletz, A., Heikamp, T., Trommsdorff, G., & Gollwitzer, P. M. (2011). If–then planning helps school-aged children to ignore attractive distractions. *Social Psychology, 42,* 39–47.

CHAPTER 5

The Future Self

Hal E. Hershfield
Daniel M. Bartels

Whether it is the choice between spending and saving, eating a tempting dessert versus maintaining one's diet, or sinning rather than acting in a less exciting but more morally upstanding way, many decisions require making tradeoffs between the present and the future. Sometimes, a choice poses short-term rewards that could have detrimental effects in the long run (e.g., "That trip to Paris would be fun right now, but I will be paying it off for months"), whereas the future-oriented option brings with it a present sacrifice but heightened well-being in the long run (e.g., "Staying in Cleveland isn't as much fun right now, but I can have a more comfortable retirement with my extra savings"). Given the serious costs that such choices can impose on both people and societies, it is perhaps not surprising that much work in behavioral science (e.g., psychology, economics, marketing, behavioral economics) is dedicated to understanding how people make these sorts of tradeoffs and how decision making in these domains can be improved.

A large body of literature has examined such tradeoffs through the lens of temporal discounting (i.e., how much people devalue delayed rewards and why; see Frederick, Loewenstein, & O'Donoghue, 2002; Scholten & Read, 2010; Urminsky & Zauberman, 2016). Related lines of research examine the ways in which people fail to adequately account for the emotions that they will experience over time (affective forecasting; e.g., Wilson & Gilbert, 2005), fail to delay gratification (e.g., Metcalfe & Mischel, 1999), overweigh present emotions and outcomes (e.g., Loewenstein, O'Donoghue, & Rabin, 2003), and adequately or inadequately consider and weigh properties of present and future rewards (e.g., Soman et al., 2005). Although a variety of perspectives have been applied to study these intertemporal tradeoffs, in this chapter we focus on research that examines how thoughts about one's future self affect decisions with delayed consequences. To do so, we discuss three theoretical perspectives on the future self, the future self as another, continuity between selves, and failures of imagination. Throughout, we examine the myriad considerations that influence decisions made on behalf of the future self in many domains (including finance, health, ethical decision making, and child development), as well as interventions that have been shown to change the way that people think about the future self and potentially promote more prudent-seeming behavior. We close by proposing several questions for future research to tackle. Although researchers have been examining the ways that people think about and treat the future self for a long while (e.g., Markus & Oyserman, 1989), we focus here on studies conducted over the last 10 years, with occasional mentions of earlier research where necessary.

THEORETICAL BACKGROUND

Most decisions entail delayed consequences and, as such, can pose challenging cognitive and emotional hurdles for the decision maker. To consider a few examples, decision makers must grapple with the uncertainty of future states of the world, their comfort with various levels of risk, and an inability to fully understand how present-day decisions will affect them later on. There are also a large number of challenges that specifically involve conceptualizations of the self over time. For instance: (1) How much do we or should we care about that future self who stands to benefit or suffer from actions taken by the present self? (2) What is the planning horizon, and are we thinking about the future consequences of our actions at all? (3) Can we even imagine a future self that doesn't exist (yet)? (4) Can we integrate our image of the future self with all these other complexities to imagine the future state that the future self will find him- or herself in as a result of the current self's decisions?

Even decisions with relatively short time frames can be challenging for various reasons. For example, sleeping in and having 30 minutes of extra sleep but feeling regretful later for skipping a gym class could reflect a lack of projection to the future (i.e., only thinking about the next 30 minutes of one's life and neglecting the rest of the day), an underweighing of concern for the future self (which might or might not be justified), or an underappreciation of just how crummy we will later feel about skipping the gym. And, of course, when the choices involve much longer frames (e.g., retirement decisions), these issues are all the more challenging, with the current self sometimes completely ignoring the interests and feelings of a future self who may desire to be more physically healthy and financially secure. Most of the literature that we review in this chapter relates to the way that people deal with these challenges (with varying degrees of effectiveness).

There have been several treatments of the tension between the present and future self in a variety of literatures, with many offering (normative) prescriptions for how to best make these kinds of choices. We briefly review this literature to frame our discussion of the last decade of research on the future self and its role in decision making.

One set of theories, mostly discussed in economics, attempts to model high-conflict choices with delayed consequences as a competition between multiple simultaneously existing selves (Alos-Ferrer & Strack, 2014; Fudenberg & Levine,

2012; O'Connor et al., 2002; Schelling, 1984; Thaler & Shefrin, 1981). Schelling (1984), for example, discusses the far-sighted self who places the alarm clock across the room, anticipating that tomorrow morning's myopic self will hit the snooze button. And Elster (1977) points to the case of Ulysses, who had the sophisticated insight that his future self would possess different preferences than his current self: By having his shipmates tie him to the ship's mast, he was able to listen to the songs of the Sirens (something his current self desired), while refraining from jumping overboard to his death (something his future self would want to avoid; Homer, trans. 1997). Within these "multiple-selves" models, there can be an ongoing negotiation between the current self and the future self, and "self-control failures" or "failures to defer gratification" are usually attributed to the future self's less powerful status in such negotiations (Bazerman, Tenbrunsel, & Wade-Benzoni, 1998; cf. Bartels & Rips, 2010).

A separate body of ideas is discussed in philosophy, in which theorists have been arguing over when, why, and how much we ought to care about the future self based on determining what it means for a person to continue existing over time or go out of existence (see, e.g., Martin & Barresi, 2002). These are normative rather than descriptive theories, describing how we ought to think about the self over time, rather than how we actually think about the self over time. This literature offers a vast diversity of perspectives, and some views argue that there is no such thing as personal identity over time (i.e., that we do not exist at all; Unger, 1979).

Another group of theories, which we term "future self as other" theories, argue that what matters is the degree to which the future self deserves resources (and thus should be awarded those resources; Brink, 1997) or that our concern for our future selves should be driven by the kinds of care that we show for our loved ones, such as our children (Whiting, 1986).

Other views, which we call "continuity theories," specify what should determine our level of concern for the future self (e.g., continuity of the body, Thomson, 1997; psychological features, Parfit, 1984; consciousness, Locke, 1975).

A final group of more behaviorally informed theories references the myriad ways in which people do not adequately project into the future or mispredict aspects of the future. This is a widely varied group of less comprehensive frameworks—usually developed to characterize one or a few such misprojections—and we refer to a selection of these theories when we discuss failures of imagination.

Three of these approaches have been subjected to empirical examination in recent years, and, as a result, we next discuss research on (1) the future self as another, (2) continuity between selves over time, and (3) failures of imagination, noting some connections between them, and then discuss directions for future research.

THE FUTURE SELF AS ANOTHER

Theorists have suggested that the future self may *feel* like, may be *treated* like, or may actually *be* a distinctly different person from the current self (see, e.g., Parfit, 1971). Parfit (1971) considers a young boy who starts to smoke, knowing that doing so will negatively affect the health of his future self but having no self-interested reason to care from the perspective of the current self. Others have pointed to the idea that overspending in the present and failing to save for one's future retirement might be linked to a person's view of his or her future self as another, different person altogether (Diamond & Koszegi, 2003).

Some research suggests that people view the future self much as they view other persons. In early work, Pronin and Ross (2006) found that research participants were more likely to take an observer's viewpoint when mentally picturing a future self (a perspective that is also taken for past selves; Libby & Eibach, 2009) but a first-person perspective when thinking about actions occurring to the present self. Participants also perceived a future self's actions in terms of that self's traits and dispositions, much the same way that observers do for others in the present. Other work has found that people are more likely to think of the future self in abstract rather than concrete terms, as they tend to do for other people in the present (Wakslak, Nussbaum, Liberman, & Trope, 2008). Further, Ersner-Hershfield, Wimmer, and Knutson (2009) found that neural activation patterns elicited by thinking about a future self in 10 years' time were actually more similar to the activation patterns that result from thinking about others than to the patterns that are elicited by thinking about the self today (see also Mitchell, Schirmer, Ames, & Gilbert, 2011). A distant future self, in other words, may be viewed in ways that are similar to how we see others.

This tendency to see the future self as another can alter intertemporal decisions. If the future self really is seen as another person, then we might feel no more obligated to make sacrifices for our distant selves than we are to sacrifice for others today (Parfit, 1984). Saving money for future selves and forgoing delicious but fattening desserts today may be similar, in some ways, to giving our hard-earned dollars and future health benefits to other people with whom we share little connection. If people were exclusively self-interested (which is to say "other-disinterested"), then this lack of connection to future selves would undermine our generosity toward them. Yet, as Whiting (1986) points out, we often make sacrifices for others (particularly close others) and do not always act in self-interested ways. Parents regularly give up aspects of their lives to ensure that their children are better off now and in the future, adult children make sacrifices for their aging parents, and healthy marriages often entail the partners giving up something for each other.

These observations suggest that treating the future self as another person might facilitate providing for that future self in some contexts. Consider the categories of relationships that people can form with others and the dimensions on which these relationships may vary. If the future self were to be thought of as another person, then what is crucial for understanding how people make intertemporal tradeoffs is knowing the category of "other" to which the future self belongs. If the future self is perceived more like another person with whom one shares few common bonds—more like a distant coworker or even a stranger—then people might serve the wishes of the current self. If, instead, the future self is perceived as a close other—for example, an other with whom there is a shared emotional bond—then, in some cases, the current self might make sacrifices today for the future self's well-being (even if that emotional bond is to some extent imaginary, in the way that one might still feel an emotional connection to a loved one who is no longer alive or not yet born).

So it is possible that one way of promoting the wishes of the future self might be to treat that self like a close other, one for whom present sacrifices are encouraged. And in some cases, a separation between selves might possibly help people behave more prudently, although this conjecture deserves more empirical scrutiny (cf. Peetz & Wilson, 2013). The notion is that it might be easier to maintain your bad habits if you think you are only hurting yourself. People might have an easier time subjecting themselves to negative events than they would subjecting others to negative events. We could imagine that the lack of harmful externalities might undercut one's attempt at changing his or her behavior for the better, as in the case of smokers who quit smoking to benefit their family members' health, or health care staff members who are more likely to maintain good hygiene practices when they are reminded that they are in a hospital to take care of others (Grant & Hofmann, 2011). People may be willing, in other words, to take risks with themselves that they would not take with others.

Recent work suggests that thinking of the future self as at least separate from the current self can affect intertemporal decision making. Peetz and Wilson (2013), for example, found that people classify themselves on either side of a temporal divide (e.g., New Year's Day) as belonging to different categories and that they do so spontaneously in an effort to create distance between selves over time (Peetz & Wilson, 2014). Importantly, when a temporal landmark such as a birthday parses the current self from the future self, research participants are more likely to take the actions necessary to create a better future self. In other words, the temporal barrier allowed people to see a contrast between present and future selves, and this contrast was more likely to activate self-improvement processes (Peetz & Wilson, 2013).

Other research has shown that temporal landmarks—such as the start of a new year, new month, or even new week—help separate the past self from the present self, allowing people to relegate imperfections into earlier time periods and plan aspirational behaviors for selves that exist on the other side of the temporal divide (e.g., dieting; Dai, Milkman, & Riis, 2014, 2015). Theorists have also suggested that as a new temporal divide approaches—in the form of a major milestone birthday—people may be more likely to take stock of their lives (Neugarten & Hagestad, 1976). In fact, Alter and Hershfield (2014) suggest that taking stock of one's life at a time before the present self—for example, at age 39—becomes a seemingly older future self—for example, a 40-year-old—can lead to a search for meaning, a pursuit that can result in positive outcomes (signing up to run a marathon) or negative ones (signing up for a dating website that specializes in extramarital affairs).

In the work we just reviewed, the future self is seen as separated from the current self, but this is not the same as viewing the future self as an explicitly different person altogether. A recent study on university employees comes closer to treating the future self as another person. Namely, Bryan and Hershfield (2012) found that a retirement appeal that explicitly mentioned one's responsibility toward the future self (e.g., "Your future self is completely dependent on you") increased retirement saving more than a traditional self-interested appeal (e.g., "It is in your long-term interest to save for the future") did. The mention of the future self produced changes in saving only when employees already noted that they felt similar and connected to their future selves. It was helpful to see the future self as another person, but only if it was another person to whom respondents felt a sense of emotional connection.

Nonetheless, Bryan and Hershfield (2012) never explicitly tested whether mentions of the future self as another person were the motivating force behind their results. Future work may thus want to further investigate whether messages that frame the future self as an other are more effective at changing saving behavior than messages that take a different frame (e.g., the future self as a continuation of the present self).

Taken together, the "future self as another" perspective considers the ways in which the future self may be thought of as another person altogether (either metaphorically or literally) and how such thoughts can affect intertemporal decision making. In the next section, we discuss a different theoretical perspective, one in which what matters for intertemporal decision making is the sense of continuity between selves over time.

CONTINUITY BETWEEN SELVES OVER TIME

Many philosophers have theorized about how we ought to think about the future self and how we should conceptualize what is meant by a lifetime. Whereas much of this (normative) argumentation can seem somewhat abstract, the practical consequences of our representations of what makes a person or a lifetime can be significant. For example, the specific view of what constitutes continuity over a lifetime ought to influence the way one thinks about beginning-of-life issues (e.g., abortion), end-of-life issues (e.g., right to die, estate planning), or whether a future version of someone should be held responsible for a previous person's actions. Philosophers have posed thought experiments that invite the reader to consider whether a person persists over the course of transformations and how this is affected by the kinds of transformations the person experiences (see, e.g., Lewis, 1976; Nozick, 1981). Parfit (1984) questions which features of a person have to be sustained to support the continuity of a person and how numerous and strong the connections between those features have to be for a later person to count as being the same as the original person. He maintains that a reduction in the number and strength of connections between psychological aspects of a person can warrant a reduction in concern for one's future self (Parfit, 1971). Put another way, when deciding whether to allocate a set of resources to the current self or a set of resources to the future self, what should matter is the "psychological connectedness"—or overlap in personality, beliefs, ideals, preferences, and so forth (Perry, 1972; Unger, 1991)—between these selves. With enough overlap, all else being equal, one should be willing to delay commensurate rewards to a future self. But with sufficiently less psychological overlap between selves, one should consume now and ignore the interests of the future self. (Parfit's normative arguments are controversial; see Dancy, 1997, for an edited volume presenting some opposing views.)

Notably, this perspective on current and future selves does not state that the future self must be seen as another person. Rather, the future self is viewed as a continuation of the current self, but with varying degrees of overlap. Future versions of the self may seem almost identical to the current self, or they may be quite different; what matters for patience over time is the degree of continuity that is felt (Bartels & Rips, 2010; Bartels & Urminsky, 2011). In our work, we have often used the terms *connectedness* and *continuity* almost interchangeably, because for the majority of contexts we test, they are almost synonymous. But one way to characterize the difference is that connectedness can be assessed between any two stages of a person (e.g., how much overlap is there in the important psychological characteristics between the 18-year-old and 50-year-old version of some person?), whereas continuity can be assessed over all adjacent stages of a person (e.g., the proportion of those characteristics that are maintained between the 18- and 19-year-old persons, the 19- and 20-year-old persons, continuing through the 49- and 50-year-old versions).

Measuring and Manipulating the Link between Continuity and Patience

Early work by Frederick (2003) investigated the link between psychological connectedness and discounting of financial rewards by asking research participants to rate how connected they felt to future versions of themselves via a numerical scale (0 = completely different; 100 = exactly the same) and then to complete a *temporal discounting* task, in which participants had to make choices between smaller amounts of money that they could receive immediately versus larger amounts of money that would arrive at a delay. This initial examination found no link between perceived connectedness and patience for financial rewards. But, using a different measure of connectedness—one that used pairs of successively overlapping circles to represent continuity with future selves (see Figure 5.1 for various measures of continuity and connectedness)—Ersner-Hershfield, Garton, Ballard, Samanez-Larkin, and Knutson (2009) found a correlation between ratings of connectedness and patience on an incentive-compatible temporal discounting task, with higher levels of connectedness being positively linked to more patience: Participants who felt a greater sense of connection with a future self in 10 years were more willing to wait for larger financial rewards. Respondents who reported greater connection to their future selves had also accumulated more financial assets over time, a relationship that held when controlling for age (which has been found to correlate positively with future self-continuity; Rutt & Löckenhoff, 2016), income, and education.

At the same time, Bartels and Rips (2010) ran experiments to determine whether changes in perceived connectedness can cause changes in temporal discounting of financial rewards. In some studies, when research participants read vignettes about third parties—hypothetical people who had undergone identity-altering events (e.g., a cross-country move)—participants allocated more funds to the person before rather than after such connectedness-reducing events, providing the first experimental evidence that changes in connectedness causes changes in time preferences. People were less willing to provide benefits to someone else's "future self " when the target had undergone a large change indicating a significant discontinuity in the person's life. Bartels and Rips (2010) also found that people discount the value of rewards more over those periods in which they perceive more personal change (larger decreases in connectedness) as a result of the experimental manipulations.

Further evidence for the link between connectedness and patience comes from social neuroscience research. As mentioned earlier, Ersner-Hershfield, Wimmer, and colleagues (2009) found that neural patterns for thoughts about the future self more closely mimicked neural patterns for thoughts about other people (rather than the neural patterns elicited by thinking about the present self). But there was individual variability in these neural differences: For some participants, thinking about the future self caused neural activation patterns that were almost exactly like patterns that were caused by thinking about another person; for other participants, thinking about the future self showed neural activation patterns that were more or less in line with patterns caused by thinking about the current self. Because other research has shown that a similar region of the brain (i.e., the ventral medial prefrontal cortex) was more strongly active when participants made judgments about the mental states of others who were perceived to be similar to oneself (Mitchell, Macrae, & Banaji, 2006), we interpret variability in neural activation patterns between the current self and the future self to be suggestive of variations in continuity. Along these lines, participants who showed the biggest differences between activation elicited by the current self and activation elicited by the future self (suggesting that they perceived a relative lack of self-continuity over time) were the least patient when it came to waiting for financial rewards (Ersner-Hershfield, Wimmer, et al., 2009).

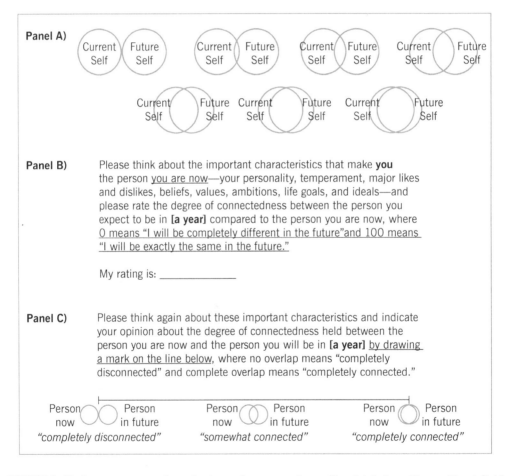

FIGURE 5.1. Various measures of continuity and connectedness. Panel A is from Ersner-Hershfield et al. (2009) and others; Panel B from Frederick (2003), Bartels and Rips (2010), and others; Panel C from Bartels and Urminsky (2011) and others. Reprinted by permission. Available at *https://creativecommons.org/licenses/by/3.09/us/.*

Recent research has found similar relationships between perceived self-continuity and decision making in other contexts. For example, higher levels of continuity can help explain the link between power and lower discount rates (Joshi & Fast, 2013; see also Garbinsky, Klesse, & Aaker, 2014). Other work has found that higher levels of self-continuity are positively correlated with better academic performance (Adelman et al., 2017), a lower likelihood of procrastination in the completion of immediately undesirable tasks (Blouin-Hudon & Pychyl, 2015), a higher likelihood of saving money for the future self rather than giving it to others (Bartels, Kvaran, & Nichols, 2013), and the tendency to forgo immediately rewarding but ethically dubious courses of action (Hershfield, Cohen, & Thompson, 2012), a relationship that was distinct from trait levels of self-control (Tangney, Baumeister, & Boone, 2004). In a consumer behavior context, elevated self-continuity is correlated with evaluations of products, brands, and charitable causes meant to be consumed by distant selves (Zhang & Aggarwal, 2015). Conversely, anthropological research found that young people in Canada who had disrupted perceptions of personal identity over time (e.g., because they were part of cultural groups that lacked a sense of cultural continuity) showed dramatically elevated suicide risk (Chandler & Lalonde, 1998). Although these grave events have many causes, Chandler and Lalonde (1998) suggest that these young people, who had a difficult time envisioning, explaining, and empathizing with what they'd be like in the future, were less likely to realize their futures, engaging in behaviors that could be interpreted as extreme expression of alienation from and disregard for the future self.

Recent research has investigated whether manipulating perceived connectedness in a person can also change his or her level of patience about outcomes he or she will receive. Using a variety of methods to alter perceived connectedness (e.g., by telling research participants that research has found that identity is relatively stable or unstable over time), Bartels and Urminsky (2011) found that increasing a person's sense of connection with his or her future self makes the person more patient in awaiting financial rewards and consumption experiences. Importantly, the researchers showed that this relationship between connectedness and patience was distinct from other related constructs, such as uncertainty of future preferences, predicted change in spending money and free time, positive and negative affect, abstract construal, future time perspective, and self-control. Manipulating levels of connectedness to future selves has also been linked to more ethical decision making (Hershfield et al., 2012; Sheldon & Fishbach, 2015), higher grade point averages among children (Nurra & Oyserman, 2015), and personal giving, with lower levels of connectedness leading to more generosity to others with future allocations of money (Bartels et al., 2013).

What Is Meant by Continuity?

Although this work has established that there is an important relationship between self-continuity and intertemporal decisions, there has been debate in the literature regarding what exactly continuity entails. This debate has only recently motivated empirical investigations. Theorists disagree about what kind of continuity matters the most. Some philosophers argue that what is most important for the continuity of a person over time is continuity with respect to his or her consciousness (e.g.,

Locke, 1975), his or her body (e.g., Olson, 1997), or various aspects of his or her psychology (e.g., Johnston, 1987). The following thought experiment was designed to examine what comprises continuity: In which of the following two cases is the self preserved? In one case, one's brain is transplanted to a new body and all memories remain intact, and in the other case, all memories are lost. Intuitively, it seems as if the "self" is preserved when memories are left intact but not when they are destroyed (an intuition that is at the heart of many science fiction stories, e.g., Saunders, 1992). Indeed, a recent study found that people believed a hypothetical character would be less himself if his memories were erased compared with a situation in which they were preserved (Blok, Newman, & Rips, 2005). And yet, consider another thought experiment in which you will be tortured tomorrow, but beforehand complete amnesia will be induced (Nichols & Bruno, 2010; Williams, 1970). None of your memories will survive, but what is the response to the prospect of this torture? If it is fear, then that suggests that you believe that *you* will still feel pain, despite the fact that your memories have been demolished. Such thoughts represent an obvious contradiction to the results of the earlier thought experiment.

Apparent contradictions about which kinds of continuity are important have given rise to research asking what laypeople think matters most for continuity. Is it more physical or psychological in nature? In recent work, Nichols and Bruno (2010) examined this question and found that when psychological versus physical continuity are pitted against each other, a majority of people felt that a person's psychology—particularly, their memories—was more important for the continuity of identity.

Other research has examined in more detail which aspects of psychological continuity matter. Specifically, Strohminger and Nichols (2014) found that moral traits (e.g., empathy for the suffering of others) were most central to perceptions of self-continuity, followed by memory (especially emotional and autobiographical memory). Perceptual traits such as the ability to feel pain or see color were most weakly linked to the preservation of identity over time. In follow-up research, Strohminger and Nichols (2015) asked family members of patients with frontotemporal dementia (FTD), Alzheimer's disease (AD), and amyotrophic lateral sclerosis (ALS) to rate the extent to which the patients' identities had remained stable since the onset of disease (e.g., "regardless of the severity of the illness, how much do you sense that the patient is still the same person underneath?"). Patients with FTD, the disease that affects moral traits the most (e.g., decreased inhibition and decreased warmth toward others) were rated as having experienced the most disrupted identity. Taken together, it seems that what matters when considering continuity between successive selves is a sense that a person's core identity is preserved, and different categories of features are given different weight, in the following order: morality, then personality, then preferences, experiences, and memories (Strohminger & Nichols, 2014).

Adding another layer to this work, Molouki and Bartels (2016) examined whether specific kinds of changes to these various categories of features were especially threatening to self-continuity. In their experiments, they asked participants to imagine that a specific feature (drawn from the categories of morality, personality, etc.) would change over the next year and then to consider whether, after the change, they would still be substantially the same persons they were now, or whether they would be different persons. Crucially, they found that *improvements* in such features do not undermine a perception of self-continuity, arguing that people generally expect and desire improvement, and changes consistent with these expectations promote self-continuity.

People appear to have theories of how their lives will play out, and future scenarios that differ from those ideas cause a sense of discontinuity. People also have theories of how they came to be the persons they are—they have ideas about how the features in their self-concepts (e.g., memories, moral qualities, personality traits) are causally linked. For instance, they have theories about how their memories might have caused their personality traits, and these theories contribute to their sense of continuity as persons. Chen, Urminsky, and Bartels (2016) found that some features are perceived to be more causally central than others and that changes in such causally central features are believed to be more disruptive to one's continuity.

Taken together, a sense of connection between selves over time is causally related to patience over time. Moreover, research in this area has suggested (1) that people place a special emphasis on psychological continuity, (2) that some kinds of psychological features tend to contribute more to continuity than others (e.g., moral qualities vs. other personality traits), and that (3) people's ideas about the future (i.e., their desires and expectations for positive changes on some features), as well as (4) their ideas about their past (i.e., how some of their features cause or are affected by others) all have an important role to play in determining how we see continuity in our lives and in the lives of others. We next turn to a final grouping of theories that discuss the ways in which failures to fully imagine the future self can influence decision making.

FAILURES OF IMAGINATION

An inability to fully think through the implications of one's choices can complicate intertemporal choices. For example, some research suggests that people don't often account for even the very temporally near opportunity costs presented by their choices—that is, that not buying a $15 item at a store leaves you with $15 to be used for other purposes (Frederick, Novemsky, Wang, Dhar, & Nowls, 2009; Spiller, 2011; Bartels & Urminsky, 2015). Of course, the difficulties get even more complicated for choices with more distant future outcomes, as even the most earnest attempts to imagine what the future will be like will engender representations of future situations that miss (sometimes important) details. Along these lines, Plato (trans. 2008) and Pigou (1932) note that distant future experiences may be imagined less vividly and seem less real. Because the future self can only be accessed via imagination, the ability to vividly represent the future self—that is, the ability to not succumb to failures of imagination—may help explain why some people give more or less weight to the concerns of the future self (Blouin-Hedon & Pychyl, 2015).

Vivid perceptions of the future could be crucial for making decisions that have different consequences over time. Vivid examples are often processed more emotionally, and this can affect generosity. For example, the literature on charitable giving suggests that vivid appeals are more likely to evoke sympathy and subsequent donations than ones that are "colder"—more pallid and/or less emotional appeals.

A picture of one starving child can increase generosity more than a passage detailing the number of children who have been affected by malnourishment (Slovic, Västfjäll, Gregory, & Olson, 2016). For this reason, when making intertemporal decisions, the present self may be theoretically favored over the future self if the future self—and its wants, desires, and emotions—is not represented vividly.

Failures of imagination can have many causes. When imagining a future situation, greater temporal distance can result in perceptions of a future self that is more abstract and less detailed (e.g., Trope & Liberman, 2010). With more abstraction, it can be more difficult to fully imagine the emotional experiences of a future self. And, when imagining emotional reactions to future events, people believe that their responses will be less extreme. That is, participants believe that future events will produce less intense pains and pleasures than if the same event were to occur in the present (Kassam, Gilbert, Boston, & Wilson, 2008). The reverse has also been demonstrated: Events that are described as being more intensely emotional are also perceived as less psychologically distant (Van Boven, Kane, McGraw, & Dale, 2010). As a result, the future self tends to be "dehumanized" and stripped of the warmth and human nature that one might ascribe to the current self (Haslam & Bain, 2007).

Even when people do understand the idea that future events may provoke emotional reactions similar to ones felt in the present, it can nonetheless be challenging to fully understand the future self's preferences, opinions, and feelings precisely because such feelings and preferences may change once one *becomes* one's future self. Paul (2015), for example, proposes a thought experiment wherein all of one's close friends and family members have decided to become vampires, claiming that it is the best decision they've made. The available data suggest that you will also enjoy the life of a vampire (e.g., the nightlife and the fashionable capes), but the catch is that once you decide to make this transformation, you can never undo it. As is the case with many major life choices, this decision carries with it a great deal of weight: Once you become your future self—in this case, a vampire (or a parent)—the preferences that you hold may be fundamentally different from the ones held by the present self. A failure of imagination, then, can occur simply because it can be impossible to know how future tastes may change once the future arrives. So transformative experiences represent one set of experiences in which failures of imagination are inevitable.

But there may be other, more banal situations in which failures of imagination also arise. Given the many ways that contextual factors influence identity, people may have a difficult time imagining which future self—among many possible future selves—will arise (e.g., Oyserman, 2015; Oyserman, Elmore, & Smith, 2012). And, when it comes to imagining much older selves, people may simply be unmotivated to fully engage, due to the negative stereotypes that are associated with the aging process (Levy, Slade, Kunkel, & Kasl, 2002), older people in general (North & Fiske, 2012), and a desire to avoid thinking about death (e.g., Pyszczynski, Solomon, & Greenberg, 2015).

As failures of imagination can reduce the concern afforded to future selves in intertemporal decision-making contexts, recent research has attempted to aid people in the exercise of imagining future selves. For example, Lewis and Oyserman (2015) found that when research participants were asked to think about the distance between now and some future event in a granular metric (such as days), they were more likely to want to take action (e.g., think that they need to start saving sooner for retirement or for their child's education) than when they thought about that distance in a less granular way, such as months or years. The granular metric made the future self seem like it was temporally closer (Zauberman, Kim, Malkoc, & Bettman, 2009) to the current self (and presumably more detailed, though the authors did not explicitly test this possibility). More directly, Hershfield et al. (2011) found that research participants who had been exposed to age-progressed avatars expressed more financial patience on a variety of laboratory decision-making tasks. Exposure to such images also resulted in a decreased likelihood of cheating in a laboratory setting (van Gelder, Hershfield, & Nordgren, 2013) and lower levels of delinquent behavior among adolescents in a longitudinal study (van Gelder, Luciano, Kranenberg, & Hershfield, 2015). In the health domain, participants who saw a weight-reduced future self ate less ice cream in an ostensible taste test and were also significantly more likely to try a sugar-free drink as a reward (Kuo, Lee, & Chiou, 2016).

Finally, there may be times that people do attempt to imagine the future but fail to do so in a realistic, grounded way. A recent body of research, for example, has examined how indulging in positive thoughts and images about the future (and the future self) versus grounded expectations about the future affects behavior over time. Oettingen (2012) and colleagues have found that positively daydreaming and fantasizing about the future can lead to worse future outcomes than allowing also for negative thoughts and images; in contrast, judging the future as likely to be positive, as in people's positive expectations, predicted better future outcomes than judging the future to become bleak (Oettingen & Mayer, 2002). Positive fantasies about idealized futures can sap the energy and motivation needed to pursue that fantasized future (Kappes & Oettingen, 2011). Such positive fantasies have predicted subsequent low effort and low success in a variety of different outcome domains, including weight loss, academic performance, romantic relationships, and job pursuit (Oettingen & Mayer, 2002; Oettingen & Wadden, 1991). For example, among students of low socioeconomic status, positive fantasies predicted more days absent and lower grades by the end of a vocational education program (even when controlling for initial academic performance; Kappes, Oettingen, & Mayer, 2012). In the mental health domain, a recent paper found that engaging in positive fantasies about the future was related to increased depressive symptoms for up to 7 months after measurement (Oettingen, Mayer, & Portnow, 2016). And positive fantasies seem particularly likely to arise when people have a strong need that is currently unmet (Kappes, Schwörer, & Oettingen, 2012).

Taken together, this grouping of theories and empirical papers suggests that one cause of impoverished intertemporal decision making is the inability to fully and vividly imagine a realistic future self. We next discuss some avenues for potential future research.

REMAINING QUESTIONS AND AREAS FOR FUTURE EXPLORATION

Although some progress has been made, there are many avenues for future research that will help to clarify and extend some of the ideas above as well as to open up new areas of research on the future self. Here we highlight a few promising directions.

Naturally Occurring Differences in Imaginative Capabilities

Notably, although previous studies have demonstrated that imagination aids reduced discounting (e.g., Hershfield et al., 2011), no research has directly examined whether people with better imaginations are also naturally more patient. To some extent, a recent neuroimaging study suggests that a failure of imagination is related to discounting (Cooper, Kable, Kim, & Zauberman, 2013). Could it also be the case that people with more vivid imaginations, that is, more of an ability to conjure the future self, are also more likely to be patient with future rewards?

End-of-Life Decision Making

Many policy issues concern end-of-life decisions, such as the selection of medical care plans and beneficiaries. Although there is debate about what the optimal choice might be, many policymakers would prefer that people make well-informed choices about alternative courses of actions in these contexts, rather than end up in a given situation because it was the default course of action. Yet recent work suggests that people may fail to spend the time required to make difficult end-of-life decisions because of the aversive nature of thinking about one's death (Salisbury & Nenkov, 2016). Death, however, represents another temporal landmark that brings with it its own complicated philosophical issues (Newman, Blok, & Rips, 2006). It could be valuable to learn more about whether, for example, a belief in the afterlife— believing that some version of the self exists after biological death—affects the ease with which people make (or the unease they feel about making) end-of-life decisions (which might be believed to affect a version of the self that exists in the afterlife). Further, could a sense of connection with one's offspring relate to how much one wants to promote their interests after death, much as connectedness to one's future self might promote the interests of the future self during one's life?

Calibration Regarding How Much the Future Self Will Resemble the Current Self

Much of this chapter has focused on the ways in which the interests of the current self can at times outweigh those of the future self, with a large focus on how failing to fully consider the future self can lead to suboptimal situations for that distant self. For example, the current self may want to spend money and assume that the future self will be comfortable leading a more frugal life (when in fact she or he may not be). It's also possible—and quite plausible, actually—that people project more continuity than they will obtain. That is, we may overweigh the extent to which our current self's interests extend to the future self (e.g., "The meaning of the tattoo I am about to get will always be important to me"). There might be motivational reasons for this expectation of constancy, which might be an overestimation of actual constancy (Quoidbach, Gilbert, & Wilson, 2013). Recognizing that tastes and other characteristics will change can be akin to recognizing that the current self is not as constant as we normally assume it to be, which could be anxiety-inducing (Proust, 1949; Pyszczynski et al., 2015). If people predict more (or less) constancy in their selves than actually obtains, how might this affect the quality of the choices they make for those future selves? There are a host of questions left to be explored here.

Empirical Links between Various Theories

In reviewing the literature, we have noticed that the various distinctions between future self as another, continuity, and failure of imagination research traditions can often be blurred and overlapping. Questions arise regarding what exactly the links are between the various lines of research referenced in this chapter. A previous review (Hershfield, 2011) suggested that there might in fact be bidirectional links between connectedness, liking, and vividness. And as an example of how these ideas might come together, Hershfield and colleagues (2011) found that viewing age-progressed images (thus increasing vividness of imagination) also increased perceived continuity with a retirement-age self. Bartels and Urminsky (2015) orthogonally manipulated (1) psychological connectedness and (2) factors relating to failures of imagination—namely, the salience of tradeoffs inherent in spending versus saving decisions—and found that the two factors jointly determined people's choices. We noted earlier that sometimes people fail to think through the opportunity cost of their choices—that spending $15 on this item means not having that $15 available to spend on something else or to save for the future. It turns out that in order for people's feelings of connectedness to the future self (which affect their valuation of that future self's outcomes) to influence their decisions in the present, people need to be thinking through these tradeoffs. In these studies, people reduced their discretionary spending (to save for the future self) only when made to feel highly connected to the future self (i.e., causing them to value their future outcomes more) and when the opportunity costs of present spending—that is, the tradeoffs posed by these decisions—were highlighted.

   More work should be done to investigate the relationships between the many factors noted in this review. For example, when might *continuity of the self* versus the (perceived) *otherness of the future self* affect decision making differently? Here, we suggest that an important factor is the time scale of intertemporal decisions. It seems likely that there is a high degree of psychological continuity between the nighttime self who stays up late watching old episodes of *Law and Order* and the morning self who is exhausted and groggy from only getting 5 hours of sleep (Gammill & Pross, 1993). There is, in other words, no good reason to suspect that these two particular selves do not share the types of things that promote psychological continuity over time (e.g., moral values), though of course other things may differ between these selves, such as their goals and desires. So, in order to produce good outcomes for both of these selves (e.g., to smooth utility across them, rather than slighting either one), it could be useful to view the future self (tomorrow morning) as another person with whom one has a close emotional bond. That is, in the short term, "other person" or "simultaneously existing, competing selves" theories of the future self might tell us the most about how to promote prudence. In contrast, over longer periods of time in which greater personal change might occur (e.g., between an earlier time point and retirement), theories about psychological continuity and/

or the nature of our relationship with the future self (close or distant) may be most informative.

Future work may also help us better understand the link between future self-continuity and delay of gratification. At first glance, continuity with one's future self may be a necessary precursor to the ability to delay gratification in general. Yet, in the traditional empirical contexts in which delay of gratification has been investigated (e.g., children choosing between one treat now vs. two after a 10–15 minute delay; Metcalfe & Mischel, 1999), it is hard to imagine that there could be measurable discontinuities between selves over a 15-minute delay. Rather, what may matter more in such short-term contexts is whether the current self can accurately anticipate the feelings of the future self.

Another important direction for future research is to understand what underlies concern for a future self. Some minimalist accounts, such as Parfit's (1984), argue that concern for the future self should be tied almost exclusively to psychological connectedness. It seems quite possible, however, that the ability to imagine the future self, independent from feelings of connectedness, may promote concern. For example, prompts to consider the existence of the future self may increase concern, particularly where those prompts increase the vividness of the representation of that future self. Additionally, if one does not have an ability to adequately imagine the future self, connectedness may impair one's ability to make decisions that are in the best interest of the future self. For example, if a person believes that she will remain mostly the same over time—that is, is highly connected to the future self—her simulations of her future self may be overly similar to what her current self looks like and lead to decisions that undermine the future self's well-being. For example, putting off a rock-climbing vacation so that a future self can enjoy it may not be a good idea if that future self doesn't have the abilities and preferences of the current self. We leave it to future (and ongoing) work to examine these interesting possibilities.

CONCLUSION

People must regularly trade off present wants and desires against future ideals and hopes. Previous research has gone a long way toward understanding some of the antecedents and consequences of such intertemporal choices. Here, we take a slightly different approach and focus on the thoughts that people have about their selves over time and how such thoughts can affect the decisions that they make. We have discussed three groups of theoretical perspectives that have received empirical attention over the last several years. First, "future self as another" theories examine the extent to which the future self is seen as a separate, different person from the current self. Second, "continuity" theories focus on the degree of psychological overlap that is perceived between selves over time. Third, "failures of imagination" theories look at how vividly people are able to represent their future selves. This research has used both measurement of individual differences and experimental designs to better understand how considerations of the future self affect the propensity to make prudent long-term decisions. Although this recent research has made impressive strides, much still remains to be done. We leave it to your future selves and ours to push this body of work further along.

References

Adelman, R. M., Herrmann, S. D., Bodford, J. E., Barbour, J. E., Graudejus, O., Okun, M. A., & Kwan, V. S. Y. (2017). Feeling closer to the future self and doing better: Temporal psychological mechanisms underlying academic performance. *Journal of Personality, 85,* 398–408.

Alos-Ferrer, C., & Strack, F. (2014). From dual processes to multiple selves: Implications for economic behavior. *Journal of Economic Psychology, 41,* 1–11.

Alter, A. L., & Hershfield, H. E. (2014). People search for meaning when they approach a new decade in chronological age. *Proceedings of the National Academy of Sciences of the USA, 111,* 17066–17070.

Bartels, D. M., Kvaran, T., & Nichols, S. (2013). Selfless giving. *Cognition, 129,* 392–403.

Bartels, D. M., & Rips, L. J. (2010). Psychological connectedness and intertemporal choice. *Journal of Experimental Psychology: General, 139,* 49–69.

Bartels, D. M., & Urminsky, O. (2011). On intertemporal selfishness: How the perceived instability of identity underlies impatient consumption. *Journal of Consumer Research, 38,* 182–198.

Bartels, D. M., & Urminsky, O. (2015). To know and to care: How awareness and valuation of the future jointly shape consumer spending. *Journal of Consumer Research, 41,* 1469–1485.

Bazerman, M. H., Tenbrunsel, A. E., & Wade-Benzoni, K. (1998). Negotiating with yourself and losing: Making decisions with competing internal preferences. *Academy of Management Review, 23,* 225–241.

Blok, S., Newman, G., & Rips, L. J. (2005). Individuals and their concepts. In W.-K. Ahn, R. L. Goldstone, B. C. Love, A. B. Markman, & P. Wolff (Eds.), *Categorization inside and outside the laboratory: Essays in honor of Douglas L. Medin* (pp. 127–149). Washington, DC: American Psychological Association.

Blouin-Hudon, E. M. C., & Pychyl, T. A. (2015). Experiencing the temporally extended self: Initial support for the role of affective states, vivid mental imagery, and future self-continuity in the prediction of academic procrastination. *Personality and Individual Differences, 86,* 50–56.

Brink, D. O. (1997). Rational egoism and the separateness of persons. In J. Dancy (Ed.), *Reading Parfit* (pp. 96–134). Oxford, UK: Blackwell.

Bryan, C. J., & Hershfield, H. E. (2012). You owe it to yourself: Boosting retirement saving with a responsibility-based appeal. *Journal of Experimental Psychology: General, 141,* 429–432.

Chandler, M. J., & Lalonde, C. (1998). Cultural continuity as a hedge against suicide in Canada's First Nations. *Transcultural Psychiatry, 35,* 191–219.

Chen, S. Y., Urminsky, O., & Bartels, D. M. (2016). Beliefs about the causal structure of the self-concept determine which changes disrupt personal identity. *Psychological Science, 27,* 1398–1406.

Cooper, N., Kable, J. W., Kim, B. K., & Zauberman, G. (2013). Brain activity in valuation regions while thinking about the future predicts individual discount rates. *Journal of Neuroscience, 33,* 13150–13156.

Dai, H., Milkman, K. L., & Riis, J. (2014). The fresh start effect: Temporal landmarks motivate aspirational behavior. *Management Science, 60,* 2563–2582.

Dai, H., Milkman, K. L., & Riis, J. (2015). Put your imperfections behind you: Temporal landmarks spur goal initiation when they signal new beginnings. *Psychological Science, 26,* 1927–1936.

Dancy, J. (1997). *Reading Parfit.* Oxford, UK: Blackwell.

Diamond, P., & Koszegi, B. (2003). Quasi-hyperbolic discounting and retirement. *Journal of Public Economics, 87,* 1839–1872.

Elster, J. (1977). Ulysses and the sirens: A theory of imperfect rationality. *Social Science Information, 16,* 469–526.

Ersner-Hershfield, H., Garton, M. T., Ballard, K., Samanez-Larkin, G. R., & Knutson, B. (2009). Don't stop thinking about tomorrow: Individual differences in future self-continuity account for saving. *Judgment and Decision Making, 4,* 280–286.

Ersner-Hershfield, H., Wimmer, G. E., & Knutson, B. (2009). Saving for the future self: Neural measures of future self-continuity predict temporal discounting. *Social Cognitive and Affective Neuroscience, 4,* 85–92.

Frederick, S. (2003). Time preference and personal identity. In G. Loewenstein, D. Read, & R. Baumeister (Eds.), *Time and decision: Economic and psychological perspectives on intertemporal choice* (pp. 89–113). New York: Russell Sage Foundation.

Frederick, S., Loewenstein, G., & O'Donoghue, T. (2002). Time discounting and time preference: A critical review. *Journal of Economic Literature, 40,* 351–401.

Frederick, S., Novemsky, N., Wang, J., Dhar, R., & Nowlis, S. (2009). Opportunity cost neglect. *Journal of Consumer Research, 36,* 553–561.

Fudenberg, D., & Levine, D. K. (2012). Fairness, risk preferences and independence: Impossibility theorems. *Journal of Economic Behavior and Organization, 81,* 606–612.

Gammill, T., & Pross, M. (1993). The glasses (Television series episode). *Seinfeld.* New York: Sony Pictures.

Garbinsky, E. N., Klesse, A. K., & Aaker, J. (2014). Money in the bank: Feeling powerful increases saving. *Journal of Consumer Research, 41,* 610–623.

Grant, A. M., & Hofmann, D. A. (2011). It's not all about me: Motivating hand hygiene among health care professionals by focusing on patients. *Psychological Science, 22,* 1494–1499.

Haslam, N., & Bain, P. (2007). Humanizing the self: Moderators of the attribution of lesser humanness to others. *Personality and Social Psychology Bulletin, 33,* 57–68.

Hershfield, H. E. (2011). Future self-continuity: How conceptions of the future self transform intertemporal choice. *Annals of the New York Academy of Sciences, 1235,* 30–43.

Hershfield, H. E., Cohen, T. R., & Thompson, L. (2012). Short horizons and tempting situations: Lack of continuity to our future selves leads to unethical decision making and behavior. *Organizational Behavior and Human Decision Processes, 117,* 298–310.

Hershfield, H. E., Goldstein, D. G., Sharpe, W. F., Fox, J., Yeykelis, L., Carstensen, L. L., & Bailenson, J. N. (2011). Increasing saving behavior through age-progressed renderings of the future self. *Journal of Marketing Research, 48,* S23–S37.

Homer. (1997). *The Odyssey.* New York: Penguin Books.

Johnston, M. (1987). Human beings. *Journal of Philosophy, 84,* 59–83.

Joshi, P. D., & Fast, N. J. (2013). Power and reduced temporal discounting. *Psychological Science, 24,* 432–438.

Kappes, H. B., & Oettingen, G. (2011). Positive fantasies about idealized futures sap energy. *Journal of Experimental Social Psychology, 47,* 719–729.

Kappes, H. B., Oettingen, G., & Mayer, D. (2012). Positive fantasies predict low academic achievement in disadvantaged students. *European Journal of Social Psychology, 45,* 218–229.

Kappes, H. B., Schwörer, B., & Oettingen, G. (2012). Needs instigate positive fantasies of idealized futures. *European Journal of Social Psychology, 42,* 299–307.

Kassam, K. S., Gilbert, D. T., Boston, A., & Wilson, T. D. (2008). Future anhedonia and time discounting. *Journal of Experimental Social Psychology, 44,* 1533–1537.

Kuo, H. C., Lee, C. C., & Chiou, W. B. (2016). The power of the virtual ideal self in weight control: Weight-reduced avatars can enhance the tendency to delay gratification and regulate dietary practices. *Cyberpsychology, Behavior, and Social Networking, 19,* 80–85.

Levy, B. R., Slade, M. D., Kunkel, S. R., & Kasl, S. V. (2002). Longevity increased by positive self-perceptions of aging. *Journal of Personality and Social Psychology, 83*, 261–270.

Lewis, D. (1976). Survival and identity. In A. Rorty (Ed.), *The identities of persons* (pp. 17–40). Berkeley: University of California Press.

Lewis, N. A., & Oyserman, D. (2015). When does the future begin?: Time metrics matter, connecting present and future selves. *Psychological Science, 26*, 816–825.

Libby, L. K., & Eibach, R. P. (2009). Seeing the links between the personal past, present, and future: How imagery perspective in mental simulation functions in defining the temporally extended self. In K. D. Markman, W. M. P. Klein, & J. A. Suhr (Eds.), *Handbook of imagination and mental simulation* (pp. 359–372). New York: Psychology Press.

Locke, E. A. (1975). Personnel attitudes and motivation. *Annual Review of Psychology, 26*, 457–480.

Loewenstein, G., O'Donoghue, T., & Rabin, M. (2003). Projection bias in predicting future utility. *Quarterly Journal of Economics, 118*, 1209–1248.

Markus, H., & Oyserman, D. (1989). Gender and thought: The role of the self-concept. In M Crawford & M. Gentry (Eds.), *Gender and thought: Psychological perspectives* (pp. 100–127). New York: Springer.

Martin, R., & Barresi, J. (2002). *Personal identity*. Malden, MA: Blackwell.

Metcalfe, J., & Mischel, W. (1999). A hot/cool-system analysis of delay of gratification: Dynamics of willpower. *Psychological Review, 106*, 3–19.

Mitchell, J. P., Macrae, C. N., & Banaji, M. R. (2006). Dissociable medial prefrontal contributions to judgments of similar and dissimilar others. *Neuron, 50*, 655–663.

Mitchell, J. P., Schirmer, J., Ames, D. L., & Gilbert, D. T. (2011). Medial prefrontal cortex predicts intertemporal choice. *Journal of Cognitive Neuroscience, 23*, 857–866.

Molouki, S., & Bartels, D. M., (2016). Personal change and the continuity of identity. Available at *https://mindmodeling.org/cogsci2015/papers/0282/paper0282.pdf*.

Newman, G. E., Blok, S. V., & Rips, L. J. (2006). Beliefs in afterlife as a by-product of persistence judgments. *Behavioral and Brain Sciences, 29*, 480–481.

Neugarten, B. L., & Hagestad, G. O. (1976). Age and the life course. In B. B. Binstock & E. Shanas (Eds.), *Handbook of aging and the social sciences* (pp. 626–649). New York: Van Nostrand Reinhold.

Nichols, S., & Bruno, M. (2010). Intuitions about personal identity: An empirical study. *Philosophical Psychology, 23*, 293–312.

North, M. S., & Fiske, S. T. (2012). An inconvenienced youth? Ageism and its potential intergenerational roots. *Psychological Bulletin, 138*, 982–997.

Nozick, R. (1981). *Philosophical explanations*. Cambridge, MA: Harvard University Press.

Nurra, C., & Oyserman, D. (2015). *From future self to current action* (Working paper). Los Angeles: University of Southern California.

O'Connor, K. M., De Dreu, C. K., Schroth, H., Barry, B., Lituchy, T. R., & Bazerman, M. H. (2002). What we want to do versus what we think we should do: An empirical investigation of intrapersonal conflict. *Journal of Behavioral Decision Making, 15*, 403–418.

Oettingen, G. (2012). Future thought and behaviour change. *European Review of Social Psychology, 23*, 1–63.

Oettingen, G., & Mayer, D. (2002). The motivating function of thinking about the future: Expectations versus fantasies. *Journal of Personality and Social Psychology, 83*, 1198–1212.

Oettingen, G., Mayer, D., & Portnow, S. (2016). Pleasure now, pain later: Positive fantasies about the future predict symptoms of depression. *Psychological Science, 27*, 345–353.

Oettingen, G., & Wadden, T. A. (1991). Expectation, fantasy, and weight loss: Is the impact of positive thinking always positive? *Cognitive Therapy and Research, 15*, 167–175.

Olson, E. T. (1997). Was I ever a fetus? *Philosophy and Phenomenological Research: A Quarterly Journal, 57*, 95–110.

Oyserman, D. (2015). Identity–based motivation. In R. Scott & S. Kosslyn (Eds.), *Emerging trends in the behavioral and social sciences* (pp. 1–11). Hoboken, NJ: Wiley.

Oyserman, D., Elmore, K., & Smith, G. (2012). Self, self-concept and identity. In M. Leary & J. Tangney (Eds.), *Handbook of self and identity* (2nd ed., pp. 69–104). New York: Guilford Press.

Parfit, D. (1971). Personal identity. *Philosophical Review, 80,* 3–27.

Parfit, D. (1984). *Reasons and persons.* Oxford, UK: Oxford Paperbacks.

Paul, L. A. (2015). *Transformative experience.* London: Oxford University Press.

Peetz, J., & Wilson, A. E. (2013). The post-birthday world: Consequences of temporal landmarks for temporal self-appraisal and motivation. *Journal of Personality and Social Psychology, 104,* 249–266.

Peetz, J., & Wilson, A. E. (2014). Marking time: Selective use of temporal landmarks as barriers between current and future selves. *Personality and Social Psychology Bulletin, 40,* 44–56.

Perry, J. (1972). Can the self divide? *Journal of Philosophy, 69,* 463–488.

Pigou, A. C. (1932). *The economics of welfare.* London: Macmillan.

Plato. (2008). *Protagoras.* New York: Cambridge University Press.

Pronin, E., & Ross, L. (2006). Temporal differences in trait self-ascription: When the self is seen as an other. *Journal of Personality and Social Psychology, 90,* 197–209.

Proust, M. (1949). *Within a budding grove* (C. K. Scott-Moncrieff, Trans.) London: Chatto & Windus.

Pyszczynski, T., Solomon, S., & Greenberg, J. (2015). Thirty years of terror management theory: From genesis to revelation. *Advances in Experimental Social Psychology, 52,* 1–70.

Quoidbach, J., Gilbert, D. T., & Wilson, T. D. (2013). The end of history illusion. *Science, 339,* 96–98.

Rutt, J. L., & Löckenhoff, C. E. (2016). From past to future: Temporal self-continuity across the life span. *Psychology and Aging, 31,* 631–639.

Salisbury, L. C., & Nenkov, G. Y. (2016). Solving the annuity puzzle: The role of mortality salience in retirement savings decumulation decisions. *Journal of Consumer Psychology, 26,* 417–425.

Saunders, G. (1992, October 5). Offloading for Mrs. Schwartz. *The New Yorker,* pp. 148.

Schelling, T. C. (1984). Self-command in practice, in policy, and in a theory of rational choice. *American Economic Review, 74,* 1–11.

Scholten, M., & Read, D. (2010). The psychology of intertemporal tradeoffs. *Psychological Review, 117,* 925–944.

Sheldon, O. J., & Fishbach, A. (2015). Anticipating and resisting the temptation to behave unethically. *Personality and Social Psychology Bulletin, 41,* 962–975.

Slovic, P., Västfjäll, D., Gregory, R., & Olson, K. G. (2016). Valuing lives you might save: Understanding psychic numbing in the face of genocide. In C. H. Anderton & J. Brauer (Eds.), *Economic aspects of genocides, other mass atrocities, and their prevention* (pp. 613–638). New York: Oxford University Press.

Soman, D., Ainslie, G., Frederick, S., Li, X., Lynch, J., Moreau, P., . . . Zauberman, G. (2005). The psychology of intertemporal discounting: Why are distant events valued differently from proximal ones? *Marketing Letters, 16,* 347–360.

Spiller, S. A. (2011). Opportunity cost consideration. *Journal of Consumer Research, 38,* 595–610.

Strohminger, N., & Nichols, S. (2014). The essential moral self. *Cognition, 131,* 159–171.

Strohminger, N., & Nichols, S. (2015). Neurodegeneration and identity. *Psychological Science, 26,* 1469–1479.

Tangney, J. P., Baumeister, R. F., & Boone, A. L. (2004). High self-control predicts good adjustment, less pathology, better grades, and interpersonal success. *Journal of Personality, 72,* 271–324.

Thaler, R. H., & Shefrin, H. M. (1981). An economic theory of self-control. *Journal of Political Economy, 89,* 392–406.

Thomson, J. J. (1997). People and their bodies. In J. Dancy (Ed.), *Reading Parfit* (pp. 202–229). Oxford, UK: Blackwell.

Trope, Y., & Liberman, N. (2010). Construal-level theory of psychological distance. *Psychological Review, 117,* 440–463.

Unger, P. (1979). There are no ordinary things. *Synthese, 41,* 117–154.

Unger, P. (1991). *Identity, consciousness, and value.* New York: Oxford University Press.

Urminsky, O., & Zauberman, G. (2016). The psychology of intertemporal preferences. In G. Wu & G. Keren (Eds.), *Blackwell handbook of judgment and decision making* (pp. 141–181). Hoboken, NJ: Wiley-Blackwell.

Van Boven, L., Kane, J., McGraw, A. P., & Dale, J. (2010). Feeling close: Emotional intensity reduces perceived psychological distance. *Journal of Personality and Social Psychology, 98,* 872–885.

van Gelder, J. L., Hershfield, H. E., & Nordgren, L. F. (2013). Vividness of the future self predicts delinquency. *Psychological Science, 24,* 974–980.

van Gelder, J. L., Luciano, E. C., Weulen Kranenbarg, M., & Hershfield, H. E. (2015). Friends with my future self: Longitudinal vividness intervention reduces delinquency. *Criminology, 53,* 158–179.

Wakslak, C. J., Nussbaum, S., Liberman, N., & Trope, Y. (2008). Representations of the self in the near and distant future. *Journal of Personality and Social Psychology, 95,* 757–773.

Whiting, J. (1986). Friends and future selves. *Philosophical Review, 95,* 547–580.

Williams, B. (1970). The self and the future. *Philosophical Review, 79,* 161–180.

Wilson, T. D., & Gilbert, D. T. (2005). Affective forecasting: Knowing what to want. *Current Directions in Psychological Science, 14,* 131–134.

Zauberman, G., Kim, B. K., Malkoc, S. A., & Bettman, J. R. (2009). Discounting time and time discounting. *Journal of Marketing Research, 46,* 543–556.

Zhang, M., & Aggarwal, P. (2015). Looking ahead or looking back: Current evaluations and the effect of psychological connectedness to a temporal self. *Journal of Consumer Psychology, 25,* 512–518.

CHAPTER 6

>>>>>>>>>>>>>>>

Counterfactual Thinking

Kai Epstude

It is true that in retrospect . . . every sequence of events looks as though it could not have happened otherwise, but this is an optical, or, rather, an existential, illusion: nothing could ever happen if reality did not kill, by definition, all the other potentialities originally inherent in any given situation.
—HANNAH ARENDT (1967, p. 56)

When Hannah Arendt wrote this, she was discussing philosophers' conceptions of truth and factuality in the context of lies in politics. Her goal was to show that whatever reality we are faced with exists only because other options did not occur. However, the options that did not become reality might still contain valid information relevant for the future. Arendt also knew that these alternative trajectories of the past might have a dangerous side. The mere fact that they did not happen (even though they were very likely) might make them seem unimportant, uninformative, or in some cases even wrong. The present chapter aims to show the function of such alternatives to past events for self-regulation and future goal pursuit.

One might wonder why a volume focusing on the psychology of future thinking includes a chapter focusing on mental simulation of past events. The reason for this is the simple fact that humans are able to reflect on past events. They can evaluate the facts in relation of the past event, and they are able to imagine how things could have turned out differently. This represents a fundamental capacity of human cognition (Baumeister & Masicampo, 2010), and it has consequences for our affective experiences in the present, as well for adjusting our behavior in the future (Byrne, 2016; Epstude & Roese, 2008). Even though few would deny that the past may be informative for future situations, it may still appear somewhat vague how that could actually work. The present chapter will give an overview of theories and research on counterfactual thoughts—mental simulations of alternatives to past events—and will outline how this type of thinking affects the formation of intentions and actual future behavior.

WHAT IS COUNTERFACTUAL THINKING?

Although research on counterfactual thoughts is diverse, there is a pretty solid consensus on how the concept is defined. Mental simulations of alternatives to past behavior or its outcomes are defined as counterfactual thoughts (e.g., Epstude & Roese, 2008, 2011; Kahneman & Miller, 1986). They oftentimes have an if–then structure, consisting of an antecedent (i.e., the *if* part) and a consequence (i.e., the *then* part). Even though both are connected by a logical conditional, the truth value of this logical link can vary. It is possible to imagine highly likely alternatives to a past event (e.g., "If I had studied harder, I would not have failed the test"), as well as highly unrealistic alternatives (e.g., "If my mind were a computer, I would not have failed a test"). The content of a counterfactual depends on the specific circumstances and motivational aspects of a given situation. Oftentimes, emotions such as regret are studied in relation to counterfactual thoughts.

Counterfactuals may involve simulations about how an outcome could have been better (e.g., "If I had run faster, I would have caught the train"; upward counterfactual) or worse (e.g., "If I had waited for him, I would have missed my train"; downward counterfactual). This dimension is usually referred to as the *direction* of counterfactual thoughts. In addition, individuals can simulate events that could or should have happened (e.g., "If I had responded to his message, he would not be mad at me"; additive counterfactual) or events that could or should not have happened (e.g., "If I hadn't said what said, the situation would not escalated"; subtractive counterfactuals). This dimension refers to the *structure* of the counterfactual. Counterfactuals may also vary in terms of their *targets*. They can focus on an individual's own actions ("If I hadn't forgotten to buy tickets . . .") or the actions of someone else ("If she had reminded me to buy tickets . . .").

Different schools of thought have focused on different qualities of counterfactuals. This is not only true for psychology but also for researchers in neighboring fields. The next section presents a short overview of two key approaches, which have delivered valuable insights in recent decades.

PERSPECTIVES ON COUNTERFACTUAL THINKING

Drawing Inferences from Counterfactuals

Cognitive psychologists focus on the fact that counterfactuals are conditionals (e.g., Byrne, 2005, 2016). The fact that they consist of a consequence that is dependent on an antecedent leads to the question of how such conditionals are processed. Oftentimes phrases such as "would have" or "should have" are seen as markers for counterfactuals (Byrne, 2016). In order to understand such a counterfactual, several possibilities have to be kept in mind. A counterfactual such as "If the car was out of petrol, it would have stalled" can have two implications: The car was out of petrol and therefore stalled, or the car was not out of petrol and therefore did not stall. Santamaria, Espino, and Byrne (2005) presented their participants with such counterfactual statements and measured the reading times for the different implications such a statement might have. They found that a counterfactual seems to activate both types of implications. This finding indicates that participants keep those two possibilities in mind when interpreting a counterfactual. However, this is not always the case. A threat to another person formulated as a counterfactual (e.g., "If you had done *X,* then I would have done *Y*") immediately leads to the conclusion that *X* hasn't happened. Interestingly, such threats are interpreted as a way to induce future behavior (Egan & Byrne, 2012).

How causal inferences are linked to counterfactuals is another central question (e.g., Spellman & Mandel, 1999). One key finding is that counterfactuals tend to focus on features of the situation that could have prevented the outcome. This is especially true for those aspects of the situation that are perceived as mutable (e.g., Wells & Gavanski, 1989). However, causal inferences take into account other features of the situation. Consider a car accident that occurred after Mr. Jones voluntarily decided to take a detour. He crashed with a truck driven by Mr. Smith, who was slightly drunk at the time of the accident. Participants focusing on Mr. Jones do indeed generate counterfactuals about the unusual and mutable feature of the situation, namely, his decision to take an uncommon route (i.e., how the accident could have been prevented). However, when looking for a specific cause for the accident, participants also take into account the fact Mr. Smith was drunk (Mandel & Lehman, 1996). In light of such distinct patterns of counterfactuals and causal judgments, Spellman and Mandel (1999) conclude that counterfactuals are just one aspect of cognition influencing causal inferences. The link between counterfactuals and causal inferences has important consequences when it comes to blame and responsibility assignment in legal decision making (Spellman & Kincannon, 2001).

The Development of Counterfactuals

Developmental psychologists examine reasoning processes behind counterfactual thoughts with a focus on the age by which children are able to process counterfactual information (e.g., Beck, Robinson, Carroll, & Apperly, 2006; Ferrell, Guttentag, & Gredlein, 2009). Two lines of research can be distinguished in that respect: one focusing on the inference processes that enable children to draw the right conclusions from counterfactuals and another focusing on the experience of counterfactual emotions such as regret and the occurrence of potential behavioral consequences.

Drawing correct inferences from a counterfactual is a complex endeavor for a child. A key paradigm for the investigation of these inferences is the false-belief task (e.g., Riggs, Peterson, Robinson, & Mitchell, 1998; Wimmer & Perner, 1983). Children hear a story in which, unbeknownst to an actor A, an item (e.g., chocolate) is misplaced by actor B. They have to decide where actor A would search for the item. In adapted versions, a counterfactual element is introduced by asking questions implying an alternative scenario (i.e., "What if it wasn't the actor A who would search for the chocolate but actor B?"; e.g., Rafetseder, Cristi-Vargas, & Perner, 2010). The counterfactual version is difficult to answer for children around the age of 6. Later research showed that even 12-year-olds still perform worse than adults in a slightly more complex version of this task (Rafetseder, Schwitalla, & Perner, 2013). Imagining that events could unfold in multiple different ways in the future seems to be an equally complex process. Beck and her colleagues (2006) asked their participants to predict the pathway of a toy mouse falling through a set of tubes and to make sure that the mouse lands safely on a cushion. In order to correctly place the cushion, the children had to take into account alternative pathways through the tube system and had to act upon the respective conclusions by correctly placing the cushion. In that paradigm, children of age 3 or 4 have difficulties in grasping the various options as a set of actual possibilities that may occur in the future. These results illustrate that the reasoning processes underlying counterfactual thoughts are complex and that they take time to develop.

For the present chapter, it is also relevant to examine whether children are able to adjust their future behavior based on a counterfactual or a related affective experience. Upon learning that they chose the less valuable prize hidden in one of two boxes, children around the age of 6 experience regret. Importantly, when having the chance to adjust their decision in the same situation 1 day later, children indeed choose a different box (O'Connor, McCormack, & Feeney, 2014). This result illustrates that those children actually experience regret and point to effects of this emotion on a behavioral level. An interesting dissociation was reported by McCormack and Feeney (2015). They show that, although children around the age of 6 or 7 do understand the counterfactual emotion of relief, they are not yet able to anticipate its occurrence. Comparing the results of this kind of study to those derived from the false-belief paradigms, one can conclude that drawing the correct logical conclusions from scenarios versus making decisions in more play-oriented paradigms leads to slightly different results. Correctly responding to relatively complex counterfactual situations seems to be a skill that develops relatively late. However, gaining emotional insights from a suboptimal decision seems to emerge much earlier. Future research needs to examine these differences in the developmental pattern in experiencing versus anticipating counterfactual emotions in more detail.

WHAT TRIGGERS COUNTERFACTUAL THOUGHTS?

When studying counterfactuals, we also have to examine *when* they do occur. Unexpected events elicit more counterfactuals than expected ones (Kahneman & Miller, 1986). Situations in which the actor engaged in an action elicit more counterfactuals than situations in which the actor remained passive (Byrne & McEleney, 2000). More recent events are more likely to elicit counterfactuals than events that are temporally distant. The latter is especially relevant when considering a chain of events leading to a critical outcome. Individuals tend to focus on features of the event chain that are closer to the outcome (Kahneman & Miller, 1986; Miller & Gunasegaram, 1990). Furthermore, events that were controllable elicit more counterfactuals than uncontrollable events (Girotto, Legrenzi, & Ritto, 1991). Although the latter finding seems very straightforward, it needs be considered with caution. The subjective nature of control perceptions has potentially harmful consequences in the context of counterfactual thinking. Individuals might perceive a situation as subjectively controllable when objectively it was not (e.g., Markman & Miller, 2006).

What can we conclude from the findings on conditions facilitating counterfactuals? All of the situations mentioned above point to instances in which an expected (or aspired) outcome was not achieved. However, the original goal may still be active, and the original path of action might still be seen as informative. This is especially true if the event happened more recently and individuals think they had some kind of influence over the outcome. Subjectively, such situations might appear more manageable compared with various other constellations (e.g., an expected failure, or an event that is perceived to beyond personal control). Therefore, counterfactuals may be not just one way to reflect on the past. Instead, they might have systematic functions for the regulation of future behavior.

The potential of counterfactuals to inform future behavior is, of course, dependent on whether the situation can still be fixed. The literature on the experience of regret provides evidence for such situations. Roese and Summerville (2005) showed that regrets are especially likely in situations in which the future may hold the possibility to "repair" the situation or to act in a different manner than before. They termed this the *opportunity principle*. The idea is that counterfactuals may be especially useful in such cases because they provide insights into how to potentially adjust behavior in similar situations, thereby increasing the chance of successful future goal pursuit. This is another indication for the assumption that counterfactuals (and regrets) prepare individuals for future situations and actions.

In light of the evidence from these different lines of research suggesting a functional role of counterfactual thoughts in behavior regulation, one might wonder exactly how counterfactuals can facilitate behavior. Functionality, in the context of this chapter, is characterized by the idea that counterfactuals are linked to the pursuit of a specific goal. The term *functional counterfactual* should therefore not be equated with being positive or negative according to a normative perspective. Rather, it should simply be understood as facilitating the pursuit of an attainable goal. Conversely, if a goal cannot be attained anymore or if individuals infer the incorrect reason for their initial failure, counterfactuals gain a dysfunctional quality (see also Sherman & McConnell, 1995).

A FUNCTIONAL APPROACH TO COUNTERFACTUAL THINKING

Counterfactual thinking can influence behavior in two different ways: directly, by affecting behavior related to the specific problem, or indirectly, via broader consequences on information processing and motivation (independent of the respective problem). These two distinct ways of influence on future behavior were described in the functional approach to counterfactuals (Epstude & Roese, 2008; Roese & Epstude, 2017).

The Content-Specific Pathway

The influence of counterfactuals on behavior directly linked to the specific problem on which they are focused is the subject of the content-specific pathway. Within the content-specific pathway, we assume three distinct steps linking a counterfactual to a specific behavior: the recognition of a problem, the formation of an intention, and the transformation of an intention to a behavior. In addition, we propose a feedback loop involving a comparison between the original goal and the actual outcome.

Recognizing a Problem

As already outlined, the trigger for counterfactual thoughts is often an unexpected event. In the case of a mishap or an unfortunate event, we are likely to imagine how things could have gone better. Those events oftentimes also elicit negative affect, which might have a signaling function indicating a problem. Crucial evidence for this part of the model comes from research comparing counterfactual thinking after unexpected positive versus negative events. For example, losing, compared with winning, after betting on the outcome of a football match led to more counterfactual thoughts (Gilovich, 1983). When asked for counterfactuals using an open-end format, participants report more counterfactuals after failure than after success (Roese & Hur, 1997).

Forming an Intention

Once a counterfactual occurs, an intention will likely be formed. Smallman and Roese (2009) demonstrated this step in a set of studies using a serial priming procedure. They asked their participants to read statements that described mishaps (e.g., getting a sunburn). In the next step, participants had to respond to either a counterfactual on how this situation could have been prevented or a statement of how they had responded to such an event in the past (control condition). In the sunburn example, the counterfactual statement was "It is possible to have worn sunscreen." In the control condition, participants read "In the past have worn sunscreen." The task was to respond to this type of statement in terms of whether it would have prevented the situation (*yes* vs. *no*). Next, participants received a cue for the formation of the intention (i.e., "In the future I will _____"). Finally, participants responded to a complete intention in a *yes/no* format (e.g., "In the future I will wear sunscreen"). For the latter part, response times were recorded. Smallman and Roese (2009) found that the counterfactual statements compared with the control statements in the earlier part of the priming sequence facilitated the response to the intention. This result indicates that counterfactuals do indeed prepare individuals to act differently in a similar situation in the future. Smallman and McCulloch (2012) found that this effect is particularly strong when the mishap occurred in the recent (vs. the distant) past and when the future event occurs in the near (vs. the distant) future. Furthermore, recent research demonstrated that the more specific the counterfactual information is, the stronger the facilitation effect on intention formation is (Smallman, 2013). These findings were all obtained within variations of the same sequential priming paradigm. They provide the clearest evidence so far of counterfactuals influencing the formation of intentions and give an indication of how this process works. Similar to findings from the general literature on intention formation, specificity and temporal proximity seem to be key ingredients for the impact on intentions for future behavior (see also Bandura, 1991; Gollwitzer & Brandstätter, 1997; Liberman, Trope, McCrea, & Sherman, 2007). It is important to keep in mind that not every counterfactual may lead to an intention. In line with research on fantasy realization theory (e.g., Oettingen, 2012), one can assume that specifically those counterfactuals highlighting the desired future outcome in relation to the obstacle that needs to be overcome lead to an actual intention. This process of mental contrasting (i.e., contrasting the desired future with obstacles of present reality) will likely lead to the formation of a binding future intention.

Research from the broader literature on counterfactuals and regret corroborates the beneficial effects of counterfactuals on intention formation. For example, Epstude and Jonas (2015) studied HIV+ individuals with regard to counterfactuals about the circumstances of the infection (e.g., "I wish I had used a condom"). Individuals who reported actually having counterfactual thoughts reported a higher intention to use a condom in the future. Similarly, Gleicher et al. (1995) report that participants who imagined having contracted HIV (compared with just receiving information about the virus) had higher safe-sex intentions for the future. Although both studies were conducted with very different samples, they illustrate the beneficial nature of counterfactuals for intention formation.

Regulating Behavior

The step from an intention to the respective behavior is the final part of the content-specific pathway. Abundant research exists on the link between intentions and behavior (for reviews, see Gollwitzer & Sheeran, 2006; Webb & Sheeran, 2006). For the present purpose, studies looking at a direct effect of counterfactuals on the respective behaviors are especially interesting. Morris and Moore (2000, Study 2a) asked aviation students to generate self-focused upward or downward counterfactual thoughts in between various landing attempts in a flight simulator. Independent judges rated the quality of the landing attempts afterward. The results showed that, over the course of the various landing attempts, participants who generated self-focused upward counterfactuals (i.e., "If I only had done X, then the landing would have been better") performed better than those who generated self-focused downward counterfactuals.

Feedback Loop

Once an action has occurred, individuals will compare the achieved outcome to their initial expectations. If the comparison is unsatisfactory, it can elicit new counterfactuals, and the described process starts over. This type of feedback loop is not unique to our model. Similar ideas have been proposed in other theories of behavior regulation (e.g., Carver & Scheier, 1998). However, in the context of counterfactual thoughts and their role in behavior, it is important to keep in mind that this loop exists. It takes into account the fact that counterfactuals do not occur in isolation but are part of the broader goal-related cognition. When a goal remains unfulfilled, the respective cognitive content remains active (Förster, Liberman, & Higgins, 2005; Zeigarnik, 1927). In that sense, the counterfactual is one expression of a *current concern* (Klinger & Cox, 2004). The individual can decide either to remain committed to the goal or to simply disengage from the goal and give up (see also Epstude & Roese, 2011).

The Content-Neutral Pathway

In addition to very specific effects tied to a problem, much broader effects of counterfactuals on behavior have been demonstrated. Galinsky and Moskowitz (2000) asked their participants to engage in counterfactual versus factual thinking about a hypothetical scenario. In an ostensibly unrelated part of their study, they measured participants' performance in a creative insight task (i.e., the Duncker candle problem). They found that participants who engaged in counterfactual thoughts performed better than those who simply engaged in factual thinking. Thus, in this study, counterfactuals seemed to have had a very general effect on behavior that was independent of the content of the thoughts. Galinsky and Moskowitz (2000) called this the *counterfactual mindset*. Markman, Lindberg, Kray, and Galinsky (2007) adjusted the original manipulation of a counterfactual mindset in a way that allows a comparison between mindsets elicited by additive versus subtractive counterfactuals. Some participants imagined a situation in which an action should not have occurred (subtractive mindset); other participants imagined a situation in which an action should have occurred (additive mindset). The results show that the creativity effects were mostly driven by an additive counterfactual mindset. In contrast, a subtractive counterfactual mindset seems to facilitate the performance on analytic tasks (Markman et al., 2007). McCulloch and Smallman (2014) examined how the counterfactual mindset affects intention formation (a process that is often examined independent of such content-neutral effects). They found that specifically those participants who were in a subtractive counterfactual mindset benefited from implementation intentions, whereas the additive mindset helped participants who formed goal intentions. This can be interpreted as a compatibility effect. Relatively focused information processing is a characteristic of both the subtractive mindset and implementation intentions. Broader information processing is characteristic of an additive mindset, as well as goal intentions.

There are several other domains that profit from counterfactual thinking in a broader manner, such as perceived control (Nasco & Marsh, 1999) or motivational orientation (i.e., regulatory focus; Roese, Hur, & Pennington, 1999). Although the role of these mechanisms in regulating behavior has been widely demonstrated, research still needs to examine how such content-neutral effects influence the content-specific pathway. It might well be the case that different features of the content-specific pathway are affected by content-neutral effects in specific ways. However, so far no research has targeted this question in a systematic manner.

SPECIFIC PROBLEMS WITHIN THE FUNCTIONAL APPROACH

Although this general model of how a counterfactual may influence behavior is relatively straightforward, some aspects of this model are quite specific to research on counterfactuals. The idea of a functional counterfactual crucially relies on the assumption that individuals know what exactly caused the suboptimal outcome and how they may adjust their behavior to achieve it; a causal inference is therefore crucial for the functionality of a counterfactual thought. A second question is whether mental simulations of alternative events or their outcomes necessarily focus on events in the past, or whether a similar type of reflection is possible with regard to events in the future. In the next section, both questions are outlined, and their implications for future behavior are discussed.

Inferences and Goals Determine Functionality

Upon failing an exam, one can draw different kinds of inferences. The exam might have been too hard, the teacher might not have been very good, one might not have prepared well enough, or partying the night before the exam might not have been such a good idea. These different kinds of inferences vary in their functionality for future behavior. In order to be informative for successful future goal pursuit, a counterfactual must involve an accurate causal inference. In other words, one needs to draw the right conclusions in order to succeed in a similar future situation. The inference process underlying counterfactual thoughts is complex and highly dependent on situational factors (Alicke, Mandel, Hilton, Gerstenberg, & Lagnado, 2015; Hilton, 2007; Mandel & Lehman, 1996). The outcome of this process is subject to various potential biases. For example, Knobe and Fraser (2008) found that identical behaviors led to different attributions n in two situations: (1) a social norm was violated; (2) a social norm was not violated. For example, if a computer crashes when a person who was not permitted to work on it does so (compared with a person who has permission), the person is seen as the cause of the crash. Another example, mentioned above, is the temporal order effect (e.g., Miller & Gunasegaram, 1990). To illustrate, when asked why they weren't successful at an exam, individuals would give a higher weight to the lack of effort on the day before the exam compared with the fact that they did not invest sufficient time 3 weeks earlier. Those examples illustrate that actual inferences do not necessarily correspond to logical inferential processes. Even when an inference is drawn that is not accurate according to formal logic but works in a given situation, it may still affect behavior. This so-called pragmatic accuracy simply assumes that individuals will make the inference that works best for them according to their understanding of reality, thereby making counterfactual thoughts functional (Epstude & Roese, 2008; Swann, 1984). An illustration of a similar "illogical" type of inference process is a recent finding we obtained when studying individuals who engage in risky sexual behavior (Jonas & Epstude, 2017). We contacted participants after they attended a sex party and asked them to reflect on their own behavior. Instead of focusing on safe-sex behavior, most participants formed counterfactuals about things they wished they had done during the party (i.e., more sexual encounters). This finding shows that in a context in which a health goal is not necessarily central, counterfactuals can be determined by different goals. In the present case, a more hedonic goal was central. Thus counterfactuals focus on hedonic aspects of the situation.

The downside of the functional quality of the inference process is that it carries the danger of becoming dysfunctional. Wrongly assuming that one could have saved a loved one from becoming ill can have dramatic consequences for well-being (Davis, Lehman, Wortman, Silver, & Thompson, 1995). Therefore, the inference process is one of the key features of counterfactuals, determining their functional, as well as dysfunctional, qualities.

Prefactual Thoughts

So far, I have outlined the functions of mental simulations of alternatives to past events and their value for future behavior. Although counterfactuals, per definition, focus on the past, that does not mean that individuals are not able to imagine various if–then scenarios with regard to the future. This type of thinking has been labeled *prefactual* (e.g., McConnell et al., 2000; Sanna, 1996; Scholl & Sassenberg, 2014). There is little systematic research on the concept. Moreover, definitions tend to vary. In an attempt to outline a more systematic approach to the concept, we recently defined prefactuals as conditional propositions involving an action–outcome relation that may or may not occur in the future (Epstude, Scholl, & Roese, 2016). For example, upon being faced with the task of deciding what to do during a first date, one could mentally simulate various behaviors and the respective responses they may elicit in the other person ("If we go to the cozy restaurant, then we will most likely go for a drink afterward"). Importantly, the central feature of the prefactual construct is the belief that an antecedent is linked to an outcome with a certain likelihood. This likelihood can be high or low. In the date night example, one could also imagine surprising the date by going to a 5-hour opera performance and the respective consequences for the remainder of the evening. As it becomes apparent from these examples, prefactuals are distinct from the broader concept of expectancies. They do not necessarily concern a future scenario one actually anticipates to occur. In order to become an expectancy, a specific prefactual needs to be selected. An intention will be formed afterward. Just like counterfactuals, prefactuals may vary in their direction (i.e., upward vs. downward) and their structure (i.e., additive vs. subtractive).

Research systematically examining prefactual thoughts is sparse. For the present purpose, it is especially interesting to look at the function of those future-oriented thoughts. Interestingly, the motivational effects of prefactuals are assumed to be similar to those of counterfactuals. Individuals tend to be more motivated by upward counterfactuals which are focused on the self (compared with downward counterfactuals). Scholl and Sassenberg (2015, Study 3) examined that question in the context of power. Their participants were assigned either a manager's or a subordinate's role in an anticipated dyadic interaction. The anticipated task was either a task that benefited from forethought (i.e., recalling the names of U.S. states) or was independent of forethought (i.e., a letter speed counting task involving the names of U.S. states). Participants were asked to list prefactual thoughts regarding these tasks. Powerful individuals produced more prefactuals when they were beneficial for the solution of a task compared with when they were not beneficial. No such difference emerged for powerless individuals (Scholl & Sassenberg, 2015). These findings indicate that prefactuals are very pragmatically used in situations in which individuals have the option to act.

Prefactuals may also have dysfunctional effects. McCrea and Flamm (2012) showed that the tendency to self-handicap is linked to the occurrence of downward prefactuals. Imagining how things could go wrong increases self-handicapping. Although those individuals might also have goals to succeed at certain tasks, the prefactuals generated interfere with those goals. Sanna (1996) demonstrated similar findings with regard to defensive pessimists. Both lines of research indicate that prefactuals affect behavior. However, the resulting behavior is suboptimal when it comes to pursuing the actual goal.

Many aspects of the prefactual construct are still underexplored. Specifically, the idea of content-neutral effects, which was outlined above for counterfactuals, has not been tested yet. Some of the findings on the mindset for counterfactuals might easily extend to prefactuals. However, the broader motivational consequences still need to be examined in more detail.

When it comes to prefactual thoughts, it is important to keep in mind that those are only one type of mental simulations about the future. There are, of course, various other theoretical approaches dealing with related concepts. A common theme is that the more realistic and specific those mental simulations are, the higher is the likelihood that the respective behavior will be successful. For example, Pham and Taylor (1999) showed that mentally simulating the process of pursuing a goal leads to better results than mentally simulating the desired outcome. Similarly, many studies showed that forming an implementation intention is a better predictor of future behavior than the formation of simple goal intentions, even in the light of factors that hinder goal pursuit (e.g., Gollwitzer, 2014).

Our approach to prefactuals also shares similarities with Oettingen's work on the distinct effect of future fantasies and expectancies (e.g., Oettingen, 2012). Future fantasies refer to positive thoughts and images about a desired future that are facilitated by an individual's current or long-term needs (Oettingen & Mayer, 2002; Kappes, Schwörer, & Oettingen, 2012). Expectancies, on the contrary, are judgments about the probabilities that the desired future will actually come about. They are grounded in people's past experiences rather than in their personal needs. Importantly, expectancies and fantasies differ in their motivational impact. Whereas positive expectancies about attaining future success predict effort and actual success, the opposite is true for positive fantasies. The more people generate positive fantasies about the future, the less effort they exert, and the less successful they are in bringing about the desired future (e.g., Oettingen, 2012; Oettingen & Mayer, 2002; Oettingen & Schwörer, 2013).

Prefactuals are often very specific, but they vary in their degree of realism. One can form very specific prefactuals that are still very unlikely to become reality (e.g., "If I win the lottery, I will buy the mansion at the lake outside of the city"). It is unlikely that such prefactuals will have an effect of behavior. However, with an increase of the degree of realism, the likelihood that the prefactual affects behavior also increases. At times, prefactuals may also highlight the fact that the thought content is unrealistic and thereby eliminate such thoughts from the list of potential behavioral options. The selected option can then be transformed into a binding goal through the process of mental contrasting (e.g., Oettingen, Pak, & Schnetter, 2001).

Epstude and colleagues (2016) briefly describe the curious example of thought protocols in Mahler's (1933) research on magical thinking. One can find examples of very unrealistic prefactuals during the solution attempts (i.e., blowing on a knot in a rope to make it disappear). When the task cannot be solved by logical reasoning alone, such prefactuals actually enhance motivation, possibly by eliminating unrealistic options. In this respect, prefactuals may serve as a tool to distinguish useful from less useful behavior options. Moreover, prefactuals may also help to adjust expectancies by highlighting the degree of realism of the specific action–outcome contingency.

MOTIVATIONAL ASPECTS OF COUNTERFACTUALS

It was mentioned previously that especially unexpected negative events are key triggers of counterfactual thoughts (e.g., Kahneman & Miller, 1986). However, a number of additional factors have been identified, too. One intriguing example from the literature on regret points to the fact that an unfulfilled need to belong might trigger the emotion of regret (Morrison, Epstude, & Roese, 2012). Participant's regrets generally center on aspects of their social lives (romance, family), or on aspects of their careers (work, education). The need to belong is crucially linked to social regrets. Therefore, threats to the need to belong lead to much more intense feelings of regret than threats in other life domains. One can also assume that more counterfactuals arise in such situations. This domain-specific pattern of regret (and potentially counterfactual thoughts) points to the possibility that violations of specific needs differentially affect the occurrence of counterfactuals. The violation of a basic motive (i.e., belongingness; Fiske, 2009) elicit regrets and motivation focusing on "fixing" the situation. This finding is currently still unique in the literature on regret. When it comes to mental simulations of future events, research has already demonstrated that people readily and positively fantasize about stimuli that address an activated need (Kappes et al., 2012). Therefore, examining domain-specific patterns of counterfactuals and regrets is essential in order to study their functionality for future behavior (Roese & Epstude, 2017).

When individuals reflect on major events that in retrospect served as turning points in their lives (e.g., entering college), counterfactuals play another important role (Kray et al., 2010). Upon reflecting on how things could have turned out differently, individuals report the perception that the actual event was meant to happen. In other words, they perceive that it was fate. Furthermore, counterfactual reflection facilitates the perception that the event was beneficial for the individual. Both of these factors lead to an increased perception of the event as being meaningful (Kray et al., 2010). Experiencing life as meaningful has a range of positive consequences. The motivation to find meaning is a crucial driving force in human life. Successfully finding meaning is oftentimes seen as a key condition for a good life (King & Napa, 1998). Imagining how things could have been different can make individuals more content with their lives, and thereby also help them to cope with difficulties in the future (see also King & Hicks, 2007).

AFFECTIVE CONSEQUENCES OF COUNTERFACTUALS

Much of the research outlined above concerned situations in which individuals imagine how things could have been better. When it comes to affective consequences of these thoughts, regret has received considerable attention as the prototypical counterfactual emotion (Kahneman & Miller, 1986). However, various other emotions may also be triggered by upward counterfactuals. For example, guilt, shame, and disappointment have all been studied in that context (e.g., Niedenthal, Tangney, & Gavanski, 1994; Zeelenberg et al., 1998). When it comes to positive emotions, not upward but downward counterfactuals are crucial determinants. Sweeny and Vohs (2012) showed that a specific type of relief is linked to counterfactual thoughts. They demonstrated that in situations in which individuals narrowly avoid an embarrassing situation (i.e., singing in front of a crowd), downward counterfactuals elicit (near-miss) relief. No link between counterfactuals and (task-completion) relief was found for situations in which individuals experienced the embarrassing situation and were just glad that it was over. In this type of setting, counterfactuals take on the form of appraisals eliciting specific emotions. The future behavioral consequences of such appraisals and the respective emotions have been widely studied in emotion research (e.g., Frijda, 1986).

Besides such very specific patterns of counterfactuals leading to specific emotions, there are also more general links of counterfactuals and affective responses. Regret and counterfactuals are linked to depressive symptoms (Markman & Miller, 2006), to general distress (Roese et al., 2009), and to self-blame (Davis et al., 1995). In the context of an HIV infection, Epstude and Jonas (2015) showed that health-related counterfactuals can lead to a lower satisfaction with life. These broader affective consequences of counterfactuals influence how individuals approach the future. However, depending on the specific context, counterfactuals may also provide an opportunity to target specific negative thoughts in a therapeutic manner.

CONCLUSIONS: COUNTERFACTUALS AND THE FUTURE

When focusing on the question of how individuals think about the future, it is useful to keep in mind that some aspects of future-related cognition are determined by the way we think about the past. Counterfactuals represent a bridge between past possibilities and future opportunities. Reflecting on situations in the past can help to avoid suboptimal behavior in the future and helps individuals to prepare for similar situations. It is, however, crucial to keep in mind that the consequences of counterfactual thoughts depend on the goals an individual has in a given situation. Much of the theorizing on counterfactual thoughts was developed independent of research on future thinking. Therefore, the terminology and also the research paradigms sometimes differ. However, counterfactuals are a crucial part of temporal cognition. In line with the opening quote by Hannah Arendt, we can conclude that the fact that counterfactuals and future cognition have oftentimes been seen as independent lines of research in the past does not mean that this distinction is logical or useful. Both areas of research have much to contribute to each other.

REFERENCES

Alicke, M. D., Mandel, D. R., Hilton, D. J., Gerstenberg, T., & Lagnado, D. A. (2015). Causal conceptions in social explanation and moral evaluation: A historical tour. *Perspectives on Psychological Science, 10,* 790–812.

Arendt, H. (1967, February 25). Truth and politics. *The New Yorker,* pp. 59–88.

Bandura, A. (1991). Social cognitive theory of self-regulation. *Organizational Behavior and Human Decision Processes, 50,* 248–287.

Baumeister, R. F., & Masicampo, E. J. (2010). Conscious thought is for facilitating social and cultural interactions: How mental simulations serve the animal–culture interface. *Psychological Review, 117,* 945–971.

Beck, S. R., Robinson, E. J., Carroll, D. J., & Apperly, I. A. (2006). Children's thinking about counterfactuals and future hypotheticals as possibilities. *Child Development, 77,* 413–426.

Byrne, R. M. J. (2005). *The rational imagination: How people create alternatives to reality.* Cambridge, MA: MIT Press.

Byrne, R. M. J. (2016). Counterfactual thought. *Annual Review of Psychology, 67,* 135–157.

Byrne, R. M. J., & McEleney, A. (2000). Counterfactual thinking about actions and failures to act. *Journal of Experimental Psychology: Learning Memory, and Cognition, 26,* 1318–1331.

Carver, C. S., & Scheier, M. F. (1998). *On the self-regulation of behavior.* New York: Cambridge University Press.

Davis, C. G., Lehman, D. R., Wortman, C. B., Silver, R. C., & Thompson, S. C. (1995). The undoing of traumatic life events. *Personality and Social Psychology Bulletin, 21,* 109–124.

Egan, S. M., & Byrne, R. M. (2012). Inferences from counterfactual threats and promises. *Experimental Psychology, 59,* 227–235.

Epstude, K., & Jonas, K. J. (2015). Regret and counterfactual thinking in the face of inevitability: The case of HIV positive men. *Social Psychological and Personality Science, 6,* 157–163.

Epstude, K., & Roese, N. J. (2008). The functional theory of counterfactual thinking. *Personality and Social Psychology Review, 12,* 168–192.

Epstude, K., & Roese, N. J. (2011). When goal pursuit fails: The functions of counterfactual thought in intention formation. *Social Psychology, 42,* 19–27.

Epstude, K., Scholl, A., & Roese, N. J. (2016). Prefactual thoughts: Mental simulations about what might happen. *Review of General Psychology, 20,* 48–56.

Ferrell, J. M., Guttentag, R. E., & Gredlein, J. M. (2009). Children's understanding of counterfactual emotions: Age differences, individual differences, and the effects of counterfactual-information salience. *British Journal of Developmental Psychology, 27,* 569–585.

Fiske, S. T. (2009). *Social beings: Core motives in social psychology.* New York: Wiley.

Förster, J., Liberman, N., & Higgins, E. T. (2005). Accessibility from active and fulfilled goals. *Journal of Experimental Social Psychology, 41,* 220–239.

Frijda, N. H. (1986). *The emotions.* New York: Cambridge University Press.

Galinsky, A. D., & Moskowitz, G. B. (2000). Counterfactuals as behavioral primes: Priming the simulation heuristic and the consideration of alternatives. *Journal of Experimental Social Psychology, 36,* 357–383.

Gilovich, T. (1983). Biased evaluation and persistence in gambling. *Journal of Personality and Social Psychology, 44,* 1110–1126.

Girotto, V., Legrenzi, P., & Rizzo, A. (1991). Counterfactual thinking: The role of event controllability. *Acta Psychologica, 78,* 111–133.

Gleicher, F., Boninger, D., Strathman, A., Armor, D., Hetts, J., & Ahn, M. (1995). With an eye toward the future: The impact of counterfactual thinking on affect, attitudes, and behavior. In N. J. Roese & J. M. Olson (Eds.), *What might have been: The social psychology of counterfactual thinking* (pp. 283–304). Mahwah, NJ: Erlbaum.

Gollwitzer, P. M. (2014). Weakness of the will: Is a quick fix possible? *Motivation and Emotion, 38,* 305–322.

Gollwitzer, P. M., & Brandstätter, V. (1997). Implementation intentions and effective goal pursuit. *Journal of Personality and Social Psychology, 73,* 186–199.

Gollwitzer, P. M., & Sheeran, P. (2006). Implementation intentions and goal achievement: A meta-analysis of effects and processes. *Advances in Experimental Social Psychology, 38,* 69–119.

Hilton, D. (2007). Causal explanation. In A. W. Kruglanski & E. T. Higgins (Eds.), *Social psychology: Handbook of basic principles* (2nd ed., pp. 232–253). New York: Guilford Press.

Jonas, K. J., & Epstude, K. (2017). *The goal-dependent functions of counterfactuals in a sexual context.* Manuscript in preparation.

Kahneman, D., & Miller, D. T. (1986). Norm theory: Comparing reality to its alternatives. *Psychological Review, 93,* 136–153.

Kappes, H. B., Schwörer, B., & Oettingen, G. (2012). Needs instigate positive fantasies of idealized futures. *European Journal of Social Psychology, 42,* 299–307.

King, L. A., & Hicks, J. A. (2007). Whatever happened to "what might have been"?: Regret, happiness, and maturity. *American Psychologist, 62,* 625–636.

King, L. A., & Napa, C. K. (1998). What makes a life good? *Journal of Personality and Social Psychology, 75,* 156–165.

Klinger, E., & Cox, W. M. (2004). Motivation and the theory of current concerns. In W. M. Cox & E. Klinger (Eds.), *Handbook of motivational counseling: Concepts, approaches, and assessment* (pp. 3–27). Chichester, UK: Wiley.

Knobe, J., & Fraser, B. (2008). Causal judgment and moral judgment: Two experiments. In W. Sinnott-Armstrong (Ed.), *Moral psychology: Vol. 2. The cognitive science of morality* (pp. 441–447). Cambridge, MA: MIT Press.

Kray, L. J., George, L. G., Liljenquist, K. A., Galinsky, A. D., Tetlock, P. E., & Roese, N. J. (2010). From what might have been to what must have been: Counterfactual thinking creates meaning. *Journal of Personality and Social Psychology, 98,* 106–118.

Liberman, N., Trope, Y., McCrea, S. M., & Sherman, S. J. (2007). The effect of level of construal on the temporal distance of activity enactment. *Journal of Experimental Social Psychology, 43,* 143–149.

Mahler, W. (1933). Ersatzhandlungen verschiedenen Realitätsgrades [Compensatory actions based on different degrees of reality]. *Psychologische Forschung, 18,* 27–89.

Mandel, D. R., & Lehman, D. R. (1996). Counterfactual thinking and ascriptions of cause and preventability. *Journal of Personality and Social Psychology, 71,* 450–463.

Markman, K. D., Lindberg, M. J., Kray, L. J., & Galinsky, A. D. (2007). Implications of counterfactual structure for creative generation and analytical problem-solving. *Personality and Social Psychology Bulletin, 33,* 312–324.

Markman, K. D., & Miller, A. K. (2006). Depression, control and counterfactual thinking: Functional for whom? *Journal of Social and Clinical Psychology, 25,* 210–227.

McConnell, A. R., Niedermeier, K. E., Leibold, J. M., El-Alayli, A. G., Chin, P. P., & Kuiper, N. M. (2000). What if I find it cheaper someplace else?: Role of prefactual thinking and anticipated regret in consumer behavior. *Psychology and Marketing, 17,* 281–298.

McCormack, T., & Feeney, A. (2015). The development of the experience and anticipation of regret. *Cognition and Emotion, 29,* 266–280.

McCrea, S. M., & Flamm, A. (2012). Dysfunctional anticipatory thoughts and the self-handicapping strategy. *European Journal of Social Psychology, 42,* 72–81.

McCulloch, K. C., & Smallman, R. (2014). The implications of counterfactual mind-sets for the functioning of implementation intentions. *Motivation and Emotion, 38,* 635–644.

Miller, D. T., & Gunasegaram, S. (1990). Temporal order and the perceived mutability of events: Implications for blame assignment. *Journal of Personality and Social Psychology, 59,* 1111–1118.

Morris, M., & Moore, P. C. (2000). The lessons we (don't) learn: Counterfactual thinking and organizational accountability after a close call. *Administrative Science Quarterly, 45,* 737–765.

Morrison, M., Epstude, K., & Roese, N. J. (2012). Life regrets and the need to belong. *Social Psychological and Personality Science, 3*, 675–681.

Nasco, S. A., & Marsh, K. L. (1999). Gaining control through counterfactual thinking. *Personality and Social Psychology Bulletin, 25*, 556–568.

Niedenthal, P. M., Tangney, J. P., & Gavanski, I. (1994). "If only I weren't" versus "If only I hadn't": Distinguishing shame and guilt in counterfactual thinking. *Journal of Personality and Social Psychology, 67*, 584–595.

O'Connor, E., McCormack, T., & Feeney, A. (2014). Do children who experience regret make better decisions?: A developmental study of the behavioral consequences of regret. *Child Development, 85*, 1995–2010.

Oettingen, G. (2012). Future thought and behaviour change. *European Review of Social Psychology, 23*, 1–63.

Oettingen, G., & Mayer, D. (2002). The motivating function of thinking about the future: Expectations versus fantasies. *Journal of Personality and Social Psychology, 83*, 1198–1212.

Oettingen, G., Pak, H. J., & Schnetter, K. (2001). Self-regulation of goal-setting: Turning free fantasies about the future into binding goals. *Journal of Personality and Social Psychology, 80*, 736–753.

Oettingen, G., & Schwörer, B. (2013). Mind wandering via mental contrasting as a tool for behavior change. *Frontiers in Psychology, 4*, 562.

Pham, L. B., & Taylor, S. E. (1999). From thought to action: Effects of process- versus outcome-based mental simulations on performance. *Personality and Social Psychology Bulletin, 25*, 250–260.

Rafetseder, E., Cristi-Vargas, R., & Perner, J. (2010). Counterfactual reasoning: Developing a sense of "nearest possible world." *Child Development, 81*, 376–389.

Rafetseder, E., Schwitalla, M., & Perner, J. (2013). Counterfactual reasoning: From childhood to adulthood. *Journal of Experimental Child Psychology, 114*, 389–404.

Riggs, K. J., Peterson, D. M., Robinson, E. J., & Mitchell, P. (1998). Are errors in false belief tasks symptomatic of a broader difficulty with counterfactuality? *Cognitive Development, 13*, 73–90.

Roese, N. J., & Epstude, K. (2017). The functional theory of counterfactual thinking: New evidence, new challenges, new insights. *Advances in Experimental Social Psychology, 56*, 1–79.

Roese, N. J., Epstude, K., Fessel, F., Morrisson, M., Smallman, R., Summerville, A., . . . Segerstrom, S. (2009). Regret predicts depression but not anxiety: New findings from a nationally representative sample. *Journal of Social and Clinical Psychology, 28*, 671–688.

Roese, N. J., & Hur, T. (1997). Affective determinants in counterfactual thinking. *Social Cognition, 15*, 274–290.

Roese, N. J., Hur, T., & Pennington, G. L. (1999). Counterfactual thinking and regulatory focus: Implications for action versus inaction and sufficiency versus necessity. *Journal of Personality and Social Psychology, 77*, 1109–1120.

Roese, N. J., & Summerville, A. (2005). What we regret most . . . and why. *Personality and Social Psychology Bulletin, 31*, 1273–1285.

Sanna, L. J. (1996). Defensive pessimism, optimism, and stimulating alternatives: Some ups and downs of prefactual and counterfactual thinking. *Journal of Personality and Social Psychology, 71*, 1020–1036.

Santamaria, C., Espino, O., & Byrne, R. M. J. (2005). Counterfactual and semifactual conditionals prime alternative possibilities. *Journal of Experimental Psychology: Learning, Memory, and Cognition, 31*, 1149–1154.

Scholl, A., & Sassenberg, K. (2014). Where could we stand if I had . . . ?: How social power impacts counterfactual thinking after failure. *Journal of Experimental Social Psychology, 53*, 51–61.

Scholl, A., & Sassenberg, K. (2015). Better know when (not) to think twice: How social power impacts prefactual thought. *Personality and Social Psychology Bulletin, 41,* 159–170.

Sherman, S. J., & McConnell, A. R. (1995). Dysfunctional implications of counterfactual thinking: When alternatives to reality fail us. In N. J. Roese & J. M. Olson (Eds.), *What might have been: The social psychology of counterfactual thinking* (pp. 199–231). Mahwah, NJ: Erlbaum.

Smallman, R. (2013). It's what's inside that counts: The role of counterfactual content in intention formation. *Journal of Experimental Social Psychology, 49,* 842–851.

Smallman, R., & McCulloch, K. C. (2012). Learning from yesterday's mistakes to fix tomorrow's problems: When functional counterfactual thinking and psychological distance collide. *European Journal of Social Psychology, 42,* 383–390.

Smallman, R., & Roese, N. J. (2009). Counterfactual thinking facilitates behavioral intentions. *Journal of Experimental Social Psychology, 45,* 845–852.

Spellman, B. A., & Kincannon, A. (2001). The relation between counterfactual ("but for") and causal reasoning: Experimental findings and implications for jurors' decisions. *Law and Contemporary Problems, 64,* 241–264.

Spellman, B. A., & Mandel, D. R. (1999). When possibility informs reality: Counterfactual thinking as a cue to causality. *Current Directions in Psychological Science, 8,* 120–123.

Swann, W. B., Jr. (1984). The quest for accuracy in person perception: A matter of pragmatics. *Psychological Review, 91,* 457–477.

Sweeny, K., & Vohs, K. D. (2012). On near misses and completed tasks: The nature of relief. *Psychological. Science, 23,* 464–468.

Webb, T. L., & Sheeran, P. (2006). Does changing behavioral intentions engender behavior change?: A meta-analysis of the experimental evidence. *Psychological Bulletin, 132,* 249–268.

Wells, G. L., & Gavanski, I. (1989). Mental simulation of causality. *Journal of Personality and Social Psychology, 56,* 161–169.

Wimmer, H., & Perner, J. (1983). Beliefs about beliefs: Representation and constraining function of wrong beliefs in young children's understanding of deception. *Cognition, 13,* 103–128.

Zeelenberg, M., van Dijk, W. W., Van der Pligt, J., Manstead, A. S., Van Empelen, P., & Reinderman, D. (1998). Emotional reactions to the outcomes of decisions: The role of counterfactual thought in the experience of regret and disappointment. *Organizational Behavior and Human Decision Processes, 75,* 117–141.

Zeigarnik, B. (1927). On finished and unfinished tasks. In W. D. Ellis (Ed.), *A source book of Gestalt psychology* (pp. 300–314). New York: Harcourt Brace.

CHAPTER 7

Fantasy about the Future as Friend and Foe

Gabriele Oettingen
A. Timur Sevincer

"I wish that my SAT scores would finally arrive. My score will definitely be over 1200; I will be in the 80th percentile! I'll get into all my favorite colleges. My parents and I will tour schools, and in the fall my best friend and I will enroll in our favorite one together. Finally, I'll start living my own life, separate from my parents, in college—a dream comes true!"

What will happen to our prospective college student when the actual scores become available online? Will they match up with his expectations? How will he feel, what will he tell his friends, and what will he tell his family? Did the positive thinking help him study hard for the test? Will they help him enjoy the feeling of accomplishment if his scores are high, and attenuate the negative feelings if his scores are low? Or will the opposite happen—did his positive fantasies about the future hamper his efforts to study? And will they detract from his joy in the case of good news and heighten the negative feelings if the news is dire?

In the present chapter, we attempt to answer these questions for our hypothetical student, investigating the role of positive future fantasies in situations in which we need only to wait (e.g., for our SAT scores), as well as in situations in which we must take action to achieve our goals. As pleasant as they feel in the moment, positive fantasies can be a substantial handicap when it comes to realizing these fantasies in actuality. Such flights of fancy bring up feelings of accomplishment that mimic the real thing, in turn prompting feelings of relaxation and sapping the energy needed to achieve the fantasies in the first place. Why, then, are humans so prone to fantasizing about the future, if doing so in fact reduces the chances of achieving our fantasies, as well as harming our future well-being? In an attempt to answer this question, we must look at the roots of positive fantasies. Our dreams about the future stem largely from our needs—whether physiological or psychological.

Turning to Fantasy Realization Theory, we then describe a self-regulation strategy and its underlying mechanisms and processes, which, when put into practice, has been found to counterbalance the energy-sucking effect of positive fantasies and translate them into action. The primary facet of this strategy is called *mental contrasting*, which juxtaposes future fantasies with thoughts about the real, current obstacles in their way, in such a fashion that highlights the direction in which to act and at the same time energizes people to take the steps needed to fulfill their fantasies. The technique of mental contrasting has been found to affect behavior change in various life domains (e.g., achievement, health, interpersonal relations). We discuss the theoretical basis for and research behind mental contrasting, as well as the nonconscious mechanisms mediating its effects. A large body of research has accumulated showing that mental contrasting, with and without the supplemental strategy of if–then plans (also known as implementation intentions) has substantial short-term and long-term effects, helping people gain insight into their lives and constructively shape their long-term development without outside guidance from coaches and counselors, drawing only from what is within themselves.

POSITIVE FANTASIES ABOUT THE FUTURE

Positive fantasies about the future are defined as thoughts and images arising in the mind's eye depicting desired future events (Oettingen & Mayer, 2002; Oettingen, 2012). They are different from beliefs and expectations, as clearly articulated by William James (1890/1950): "Everyone knows the difference between imagining a thing and believing in its existence, between supposing a proposition and acquiescing in its truth" (p. 283). James's distinction between believing and imagining pertained to events of the past or the present. Following his reasoning, Oettingen and Mayer (2002) have differentiated between two kinds of thinking about the future: beliefs (expectancy judgments) that assess the likelihood of an event's occurrence and images (fantasies) that portray future events themselves as they appear in the mind. Positive expectancy judgments are beliefs that a desired event is likely to occur or an undesired event will not occur. Positive fantasies about the future, in contrast, are mental images of desired future events occurring or of undesired events not occurring. Positive fantasies differ from what Lewin (1926) and Mahler (1933) called *Zauberdenken* (i.e., thoughts depicting actions and events that violate known natural laws). Under this distinction, a positive future fantasy would not include the ability to fly or have other supernatural powers, for example. They are ultimately grounded in what is generally possible and, instead, more closely resemble what Klinger (1971, 1978) named "daydreams," that is, thoughts pertaining to immediate or longer range desires, including activities instrumental to attaining that desired future (Oettingen & Mayer, 2002).

The first type of future-oriented thinking, beliefs in the form of expectations or judgments of future probability, can be further separated into several different categories: self-efficacy expectations (beliefs or judgments that one will be able to perform a certain behavior leading to a desired outcome; Bandura 1977), outcome expectations (that a certain behavior will lead to the desired outcome; Bandura, 1977), general expectations (that a certain outcome will be achieved; Oettingen &

Mayer, 2002), and generalized optimism (the belief that one's own future will be positive; Scheier & Carver; 1985; Carver & Scheier, Chapter 11, this volume). Each kind of positive expectation about the future has been found to predict high effort and success in attaining future goals across a wide variety of life domains (e.g., Maddux & Kleiman, Chapter 9, this volume; Schunk & DiBenedetto, Chapter 8, this volume). Positive expectations have also been linked to greater well-being (Carver & Scheier, Chapter 11, this volume). The reason for this predictive relationship is that people calculate their expectations about the future based greatly on their past experiences. A student who has passed a difficult exam, for example, is likely to expect that she or he can pass similar exams in the future as well.

In contrast to positive expectations, the second type of future-oriented thinking, fantasies, are detached from an individual's past experiences (Oettingen & Mayer, 2002). An aspiring musician may, for example, vividly dream about giving an excellent performance in front of a packed audience despite never having done so before.

Positive fantasies about the future also differ from goals and plans, which involve a commitment or intention to act or behave in a way that moves one toward attainment of one's desired future state (Gollwitzer, 1999; Ajzen & Fishbein, 1969; Klinger, 1975; Locke, Shaw, Saari, & Latham, 1981). For goals and plans to emerge, people must judge an envisioned future to be attainable or avoidable (Atkinson, 1957; Gollwitzer, 1990; Kruglanski et al., 2015). The formation of goals and plans greatly fosters effort, increasing the likelihood of successfully attaining those goals (Gollwitzer, 1999; A. Kappes & Oettingen, 2014), benefiting people's well-being (Emmons, 1996). In contrast, positive fantasies do not involve a commitment or intention to act or behave in a certain way. They also do not necessarily require a judgment that the imagined future is attainable.

Thus defined, positive future fantasies resemble other terms in other chapters of this volume and elsewhere, including episodic future thinking (Atance, Chapter 4, this volume), mental simulations of future events (Szpunar & Schacter, Chapter 3, this volume; Taylor, Pham, Rivkin, & Armor, 1998), mind-wandering into the future (task-unrelated thoughts; Smallwood & Schooler, 2006), and prospection (Gilbert & Wilson, 2007), in that they all describe vivid, detailed depictions of personally relevant future events in one's conscious stream of thought. Positive future fantasies differ from these concepts, however, in that they exclusively depict the future in a positive and idealized way.

Positive Future Fantasies and Emotion

Waiting for Good News: Happy Now, Disappointed Later

When required to wait for an important unknown outcome, positive thoughts and images make people feel worse in the case of unfortunate news and less happy if the news is good. Indeed, in a recent study, law students who displayed more positive emotions and foresaw a better outcome while awaiting their results on the bar exam experienced greater denial and were more devastated when they later found out they had failed. They were also less happy when they received good news. If the news was bad, the students were also less ready to remedy their low scores—another way positive fantasies can be harmful (Sweeny, Reynolds, Falkenstein, Andrews, & Dooley,

2016). In a study of elderly adults, those who envisioned their future selves as more happy than their present selves similarly reported being less happy when assessed later on, potentially because they did not consider the inevitable uncomfortable realities of aging and were thus unprepared and consequently more disappointed when they hit (Cheng, Fung, & Chan, 2009). Another study of elderly adults likewise found a predictive relationship between foreseeing future happiness and worse health and lowered longevity in the future (Lang, Weiss, Gerstorf, & Wagner, 2013).

Even when positive fantasies reference a future that does not affect one's own life and are not influenced by one's actions, they still predict more disappointment later on. In a study of soccer fans, for instance, when participants positively fantasized about their favorite team winning the next game, they were more disappointed when the team lost than fans who entertained thoughts of a possible defeat. When participants' favorite team won, those fans who had positively fantasized and those who allowed for negative fantasies showed no difference in their levels of happiness or relief (Wagner, Sevincer, & Oettingen, 2017).

It therefore makes sense that, when required to wait for an important but unknown outcome (e.g., awaiting the answer to a job interview), people consciously desire to cultivate ambivalence (having both positive and negative thoughts and feelings toward the same event or outcome). Strategically generating ambivalence over future outcomes rather than swinging into sheerly positive or sheerly negative thoughts is a way to protect ourselves from suffering ill emotions in case of failure (Reich & Wheeler, 2016). Ambivalence as a strategic protection is particularly pronounced when uncertainty is high. In the case of the law students in the study by Sweeny and colleagues (2016), attenuating purely positive thoughts about the future and increasing thoughts of ambivalence, though uncomfortable in the moment, may have resulted in less painful emotions when the hoped-for future failed to materialize.

Why do positive fantasies about the future predict high disappointment and little remedial action when the eventual outcome is revealed to be negative? Primarily because such exclusively positive thoughts and images lull us into a false sense of security. We mentally experience the future success, even if not yet achieved, much the same way as the success itself. But while doing so eases the agony of the uncertain present and relieves us of having to contemplate potential defeat, when defeat then occurs, people may be even more devastated and respond with disbelief and denial instead of taking the necessary steps to remedy the situation. This assessment is backed up by previous research showing that people often brace themselves to prevent from being taken aback by unforeseen failure (Sweeny, Carroll, & Shepperd, 2006; Shepperd, Falkenstein, & Sweeny, Chapter 12, this volume). The pain associated with waiting pays off once the news arrives, whether negative or positive, either through lowering disappointment or heightening relief, respectively.

Waiting for Better Times: Pleasure Now, Depression Later

Positive fantasies about the future not only result in negative emotions in the moment when the outcome is eventually revealed but also predict harm in overall mental health. In recent studies, the more positive people's fantasies were, the less depressed they were in that moment, but the more depressed they became over time (Oettingen, Mayer, & Portnow, 2016). These predictive relations, which held for up to 7 months, have been found in adults and in children, measured both through semiprojective methods, in which researchers prompt study participants to imagine the future after being given the first lines of a scene, and through diary methods, in which participants must pause throughout the day when beeped and record their spontaneous thoughts and images of the future and their valence. The results also suggest that positive fantasies about the future relate to low mental health by predicting lower effort and, therefore, lower success, which in turn predicted greater depressive affect.

So far, we have focused on consequences of positive fantasies about the future, both emotional and behavioral, in situations in which people had to wait for something largely or entirely out of their control such as waiting for results of an exam (after having taken the test), waiting to get older, waiting for the final score of a soccer game, or waiting to hear back from a potential employer after a job interview. It is clear that in such situations that are out of one's control, positive thinking comes at a cost. Although pleasant in the moment, when negative feedback or an undesirable outcome hits, positive fantasies result in heightened negative affect and less engagement in efforts to remedy the situation.

Positive Future Fantasies and Action

Are positive fantasies about the future similarly detrimental when it comes to situations in which one's actions can influence the outcome? The power of positive thinking is a popular topic in the self-help literature, a large body of which asserts that positive thinking alone is predictive of success in any situation (Byrne, 2006; Galvan, 2012). This potent message has permeated society: Wishing, willing, and doing are seen as intrinsically linked, with positive visualization inciting us to action, ultimately solving our concerns and fulfilling our deepest fantasies (Carnegie, 1948/1984).

Despite what popular culture tells us, a multitude of studies shows that positive thinking alone is detrimental in terms of what action we take (or do not take), as well as how we cope with negative feedback. In a study of women enrolled in a weight-reduction program, for example, Oettingen and Wadden (1991) found that the more positive the participants' fantasies of success were, the less weight they lost when assessed 3 months and 1 year later. In fact, participants with the most highly positive fantasies—those who pictured themselves looking ideally slim and beautiful, or who dreamed about easily resisting temptation—lost 24 pounds less than those who also allowed negative images to surface. The researchers used a semiprojective method to measure the level of positivity of the women's fantasies, asking participants to complete short stories that could turn out either negatively or positively. After filling in the story with their projections about the future, participants then estimated how positive or negative their projections made them feel. Importantly, participants' positive expectations of weight loss based on past dieting experience predicted more success in losing weight, speaking to the distinction between positive fantasies and expectations and their different relationships with the future. Other studies of health have produced similar results, such as one finding that the more positively hip replacement surgery patients fantasized about a swift recovery, the less well they were able to move their new joints, the fewer stairs they could walk, and the less well their general recoveries went as judged by the physical therapists (Oettingen & Mayer, 2002).

Findings about the deleterious predictive relation of positive fantasies and health outcomes extend to the realm of academics. In one study, the more positively college students fantasized about getting a good grade on an exam, as measured via a semiprojective method, the worse they actually performed (Oettingen & Mayer, 2002). It's not just college students, either. In another set of studies, participants included a group of ethnically diverse, economically disadvantaged women enrolled in a business skills program at a vocational school in New York City, displayed similar patterns of behavior (H. B. Kappes, Oettingen, & Mayer, 2012). Expectations of success and achievement fantasies were assessed via an adapted version of the semiprojective method used in the earlier study of college students (Oettingen & Mayer, 2002). Participants were provided with the beginning lines of four scenarios and asked to imagine themselves in these situations. One scenario, for instance, read: "You took your first test as a Business Skills Program student, and your teacher graded them last night. Now you're sitting in class, the teacher walks in and starts to hand the tests back. She puts your test in front of you . . . " Participants wrote down all the thoughts and images that sprang to mind and answered questions gaging the general positivity of their responses. Fantasies and expectations predicted grade-point average (GPA) and attendance, albeit in opposite directions. That is, positive fantasies predicted a lower GPA and more days absent, whereas positive expectations predicted a higher GPA and fewer days absent. Attendance significantly mediated GPA, such that women who missed more days of class also received a worse GPA. Two further studies teased apart these results, involving similar samples of students enrolled in vocational education programs. In these studies, students' expectations were "empty"—that is, students had just entered the program and had no experience on which to base their expectations about how well they might do. Unlike in the first study, expectations predicted performance only when participants were able to look back at relevant past performance. Positive fantasies, free thoughts and images independent of one's past experiences, in contrast, were a predictor of low effort and success across all three studies.

Unsurprisingly, the effects of positive fantasies in health and academic contexts also seem to apply to interpersonal relationships. In a study involving students with crushes on another student, Oettingen and Mayer (2002) found that the more positively students fantasized about getting together with the person of their desire, the less likely they were to actually start a romantic relationship with that person. In the professional sphere, university graduates who fantasized about an easy transition into work life earned less money and received fewer job offers 2 years later. Tellingly, the more positive their fantasies, the fewer job applications they had sent out, suggesting that positive future fantasies lead to low success via reduced effort.

Perhaps most interestingly, the observed effects of positive future fantasies appear to play out not just in individuals, but also on a societal level. A content analysis study revealed that high concentrations of positive fantasies about the future contained in presidential addresses and newspaper articles strongly predicted later economic downturn, as indicated by decreases in the gross domestic product, employment rate, and the Dow Jones Industrial Average (Sevincer, Wagner, Kalvelage, & Oettingen, 2014).

Mechanisms

How could this be? Why are positive fantasies detrimental to future actions and outcomes, despite being so pleasant and comforting in the moment? Reframing the question may reveal the answer. That is, are positive fantasies a barrier to action precisely because they are so pleasant and comforting? Indeed, this appears to be the case: Positively fantasizing about a desired future may make people feel accomplished temporarily, the fantasy coming replete with all the emotional, cognitive, and behavioral consequences of achievement in one's mind. The premature experience of success diminishes the drive to translate fantasy into reality through action.

MENTAL ATTAINMENT

The energy-sapping effects of positive future fantasies are not necessarily always a problem. In two experiments (Sciarappo, Norton, Oettingen, & Gollwitzer, 2015), college students were instructed to fantasize positively about a hypothetical scenario: being rewarded with a large sum of money. In the two control groups, participants either did not receive any fantasy inductions or were instructed to question whether receiving the money would in fact be so pleasurable after all. Afterward, the students had to choose between receiving a small sum of money right away versus a larger sum later on. Students in the positive fantasy group volunteered to wait for the larger sum more happily than students in both control groups. The results suggest that positive fantasies made students more patient and able to wait for their wished-for future. This is likely because they had already attained their wish, if only in their minds, and thus acted as if they had already received a large sum of money. Indeed, this appeared to be the case when researchers measured nonconscious affect as an indicator of mental attainment (H. B. Kappes, A. Kappes, & Oettingen, 2015).

RELAXATION

Positive fantasies about the future are relaxing. Unfortunately for daydreamers, however, relaxation is not conducive to fulfilling one's fantasies and aspirations (Brehm & Self, 1989; Oettingen, 2012). In a study attempting to determine whether positive fantasies indeed lower people's energy, researchers induced two groups of women to generate either positive or questioning fantasies about how cool it would be to wear exciting high-heeled shoes (H. B. Kappes & Oettingen, 2011). Participants in the positive fantasy group were subsequently less energized physically, as measured by their systolic blood pressure (SBP; Wright, 1996) than those in the questioning condition. These findings showing direct physiological effects of positive fantasies were bolstered by two further experiments measuring energy subjectively via questionnaires.

CHALLENGE

When wish fulfillment is easy (e.g., people living in a large city choosing to dine at an Italian rather than a French restaurant), it doesn't take much investment of time and energy to fulfill one's fantasies. People can follow their whims, guiding them in the moment (i.e., ideo-motor action; James, 1890/1950). When wishes are complex and harder to realize, however, positive fantasies become a problem due to their energy-sapping effects. In support of this hypothesis, H. B. Kappes, Sharma, and Oettingen (2013) found that positive fantasies did not influence people's charitable behavior when giving was easy (low resources were requested) but did when giving was hard (high resources were requested). When giving was hard, requiring substantial resources, positive fantasies (vs. control thoughts) caused participants to interpret the request as overly demanding, making college students more stingy, whether the donation was one of time, energy, or money. No such response was observed when giving was easy and few resources were requested.

Origins of Positive Future Fantasies

Positive expectations are based on people's past experiences (Bandura, 1977; Oettingen & Mayer, 2002; H. B. Kappes, Oettingen, & Mayer, 2012). Where do positive fantasies come from then? H. B. Kappes, Schwörer, and Oettingen (2012) reasoned that the function of positive fantasies is to fulfill deficient states when these deficiencies cannot be easily reached or remedied. That fantasy in general stems from a state of deficiency or deprivation, which triggers behavior to remedy the deprivation, has long been established (Hull, 1943; McClelland, 1985). Thus one might argue that one function of positive future fantasies is to end a state of deprivation by satisfying a need. If positive fantasies are about fulfilling needs, then instilling a state of deficiency, and along with it the concordant need to fill that deficiency, should induce positive fantasies revolving around filling the deficiency and eliminating the need.

Under that premise, H. B. Kappes, Schwörer, and Oettingen (2012) set out to test the idea that positive future fantasy arises out of deficiency or need. The researchers induced thirst by offering student participants dry salty crackers to eat under the guise of participating in a taste test. Half of the participants were kept thirsty; the other half were allowed to satisfy their need by drinking water. All participants were then asked to fantasize about the ending of a relevant scenario about drinking water, as well as about the ending of an irrelevant control scenario about giving advice to a friend. Semiprojective measures were used. Results showed that in the thirst condition versus the no-thirst condition, in which participants had access to plenty of water, participants fantasized more positively about quenching their thirst in their responses to the relevant scenario. In the irrelevant scenario, the positivity of the fantasies did not differ between conditions.

This pattern has also been found for psychological needs, including the desire for meaning in life, relatedness, and power. People with a stronger need generated more positive fantasies about the future in response to relevant scenarios than participants with weakly felt needs, regardless of what need was assessed. Content analyses of participants' responses also supported Oettingen and Mayer's (2002) contention that the self-reported positivity of generated fantasies closely relates to the degree to which people idealize the content of those fantasies (H. B. Kappes, Schwörer, & Oettingen, 2012).

Positive fantasies thus appear to keep people "in the field" (Lewin, 1926) when a need cannot be satisfied at the present moment. This supposition was further supported by Oettingen and Mayer (2002), who found that students who indulged in positive fantasies about getting together with their "crush" were more likely to passively wait until the crush discovered them rather than actively approach the adored persons; that way, they silently nourished their positive fantasies instead of getting involved and risking a definite, potentially negative answer in which their love is not reciprocated. Positive fantasies are seductive. But like temptresses of myth, they sap the hero's energy and waylay him on the path to his desire.

Positive Future Fantasies: Summary

The difference in the effects of positive thinking about the future in terms of positive expectations versus positive fantasies can be illustrated by their different origins: Whereas expectations are based on a person's performance history, the roots of fantasies lie in a person's needs, stemming from states of deficiency. Although such fantasies can ward off depressive symptoms in the short term, sustained over time they can lead to low energy and effort, rendering them a risk factor for depression in the long term, as people withdraw from the world and retreat entirely into fantasy. This state of cycling into extended fantasy and depression is not inevitable or irreversible, however. Positive fantasies can even become a protective factor against depression in the long run, when supplemented with a healthy dose of reality.

MENTAL CONTRASTING OF POSITIVE FUTURE FANTASIES

Mental Contrasting: Principle

Ironically, positive fantasies sap the energy needed to fulfill them. But fantasies aren't entirely worthless: They give us something to strive for and provide direction for our actions. We wanted to find a strategy that allows people to harness their fantasies and that, instead of sapping their willpower, fosters the energy needed to bring those fantasies to life. Fantasy Realization Theory (FRT; Oettingen, 1997, 2000, 2012) proposes mental contrasting as such a strategy. Mental contrasting triggers active goal pursuit by juxtaposing positive future fantasies with potential obstacles of present reality. When positive fantasies are mentally contrasted with current obstacles in this way, instead of producing feelings of relaxation, they trigger the energy needed to overcome the identified obstacles standing in the way of the desired future, increasing their likelihood of attainment. When an obstacle can potentially be overcome, people become energized and put in the effort needed to fulfill their wishes. When an obstacle cannot be overcome, people have different options: They can attenuate their wish, delegate actions to others or to a more opportune time, or let go of the fantasy and refocus their efforts elsewhere. All of these options help people to invest their energy in more promising endeavors in light of insurmountable odds.

Mental contrasting involves three steps: (1) defining an important wish; (2) engaging in the fantasy by specifying and imagining the best possible outcome, and (3) identifying a central inner obstacle standing in the way of that outcome and imagining that obstacle. For example, a person might identify a wish to jog vigorously 7 days a week. After completing that first step of wish identification, second she would imagine herself fulfilling that scenario and the great feelings of fitness that come with it. Third, she would identify and imagine her tiredness after work as her own personal obstacle. If she perceives her after-work tiredness as surmountable, she will stick to the exercise schedule she set for herself; if she perceives it as insurmountable, she can modify her wish (e.g., "exercise over the weekend when I am less tired"), tackle it at a later time (e.g., "when I have finished my paper"), or let go of that particular wish and redirect her efforts (e.g., switching to yoga at home). She can also attempt to circumvent the obstacle entirely by preventing it from occurring (e.g., "I will refrain from watching shows at night to get to bed in time"). Mental contrasting thus supports individuals in prioritizing their pursuits, helping them pursue wishes that are desirable and feasible and tackle the obstacles in their way, and adjust or let go of those wishes that are less desirable, have too many costs, or are simply unrealizable.

Three Further Modes of Thought

Despite its utility, the vast majority of people do not use mental contrasting as their predominant mode of thought in daily life (Sevincer & Oettingen, 2013). FRT describes three other, less desirable modes of thought: reverse contrasting, indulging in future fantasies, and dwelling on present obstacles. Reverse contrasting, as the name implies, means the opposite of mental contrasting; that is, imagining reality and its attendant obstacles first, then fantasizing about the desired future. Switching the order of imagined scenarios fails to anchor positive fantasies with the subsequent images of reality and prevents people from accurately recognizing the obstacles in the way of their dreams. This mode of thought, therefore, does not lead to behavior change, even though the content is the same as in mental constrasting. Indulging in fantasies and dwelling on obstacles also predictably do not lead to behavior change, as indulging ignores the obstacles that energize the person, whereas dwelling ignores the positive fantasies that provide the direction to act.

Mental Contrasting and Behavior Change

Achievement, Health, and Interpersonal Relations

Studies have shown that mental contrasting fosters behavior change across life domains, including academic and professional achievement, health, interpersonal relationships, and physical and mental well-being. Mental contrasting has been used as a highly effective strategy enabling students to learn a foreign language (Oettingen, Hönig, & Gollwitzer, 2000; A. Gollwitzer, Oettingen, Kirby, Duckworth, & Mayer, 2011), to improve in math (Oettingen et al., 2001), to study abroad (Oettingen et al., 2001), and to enroll in vocational training (Oettingen, Mayer, Thorpe, Janetzke, & Lorenz, 2005). Mental contrasting also heightened the odds of finding integrative (win–win) solutions (Kirk, Oettingen, & Gollwitzer, 2011), and successful decision making in everyday life (Oettingen, Mayer, & Brinkmann, 2010). In the domain of health, mental contrasting has helped students take steps toward reducing or stopping smoking (Oettingen, Mayer, & Thorpe, 2010), increased physical exercise in overweight men of low socioeconomic status (SES; Sheeran, Harris, Vaughan, Oettingen, & Gollwitzer, 2013), and helped patients with Type 2 diabetes cope with daily life (Adriaanse, de Ridder, & Voorneman, 2013). In the social realm, mental contrasting has been found to foster interpersonal relations and lead to effective conciliation (Oettingen et al., 2001; Schrage, Schwörer, & Oettingen, 2017). It facilitated getting to know an attractive stranger, heightened tolerance, and taking responsibility for members of an outgroup (Oettingen et al., 2005). In addition, it promoted help seeking in college students and help giving in emergency care nurses (Oettingen, Stephens, Mayer, & Brinkmann, 2010).

Mechanisms

Mental contrasting is a conscious imagery strategy that affects nonconscious cognitive processes, motivation, and responses to feedback. By instigating these processes, mental contrasting fosters behavior change outside of conscious awareness, sidestepping the difficult task of conscious self-regulation.

NONCONSCIOUS COGNITION

The success of mental contrasting is undergirded by three cognitive processes taking place outside of awareness, which in turn predict its behavioral effects. First, mental contrasting induces people to interpret reality as an obstacle when the obstacles are perceived as surmountable. Two studies, using a task-switching paradigm (Kiesel et al., 2010), showed that mental contrasting led participants to nonconsciously recategorize their self-generated words of present reality as obstacles, an effect not seen in other thought modes such as reverse contrasting. This recategorization of reality words as obstacles predicted heightened effort and success in participants' attainment of their desires. In a third study, the authors found that mental contrasting of feasible wishes facilitates the discovery of other relevant obstacles on the way (A. Kappes, Wendt, Reinelt, & Oettingen, 2013).

At the same time, mental contrasting strengthens the associative links between the desired future and reality and the obstacles therein, an effect that again manifests in behavior. A. Kappes and Oettingen (2014) asked students to give a video presentation describing the professional and personal attributes they believed made them successful job candidates and were told that human resource experts would later judge the quality of their presentations. Before the students started to present, the researchers instructed them to either mental contrast, reverse contrast, or think about irrelevant content, and then measured their nonconscious associative links via a primed lexical decision task (Neely, 1977). More than the participants in the control groups, those in the mental contrasting condition evinced strong future-reality associative links when they saw their obstacles as surmountable and weak links when they saw their obstacles as insurmountable. Importantly, the strength of these nonconscious associative links predicted the quality of participants' performances in their presentations.

In another study, A. Kappes and Oettingen (2014) induced in participants a wish to excel on an upcoming creativity test, after which half received positive feedback and the other half received negative feedback. All participants engaged in mental contrasting. In participants who received positive feedback, mental contrasting lost its energizing power, and the participants no longer showed the strong implicit associative links because the wish had been fulfilled. The results are in line with past studies showing that when people are under the impression that they have achieved their desires, they stop striving (Masicampo & Baumeister, 2011; McCulloch, Fitzsimons, Chua, & Albarracin, 2011).

Finally, mental contrasting strengthens the associative link between one's obstacle and the behavior instrumental to overcoming that obstacle. This linkage between the obstacle and the behavior related to overcoming it predicted increased fantasy-directed action. A. Kappes, Singmann, and Oettingen (2012) showed that, when obstacles were seen as surmountable, mental contrasting facilitated a strong associative link between obstacle and action. When obstacles were seen as insurmountable, mental contrasting weakened the associative link. The mental link between obstacle and action induced by mental contrasting manifested behaviorally in action and successful performance—in this particular study, by participants' choosing to use stairs instead of the elevator to fulfill their wish of becoming fitter.

NONCONSCIOUS ENERGY

Alone, positive future fantasies engender relaxation and low energy (H. B. Kappes & Oettingen, 2011). After employing mental contrasting, the level of subsequent energization depends on the obstacle and whether it is surmountable or not; that is, whether expectations of success are high or low (Oettingen et al., 2009). Energization level, as measured by SBP (Wright, 1996) and by subjective reports of energy, mediated the effects of mental contrasting on efforts for wish fulfillment. A series of other experimental studies measuring SBP supported the described pattern of results (Sevincer, Busatta, & Oettingen, 2014; Sevincer & Oettingen, 2015).

COPING WITH SETBACKS

Dealing with setbacks in a way that fosters resilience is pivotal to leading a happy and constructive life (Nussbaum & Dweck, 2008; Dweck & Yeager, Chapter 18, this volume). However, people often interpret setbacks as failure and resist processing the important information contained in negative feedback. Mental contrasting helps people to constructively deal with setbacks in two ways: It fosters the processing of information contained in setbacks, and it protects against a loss of subjective competence.

When university students participating in a study saw obstacles as surmountable (high expectations of success), students who engaged in mental contrasting readily processed the valuable information inherent in negative feedback after encountering a setback and used the information learned to calibrate and reform plans to help them reach their desire (A. Kappes, Oettingen, & Pak, 2012). Students' subjective sense of competence was also sustained. In contrast, when students viewed obstacles as insurmountable, they distanced themselves from negative feedback, and their sense of competence diminished, freeing them up to engage in more promising endeavors. No such effects were observed in the control groups of students who engaged in other relevant modes of thinking about the future, such as indulging in fantasies and dwelling on obstacles. Positive feedback was not found to have any effect across conditions, on either information processing or subjective confidence level.

Mental Contrasting of Negative Future Fantasies

So far, we have almost exclusively dealt with positive fantasies about the future, reporting studies showing that mentally contrasting positive future fantasies with potential obstacles of present reality helps promote effort and success in a variety of life domains. Frequently, however, people also harbor negative fantasies about futures they fear. Sometimes these fears may be justified, whereas other fears may be unjustified. Studies have shown that mental contrasting can be applied to affect behavior change also in the case of such negative fantasies, helping people overcome both justified and unjustified fears. In a study of people whose fears were justified—in this case, regular smokers afraid of dying from lung cancer—mentally contrasting negative visions of the future with positive aspects of reality helped them confront that fear and resulted in more immediate efforts to stop smoking (Oettingen, Mayer, & Thorpe, 2010). In a study of people with the unjustified fear of losing job opportunities to immigrants, mentally contrasting enabled them to lose that fear, leading to more tolerance and willingness to integrate with immigrants (Oettingen et al., 2005).

Spontaneous Mental Contrasting

To measure whether people spontaneously use mental contrasting when thinking about the future, Sevincer and Oettingen (2013) asked participants to freely think about an important personal wish and to write down their thoughts and images. Using content analysis, participants who wrote about the desired future followed by the present reality were classified as mentally contrasting, those who wrote about the future only as indulging, those who wrote about the present reality only as dwelling, and those who wrote about the reality followed by the future as reverse contrasting. Just as participants who were instructed to mentally contrast, those who engaged in mental contrasting spontaneously scored higher on selective goal pursuit as measured by self-reported commitment and observed performance. In line with prior research showing that people tend to think positively about the future (Shepperd, Falkenstein, & Sweeny, Chapter 12, this volume), indulging in fantasies was the predominant mode of thought, and only a minority of participants (10–20%) used mental contrasting spontaneously.

The variation in spontaneous thought mode depends on a combination of situational and person variables. Situational variables include cognitive fatigue (Muraven & Baumeister, 2000), which, studies have shown, decreases the likelihood of mental contrasting (Sevincer, Schlier, & Oettingen, 2015), potentially because of the tactic's high cognitive demands (Achtziger, Fehr, Oettingen, Gollwitzer, & Rockstroh, 2009). Mood has also been shown to affect the likelihood of spontaneous mental contrasting. H. B. Kappes, Oettingen, Mayer, and Maglio (2011) hypothesized that because sad mood indicates the presence of a problem (Schwarz & Bless, 1991), and because mental contrasting has been found to be an effective problem-solving strategy, participants in a sad (vs. happy and neutral) mood should be more likely to mentally contrast, which was borne out in the study results.

Mental contrasting has been associated with specific person attributes relating to how people think about and consider the future. For example, people who view the future as something that can be changed and improved (those with an incremental vs. entity theory; Dweck, 1999) were more likely to use mental contrasting (and indulging; Sevincer, Kluge, & Oettingen, 2014). In addition, people who are well self-regulated in their academic pursuits and in everyday life in general, as indicated by their high self-reported self-regulation skills, above-average school grades, high need for achievement, and high need for cognition, have been found to be more likely to engage in mental contrasting (Sevincer, Mehl, & Oettingen, in press). Taken together, the findings suggest that people who see the future as malleable and worthwhile and those who are well self-regulated use mental contrasting, which likely has a reciprocal effect, in turn allowing them to attain their goals and master their everyday lives.

Mental Contrasting as an Intervention

The evidence thus far presented has established mental contrasting as a promising intervention that can translate to realizing wishes of any kind. When applied as a metacognitive strategy, that is, one inducing people to think about their own thoughts (Flavell, 1979), mental contrasting (vs. indulging) has been shown to foster effective and easy decision making that experimental participants have brought back to improve their everyday lives. In a study involving middle managers, followed up after being taught the strategy, managers in the mental contrasting group described their daily lives as easier when it came to making their decisions, managing their time, completing some tasks, and delegating or letting go of others (Oettingen, Mayer, & Brinkmann, 2010). In another study, researchers instructed student participants in mental contrasting (vs. indulging, dwelling, or no instructions) before having them play a game (borrowed from behavioral economics) involving negotiating the selling and buying of a car. Participants who engaged in mental contrasting found more win–win solutions as a team and treated their negotiation partners more fairly (Kirk et al., 2011). Other studies involve behavior change in health (e.g., Sheeran et al., 2013; Adriaanse et al., 2013) and education (e.g., A. Gollwitzer et al., 2011; see Oettingen, 2012, 2014, for summaries).

Most of the intervention research discussed thus far has involved mental contrasting of a variety of wishes, those possible to fulfill and those that involved insurmountable obstacles. By mental contrasting, people figured out which wishes were desirable and feasible and thus which to pursue and which ones to let go. Sometimes, however, there are few opportunities for wish fulfillment but also no alternative options. For example, a person might be asked to change his or her health habits for medical reasons, a schoolchild needs to learn basic math, or a family member needs to take care of his or her relative. In such cases, in which disengagement is not possible or advisable, the only option is to forge ahead with the task. Intervention strategies should aim to teach people to find a wish that is feasible and an obstacle that is surmountable, fostering pursuit of rather than letting go of their desired futures. Thus the first step in teaching people to mentally contrast in the real world is to select those wishes that are feasible, but still challenging.

Establishing High Expectations of Success

High expectations of success are found in feasible wishes and surmountable obstacles. Because expectations of success are grounded in past performance, they should be easily movable in domains in which people do not have much prior experience (Bandura, 1977; H. B. Kappes, Oettingen, & Mayer, 2012). In two experiments, Oettingen, Marquardt, and Gollwitzer (2012) told students that their creative potential was either high or moderate prior to the participants' taking a creativity test that they had been primed to want to do well on. After they were told their (bogus) potential but before taking the test, students were randomly assigned to a mental contrasting, indulging, or dwelling group. Students in the mental contrasting group who were told that they had high creative potential and thus had high expectations of success performed more creatively on the test compared with students told they had moderate potential. Students in the mental contrasting condition also scored as more creative compared with those in the indulging, dwelling, and content control conditions, irrespective of whether they were told their creative potential was high or moderate.

In a group context, high expectations of success can be instilled if participants are given tasks solvable by all members of the group. A. Gollwitzer et al. (2011) employed this premise with second and third graders at a German elementary school from low-income families to help them learn English. Students were given a list of English words and asked to learn them over the next 2 weeks, when there would be a short quiz with prizes. The children were then taught how to mentally contrast or to merely think positively about excelling in the quiz. Mental contrasting (vs. indulging) led to better performance on the language quiz.

Another strategy for eliciting high expectations of success is instructing people to identify not just any important wish, but an important wish that they can fulfill. That way people will be able to generate only an internal personal obstacle that is controllable. In a study of students who wished to eat more healthily, for instance, students were instructed to mentally contrast an attainable but challenging wish related to dietary changes and a specific obstacle within their control—such as the urge to eat chocolate cake rather than an uncontrollable obstacle such as the presence of cake at a friend's birthday party. In this way mental contrasting cuts through excuses. In this particular study, participants in the mental contrasting group ate fewer calories and exercised more than those in the control groups. The effects of the mental contrasting intervention focusing on diet spontaneously transferred to exercising behavior (Johannessen, Oettingen, & Mayer, 2012).

Mental Contrasting: Summary

In mental contrasting, combining positive future fantasies with images of the obstacles standing in the way of realizing the future triggers nonconscious cognitive and motivational processes, as well as response to negative feedback, which then predicts prioritization and sustained behavior change (see Oettingen, 2012, 2014, for summaries). People rarely engage in mental contrasting spontaneously. Instead, they use other, one-sided modes of thought and especially prefer to indulge in positive fantasies about the future. Mental contrasting interventions have been shown to improve people's time management and to help them deal better and more effectively with chronic illnesses, achieve higher academic and professional success, and increase commitment to romantic relationships.

MENTAL CONTRASTING WITH IMPLEMENTATION INTENTIONS

Sometimes people have obstacles that are surmountable but are particularly hard to deal with (e.g., impulsive behavior, strong emotions, an ingrained habit). Although mental contrasting builds nonconscious associative links between the obstacle and the behavior instrumental to overcoming the obstacle (A. Kappes, Singmann, & Oettingen, 2012), it might be helpful to add a complementary strategy that strengthens this associative link even further.

Implementation intentions, also known as if–then plans, have been found to be such a strategy (Gollwitzer, 1999, 2014; Gollwitzer & Crosby, Chapter 17, this volume), strengthening the association between a specific obstacle and the relevant goal-directed action instrumental to overcoming it. Implementation intentions provide specific instructions to oneself in the form: "If situation X, then I will perform goal-directed behavior Y!" plans.

Research has shown that implementation intentions effectively foster goal pursuit ($d = 0.65$; meta-analysis by Gollwitzer & Sheeran, 2006). However, there are prerequisites for the strategy to be effective. First, people must be firmly committed to the overarching goal (Sheeran, Webb, & Gollwitzer, 2005). The situation in the *if* part of the construction must also describe a situation relevant to goal pursuit (e.g., an obstacle), and the behavior in the *then* part must support goal attainment. Research thus far has examined the effects of implementation intentions, whereby participants received instruction from researchers who guided them to enter relevant content in the *if* parts and *then* parts of their if–then plans (e.g., Gollwitzer, 2014; Gollwitzer & Sheeran, 2006; Armitage, 2004). But the strategy of implementation intentions should be of even greater importance if it could be implemented by participants independently. To do so, people need to be able to identify the content of the *if* part and the *then* part on their own, and they need to satisfy the necessary conditions on their own. That is where mental contrasting comes in. The strategy, as described earlier in this chapter, instigates determined goal commitment and pursuit. It also helps identify the situation for the *if* part (obstacle) of implementation intentions, as well as helping people identify the instrumental action for the *then* part of the plan (behavior necessary to overcome the obstacle) in promoting visualization of the obstacle. Therefore, mental contrasting was combined with implementation intentions into a strategy called MCII (Oettingen, 2012, 2014; Oettingen & Gollwitzer, 2010).

MCII as an Intervention

To test the additive value of combining mental contrasting with implementation intentions, as opposed to using the strategies by themselves, Kirk, Oettingen, and Gollwitzer (2013) conducted an experiment again using a negotiation game borrowed from behavioral economics to measure success. Students taught how to use MCII generated more integrative or win–win solutions than those who used mental contrasting or implementation intentions alone. Students in the MCII condition also demonstrated more perspective taking and cooperation. In other studies testing the strategy in the health domain, MCII enabled students to get rid of bad snacking habits more effectively than mental contrasting or implementation intentions alone. By creating insight into their wishes, outcomes, and obstacles, mental contrasting prepared people to generate valid if–then plans (Adriaanse et al., 2010).

Studies in diverse groups of participants, using a variety of controls, have repeatedly demonstrated the effectiveness of MCII as an intervention that works across a wide array of life domains. In the domain of fitness, participants who employed MCII engaged in regular physical exercise over a period of 4 months (Stadler, Oettingen, & Gollwitzer, 2009), consumed more fruits and vegetables over a period of 2 years (Stadler, Oettingen, & Gollwitzer, 2010), and ate less red meat over 5 weeks (Loy, Wieber, Gollwitzer, & Oettingen, 2016). MCII also helped increase physical exercise and weight reduction in patients who had had strokes over a period of 1 year (Marquardt, Oettingen, Gollwitzer, Sheeran, & Liepert, in press), and increased physical capacity in patients with chronic back pain over 3 months (Christiansen, Oettingen, Dahme, & Klinger, 2010).

In the academic domain, MCII supported medical residents in studying for their exams and helped them manage their time (Saddawi-Konefka et al., 2017). The same effects in time management and performance were observed in working mothers from low-income backgrounds instructed in MCII, who achieved success in attending vocational education (Oettingen, H. B. Kappes, Guttenberg, & Gollwitzer, 2015). Other studies have shown that the strategy increased the quality and quantity of homework as judged by the parents of children at risk for attention-deficit/hyperactivity disorder (ADHD; Gawrilow, Morgenroth, Schultz, Oettingen, & Gollwitzer, 2013) and that it helped high school students solve practice tasks over summer vacation for an upcoming standardized test (Duckworth, Grant, Loew, Oettingen, & Gollwitzer, 2011). Attendance and course grades improved in middle school children from low-income backgrounds instructed in MCII (Duckworth, Kirby, A. Gollwitzer, & Oettingen, 2013). When applied to the domain of interpersonal relationships, MCII increased commitment to the relationship and decreased insecurity-related behaviors (Houssais, Oettingen, & Mayer, 2013) and helped couples talk about sensitive topics (Oettingen & Cachia, 2016).

MCII: Summary and Dissemination

MCII has shown benefits in both children and adults and across SES and culture. Intervention studies have been conducted face-to-face or online showing benefits, irrespective of which modes of delivery were used. Indeed, two recent studies (Kizilcec & Cohen, 2017) found that MCII delivered as an 8-minute online intervention to a total of 17,983 people who had enrolled in massive open online courses (MOOC) increased completion rates by 32 and 15%, respectively. Interestingly, these effects were observed in participants of individualist, but not of collectivist, cultures, and only when the obstacle was related to an everyday obligation, but not to uncontrollable obstacles such as lack of time or practical barriers. In participants from individualist cultures who also generated controllable obstacles (everyday obligation), MCII improved the course completion rate by 78%. These findings highlight the most important takeaways for successful adoption of MCII: that the person must wholeheartedly embrace the wish and that the obstacle to overcome must be surmountable. Fulfilling an individualist wish (course completion) in a collectivist culture may present formidable obstacles and even lead to disengagement from the individualist wish rather than engagement because the chosen obstacle must also be something in one's personal control (see Oettingen, 2014). People can deploy MCII in everyday life in four simple steps, taking just a moment of calm and uninterrupted time. Once learned, it can be applied on one's own, without guidance from others, making it a self-sustainable, practical strategy to help people take control of their lives. MCII has been disseminated under the acronym *WOOP*, which stands for *Wish, Outcome, Obstacle, Plan* (for the dissemination of MCII or WOOP, see *www.woopmylife.org* and the WOOP app).

CONCLUSION

Positive fantasies can be a soothing friend in the moment, but over time and when wish fulfilment is challenging, they can easily turn into a foe by making people feel complacent and sapping the energy needed for fantasy realization. Mentally contrasting positive fantasies with a clear sense of reality can cause the foe to become a friend again, the fantasy revealing the necessary direction for acting toward wish fulfillment, and the anticipated obstacles providing energy instead of sapping it. Returning to our hopeful college student mentioned at the beginning of the chapter, considering his personal, inner obstacles would have balanced out his fantasies and spurred him to action when there was still plenty of opportunity to study and prepare. More preparation would have ensured him the best possible score, with all the beneficial consequences that go along with it, including less disappointment when the results come in.

REFERENCES

Achtziger, A., Fehr, T., Oettingen, G., Gollwitzer, P. M., & Rockstroh, B. (2009). Strategies of intention formation are reflected in continuous MEG activity. *Social Neuroscience, 4,* 11–27.

Adriaanse, M. A., de Ridder, D. T. D., & Voorneman, I. (2013). Improving diabetes self-management by mental contrasting. *Psychology and Health, 28,* 1–12.

Adriaanse, M. A., Oettingen, G., Gollwitzer, P. M., Hennes, E. P., de Ridder, D. T. D., & de Witt, J. B. F. (2010). When planning is not enough: Fighting unhealthy snacking habits by mental contrasting with implementation intentions (MCII). *European Journal of Social Psychology, 40,* 1277–1293.

Ajzen, I., & Fishbein, M. (1969). The prediction of behavioral intentions in a choice situation. *Journal of Experimental Social Psychology, 5,* 400–416.

Armitage, C. J. (2004). Evidence that implementation intentions reduce dietary fat intake: A randomized trial. *Health Psychology, 23,* 319–323.

Atkinson, J. W. (1957). Motivational determinants of risk-taking behavior. *Psychological Review, 64,* 359–372.

Bandura, A. (1977). Self-efficacy: Toward a unifying theory of behavioral change. *Psychological Review, 84,* 191–215.

Brehm, J. W., & Self, E. A. (1989). The intensity of motivation. *Annual Review of Psychology, 40,* 109–131.

Byrne, R. (2006). *The secret.* New York: Atria Book.

Carnegie, D. (1984). *How to stop worrying and start living.* New York: Simon & Schuster. (Original work published 1948)

Cheng, S.-T., Fung, H. H., & Chan, A. C. (2009). Self-perception and psychological well-being: The benefits of foreseeing a worse future. *Psychology and Aging, 24,* 623–633.

Christiansen, S., Oettingen, G., Dahme, B., & Klinger, R. (2010). A short goal-pursuit intervention to improve physical capacity: A randomized clinical trial in chronic back pain patients. *Pain, 149,* 444–452.

Duckworth, A. L., Grant, H., Loew, B., Oettingen, G., & Gollwitzer, P. M. (2011). Self-regulation strategies improve self-discipline in adolescents: Benefits of mental contrasting and implementation intentions. *Educational Psychology, 31,* 17–26.

Duckworth, A. L., Kirby, T. A., Gollwitzer, A., & Oettingen, G. (2013). From fantasy to action: Mental contrasting with implementation intentions (MCII) improves academic performance in children. *Social Psychological and Personality Science, 4,* 745–753.

Dweck, C. S. (1999). *Self-theories: Their role in motivation, personality, and development.* Philadelphia: Psychology Press.

Emmons, R. A. (1996). Striving and feeling: Personal goals and subjective well-being. In J. Bargh & P. M. Gollwitzer (Eds.), *The psychology of action: Linking motivation and cognition to behavior* (pp. 314–337). New York: Guilford Press.

Flavell, J. H. (1979). Metacognition and cognitive monitoring: A new area of cognitive-developmental inquiry. *American Psychologist, 34,* 906–911.

Galvan, V. (2012). *How to think positive: Get out of the hole of negative thinking and find your ultimate potential.* North Charleston, SC: CreateSpace.

Gawrilow, C., Morgenroth, K., Schultz, R., Oettingen, G., & Gollwitzer, P. (2013). Mental contrasting with implementation intentions enhances self-regulation of goal pursuit in schoolchildren at risk for ADHD. *Motivation and Emotion, 37,* 134–145.

Gilbert, D. T., & Wilson, T. D. (2007). Prospection: Experiencing the future. *Science, 317,* 1351–1354.

Gollwitzer, A., Oettingen, G., Kirby, T. A., Duckworth, A. L., & Mayer, D. (2011). Mental contrasting facilitates academic performance in school children. *Motivation and Emotion, 35,* 403–412.

Gollwitzer, P. M. (1990). Action phases and mind-sets. In E. T. Higgins & R. M. Sorrentino (Eds.), *The handbook of motivation and cognition: Foundations of social behavior* (Vol. 2, pp. 53–92). New York: Guilford Press.

Gollwitzer, P. M. (1999). Implementation intentions: Strong effects of simple plans. *American Psychologist, 54,* 493–503.

Gollwitzer, P. M. (2014). Weakness of the will: Is a quick fix possible? *Motivation and Emotion, 38,* 305–322.

Gollwitzer, P. M., & Sheeran, P. (2006). Implementation intentions and goal achievement: A meta-analysis of effects and processes. *Advances in Experimental Social Psychology, 38,* 69–119.

Houssais, S., Oettingen, G., & Mayer, D. (2013). Using mental contrasting with implementation intentions to self-regulate insecurity-based behaviors in relationships. *Motivation and Emotion, 37,* 224–233.

Hull, C. L. (1943). *Principles of behavior: An introduction to behavior theory.* New York: Appleton-Century-Crofts.

James, W. (1950). *Principles of psychology.* New York: Holt. (Original work published 1890)

Johannessen, K. B., Oettingen, G., & Mayer, D. (2012). Mental contrasting of a dieting wish improves self-reported health behaviour. *Psychology and Health, 27,* 43–58.

Kappes, A., & Oettingen, G. (2014). The emergence of goal pursuit: Mental contrasting connects future and reality. *Journal of Experimental Social Psychology, 54,* 25–39.

Kappes, A., Oettingen, G., & Pak, H. (2012). Mental contrasting and the self-regulation of responding to negative feedback. *Personality and Social Psychology Bulletin, 38,* 845–856.

Kappes, A., Singmann, H., & Oettingen, G. (2012). Mental contrasting instigates goal pursuit by linking obstacles of reality to instrumental behavior. *Journal of Experimental Social Psychology, 48,* 811–818.

Kappes, A., Wendt, M., Reinelt, T., & Oettingen, G. (2013). Mental contrasting changes the meaning of reality. *Journal of Experimental Social Psychology, 49,* 797–810.

Kappes, H. B., Kappes, A., & Oettingen, G. (2015). *When attainment is all in your head.* Unpublished manuscript, Department of Psychology, New York University, New York.

Kappes, H. B., & Oettingen, G. (2011). Positive fantasies about idealized futures sap energy. *Journal of Experimental Social Psychology, 47,* 719–729.

Kappes, H. B., Oettingen, G., & Mayer, D. (2012). Positive fantasies predict low academic achievement in disadvantaged students. *European Journal of Social Psychology, 42,* 53–64.

Kappes, H. B., Oettingen, G., Mayer, D., & Maglio, S. (2011). Sad mood promotes self-initiated mental contrasting of future and reality. *Emotion, 11,* 1206–1222.

Kappes, H. B., Schwörer, B., & Oettingen, G. (2012). Needs instigate positive fantasies of idealized futures. *European Journal of Social Psychology, 42,* 299–307.

Kappes, H. B., Sharma, E., & Oettingen, G. (2013). Positive fantasies dampen charitable giving when many resources are demanded. *Journal of Consumer Psychology, 23,* 128–135.

Kiesel, A., Steinhauser, M., Wendt, M., Falkenstein, M., Jost, K., Philipp, A. M., . . . Koch, I. (2010). Control and compatibility in task switching: A review. *Psychological Bulletin, 136,* 849–847.

Kirk, D., Oettingen, G., & Gollwitzer, P. M. (2011). Mental contrasting promotes integrative bargaining. *International Journal of Conflict Management, 22,* 324–341.

Kirk, D., Oettingen, G., & Gollwitzer, P. M. (2013). Promoting integrative bargaining: Mental contrasting with implementation intentions. *International Journal of Conflict Management, 24,* 148–165.

Kizilcec, R. F., & Cohen, G. L. (2017). Eight-minute self-regulation intervention improves educational attainment at scale in individualist but not collectivist cultures. *Proceedings of the National Academy of Sciences of the USA, 114,* 4348–4353.

Klinger, E. (1971). *Structure and functions of fantasy.* New York: Wiley.

Klinger, E. (1975). Consequences of commitment to and disengagement from incentives. *Psychological Review, 82,* 1–25.

Klinger, E. (1978). Modes of normal conscious flow. In K. S. Pope & J. L. Singer (Eds.), *The stream of consciousness: Scientific investigations into the flow of human experience* (pp. 225–258). New York: Plenum Press.

Kruglanski, A. W., Jasko, K., Chernikova, M., Milyavsky, M., Babush, M., Baldner, C., . . . Pierro, A. (2015). The rocky road from attitudes to behaviors: Charting the goal systemic course of actions. *Psychological Review, 122,* 598–620.

Lang, F. R., Weiss, D., Gerstorf, D., & Wagner, G. G. (2013). Forecasting life satisfaction across adulthood: Benefits of seeing a dark future? *Psychology and Aging, 28,* 249–261.

Lewin, K. (1926). Vorsatz, Wille und Bedürfnis [Intention, will, and need]. *Psychologische Forschung, 7*, 330–385.

Locke, E. A., Shaw, K. N., Saari, L. M., & Latham, G. P. (1981). Goal setting and task performance: 1969–1980. *Psychological Bulletin, 90*, 125–152.

Loy, L. S., Wieber, F., Gollwitzer, P. M., & Oettingen, G. (2016), Supporting sustainable food consumption: Mental contrasting with implementation intentions (MCII) aligns intentions and behavior. *Frontiers in Psychology, 7*, 607.

Mahler, W. (1933). Ersatzhandlungen verschiedenen Realitätsgrades [Compensatory action based on different degrees of reality]. *Psychologische Forschung, 18*, 27–89.

Marquardt, M. K., Oettingen, G., Gollwitzer, P. M., Sheeran, P., & Liepert, J. (in press). Mental contrasting with implementation intentions (MCII) improves physical activity and weight loss among stroke survivors over one year. *Rehabilitation Psychology*.

Masicampo, E. J., & Baumeister, R. F. (2011). Unfulfilled goals interfere with tasks that require executive functions. *Journal of Experimental Social Psychology, 47*, 685–688.

McClelland, D. C. (1985). How motives, skills, and values determine what people do. *American Psychologist, 41*, 812–825.

McCulloch, K. C., Fitzsimons, G. R., Chua, S. N., & Albarracin, D. (2011). Vicarious goal satiation. *Journal of Experimental Social Psychology, 47*, 685–688.

Muraven, M. R., & Baumeister, R. F. (2000). Self-regulation and depletion of limited resources: Does self-control resemble a muscle? *Psychological Bulletin, 126*, 247–259.

Neely, J. H. (1977). Semantic priming and retrieval from lexical memory: Roles of inhibitionless spreading activation and limited-capacity attention. *Journal of Experimental Psychology: General, 106*, 226–254.

Nussbaum, A., & Dweck, C. (2008). Defensiveness versus remediation: Self-theories and modes of self-esteem maintenance. *Personality and Social Psychology Bulletin, 34*, 599–612.

Oettingen, G. (1997). Culture and future thought. *Culture and Psychology, 3*, 353–381.

Oettingen, G. (2000). Expectancy effects on behavior depend on self-regulatory thought. *Social Cognition, 18*, 101–129.

Oettingen, G. (2012). Future thought and behaviour change. *European Review of Social Psychology, 23*, 1–63.

Oettingen, G. (2014). *Rethinking positive thinking: Inside the new science of motivation.* New York: Penguin/Random House.

Oettingen, G., & Cachia, J. Y. (2016). The problems with positive thinking and how to regulate them. In K. D. Vohs & R. F. Baumeister (Eds.), *Handbook of self-regulation: Research, theory, and applications* (3rd ed., pp. 547–570). New York: Guilford Press.

Oettingen, G., & Gollwitzer, P. M. (2010). Strategies of setting and implementing goals: Mental contrasting and implementation intentions. In J. E. Maddux & J. P. Tangney (Eds.), *Social psychological foundations of clinical psychology* (pp. 114–135). New York: Guilford Press.

Oettingen, G., Hönig, G., & Gollwitzer, P. M. (2000). Effective self-regulation of goal attainment. *International Journal of Educational Research, 33*, 705–732.

Oettingen, G., Kappes, H. B., Guttenberg, K. B., & Gollwitzer, P. M. (2015). Self-regulation of time management: Mental contrasting with implementation intentions. *European Journal of Social Psychology, 45*, 218–229.

Oettingen, G., Marquardt, M. K., & Gollwitzer, P. M. (2012). Mental contrasting turns positive feedback on creative potential into successful performance. *Journal of Experimental Social Psychology, 48*, 990–996.

Oettingen, G., & Mayer, D. (2002). The motivating function of thinking about the future: Expectations versus fantasies. *Journal of Personality and Social Psychology, 83*, 1198–1212.

Oettingen, G., Mayer, D., & Brinkmann, B. (2010). Mental contrasting of future and reality:

Managing the demands of everyday life in health care professionals. *Journal of Personnel Psychology, 9*, 138–144.

Oettingen, G., Mayer, D., & Portnow, S. (2016). Pleasure now, pain later: Positive fantasies about the future predict symptoms of depression. *Psychological Science, 27*, 345–353.

Oettingen, G., Mayer, D., Sevincer, A. T., Stephens, E. J., Pak, H., & Hagenah, M. (2009). Mental contrasting and goal commitment: The mediating role of energization. *Personality and Social Psychology Bulletin, 35*, 608–622.

Oettingen, G., Mayer, D., & Thorpe, J. (2010). Self-regulation of commitment to reduce cigarette consumption: Mental contrasting of future with reality. *Psychology and Health, 25*, 961–977.

Oettingen, G., Mayer, D., Thorpe, J. S., Janetzke, H., & Lorenz, S. (2005). Turning fantasies about positive and negative futures into self-improvement goals. *Motivation and Emotion, 29*, 237–267.

Oettingen, G., Pak, H., & Schnetter, K. (2001). Self-regulation of goal-setting: Turning free fantasies about the future into binding goals. *Journal of Personality and Social Psychology, 80*, 736–753.

Oettingen, G., Stephens, E. J., Mayer, D., & Brinkmann, B. (2010). Mental contrasting and the self-regulation of helping relations. *Social Cognition, 28*, 490–508.

Oettingen, G., & Wadden, T. A. (1991). Expectation, fantasy, and weight loss: Is the impact of positive thinking always positive? *Cognitive Therapy and Research, 15*, 167–175.

Reich, T., & Wheeler, S. C. (2016). The good and bad of ambivalence: Desiring ambivalence under outcome uncertainty. *Journal of Personality and Social Psychology, 110*, 493–508.

Saddawi-Konefka, D., Baker, K., Guarino, A., Burns, S. A., Oettingen, G., Gollwitzer, P. M., . . . Charnin, J. E. (2017). Changing resident physician studying behaviors: A randomized comparative effectiveness trial of goal setting versus WOOP. *Journal of Graduate Medical Education, 9*, 451–457.

Scheier, M. F., & Carver, C. S. (1985). Optimism, coping, and health: Assessment and implications of generalized outcome expectancies. *Health Psychology, 4*, 219–247.

Schrage, J., Schwörer, B., & Oettingen, G. (2017). *Mental contrasting and conciliatory behavior in romantic relationships*. Manuscript submitted for publication.

Schwarz, N., & Bless, H. (1991). *Happy and mindless, but sad and smart?: The impact of affective states on analytic reasoning*. Elmsford, NY: Pergamon Press.

Sciarappo, J., Norton, E., Oettingen, G., & Gollwitzer, P. M. (2015). *Positive fantasies of winning money reduce temporal discounting*. Unpublished manuscript, Department of Psychology, New York University, New York.

Sevincer, A. T., Busatta, P. D., & Oettingen, G. (2014). Mental contrasting and transfer of energization. *Personality and Social Psychology Bulletin, 40*, 139–152.

Sevincer, A. T., Kluge, L., & Oettingen, G. (2014). Implicit theories and motivational focus: Desired future versus present reality. *Motivation and Emotion, 38*, 36–46.

Sevincer, A. T., Mehl, P. J., & Oettingen, G. (in press). Well self-regulated people use mental contrasting. *Social Psychology*.

Sevincer, A. T., & Oettingen, G. (2013). Spontaneous mental contrasting and selective goal pursuit. *Personality and Social Psychology Bulletin, 39*, 1240–1254.

Sevincer, A. T., & Oettingen, G. (2015). Future thought and the self-regulation of energization. In G. H. E. Gendolla, M. Tops, & S. Koole (Eds.), *Biobehavioral approaches to self-regulation* (pp. 315–329). New York: Springer.

Sevincer, A. T., Schlier, B., & Oettingen, G. (2015). Ego depletion and the use of mental contrasting. *Motivation and Emotion, 39*, 876–891.

Sevincer, A. T., Wagner, G., Kalvelage, J., & Oettingen, G. (2014). Positive thinking about the future in newspaper reports and presidential addresses predicts economic downturn. *Psychological Science, 25*, 1010–1017.

Sheeran, P., Harris, P., Vaughan, J., Oettingen, G., & Gollwitzer, P. M. (2013). Gone exercising: Mental contrasting promotes physical activity among overweight, middle-aged, low-SES fishermen. *Health Psychology, 32,* 802–809.

Sheeran, P., Webb, T. L., & Gollwitzer, P. M. (2005). The interplay between goal intentions and implementation intentions. *Personality and Social Psychology Bulletin, 31,* 87–98.

Smallwood, J., & Schooler, J. W. (2006). The restless mind. *Psychological Bulletin, 132,* 946–958.

Stadler, G., Oettingen, G., & Gollwitzer, P. M. (2009). Physical activity in women: Effects of a self-regulation intervention. *American Journal of Preventive Medicine, 36,* 29–34.

Stadler, G., Oettingen, G., & Gollwitzer, P. M. (2010). Intervention effects of information and self-regulation on eating fruits and vegetables over two years. *Health Psychology, 29,* 274–283.

Sweeny, K., Carroll, P. J., & Shepperd, J. A. (2006). Thinking about the future: Is optimism always best? *Current Directions in Psychological Science, 15,* 302–306.

Sweeny, K., Reynolds, C. A., Falkenstein, A., Andrews, S. E., & Dooley, M. D. (2016). Two definitions of waiting well. *Emotion, 16,* 129–143.

Taylor, S. E., Pham, L. B., Rivkin, I. D., & Armor, D. A. (1998). Harnessing the imagination: Mental simulation, self-regulation, and coping. *American Psychologist, 53,* 429–439.

Wagner, G., Sevincer, A. T., & Oettingen, G. (2017). *Waiting for my team to win: Emotional consequences of positive fantasies.* Manuscript in preparation.

Wright, R. A. (1996). Brehm's theory of motivation as a model of effort and cardiovascular response. In P. M. Gollwitzer & J. A. Bargh (Eds.), *The psychology of action: Linking cognition and motivation to behavior* (pp. 424–453). New York: Guilford Press.

PART II

BELIEFS AND JUDGMENTS

CHAPTER 8

Expectations in the Academic Domain

Dale H. Schunk
Maria K. DiBenedetto

Individuals form many types of beliefs in educational contexts. Among the most influential for achievement-related processes (e.g., learning, motivation, achievement, self-regulation) are *academic expectations,* or individuals' beliefs and judgments about what they can learn or accomplish (Schunk, Meece, & Pintrich, 2014). Academic expectations represent future-thinking because they refer to what might happen. They contrast with beliefs and judgments about past events, such as attributions (perceived causes of outcomes).

The importance of academic expectations has been demonstrated in many research studies. Researchers have shown that (1) expectations relate positively to learning, motivation, achievement, and self-regulation (Multon, Brown, & Lent, 1991; Schunk & DiBenedetto, 2016; Schunk & Zimmerman, 2006; Wigfield & Eccles, 2002; Williams & Williams, 2010), and (2) improvements in learners' academic expectations can lead to enhanced achievement-related outcomes, such as increased choice of challenging activities, effort expended, persistence, self-regulation, and achievement (Pajares, 2008; Schunk & DiBenedetto, 2016; Schunk & Usher, 2012; Schunk & Zimmerman, 2006). These results support theoretical predictions on the positive role of academic expectations (Schunk, 2012; Zimmerman & Schunk, 2011).

The focus of this chapter is on expectations in the academic domain. We initially delineate some types of academic expectations and compare these with related constructs. We then situate these expectations within theoretical frameworks and discuss their hypothesized operation. Research studies are summarized showing the role of academic expectations in educational contexts. The chapter concludes with suggestions for future research and implications of research findings for educational policy and practice.

Background

Types of Academic Expectations

There are various types of academic expectations. We discuss self-efficacy, outcome expectations, and expectancies of success in this section and contrast these with related constructs.

Self-Efficacy

Self-efficacy refers to one's perceived capabilities for learning or performing actions at designated levels (Bandura, 1997). In Bandura's (1997) social cognitive theory, self-efficacy is hypothesized to affect various achievement-related outcomes, such as choice, effort, persistence, goal setting, and self-regulation. Researchers have substantiated these predictions (Fast et al., 2010; Schunk, 2012).

Self-efficacy can influence the choices students make (Patall, 2012). Learners are likely to select tasks and activities in which they feel self-efficacious and avoid those in which they do not. Unless they believe that their actions will produce the desired consequences, they have little incentive to engage in those actions. Self-efficacy also can help to determine how much effort learners expend on an activity, how long they persevere when confronting obstacles, and how resilient they are in the face of difficulties (Joët, Usher, & Bressoux, 2011; Moos & Azevedo, 2009).

Learners with a strong sense of self-efficacy set challenging goals and remain committed to them, heighten and sustain their efforts in the face of failure, and more quickly recover their self-efficacy after setbacks (Schunk, 2012). They also are more likely to engage in self-regulation activities (e.g., using effective learning strategies, monitoring their comprehension) and to create effective environments for learning (e.g., eliminating or minimizing distractions, finding effective study partners). Conversely, students who hold low self-efficacy beliefs may believe that learning is more difficult than it really is, which can produce anxiety and stress. Self-efficacy can lead to a self-fulfilling prophecy in which students learn only what they believe they can (Bandura, 1997).

Social cognitive theory postulates that individuals acquire information to appraise self-efficacy from their performances, vicarious (e.g., modeled) experiences, forms of social persuasion, and physiological indexes (Bandura, 1997). The most reliable influences on self-efficacy are individuals' interpretations of their performances, because performances are tangible indicators of capabilities. Performances viewed as successful should raise self-efficacy, and those deemed failures should lower it, although an occasional failure (or success) after many successes (or failures) may not have much impact on self-efficacy.

People acquire information about their capabilities vicariously through knowledge of how others perform (Bandura, 1997). Similarity to others is a cue for gauging self-efficacy (Schunk, 2012). Observing similar others succeed can raise observers' self-efficacy and motivate them to try the task when they believe that if others can do well, then they can, too. A vicarious increase in self-efficacy, however, can be negated by subsequent performance failure, because performances give the clearest interpretation about capabilities (Schunk, 2012).

People also develop self-efficacy beliefs from social persuasions they receive from others (Bandura, 1997), such as when a teacher tells a student, "I know you can do it." Social persuasions must be believable and persuaders must be credible for persuasions to develop students' beliefs that success is attainable. Positive feedback can raise learners' self-efficacy, but the increase will not persist if they subsequently perform poorly (Schunk, 2012).

Persons gain some self-efficacy information from physiological and emotional indicators such as anxiety and stress (Bandura, 1997). Strong emotional reactions to a task provide cues about an anticipated success or failure. When individuals experience negative thoughts and fears about their capabilities (e.g., feeling nervous thinking about speaking in front of a large group), those reactions can lower self-efficacy and trigger additional stress that can produce inadequate performances.

Outcome Expectations

Outcome expectations are beliefs about the anticipated outcomes of actions (Bandura, 1997; Shell, Murphy, & Bruning, 1989). Students commonly hold outcome expectations about grades; for example, "If I do well on this test I should receive an A in the course." Social cognitive theory (Bandura, 1997) predicts that individuals tend to engage in activities that they believe will result in positive outcomes and avoid actions that they believe may lead to negative outcomes. Students who feel highly efficacious about learning the content in a course may not work diligently if they believe that no matter how well they do, they will not receive a high grade (Schunk, 2012).

Self-efficacy and outcome expectations differ. Self-efficacy answers the question, "Can I do this?", whereas outcome expectations address the question, "What will happen if I do this?" Although these variables differ, they often are related (Bandura, 1997). Self-efficacy can help determine the outcomes one expects. Students who are confident in their academic capabilities expect high grades and other positive outcomes, whereas those with lower self-efficacy may expect lower grades before they begin a course. But self-efficacy can be inconsistent with expected outcomes (Bandura, 1997). High self-efficacy may not result in behavior consistent with that belief when individuals also believe that the outcome of engaging in that behavior will have undesired effects, perhaps because other variables weaken the link between behaviors and outcomes. As an example, academically self-efficacious students may not apply to universities with high entrance requirements and low acceptance rates if they expect that they will be rejected.

Expectations of Success

Expectations of success are one's beliefs about successfully completing an academic task or about how well one expects to do on a task (Wigfield & Eccles, 2002). Expectations of success derive from expectancy–value theory. Although there are different expectancy–value theories, the perspective focused on here is based on the work of Eccles, Wigfield, and their colleagues (Wigfield & Eccles, 2002; Wigfield,

Tonks, & Eccles, 2004; Wigfield, Tonks, & Klauda, 2016). This perspective has generated much research in academic settings (Schunk et al., 2014).

According to this theory, expectations of success influence achievement-related choices and performances. Another key variable is *value,* or individuals' beliefs about the reasons they might engage in tasks (Schunk et al., 2014). Theory and research support the prediction that both components are important in achievement settings (Wigfield et al., 2016). Students who believe they can successfully complete a task that they value are likely to be motivated to persist and expend effort to complete the task (Eccles & Wigfield, 1995). Learners who believe a task is too difficult or challenging to accomplish are less motivated and more likely to avoid doing the work, even when the task is highly valued.

Expectations of success and self-efficacy have similar characteristics. Students who hold high expectations of success are likely to have been influenced by previous similar accomplishments (Eccles, 1994; Zimmerman, 1995), similar to how self-efficacy builds upon previous mastery experiences (Schunk & DiBenedetto, 2014). However, expectations of success differ from self-efficacy. Expectations of success denote the likelihood of successful outcomes, whereas self-efficacy refers to perceptions of one's capabilities to produce those outcomes. One may believe that achievement is valuable and attainable but may not choose to pursue the activity because of a lack of belief in the capability to achieve (Bandura, 1991). For example, a high school student may believe that studying for a science exam will bring good grades that she values but does not study because she does not feel capable of learning the material well. Together, expectations of success and values may not be sufficient to motivate performance; self-efficacy also is necessary (Zimmerman, 1995).

Distinctions with Other Variables

Other variables bear some conceptual similarity to self-efficacy, outcome expectations, and expectations of success (Schunk & Zimmerman, 2006). *Abilities* are skills or capacities to learn or perform. Students with higher abilities tend to hold higher academic expectations, but there is no automatic relation between expectations and abilities. Pajares and Kranzler (1995) tested the joint contribution of ability and self-efficacy to mathematics performance and found that self-efficacy made an independent contribution to the prediction of performance. Collins (1982) identified high-, average-, and low-ability students in mathematics and within each of these three levels identified students with high and low self-efficacy. Students were given problems to solve and told they could rework those they missed. Across all ability levels, students with higher self-efficacy solved more problems correctly and chose to rework more problems they missed than did learners with lower self-efficacy.

Self-concept refers to one's collective self-perceptions formed through experiences with and interpretations of the environment and influenced by reinforcements and evaluations by others (Shavelson & Bolus, 1982). Theoretical models portray self-concept as multidimensional and hierarchically organized, with a general self-concept on top and subarea self-concepts below (Brunner et al., 2010; Pajares & Schunk, 2001, 2002). Academic expectations are self-perceptions of specific competencies and outcomes. Academic expectations should contribute to subarea self-concepts (e.g., history, biology; Bong & Skaalvik, 2003), which in turn combine to form the academic self-concept.

Self-esteem is a general affective evaluation of oneself that often includes judgments of self-worth (Covington, 2009). Whereas academic expectations involve questions of *can* (e.g., "Can I write this essay?"; "Can I solve this problem?"), self-esteem beliefs reflect questions of *feel* (e.g., "Do I like myself?"; "How do I feel about myself as a writer?"). One's beliefs about what one can do may not relate closely to how one feels about oneself. Some students with high self-esteem may hold doubts about their capabilities, and some students with high expectations for learning may hold lower self-esteem because their classmates view them negatively.

Many theories stress the idea of *perceived control* (or *agency*), which reflects the belief that one can exert a large degree of control over the important events in one's life (Bandura, 1997; Deci & Ryan, 2012). Perceived control is a type of general belief and is affected by expectations, although expectations are not the only aspects (Ryan, 1993). According to social cognitive theory (Bandura, 1997), students who believe they can control what they learn and perform are more apt to initiate and sustain behaviors directed toward those ends than are individuals who hold a low sense of control. However, a responsive environment is necessary for expectations to exert their effects (Bandura, 1997). Learners may believe they can control their use of learning strategies, effort, and persistence yet still hold low expectations for learning because they believe that the learning is unimportant and not worth the investment of time. Or they may hold high expectations for learning yet make little effort to learn because they believe that in their present environment learning will not be rewarded (Schunk & DiBenedetto, 2015).

THEORETICAL FRAMEWORKS

Many psychological theories include expectancy variables. In this chapter we focus on two theories that assign a prominent role to academic expectations and that address the expectation variables discussed earlier: social cognitive theory (self-efficacy, outcome expectations) and expectancy–value theory (expectations of success). These are discussed in turn.

Social Cognitive Theory

Reciprocal Influences

Expectations are key components of Bandura's (1986) social cognitive theory that postulates dynamic, reciprocal influences among three types of variables: personal (e.g., cognitions, affects), behavioral, and environmental. These reciprocal influences can be illustrated using self-efficacy as a personal variable. Researchers have shown that students' self-efficacy beliefs influence such behaviors as choice of tasks, persistence, effort, and achievement (Schunk & DiBenedetto, 2016). In turn, students' behaviors can modify their self-efficacy. For example, as students work on tasks, they note their progress toward their learning goals. Progress indicators such as assignments completed convey to students that they are capable of performing well, which enhances self-efficacy for continued learning (Schunk & DiBenedetto, 2014).

The hypothesized reciprocal influences between self-efficacy and environmental variables have been demonstrated in research on students with learning disabilities, many of whom hold low self-efficacy for learning (Licht & Kistner, 1986). Persons in their environments may react to them based on attributes typically associated with them rather than based on their behaviors. For example, teachers may judge such students as less capable than average learners and hold lower academic expectations for them, even in areas in which students with learning disabilities are performing adequately. In turn, teacher feedback can affect self-efficacy. Persuasive statements such as "I know that you can do this" can raise self-efficacy.

Social cognitive theory (Bandura, 1986) predicts that students' behaviors and environments can influence one another. When teachers present information, they may ask students to direct their attention to a slide projected on the board. Environmental influence on behaviors occurs when students attend to the visual without much conscious deliberation. Students' behaviors often alter the instructional environment. If teachers ask questions and students give incorrect answers, teachers may reteach key points rather than continue the lesson.

Social cognitive theory stresses the idea that people strive to develop a sense of *agency* (Bandura, 1997), or the belief that they can exert a large degree of control over important outcomes in their lives. Agency is similar to perceived control, and self-efficacy is an integral means for experiencing a sense of agency. Social cognitive theory (Schunk, 2012) predicts that students who feel efficacious about learning and performing well are apt to choose to engage in tasks, expend effort, and persist. Their successes bolster their beliefs that they can exert a high degree of control over the events in their lives.

Self-Regulated Learning

Self-regulated learning exemplifies many of these reciprocal influences and is also a means for students to exert control over their learning and performance. Self-regulated learning refers to one's self-generated feelings, thoughts, and behaviors directed toward goal attainment (Zimmerman, 2000). In an academic task, a self-efficacious student who is self-directed and self-reflective will perform better than students who are not strategic in their learning (DiBenedetto & Zimmerman, 2010; Schunk & Gunn, 1986).

Self-regulated learning involves three cyclical phases of learning: forethought, performance, and self-reflection (Zimmerman, 2000). The forethought phase takes place prior to learning and involves motivational beliefs such as self-efficacy, interest, outcome expectations, and goal orientations, as well as task analysis processes such as goal setting and strategic planning. Evidence shows that self-efficacy predicts the learning goals students set and the strategies they plan to use (Bandura & Schunk, 1981; Schunk, 2012).

During the performance phase, students engage in learning activities initiated by the forethought phase. By using self-observations and self-control processes, students are systematically and actively engaged in learning. Self-observation processes include self-monitoring and self-recording of progress. Through these self-observational processes, students receive feedback from their perceptions and feedback from others, such as teachers and peers (Schunk & DiBenedetto, 2014). Students engage in self-control processes such as imagery, self-instruction, attention focusing, and help seeking. Students who are self-efficacious about their capability to learn have been shown to sustain effort, persistence, and strategy use during learning (Pajares, 2008).

Learning efforts and feedback from others provide students with information to reflect upon, leading to self-judgments and self-reactions (Zimmerman, 2000). Self-judgments involve evaluating one's performance against one's goals and standards set in the forethought phase and then attributing the outcomes to strategy use, effort, or something uncontrollable, such as luck or ability. Self-reaction processes include satisfaction levels (level of contentment) and adaptive or defensive responses (emotional reactions) to performance. The three phases are cyclical and dynamic in that students' responses at the self-reflection phase affect future forethought-phase measures. Students who feel dissatisfied with their grades, for example, but are self-efficacious about their capability to learn will attribute performance to strategy use and effort and fine-tune or adapt their task analyses for future similar academic tasks (Schunk & DiBenedetto, 2014).

Self-efficacy is a critical motivational force in the three phases of self-regulated learning and develops as students become more self-regulated. Schunk and Zimmerman (1997) describe the development of self-regulatory competency in terms of a learner moving through four levels: observation, emulation, self-control, and self-regulation. In the first two levels, sources of self-efficacy are external to the student, whereas at the second two levels, self-efficacy becomes internalized. At the observational level, social models such as teachers and peers provide information on how to perform a task and how to engage in the forethought phase processes. Models provide a source of efficacy; for example, students seeing a teacher hold and blow into the recorder to make music are learning how to handle the instrument and create beautiful sounds. The teacher is demonstrating not only a technique but also self-efficacy in the capability to perform this simple task. At the emulation level, students are practicing the observed behavior. Self-efficacy is provided by the teacher, who gives feedback to students. Students are also beginning to feel self-efficacious as they practice and begin to internalize the behaviors associated with performing the task in the way in which the teacher modeled. At the self-control level, students perform several tasks related to playing the recorder according to the teacher's guidelines and demonstrations. Self-efficacy internalizes as students experience mastery and improved capabilities (Schunk & Zimmerman, 1997). At the self-regulation level, students can make adaptations and use different strategies for playing the recorder. They are self-efficacious in their capability to make behavioral adjustments independent of the teacher, and as they move through the three phases of self-regulated learning their self-efficacy continues to strengthen (Schunk & DiBenedetto, 2014).

Expectancy–Value Theory

Eccles and Wigfield (1995) formulated an expectancy–value theory of motivation to include psychological, cultural, and social factors. Two key factors are expectancies and values, which are derived from information that learners have about the nature of the task and which predict academic achievement, choice of activities, and persistence (Eccles & Wigfield, 1995). Expectancies and values are influenced by the beliefs one has about the task; for example, perceptions of ability or competence, goals, and feelings associated with past similar academic activities (Wigfield et al., 2016). In addition, cultural and social influences, such as other people's (e.g., teachers, parents, and peers) attitudes and expectations, influence learners' motivational beliefs of competence, goals, and feelings. Past academic experiences also influence expectations of success.

This expectancy–value theory provides a comprehensive account of achievement motivation in academic settings and predicts that many factors influence academic expectations for success and values, which in turn can affect students' motivation. In addition to discussing the influences on expectations for success, Eccles (1983) postulated four major components of task values: attainment value, intrinsic value, utility value, and cost. Attainment value is the importance the learner attaches to the task. Intrinsic value refers to the pleasure one obtains from performing the task. Utility value refers to how the activity fits into one's plans for the future. Cost refers to what the learner must give up to do the task. This model postulates that it is the relationship between one's expectations of success and the value placed on performing the task that motivates the learner to be engaged in the task.

RESEARCH EVIDENCE

Researchers have conducted much research in academic settings investigating the operation of academic expectations during learning, motivation, and self-regulation. In this section, we discuss some findings from correlational and experimental research.

Correlational Research

In correlational studies, researchers collect measures of academic expectations and other achievement-related variables to determine their interrelation. Given the correlational nature, no determination of causality can be made.

Many correlational studies with individuals of different ages show that self-efficacy bears a positive relation to learning and achievement (Schunk & DiBenedetto, 2014; Williams & Williams, 2010). Researchers have obtained significant and positive correlations between self-efficacy for learning or performing tasks and subsequent achievement on those tasks (Aguayo, Herman, Ojeda, & Flores, 2011; Joët et al., 2011). Correlations between academic self-efficacy and performance tend to be higher when self-efficacy measures correspond closely to the criterion task (i.e., task-specific self-efficacy). Based on a review of research, Pajares (2006) concluded that self-efficacy generally explains approximately 25% of the variance in academic achievement. Using meta-analyses, Multon et al. (1991) found that self-efficacy was related positively to academic performance and accounted for 14% of the variance. Stajkovic and Luthans (1998) found, across 114 studies, that the average correlation between self-efficacy and work-related performance was .38.

Researchers also have shown that self-efficacy correlates positively with indexes of self-regulation (McInerney, 2011; Schunk & Usher, 2011). Pintrich and De Groot (1990) found that measures of self-efficacy, self-regulation, and cognitive strategy used by middle school students were positively intercorrelated and predicted achievement. Bouffard-Bouchard, Parent, and Larivee (1991) found that high school students with high self-efficacy for problem solving displayed greater performance monitoring and persisted longer than students with lower self-efficacy. Zimmerman and Bandura (1994) showed that self-efficacy for writing correlated positively with college students' goals for course achievement, self-evaluative standards (satisfaction with potential grades), and achievement.

Many correlational studies have been conducted in different domains examining the relation of expectancies and values to achievement (Wigfield et al., 2016). Schoolchildren's experiences, including the classroom environment, teachers, peers, and academic subjects being taught, have been found to influence their expectancies and values. Longitudinal studies have been done tracking students over several years (Wigfield & Eccles, 2000). In one study, students in grades 5–12 completed surveys, once each year over a 2-year period, on expectancies and values for mathematics and English. In another study, students in the sixth grade completed surveys exploring how their expectancies and values for different academic subjects, sports, and social activities changed as they transitioned to junior high. A third study spanned a 10-year period in which students completed surveys examining how their expectancies and values for different subjects and other constructs changed through elementary and secondary schooling.

The preceding three studies revealed several important findings. Children's ability beliefs and expectancies for success were domain specific and related to one another (Wigfield & Eccles, 2000). Children had clear beliefs about the academic domains that they valued. Another finding was that learners' ability and value beliefs declined as they got older and varied across domains. These findings underscore the importance of educational contexts for motivation and suggest ways to enhance academic expectancies. Students who are in classrooms in which mastery learning is the focus and public displays of performance are absent or minimized are more likely to have positive academic and motivational outcomes (Wigfield et al., 2016; Zimmerman & DiBenedetto, 2008). Other suggestions based on these research results are that it is critical for teachers to hold and communicate high expectations for students, form positive and emotionally supportive relationships with students, teach content that is cognitively challenging and focused on higher level reasoning skills, and provide opportunities for independent, self-directed learning.

Experimental Research

Researchers have explored how instructional and social classroom variables affect academic expectations in diverse settings (Schunk & Usher, 2012), as well as how changes in expectations improve academic performances. A theoretical explanation of these effects is as follows (Schunk & DiBenedetto, 2016).

Improvement in expectancies depends on individuals deriving information that their capabilities are developing. We noted earlier four sources of self-efficacy beliefs: performances, vicarious experiences, forms of persuasion, and physiological indexes. Instructional and social variables in learning contexts provide students with cues about their learning progress (Schunk, 2012; Schunk & DiBenedetto, 2014). Expectancies are enhanced when students believe they are performing well and becoming more skillful. Lack of success or slow progress will not necessarily lower expectancies if students believe they can perform better by making adaptations (e.g., expending greater effort, using better learning strategies). In turn, strengthened expectancies promote motivation, learning, self-regulation, and achievement (Schunk, 2012).

Experimental research in educational contexts supports these hypothesized relations (Schunk, 2012; Schunk & Ertmer, 2000; Schunk & Usher, 2012). These studies have employed students in different grade levels (e.g., elementary, middle, high, postsecondary) and with diverse abilities (e.g., regular, remedial, gifted) and have investigated different content areas (e.g., reading, writing, mathematics, computer applications).

For example, some instructional and social elements identified by researchers that can raise expectancies are having students pursue proximal and specific learning goals, exposing learners to social models, providing students with performance and attributional feedback, teaching students to use learning strategies, having learners verbalize strategies while they apply them, making students' rewards contingent on their learning progress, and having students self-monitor and evaluate their progress (Schunk, 2012; Schunk & Ertmer, 2000). Although these elements differ, they all provide information to learners about their learning progress, which is necessary to raise their expectancies for success. Some sample research studies are discussed next to illustrate these variables.

In an early experimental study, Schunk (1982) tested the effects of providing learners with attributional feedback as they engaged in problem solving. Children who lacked subtraction skills received subtraction instruction and practice opportunities over multiple sessions. For the problem solving, children were assigned to one of three treatment conditions: past attribution, future attribution, monitoring. An adult teacher monitored children's problem solving by periodically asking each child individually on which page of the instructional material he or she was working. For children in the past attribution condition, the teacher linked prior achievement with effort by remarking that the child had been working hard. With children in the future attribution condition, the teacher remarked that the child needed to work hard. For those in the monitoring group, the teacher did not provide any comment after the child responded with his or her progress. The results showed that, compared with the future attribution and monitoring conditions, the past attribution treatment led to higher self-efficacy and subtraction skill and more rapid progress in mastering the training material. These results suggest that linking children's past progress with effort was a salient cue that they were making progress in learning, which exerted motivational effects on their self-efficacy and performance.

Schunk (1985) tested the hypothesis that participation in goal setting enhances self-efficacy and skills. Children with learning disabilities received instruction and practice in subtraction over sessions. Some children set proximal performance goals for each session, others had comparable proximal goals assigned, and children in a third condition received instruction and practice without goals. Proximal goals promoted task motivation more than no goals, but participation in goal setting led to the highest self-efficacy and subtraction skill. Allowing children to set goals may have yielded high initial expectations for successful goal attainment, which likely were validated as children observed their goal progress. Although children who were assigned goals performed as well during the instructional sessions, their lower initial expectancy of goal attainment may have left them in doubt about their capabilities, which can affect performance.

To explore the effects of goals and self-evaluation on self-efficacy and performance, Schunk and Ertmer (1999) conducted two studies with college students while they were learning computer applications. In the first study, students received instruction and practice during three laboratory sessions. Students were randomly assigned to a process or product goal condition. The process goal stressed learning computer applications; the product goal emphasized performing them. Half of the students in each goal condition evaluated their progress in learning the application after the second laboratory session. The process goal led to higher self-efficacy, judged learning progress, and self-regulatory competence and strategy use, whereas the self-evaluation component promoted self-efficacy. In the second study, which used the same goal conditions, self-evaluation students assessed their learning progress after each of the three sessions. The more frequent self-evaluation produced comparable results when coupled with a process or product goal. The opportunity for frequent self-evaluation may provide learners with good information on their progress in learning, which can substantiate self-efficacy and promote skill acquisition.

In addition to the influence of instructional and social variables, researchers have shown how personal and contextual variables may affect self-efficacy. One line of research has examined *implementation intentions,* which are if-then plans (e.g., "If this happens, then I will implement this goal-directed behavior") formed to assist goal intentions (e.g., "I intend to attain this goal"). Implementation intentions specify before task engagement how the individual will deal with situations that might arise while he or she is striving toward goal attainment (Wieber, Odenthal, & Gollwitzer, 2010). Compared with goal intentions alone, implementation intentions have an added effect on goal attainment (Oettingen, Hönig, & Gollwitzer, 2000; Wieber et al., 2010).

Implementation intentions have been shown to affect performance under certain self-efficacy conditions. Wieber and colleagues (2010) had college students work on difficult cognitive tasks. These researchers found that when self-efficacy was high, holding implementation intentions improved students' performances. When self-efficacy was low to medium, implementation intentions did not improve performance over that due to goal intentions.

In another study with high school students (Bayer & Gollwitzer, 2007), students set goal intentions for mathematical problem solving (e.g., "I will correctly solve as many problems as possible"), as well as self-efficacy-strengthening implementation intentions (e.g., "And if I start a new problem, then I will tell myself I can solve it"). Addition of the self-efficacy-strengthening implementation intentions improved individuals' performances beyond the effect of goal intentions. Self-efficacy-strengthening implementation intentions provide participants with persuasive self-efficacy information, which can raise self-efficacy (Bandura, 1997).

Other relevant research has been conducted in cross-cultural contexts. Factors in learners' cultures may affect their expectancies (Oettingen, 1995). For example, Oettingen, Little, Lindenberger, and Baltes (1994) assessed agency and control beliefs of East and West German elementary-age students. Control beliefs were roughly similar to expectations for success, and agency beliefs represented beliefs about whether students have access to and can apply school performance-related means (e.g., access to help of the teacher and effort and ability). Data were collected before the unification of East and West Germany, which at that time reflected different political and educational systems. Compared with West German youth, East German students showed lower agency and control beliefs, although the agency and control beliefs of East German students correlated more strongly with school grades than did those of the West German children.

In a similar study (Little, Oettingen, Stetsenko, & Baltes, 1995), agency and control beliefs were assessed among children in grades 2–6 in East Germany, West Germany, the United States, and Russia. The results showed that the U.S. children had the highest levels of agency and control beliefs but also the lowest belief–performance correlation. Although the U.S. children were the most optimistic, their beliefs were the most unrealistic compared with their academic performances.

The concept-oriented reading instruction (CORI) program incorporates motivational practices that are grounded in theory and research on expectancies and values (Schunk & Bursuck, 2016). In CORI science classrooms, teachers provide a variety of expository and narrative books on a topic and allow students to select the ones they want to read. Teachers also provide several hands-on activities that complement the reading. For example, in one study, third graders dissected owl pellets (Wigfield, Guthrie, Tonks, & Perencevich, 2004). In doing so, they observed that some of the pellets had fish scales, whereas others did not. This sparked an interest in understanding what foods owls ate and whether where the owls lived influenced their food sources. The hands-on activities motivated students' interest such that they wanted to read about owls. Providing students with choices in the books to read gave the learners a sense of autonomy, which also was found to increase their self-efficacy for reading the science content. Although CORI strategies are typically taught to improve reading comprehension of science content, CORI may be used with other subject areas as well (Wigfield et al., 2004).

Guthrie, McRae, and Klauda (2007) conducted a meta-analysis on CORI research, which showed that, in 11 quasi-experimental studies with students in grades 3–5, CORI had strong effects on students' expectations, intrinsic motivation, curiosity, and task orientation. In addition, students who received CORI showed an increase in reading comprehension, reading strategy use, work recognition speed, oral reading fluency, and science knowledge (Wigfield et al., 2016). These findings suggest that students' academic expectations can be enhanced when they are taught strategies for success, are motivated and engaged, and value the social interactions that are a part of CORI. Given the multiple components of CORI, it is difficult to determine the extent to which expectations influenced changes in performance; however, both social cognitive and expectancy–value theories predict that expectations play a causal role.

Several researchers have investigated the direct and indirect effects of expectations on academic outcomes, or how well changes in expectancies predict changes in performance. In an experimental study, Schunk (1981) used path analysis and found that self-efficacy exerted a direct effect on children's achievement and persistence in mathematics. Zimmerman and Bandura (1994) found that self-efficacy affected achievement directly as well as indirectly through its influence on goals (i.e., more efficacious students set more challenging goals). Schunk and Gunn (1986) found that children's long-division achievement was directly influenced by use of effective strategies and self-efficacy. Relich, Debus, and Walker (1986) also found that self-efficacy exerted a direct effect on division achievement and that instructional treatment had both a direct and an indirect effect on achievement through self-efficacy.

FUTURE RESEARCH DIRECTIONS

Researchers have explored the operation of academic expectations in diverse settings involving learning, motivation, and self-regulation. Much is known about their role in achievement contexts, but research questions remain. In this section, we make recommendations for further research on academic expectations in the following areas: their assessment, their dynamic nature, developmental changes, and their operation in groups and other educational contexts.

Assessment of Expectations

A continuing challenge is to ensure that researchers assess expectations in ways that are consistent with their conceptualizations. With respect to self-efficacy, for example, Bandura (1986, 1997) noted that context-specific judgments of self-efficacy, matched to corresponding performance outcomes, offer the best prediction of outcomes, because these judgments are the types that people make when confronted with tasks. But such correspondence is missing in many studies because researchers assess self-efficacy and performance outcomes at different levels of specificity (e.g., general self-efficacy items, specific performance items) or use self-efficacy items that more closely resemble general self-concept or self-esteem (Bandura, 2006; Bong, 2006). Self-efficacy assessments that do not mesh well with criterion tasks make determining the influence of self-efficacy problematic. To be both explanatory and predictive, expectation measures should be tailored to the domain being analyzed and reflect the various demands within that domain.

A related point is how much expectation measures generalize across domains and content areas. For example, researchers have assessed self-efficacy at levels more general than specific tasks (Zimmerman & Bandura, 1994), with items such as "How well can you get teachers to help you when you get stuck on school work?" and "How well can you study when there are other interesting things to do?" To judge self-efficacy at these general levels, students must integrate their beliefs across different situations, such as getting the teacher to help them when they need help in science, history, and mathematics.

Good alignment of self-efficacy and outcome measures allows for accurate assessment of their correspondence (agreement). Although expectations that slightly exceed what one can accomplish can enhance effort and persistence, overly high expectations may lead to insufficient preparation and poor performance

(Klassen, 2006). Researchers should determine to what degree high or low expectations in the face of incongruent performances result in higher motivation and performance. Improving correspondence will require helping students understand what they know so they can effectively use appropriate strategies to learn.

The Dynamic Nature of Expectations

Expectations are dynamic and continually capable of changing. Students' expectations at the start of a learning activity are likely to fluctuate as the activity proceeds. In many studies, however, researchers assess expectations only at fixed points in time, such as with a pretest and posttest, which does not provide a complete picture of its dynamic quality. We recommend research that better captures this dynamic quality.

Researchers also tend to use self-report measures. But to assess the dynamic nature of expectancies, other measures are needed. Some measures that are better suited to capture changes in expectancies during learning—rather than changing from before to after learning—are used in self-regulated learning research and include think-alouds, observations, traces, and microanalytic assessments.

Think-alouds require learners to verbalize aloud their thinking while engaged in learning (Greene, Robertson, & Costa, 2011). Think-alouds, which capture learners' verbalized cognitive processing, typically are recorded and transcribed. *Observations* of students while engaged in learning can occur through video and audio recording or by taking detailed notes (Perry, 1998). Observations are transcribed and coded to determine the incidence of variables of interest. *Traces* are observable measures that students create as they engage in tasks (Winne & Perry, 2000). Traces include marks students make in texts, but computer technologies have expanded the potential of traces in that researchers are able to collect measures of learners' eye movements, time spent on various aspects of material to be learned, and selections of strategies to use with content. *Microanalytic assessments* examine learners' behaviors and cognitions in real time as they engage in tasks (DiBenedetto & Zimmerman, 2010, 2013). Researchers give assessments (e.g., of expectancies, perceived progress in learning) to learners orally or in writing while they are engaged in tasks.

An example of a study using microanalytic assessments was conducted by DiBenedetto and Zimmerman (2010). High school students individually read studies and were tested on a passage on tornados. Students were asked questions specifically targeting the processes of the three phases of self-regulated learning as they engaged in the task. Thus, to capture students' self-efficacy for learning the passage, students were asked, "How confident do you feel in your capability to learn and remember all of the material on tornados for this passage?" (p. 6). The microanalytic methodology has been shown to have greater construct and predictive validity than other, more established measures and to have potential diagnostic value for guiding instruction and interventions in science learning (DiBenedetto & Zimmerman, 2013).

These assessment methods can detect moment-to-moment changes in expectations. A better understanding of their dynamic nature gained through the use of such methods will inform theory and offer suggestions for ways to help learners improve their academic expectancies.

Developmental Changes in Expectations

We recommend increased research attention to investigating developmental changes in academic expectations. Cognitive development can affect expectations. Young children often have high expectancies for performing tasks and overestimate what they can do (Wigfield, Cambria, & Eccles, 2012). The accuracy of their beliefs (i.e., how well they correspond to actual performances) typically improves with development (Davis-Kean et al., 2008; Wigfield & Eccles, 2002). As more efficient information processing develops, children become capable of engaging in increasingly complicated mental procedures (Davis-Kean et al., 2008). They are better able to weigh and combine information, assess task requirements, and compare those requirements with their perceived capabilities.

The improvement in accuracy also can result from declining expectations, which research shows often occurs with development (Lepper, Corpus, & Iyengar, 2005; Wigfield et al., 2012). In addition to developmental influences, this decline has been attributed to contextual variables such as greater competition in school, more norm-referenced grading, less teacher attention to individual learner progress, and school transitions (Wigfield et al., 2012).

The incongruence between children's expectations and their actual performances may arise because children lack task familiarity and do not fully understand what is required to perform a task well. Even when they are given feedback indicating that they have performed poorly, their expectations may not decline. As they gain experience, their accuracy improves. Children may also be unduly swayed by certain task features and decide based on these that they can or cannot perform the task (Schunk, 2012). In subtraction, for example, children may focus on how many numbers or columns the problems contain and judge problems with fewer columns as less difficult than those with more columns, even when the former are conceptually more difficult. In these cases, expectations are problematic if children are unrealistically overconfident and are not motivated to seek help and improve their skills. As children's capability to focus on multiple features improves with development, so should the accuracy of their expectations. More research is needed on ways to enhance the correspondence between expectations and performances. Researchers might explore the effects of giving children opportunities to evaluate their capabilities and instructional interventions that convey clear information to children about their skills or learning progress.

In addition, research suggests that teachers who promote a caring and nurturing classroom environment can help improve motivation and achievement scores for students (Stipek, 2006; Stipek, Feiler, Daniels, & Milburn, 1995). In a study conducted on middle-class and lower-socioeconomic-status minority students between the ages of 4 and 6 years old, differences were found in the instructional approaches for minority students compared with those for middle-class students. Instruction in the lower-class minority classrooms was often didactic in nature, by which the teachers focused on basic skills and performance learning rather than using the more student-centered method of promoting understanding, problem-solving skills, and interests. Achievement, motivation, and interest were found to be higher for students exposed to the more constructivist approach to teaching. Research suggests that the relationship between students and teachers across various grade levels is particularly important for motivation (Stipek, 2006). Teachers who convey high expectations while providing the support and encouragement needed to achieve tend to have a positive effect on students' motivation, persistence, and performance.

Operation of Expectations in Groups and Related Educational Contexts

Most research on expectations has focused on learning by individuals, even when the learners were part of a group (e.g., class). But group learning is common, as evident in the emphasis on collaborative and peer learning. Increased research attention is recommended to group expectations such as *collective self-efficacy*, or the self-efficacy of a group or larger social entity.

Such research can take different forms, one of which is exploring the operation of expectations in coregulated contexts. *Coregulation* refers to the coordination of self-regulation competencies among people in social contexts (Hadwin, Järvelä, & Miller, 2011; Järvelä & Hadwin, 2013). Learners jointly use their skills and strategies to influence one another's self-regulated learning and develop new or expanded self-regulatory capabilities that are useful in group or individual contexts. Teachers may collaborate to develop lessons and activities that they will implement in their individual classrooms.

We also recommend more research on self-efficacy in other educational contexts. Most expectancy research in education has been conducted in regular instructional settings using traditional content areas (e.g., mathematics, literacy). Examining expectancies in related educational contexts is important, because much learning takes place outside of formal instructional contexts, such as in after-school programs, homes, workplaces, and communities. Expectations are no less pertinent in these types of situations, but we know less about their operation outside of formal instructional settings.

Researchers might look, for example, at how academic expectations change as students complete homework, work in internships, and participate in mentoring interactions. In particular, we recommend research investigating the roles that other persons in these environments, such as parents, peers, mentors, and coaches, play in helping students become confident learners.

IMPLICATIONS FOR POLICY AND PRACTICE

Research on academic expectations has made tremendous advances over the past several years. Researchers have shown that expectations are positively correlated with and influence academic motivation and learning in varied domains; in turn, they are affected by social and instructional variables. Research studies are needed that shed further light on the assessment of expectations, their dynamic nature, developmental changes, and expectations in groups and in related educational contexts.

Existing research supports the point that the instructional and social conditions of schooling be examined to determine how they affect both learning and expectations. Research also is needed on the link between academic expectations and educational policies. Policies guide instructional practice by setting expectations for teachers in the form of *standards* (White & DiBenedetto, 2015), or a shared set of expectations of what students should learn and how they will demonstrate learning through assessments (Kendall, 2003). These standards represent a type of future-thinking because they include parameters for successful student performance. Their impact on education is significant because standards guide curriculum, instructional design, and assessment and provide opportunities for consistency of learning outcomes within and across states (Schmoker & Marzano, 1999). Learning standards have been developed across multiple disciplines and are established to ensure that students are learning content critical for the discipline and that assessments are aligned with the content. Further research will promote understanding of how standards affect teachers' and students' academic expectations and performances.

REFERENCES

Aguayo, D., Herman, K., Ojeda, L., & Flores, L. Y. (2011). Culture predicts Mexican Americans' college self-efficacy and college performance. *Journal of Diversity in Higher Education, 4*, 79–89.

Bandura, A. (1986). *Social foundations of thought and action: A social cognitive theory.* Englewood Cliffs, NJ: Prentice Hall.

Bandura, A. (1991). Self-regulation of motivation through anticipatory and self-regulatory mechanisms. In R. A. Dienstbier (Ed.), *Nebraska Symposium on Motivation: Vol. 38. Perspectives on motivation* (pp. 69–164). Lincoln: University of Nebraska Press.

Bandura, A. (1997). *Self-efficacy: The exercise of control.* New York: Freeman.

Bandura, A. (2006). Guide for creating self-efficacy scales. In F. Pajares & T. Urdan (Eds.), *Self-efficacy beliefs of adolescents* (pp. 307–338). Greenwich, CT: Information Age.

Bandura, A., & Schunk, D. H. (1981). Cultivating competence, self-efficacy, and intrinsic interest though proximal self-motivation. *Journal of Personality and Social Psychology, 41*, 586–598.

Bayer, U. C., & Gollwitzer, P. M. (2007). Boosting scholastic test scores by willpower: The role of implementation intentions. *Self and Identity, 6*, 1–19.

Bong, M. (2006). Asking the right question: How confident are you that you could successfully perform these tasks? In F. Pajares & T. Urdan (Eds.), *Self-efficacy beliefs of adolescents* (pp. 287–306). Greenwich, CT: Information Age.

Bong, M., & Skaalvik, E. M. (2003). Academic self-concept and self-efficacy: How different are they really? *Educational Psychology Review, 15*, 1–40.

Bouffard-Bouchard, T., Parent, S., & Larivee, S. (1991). Influence of self-efficacy on self-regulation and performance among junior and senior high-school age students. *International Journal of Behavioral Development, 14*, 153–164.

Brunner, M., Keller, U., Dierendonck, C., Reichert, M., Ugen, S., Fischbach, A., & Martin, R. (2010). The structure of academic self-concepts revisited: The nested Marsh/Shavelson model. *Journal of Educational Psychology, 102*, 964–981.

Collins, J. L. (1982, March). *Self-efficacy and ability in achievement behavior.* Paper presented at the annual meeting of the American Educational Research Association, New York.

Covington, M. V. (2009). Self-worth theory: Retrospection and prospects. In K. R. Wentzel & A. Wigfield (Eds.), *Handbook of motivation at school* (pp. 141–169). New York: Routledge.

Davis-Kean, P. E., Huesmann, L. R., Jager, J., Collins, W. A., Bates, J. E., & Lansford, J. E. (2008). Changes in the relation of self-efficacy beliefs and behaviors across development. *Child Development, 79*, 1257–1269.

Deci, E. L., & Ryan, R. M. (2012). Motivation, personality, and development within embedded social contexts: An overview of self-determination theory. In R. M. Ryan (Ed.), *Oxford handbook of human motivation* (pp. 85–107). Oxford, UK: Oxford University Press.

DiBenedetto, M. K., & Zimmerman, B. J. (2010). Differences in self-regulatory processes among students studying science: A microanalytic investigation. *Journal of Educational and Psychological Assessment, 5,* 2–24.

DiBenedetto, M. K., & Zimmerman, B. J. (2013). Construct and predictive validity of microanalytic measures of students' self-regulation of science learning. *Learning and Individual Differences, 25,* 30–41.

Eccles, J. S. (1983). Expectancies, values, and academic behaviors. In J. T. Spence (Ed.), *Achievement and achievement motives* (pp. 75–146). San Francisco: Freeman.

Eccles, J. S. (1994). Understanding women's educational and occupational choices. *Psychology of Women Quarterly, 18,* 585–609.

Eccles, J. S., & Wigfield, A. (1995). In the mind of the achiever: The structure of adolescents' academic achievement-related beliefs and self-perceptions. *Personality and Social Psychology Bulletin, 21,* 215–225.

Fast, L. A., Lewis, J. L., Bryant, M. J., Bocian, K. A., Cardullo, R. A., Rettig, M., & Hammond, K. A. (2010). Does math self-efficacy mediate the effect of the perceived classroom environment on standardized math test performance? *Journal of Educational Psychology, 102,* 729–740.

Greene, J. A., Robertson, J., & Costa, L.-J. C. (2011). Assessing self-regulated learning using think-aloud protocols. In B. J. Zimmerman & D. H. Schunk (Eds.), *Handbook of self-regulation of learning and performance* (pp. 313–328). New York: Routledge.

Guthrie, J. T., McRae, A. C., & Klauda, S. L. (2007). Contributions of concept-oriented reading instruction to knowledge about interventions for motivation in reading. *Educational Psychologist, 42,* 237–250.

Hadwin, A. F., Järvelä, S., & Miller, M. (2011). Self-regulated, co-regulated, and socially shared regulation of learning. In B. J. Zimmerman & D. H. Schunk (Eds.), *Handbook of self-regulation of learning and performance* (pp. 65–84). New York: Routledge.

Järvelä, S., & Hadwin, A. F. (2013). New frontiers: Regulating learning in CSCL. *Educational Psychologist, 48,* 25–39.

Joët, G., Usher, E. L., & Bressoux, P. (2011). Sources of self-efficacy: An investigation of elementary school students in France. *Journal of Educational Psychology, 103,* 649–663.

Kendall, J. S. (2003). Setting standards in early childhood education. *Educational Leadership, 60,* 64–68.

Klassen, R. M. (2006). Too much confidence?: The self-efficacy of adolescents with learning disabilities. In F. Pajares & T. Urdan (Eds.), *Self-efficacy beliefs of adolescents* (pp. 181–200). Greenwich, CT: Information Age.

Lepper, M. R., Corpus, J. H., & Iyengar, S. S. (2005). Intrinsic and extrinsic motivational orientations in the classroom: Age differences and academic correlates. *Journal of Educational Psychology, 97,* 184–196.

Licht, B. G., & Kistner, J. A. (1986). Motivational problems of learning-disabled children: Individual differences and their implications for treatment. In J. K. Torgesen & B. W. L. Wong (Eds.), *Psychological and educational perspectives on learning disabilities* (pp. 225–255). Orlando, FL: Academic Press.

Little, T. D., Oettingen, G., Stetsenko, A., & Baltes, P. B. (1995). Children's action-control beliefs about school performance: How do American children compare with German and Russian children? *Journal of Personality and Social Psychology, 69,* 686–700.

McInerney, D. M. (2011). Culture and self-regulation in educational contexts: Assessing the relationship of cultural group to self-regulation. In B. J. Zimmerman & D. H. Schunk

(Eds.), *Handbook of self-regulation of learning and performance* (pp. 442–464). New York: Routledge.

Moos, D. C., & Azevedo, R. (2009). Learning with computer-based learning environments: A literature review of computer self-efficacy. *Review of Educational Research, 79,* 576–600.

Multon, K. D., Brown, S. D., & Lent, R. W. (1991). Relation of self-efficacy beliefs to academic outcomes: A meta-analytic investigation. *Journal of Counseling Psychology, 38,* 30–38.

Oettingen, G. (1995). Cross-cultural perspectives on self-efficacy. In A. Bandura (Ed.), *Self-efficacy in changing societies* (pp. 149–176). New York: Cambridge University Press.

Oettingen, G., Hönig, G., & Gollwitzer, P. M. (2000). Effective self-regulation of goal attainment. *International Journal of Educational Research, 33,* 705–732.

Oettingen, G., Little, T. D., Lindenberger, U., & Baltes, P. B. (1994). Causality, agency, and control beliefs in East versus West Berlin children: A natural experiment on the role of context. *Journal of Personality and Social Psychology, 66,* 579–595.

Pajares, F. (2006). Self-efficacy during childhood and adolescence: Implications for teachers and parents. In F. Pajares & T. Urdan (Eds.), *Self-efficacy beliefs of adolescents* (pp. 339–367). Greenwich, CT: Information Age.

Pajares, F. (2008). Motivational role of self-efficacy beliefs in self-regulated learning. In D. H. Schunk & B. J. Zimmerman (Eds.), *Motivation and self-regulated learning: Theory, research, and applications* (pp. 111–139). New York: Taylor & Francis.

Pajares, F., & Kranzler, J. (1995). Self-efficacy beliefs and general mental ability in mathematical problem-solving. *Contemporary Educational Psychology, 20,* 426–443.

Pajares, F., & Schunk, D. H. (2001). Self-beliefs and school success: Self-efficacy, self-concept, and school achievement. In R. J. Riding & S. G. Rayner (Eds.), *Self-perception* (pp. 239–265). Westport, CT: Ablex.

Pajares, F., & Schunk, D. H. (2002). Self and self-belief in psychology and education: A historical perspective. In J. Aronson (Ed.), *Improving academic achievement: Impact of psychological factors on education* (pp. 3–21). San Diego, CA: Academic Press.

Patall, E. A. (2012). The motivational complexity of choosing: A review of theory and research. In R. M. Ryan (Ed.), *Oxford handbook of human motivation* (pp. 248–279). Oxford, UK: Oxford University Press.

Perry, N. E. (1998). Young children's self-regulated learning and contexts that support it. *Journal of Educational Psychology, 90,* 715–729.

Pintrich, P. R., & De Groot, E. V. (1990). Motivational and self-regulated learning components of classroom academic performance. *Journal of Educational Psychology, 82,* 33–40.

Relich, J. D., Debus, R. L., & Walker, R. (1986). The mediating role of attribution and self-efficacy variables for treatment effects on achievement outcomes. *Contemporary Educational Psychology, 11,* 195–216.

Ryan, R. M. (1993). Agency and organization: Intrinsic motivation, autonomy, and the self in psychological development. In J. E. Jacobs (Ed.), *Nebraska Symposium on Motivation 1992: Developmental perspectives on motivation* (pp. 1–56). Lincoln: University of Nebraska Press.

Schmoker, M., & Marzano, R. J. (1999). Realizing the promise of standards-based education. *Educational Leadership, 56,* 17–21.

Schunk, D. H. (1981). Modeling and attributional effects on children's achievement: A self-efficacy analysis. *Journal of Educational Psychology, 73,* 93–105.

Schunk, D. H. (1982). Effects of effort attributional feedback on children's perceived self-efficacy and achievement. *Journal of Educational Psychology, 74,* 548–556.

Schunk, D. H. (1985). Participation in goal setting: Effects on self-efficacy and skills of learning disabled children. *Journal of Special Education, 19,* 307–317.

Schunk, D. H. (2012). Social cognitive theory. In K. R. Harris, S. Graham, & T. Urdan (Eds.), *APA educational psychology handbook: Vol. 1. Theories, constructs, and critical issues* (pp. 101–123). Washington, DC: American Psychological Association.

Schunk, D. H., & Bursuck, W. D. (2016). Self-efficacy, agency, and volition: Student beliefs and reading motivation. In P. Afflerbach (Ed.), *Handbook of individual differences in reading: Reader, text, and context* (pp. 54–66). New York: Routledge.

Schunk, D. H., & DiBenedetto, M. K. (2014). Academic self-efficacy. In M. J. Furlong, R. Gilman, & E. S. Huebner (Eds.), *Handbook of positive psychology in schools* (pp. 115–130). New York: Routledge.

Schunk, D. H., & DiBenedetto, M. K. (2015). Self-efficacy: Educational aspects. In J. D. Wright (Ed.), *International encyclopedia of the social and behavioral sciences* (2nd ed., pp. 515–521). Oxford, UK: Elsevier.

Schunk, D. H., & DiBenedetto, M. K. (2016). Self-efficacy theory in education. In K. R. Wentzel & D. B. Miele (Eds.), *Handbook of motivation at school* (2nd ed., pp. 34–54). New York: Routledge.

Schunk, D. H., & Ertmer, P. A. (1999). Self-regulatory processes during computer skill acquisition: Goal and self-evaluative influences. *Journal of Educational Psychology, 91,* 251–260.

Schunk, D. H., & Ertmer, P. A. (2000). Self-regulation and academic learning: Self-efficacy enhancing interventions. In M. Boekaerts, P. R. Pintrich, & M. Zeidner (Eds.), *Handbook of self-regulation* (pp. 631–649). San Diego, CA: Academic Press.

Schunk, D. H., & Gunn, T. P. (1986). Self-efficacy and skill development: Influence of task strategies and attributions. *Journal of Educational Research, 79,* 238–244.

Schunk, D. H., Meece, J. L., & Pintrich, P. R. (2014). *Motivation in education: Theory, research, and applications* (4th ed.). Boston: Pearson Education.

Schunk, D. H., & Usher, E. L. (2011). Assessing self-efficacy for self-regulated learning. In B. J. Zimmerman & D. H. Schunk (Eds.), *Handbook of self-regulation of learning and performance* (pp. 282–297). New York: Routledge.

Schunk, D. H., & Usher, E. L. (2012). Social cognitive theory and motivation. In R. M. Ryan (Ed.), *Oxford handbook of human motivation* (pp. 13–27). New York: Oxford University Press.

Schunk, D. H., & Zimmerman, B. J. (1997). Social origins of self-regulatory competence. *Educational Psychologist, 32,* 195–208.

Schunk, D. H., & Zimmerman, B. J. (2006). Competence and control beliefs: Distinguishing the means and ends. In P. A. Alexander & P. H. Winne (Eds.), *Handbook of educational psychology* (2nd ed., pp. 349–367). Mahwah, NJ: Erlbaum.

Shavelson, R., & Bolus, R. (1982). Self-concept: The interplay of theory and methods. *Journal of Educational Psychology, 74,* 3–17.

Shell, D. F., Murphy, C. C., & Bruning, R. H. (1989). Self-efficacy and outcome expectancy mechanisms in reading and writing achievement. *Journal of Educational Psychology, 81,* 91–100.

Stajkovic, A. D., & Luthans, F. (1998). Self-efficacy and work-related performances: A meta-analysis. *Psychological Bulletin, 124,* 240–261.

Stipek, D. (2006). Relationships matter. *Educational Leadership, 64,* 46–49.

Stipek, D., Feiler, R., Daniels, D., & Milburn, S. (1995). Effects of different instructional approaches on young children's achievement and motivation. *Child Development, 66,* 209–223.

White, M. C., & DiBenedetto, M. K. (2015). *Self-regulation and the common core: Application to ELA standards.* New York: Routledge.

Wieber, F., Odenthal, G., & Gollwitzer, P. M. (2010). Self-efficacy feelings moderate implementation intention effects. *Self and Identity, 9,* 177–194.

Wigfield, A., Cambria, J., & Eccles, J. S. (2012). Motivation in education. In R. M. Ryan (Ed.), *Oxford handbook of human motivation* (pp. 463–478). Oxford, UK: Oxford University Press.

Wigfield, A., & Eccles, J. S. (2000). Expectancy-value theory of achievement motivation. *Contemporary Educational Psychology, 25,* 68–81.

Wigfield, A., & Eccles, J. S. (2002). The development of competence beliefs, expectancies for success, and achievement values from childhood through adolescence. In A. Wigfield & J. S. Eccles (Eds.), *Development of achievement motivation* (pp. 91–120). San Diego, CA: Academic Press.

Wigfield, A., Guthrie, J. T., Tonks, S., & Perencevich, K. C. (2004). Children's motivation for reading: Domain specificity and instructional influences. *Journal of Educational Research, 97,* 299–309.

Wigfield, A., Tonks, S., & Eccles, J. S. (2004). Expectancy-value theory in cross-cultural perspective. In D. M. McInerney & S. Van Etten (Eds.), *Research on sociocultural influences on motivation and learning: Vol. 4. Big theories revisited* (pp. 165–198). Greenwich, CT: Information Age.

Wigfield, A., Tonks, S., & Klauda, S. L. (2016). Expectancy-value theory. In K. R. Wentzel & D. B. Miele (Eds.), *Handbook of motivation at school* (2nd ed., pp. 55–76). New York: Routledge.

Williams, T., & Williams, K. (2010). Self-efficacy and performance in mathematics: Reciprocal determinism in 33 nations. *Journal of Educational Psychology, 102,* 453–466.

Winne, P. H., & Perry, N. E. (2000). Measuring self-regulated learning. In M. Boekaerts, P. R. Pintrich, & M. Zeidner (Eds.), *Handbook of self-regulation* (pp. 531–566). San Diego, CA: Academic Press.

Zimmerman, B. J. (1995). Self-efficacy and educational development. In A. Bandura (Ed.), *Self-efficacy in changing societies* (pp. 202–231). New York: Cambridge University Press.

Zimmerman, B. J. (2000). Attaining self-regulation: A social cognitive perspective. In M. Boekaerts, P. R. Pintrich, & M. Zeidner (Eds.), *Handbook of self-regulation* (pp. 13–39). San Diego, CA: Academic Press.

Zimmerman, B. J., & Bandura, A. (1994). Impact of self-regulatory influences on writing course achievement. *American Educational Research Journal, 31,* 845–862.

Zimmerman, B. J., & DiBenedetto, M. K. (2008). Mastery learning and assessment: Implications for students and teachers in an era of high stakes testing. *Psychology in the Schools, 45,* 206–216.

Zimmerman, B. J., & Schunk, D. H. (Eds.). (2011). *Handbook of self-regulation of learning and performance.* New York: Routledge.

CHAPTER 9

>>>>>>>>>>>>>>>>

Self-Efficacy

James E. Maddux
Evan M. Kleiman

Whether you think you can or whether you think you can't,
you're right.

—Henry Ford

People devote a lot of time, energy, and ingenuity to trying to predict and control the future—for the most part trying to achieve desirable outcomes and prevent undesirable ones. Doing this successfully depends largely on the capacity for self-regulation, which requires, among other things, a keen understanding of and confidence in one's skills and abilities. For this reason, the ability to predict and control our future depends on a robust sense of *self-efficacy*—our beliefs or expectancies about our ability to do what we believe is necessary to control our futures by achieving desired future outcomes and preventing undesirable ones. This chapter describes theory and research on how self-efficacy expectancies help us determine our futures, emphasizing outcomes relevant to psychological and physical health.

DEFINING SELF-EFFICACY EXPECTANCIES

Self-efficacy expectancies are expectancies about the ability to "organize and execute the courses of action required to produce given attainments" (Bandura, 1997, p. 3). Self-efficacy expectancies are not concerned with perceptions of skills and abilities divorced from situations; they are concerned, instead, with what people believe they can do with their skills and abilities under certain conditions. In addition, they are concerned not with expectancies about the ability to perform trivial motor acts but instead the ability to coordinate and orchestrate skills and abilities in changing and challenging situations. A good way to get a clearer sense of how self-efficacy is defined and measured is to understand how it differs from other concepts that deal with perceptions of competence and control.

Self-efficacy expectancies first need to be distinguished from *outcome expectancies* (Bandura, 1977, 1997) or *behavior-outcome expectancies* (Maddux, 1999). Self-efficacy expectancies are beliefs about how well one will be able to mobilize one's resources to perform behaviors believed necessary for attaining valued goals. An outcome expectancy is a "judgment of the likely consequence such performances will produce" (Bandura, 1997, p. 21). Thus, as people contemplate a goal and approach a task, they consider what behaviors and strategies are necessary to produce the outcome they want, and they evaluate the extent to which they are able to perform those behaviors and implement those strategies. Despite this conceptual distinction, research indicates that self-efficacy expectancies and outcome expectancies are not totally empirically independent and can influence each other in both directions (Williams, 2010) and that in some studies measures of self-efficacy expectancies may be measuring motivation to perform a behavior rather than perceived ability to perform it (Williams & Rhodes, 2014).

Self-efficacy expectancies are not *competencies*. Competencies are "the quality and range of the cognitive constructions and behavioral enactments of which the individual is capable" (Mischel, 1973, p. 266). Self-efficacy expectancies are expectancies regarding one's ability to exercise one's competencies in certain domains and situations.

Self-efficacy expectancies are not simply *predictions* about behavior. They are concerned not with what people believe they *will* do but with what they believe they *can* do under certain circumstances, especially challenging and changing circumstances.

Self-efficacy expectancies are not *intentions* to behave or intentions to attain particular goals. Intentions are what people say they are committed to doing or accomplishing—what they say they *will* do, not what they say they *can* do. Intentions are influenced by a number of factors, including self-efficacy expectancies (Maddux, 1999; Zhao, Seibert, & Hills, 2005). In addition, self-efficacy expectancies can influence behavior directly and indirectly through their influence on intentions (Bandura, 1999).

Self-efficacy is not *perceived control*. The perception of control over something depends on both self-efficacy expectancies and behavior-outcome expectancies (Kirsch, 1999; Maddux, 1999).

Finally, self-efficacy is not a *trait*. Although several measures of trait-like general efficacy expectancies have been developed (e.g., Chen, Gully, & Eden, 2001; Sherer et al., 1982) and have been used extensively in research, they generally have not demonstrated predictive value above that of domain-specific self-efficacy measures (Urdan & Pajares, 2006). In addition, a meta-analysis involving 209 studies found that correlations among various measures of general self-efficacy, locus of control, self-esteem, and neuroticism were sufficiently strong that they may be "alternative markers of a single underlying construct" (Judge, Erez, Bono, & Thoresen, 2002, p. 696; see also Windle, Markland, & Woods, 2008, for similar findings.) If our goal is to understand the role of self-efficacy expectancies in the process of self-regulation, then viewing self-efficacy as a belief or expectancy as a component of self-regulation that interacts with other components of self-regulation will be more useful than viewing it as a trait. (See Maddux & Volkmann, 2010, for a discussion of the influence of personality on the development of self-efficacy expectancies.)

MEASURING SELF-EFFICACY EXPECTANCIES

To be useful in research and practice, concepts need to be translated into operational definitions that lead to precise methods of measurement that are consistent across studies. Unfortunately, self-efficacy has been measured in such a wide variety of ways that comparing findings from one study to another often is difficult (e.g., Forsyth & Carey, 1998). For this reason, a few guidelines for measuring self-efficacy expectancies might be useful.

First, researchers should make sure that they are not inadvertently measuring one of the constructs previously described (e.g., outcome expectancies, intentions) and calling it a measure of self-efficacy. In addition, measures of self-efficacy expectancies "must be tailored to the particular domain of functioning that is the object of interest" (Bandura, 2006, pp. 307–308) (e.g., social skills, exercise, dieting, safe sex, math skills). Within a given domain, self-efficacy expectancies can be measured at varying degrees of behavioral and situational specificity, depending on what behavior or attainment one is trying to predict. Thus the measurement of self-efficacy expectancies should be designed to capture the important characteristics of the behavior and the context in which it occurs.

Specifying behaviors and contexts improves the predictive power of self-efficacy measures, but specificity can reach a point of diminishing returns if carried too far. Therefore, the researcher must have a thorough understanding of the behavioral domain in question, including the types of abilities called upon and the range of situations in which they might be used (Bandura, 1997, 2006). The information about behaviors and situations that is essential for constructing self-efficacy measures can be acquired by interviewing and surveying people who are trying to change the behavior of interest, such as people who are trying to lose weight or engage in regular exercise (Bandura, 1997, 2006). (For additional guidelines, see Bandura, 1997, pp. 42–50, and Bandura, 2006).

Measures of self-efficacy also must be concerned with gradations of challenge (Bandura, 2006). Tasks and situations differ in the degree of challenge that they present, and self-efficacy measures should reflect these differences. For example, a measure of smoker abstinence self-efficacy expectancies should include a range of situations that differ in the challenges they present to the struggling nonsmoker (e.g., after a meal, while having a drink or cup of coffee, when offered a cigarette). Self-efficacy measures can err in the direction of being not specific enough. For example, "How confident are you that you will be able to stick to your diet when tempted to break it?" is a poor measure of self-efficacy for dieting because how challenging dieting is varies from situation to situation. A good measure of self-efficacy should include a range of situations that offer a range of challenges from relatively easy to very difficult. For example, "How confident are you that you will be able to stick to your diet when watching television/when depressed/when someone offers you high-fat food/when eating breakfast at a restaurant?" is a good measure because it includes an appropriate range of situations in which dieting could be challenging. Typically, these items include a Likert-type scale (e.g., 1–7, 1–10, 1–100). Self-efficacy measures also can err in the direction of excessive specificity. For example, an assessment of self-efficacy expectancies for engaging in safe sex might include the (good) item "How confident are you that you could resist your partner's insistence that using a condom isn't necessary?" But an item that asks "How confident are you that you could open the condom wrapper?" probably is neither necessary nor useful. Likewise, a good measure of self-efficacy for exercise might include an item concerning confidence in "your ability to fit a short walk or run into a busy day," but asking about confidence in "your ability to tie your running shoes" is probably going a little too far.

ARE SELF-EFFICACY EXPECTANCIES CAUSES OF BEHAVIOR?

The importance of self-efficacy expectancies depends on the assumption that they have some causal impact on behavior. Bandura and Locke (2003) summarized the findings of nine large meta-analyses conducted on work-related performances in both laboratory and field studies (Sadri & Robertson, 1993; Stajkovic & Luthans, 1998), psychosocial functioning in children and adolescents (Holden, Moncher, Schinke, & Barker, 1990), academic achievement and persistence (Multon, Brown, & Lent, 1991), health functioning (Holden, 1991), athletic performance (Moritz, Feltz, Fahrbach, & Mack, 2000), laboratory studies in which self-efficacy expectancies were altered experimentally (Boyer et al., 2000), and collective efficacy in groups (Gully, Incalcaterra, Joshi, & Beaubien, 2002; Stajkovic & Lee, 2001). In sum, the studies reviewed by Bandura and Locke (2003) traversed various domains of functioning and types of measures of self-efficacy beliefs and used between-groups designs that compared groups of individuals experimentally raised to different levels of perceived efficacy and within-groups designs in which the same individuals were progressively raised to greater perceived self-efficacy. They concluded that "[t]he evidence from these meta-analyses is consistent in showing that efficacy expectancies contribute significantly to the level of motivation and performance" (p. 87). (See Bandura & Locke, 2003, for a more in-depth discussion of this research.)

MAJOR INFLUENCES ON SELF-EFFICACY EXPECTANCIES

Self-efficacy expectancies are the result of information integrated from five sources: performance experience, vicarious experience, verbal persuasion, imaginal experience, and affective and physiological states.

One's own *performance experiences* are the most powerful influences on self-efficacy beliefs (Bandura, 1977, 1997); expectancies about being able to perform a particular task under particular conditions are the result of past attempts at performing the task. Success that one attributes to one's own efforts will strengthen self-efficacy for performing that particular behavior under those particular circumstances. The perception that one has failed usually diminishes self-efficacy. Most experimental studies, in fact, have relied on positive or negative performance feedback to either enhance or diminish self-efficacy beliefs (e.g., Bandura & Jourden, 1991).

Self-efficacy expectancies also are influenced by *vicarious experiences*—observations of the behavior of others and the consequences of that behavior (Bandura, 1997). We see what other people are capable of doing in certain situations and form expectancies about our own capacities in those situations, depending on the extent to which we believe that we are similar to the person we observed (the "model"). The greater the perceived similarity, the greater the influence on self-efficacy beliefs. Learning by observing others is also termed *observational learning* or learning that occurs via *modeling*. In addition to the characteristics of the model, other factors that affect the impact of observational learning include how closely we observe the model, how well and accurately we remember the observed behavior, how clearly we can imagine ourselves engaging in the behavior, and how motivated we are to perform it (see also Morgenroth, Ryan, & Peters, 2015). Vicarious experiences generally have weaker effects on self-efficacy expectancy than do actual performance experiences (e.g., Ferrari, 1996).

Self-efficacy expectancies are also influenced by *verbal persuasion*—what other people tell us about our abilities and probabilities of success. The power of verbal persuasion is influenced by factors such as the expertness, trustworthiness, and attractiveness of the source, as suggested by decades of research on verbal persuasion and attitude change (Petty & Brinol, 2010). Verbal persuasion is a less powerful source of enduring change in self-efficacy than are performance experiences and vicarious experiences.

We can also influence our self-efficacy expectancies by *imagining* ourselves behaving effectively or ineffectively in hypothetical situations. Such images can be inadvertent thoughts, or they can be used as an intentional self-efficacy-enhancement strategy. These images may be derived from actual or vicarious experiences with situations similar to the one anticipated, or they may be induced by verbal persuasion, as when a psychotherapist guides a client through imagination-based interventions such as systematic desensitization and covert modeling (Williams, 2016). Images of performing successfully in challenging situations have been used to strengthen self-efficacy expectancies for a variety of tasks, athletic behaviors, and social behaviors, including job interview performance (Knudstrup, Segrest, & Hurley, 2003), golf putting (Short et al., 2002), and climbing (Jones, Mace, Bray, MacRae, & Stockbridge, 2002). In addition, *mental contrasting*—imagining having attained a goal and imagining current obstacles to the goal—can help people translate self-efficacy beliefs into actual behavior (e.g., Oettingen, 2012, 2014).

Physiological and emotional states negatively influence self-efficacy when we learn to associate poor performance or perceived failure with aversive physiological arousal. They positively influence self-efficacy when we learn to associate success with positive emotions. When we become aware of unpleasant physiological sensations (e.g., anxiety, fatigue, pain), we are more likely to doubt our competence than if our physiological sensations are pleasant or neutral (e.g., Hoeppner, Kahler, & Gwaltney, 2014). When our physiological sensations are not distracting or overwhelming, we can attend to the task at hand. Most importantly, the interpretation of physiological sensations during a task is a key contributor to self-efficacy and performance (Ciani, Easter, Summers, & Posada, 2009). For example, if I were giving a talk in front of a large audience and was pacing energetically across the stage, I might notice an increase in my heart rate. If I were to accurately attribute that increase in heart rate to my energetic pacing, I would probably not feel anxious, but if I attribute it to performance, I might be distracted from the task at hand, which might cause both an increase in anxiety and a decrease in my confidence in my ability to give the talk.

DEVELOPMENTAL ASPECTS OF SELF-EFFICACY EXPECTANCIES

Moment-to-moment learning experiences culminate over time to become well-informed self-efficacy expectancies. With each subsequent developmental period, the individual faces new demands and challenges that can build or diminish self-efficacy in various domains of life. This process begins in infancy and continues throughout the lifespan. The early development of self-efficacy expectancies is influenced by: (1) the development of the capacity for symbolic thought, (2) the development of a sense of a "self" that is separate from others, and (3) the observation of the reciprocal, cause–effect relationship between behavior and outcomes (Bandura, 1997).

As infants' capacity for symbolic thought and memory increases, they can begin to imagine and even anticipate or predict events in their environment (Mandler, 1992; Stack & Poulin-Dubois, 1998). They also realize that they are distinct from others and from objects. They develop a sense of personal agency by performing the few actions of which they are capable, such as flailing their arms and legs, cooing, and grabbing and shaking objects. With repeated observations of actions and their consequences, they learn cause–effect relationships and begin to understand that they can affect their environments. As they become increasingly aware that outcomes are contingent upon their behavior, infants will attempt novel actions and examine their outcomes. These observations provide an understanding of the control they have over their surroundings (Bandura, 1997; Berry & West, 1993).

Learning often occurs in the presence of others, either through observation or through an interaction between the child and a parent, caregiver, teacher, or peer. Observational studies of parent–child interactions in infancy show that, rather than being passive recipients of their social environment, infants anticipate, instigate, mirror, and respond to their parents' emotional expressions and behaviors (Stack & Poulin-Dubois, 1998). Caregivers' responses to children's attempts at exercising agency can play an important role in the development of children's self-efficacy expectancies and a general sense of control (Dan, Sagi-Schwartz, Bar-Haim, & Eshel, 2011; Junttila, Vauras, & Laakkonen, 2007). Caregivers can model effective self-regulation and perseverance, or they can model ineffective strategies and hasty goal abandonment. Further, by choosing tasks that are developmentally appropriate but challenging, parents can provide positive learning experiences through verbal encouragement and "scaffolding," meaning providing assistance and gradually removing it as the child learns (Mattanah, Pratt, Cowan, & Cowan, 2005).

Attending school for the first time provides new opportunities for feedback, social comparison, interpersonal interactions, and resulting self-efficacy development in academic and social domains (Urdan & Schoenfelder, 2006). Children's self-regulatory skills are tested as they struggle to wait their turn, vie for attention from the teacher and peers, try to sustain attention during class, complete tasks, and sit quietly. Interpersonal skills are developed through social interactions, as well as through imaginative or pretend play with dolls or toys and through role playing with others (Singer, 1998). Interpersonal feedback that is supportive and informative allows children to practice and improve these skills. Academic skills are similarly developed through specific feedback, modeling, encouragement, and self-observation. These early evaluative experiences contribute to academic self-efficacy, potentially influencing motivation, goal setting, expectations of success or failure, academic anxiety, academic performance, and future interpretations of feedback (Urdan & Pajares, 2006; Schunk & DiBenedetto, Chapter 8, this volume; see also Stipek, 2002). As always, context matters; differences in political systems and their respective educational contexts predicted differences among schoolchildren not only in agency beliefs but also in the relation between agency beliefs and performance (Little, Oettingen, Stetsenko, & Baltes, 1995; Oettingen, Little, Lindenberger, & Baltes, 1994)

With adolescence comes the need to manage and adapt to changes across multiple domains of life, including peer relationships, educational demands, biological changes and sexual development, romantic relationships, and demands for increasing autonomy and responsibility—such as making decisions about sex, substance use, and college or career goals. Although self-efficacy expectancies about self-regulatory abilities tend to decline during adolescence (Vecchio, Gerbino, Pastorelli, Del Bove, & Caprara, 2007), these expectancies remain strong predictors of important outcomes in many areas (Zimmerman & Cleary, 2006). For example, general life satisfaction in late adolescence is better predicted by academic and social self-efficacy expectancies in early adolescence than by popularity among peers or academic achievement (Vecchio et al., 2007). Adolescents with a stronger sense of self-efficacy to overcome peer pressure are less likely to abuse substances, engage in unsafe sexual behavior, and engage in delinquent behavior (Caprara et al., 1998; Ludwig & Pittman, 1999). In addition, self-efficacy expectancies for regulating positive and negative emotions predict self-efficacy in the domains of academics, empathy for others, and resistance of peer pressure, ultimately leading to greater prosocial behavior, less delinquent behavior, and lower risk of depression (Bandura, Caprara, Barbaranelli, Gerbino, & Pastorelli, 2003). Adolescents who are more confident that they can effectively regulate their own emotions when communicating with their parents, manage stressful or sensitive conversations, and evoke parental perspective taking report greater satisfaction with family life, more open communication with their parents, and less distrust and conflict over parental monitoring of their activities (Caprara, Pastorelli, Regalia, Scabini, & Bandura, 2005). Parental involvement and open communication, in turn, contribute positively to adolescents' self-efficacy (Bandura, 2005; Fan & Williams, 2010; Schunk & Meece, 2006; see Oettingen & Gollwitzer, 2015, for additional information about self-regulation during adolescence).

Adulthood brings additional concerns and demands, primarily in the domains of work and interpersonal roles. Expectancies about job-related abilities influence occupational choices, career paths, job-seeking behavior, job performance, salary and promotion, and job satisfaction (Abele & Spurk, 2009; see Betz, 2007, for a review). These expectancies, therefore, have the potential to greatly influence one's future in a pervasive and long-term manner. Further, job satisfaction and a sense of personal accomplishment in the realm of work predict a sense of self-worth and general well-being (Russell, 2008). Greater parenting self-efficacy is related to greater parenting competence and use of effective parenting strategies (Jones & Prinz, 2005), as well as less parenting stress and depression for both mothers and fathers (Sevigny & Loutzenhiser, 2010). In addition, parents who have higher goals for their children and who feel highly efficacious about their ability to advance their children's intellectual growth are likely to have children with higher academic self-efficacy, which fosters greater academic achievement and higher career goal setting (Bandura, Barbaranelli, Caprara, & Pastorelli, 1996, 2001).

For a variety of reasons (including declines in physical and psychological health and social support), in later life, self-efficacy often diminishes for a wide array of major life domains, including health, relationships, and cognitive tasks such as memory (McAvay, Seeman, & Rodin, 1996). Nevertheless, self-efficacy can still be improved in older age. For example, memory self-efficacy and performance on memory tasks among older adults can be improved through memory training techniques that target the factors that affect self-efficacy, including incremental (gradual, step-by-step) personal mastery experiences, vicarious learning experiences, verbal encouragement, and mitigation of anxiety (West, Bagwell, & Dark-Freudeman, 2008). Although age-related declines in efficacy expectancies may reflect actual declines in ability, providing incentives to exercise one's memory can enhance subsequent memory performance. Similarly, in order for older adults to reap the benefits of physical exercise, self-efficacy for exercise behavior should also be bolstered (McAuley, 1993). Among the infirm aged, the structure and organization of institutions (e.g., assisted living facilities and hospitals) may actually diminish self-efficacy in important domains by limiting mastery experiences (Welch & West, 1995). The children of older adults and the institutions that serve older adults should be mindful of the extent to which they provide opportunities for strengthening self-efficacy expectancies for the tasks of everyday life.

SELF-EFFICACY EXPECTANCIES AND SELF-REGULATION

The most important effects of self-efficacy expectancies on behavior result from their role in self-regulation. Research on self-efficacy has added greatly to our understanding of how people guide their own behavior in the pursuit of their goals and how they sometimes fail to do so effectively. All major theories of self-regulation (Baumeister, Vohs, & Tice, 2007; Cervone, Shadel, Smith, & Fiori, 2006; Gross, 1998; Karoly, 2010) assume that self-regulation is a complex system that consists of a set of component skills that can be learned and improved with practice. They also acknowledge the importance to successful regulation of a strong belief that one can attain the goal in question through one's own efforts.

Self-efficacy expectancies influence self-regulation in a number of ways (Bandura, 1997; Bandura & Locke, 2003). They influence the goals people choose and the tasks they decide to tackle. The higher one's self-efficacy in a specific domain is, the loftier the goals that one sets in that domain are (e.g., Tabernero & Wood, 2009).

They are an important influence on *motivational readiness*–"the willingness or inclination, whether or not ultimately realized, to act in the service of a desire" (Kruglanski, Chernikova, Rosenzweig, & Kopetz, 2014)—a precursor to self-regulation.

They influence people's choices of goal-directed activities (their plans), allocation of resources, effort, persistence in the face of challenges and obstacles, and reactions to perceived discrepancies between goals and current performance (Bandura, 1997; Bandura & Locke, 2003; Vancouver, More, & Yoder, 2008). In the face of difficulties, people with weak self-efficacy expectancies easily develop doubts

about their ability to accomplish the task at hand, whereas those with strong efficacy expectancies are more likely to continue their efforts to master a task when difficulties arise. Perseverance usually produces desired results, and this success then
strengthens the individual's self-efficacy expectancies. Motivation to accomplish
difficult tasks and accomplish lofty goals is enhanced by overestimates of personal
capabilities (i.e., positive illusions; Taylor & Brown, 1988), which then become self-
fulfilling prophecies when people set their sights high, persevere, and then surpass
their previous levels of accomplishments.

They influence *self-evaluative reactions* to feedback. People do not simply perceive information; they *interpret* it. Likewise, feedback about progress toward or
away from a goal is interpreted, and different people will interpret the same feedback in different ways and thus react to it differently. Thus *self-evaluative reactions*
are important in self-regulation because people's expectancies about the progress
they are making (or not making) toward their goals are major determinants of
their emotional reactions during goal-directed activity. These emotional reactions,
in turn, can either enhance or disrupt self-regulation (Larsen & Prizmic, 2004).
The belief that one is inefficacious and making poor progress toward a valued
goal produces distressing emotional states (e.g., anxiety, depression) that can lead
to cognitive and behavioral ineffectiveness and self-regulatory failure. The belief
that one is making good progress can be psychologically energizing and can lead
to persistence. Research suggests, in fact, not only that monitoring progress toward
a goal enhances goal attainment (Harkin et al., 2016) but also that performance
feedback moderates the relationship between self-efficacy expectancies and performance, possibly because it allows people to more accurately monitor their progress
over time (Beattie, Woodman, Fakehy, & Dempsey, 2016) or encourages people to
engage in mental contrasting of desired future goals with current obstacles (Oettingen, Marquardt, & Gollwitzer, 2012; Sevincer & Oettingen, 2013).

Self-efficacy for solving problems and making decisions influences the efficiency and effectiveness of problem solving and decision making. When faced with
complex decisions, people who have confidence in their ability to solve problems
are able to think more clearly and make better decisions than do people who doubt
their cognitive skills (e.g., Bandura, 1997). Such efficacy usually leads to better
solutions and greater achievement. In the face of difficulty, people with high self-
efficacy are more likely to remain *task diagnostic* and to search for solutions to problems. Those with low self-efficacy, however, are more likely to become *self-diagnostic*
and reflect on their inadequacies, which distracts them from their efforts to assess
and solve the problem (Bandura, 1997).

Self-efficacy expectancies can influence self-regulation through their effects
on causal attribution (i.e., explanations for causes of events, including one's own
behavior and its consequences). Self-efficacy expectancies can influence causal
attributions and vice versa because expectancies about competencies can influence
explanations of success and failure and because explanations for success and failure will, in turn, influence perceptions of competence (e.g., Stajkovic & Sommer,
2000; Tolli & Schmidt, 2008). For example, individuals with low self-efficacy for
an activity are more likely to attribute success in that activity to external factors,
whereas individuals with high self-efficacy are likely to attribute success to personal
capabilities (Bandura, 1992; Schunk, 1995). Individuals with lower self-efficacy are

also more likely to attribute failure to lack of ability than lack of skill, whereas individuals with higher self-efficacy are more likely to attribute failure to lack of effort (e.g., Sherman, 2002). In the other direction, research shows that individuals who make causal attributions for a negative event that involve stable and global causes and lead to negative future implications show decreased self-efficacy (Bennett, Adams, & Ricks, 2012; Hirschy & Morris, 2002). For example, an individual who attributes failure to his or her stable, global characteristics and has negative implications for the future (e.g., "I failed because I am dumb and will always be that way") will likely show decreased self-efficacy in the area in which he or she has failed. Finally, research also suggests that self-efficacy expectancies mediate the relationship between attributions and behavioral intentions and between attributions and behavior (Nickel & Spink, 2010; Shields, Brawley, & Lindover, 2006; Spink & Nickel, 2009).

Self-efficacy expectancies may influence *self-regulatory fatigue*. Some research suggests that self-regulation is a limited resource that is temporarily depleted when people exercise it, including when they make choices and decisions (Doerr & Baumeister, 2010; Kelley, Wagner, & Heatherton, 2015). Why this happens is unclear, but research points to fatigue in the ability to self-regulate, much like fatigue from an overused muscle (Hagger, Wood, Stiff, & Chatzisarantis, 2010; Muraven & Baumeister, 2000); a shift from engaging in effortful control to seeking reward (DeBono, Shmueli, & Muraven, 2011); or a change in preferences (Inzlicht, Legault, & Teper, 2014). A person with strong self-efficacy expectancies in a specific domain may be less likely to experience self-regulatory depletion or fatigue in that domain. People differ in the amount of effortful control they require to perform a specific activity. For example, decision making in a particular situation may require more effortful control for people with lower self-efficacy for decision making in that situation. Therefore, people with stronger self-efficacy expectancies for decision making in that situation may be less vulnerable than people with weaker self-efficacy to postdecision self-regulatory depletion. This notion is generally consistent with research suggesting that people self-regulate more effectively when they are induced to believe that self-regulation is *not* a limited resource that becomes depleted when used (Job, Walton, Bernecker, & Dweck, 2015).

People with stronger self-efficacy expectancies in a given domain are also more likely to set *learning goals* (i.e., goals concerned with improving one's skills) than *performance goals* (i.e., goals concerned with proving one's skills or avoiding looking bad) and are therefore more likely to respond resiliently to challenges and setbacks (Maddux & Goselen, 2012; see also Dweck & Yeager, Chapter 18, this volume).

The translation of self-efficacy beliefs into action can be facilitated by engaging in mental contrasting (noted previously)—imagining goal attainment and then imagining present obstacles to the goal—whereas the translation is unaffected by reverse contrasting—thinking first about obstacles and then about the goal (Kappes, Singmann, & Oettingen, 2012; Oettingen, 2012). Self-efficacy beliefs also can moderate the effect of implementation intentions ("if–then" plans) on behavior (e.g., Wieber, Odenthal, & Gollwitzer, 2010); people are more likely to implement a behavior if they believe they can. Moreover, self-efficacy expectancies can be strengthened by creating implementation intentions specifically for increasing self-efficacy prior to beginning a challenging task (Bayer & Gollwitzer, 2007).

CAN SELF-EFFICACY EXPECTANCIES SOMETIMES BE TOO STRONG?

Most of the research on the effect of self-efficacy on self-regulation suggests that "more is better"—that the stronger one's self-efficacy expectancies are, the more effective one's self-regulation in pursuit of a goal will be. But can self-efficacy expectancies be "too strong"? Perhaps so, in at least three ways.

First, as Bandura (1986) suggested, "a reasonable accurate appraisal of one's capabilities is . . . of considerable value in effective functioning" and that people who overestimate their abilities may "undertake activities that are clearly beyond their reach" (p. 393). Certainly an important feature of effective self-regulation is to know when to disengage from a goal because one's efforts are not paying off. Although strong self-efficacy expectancies usually contribute to adaptive tenacity, expectancies that are unrealistically high may result in the relentless pursuit of an unattainable goal. Thus strong self-efficacy expectancies that are not supported by past experience or rewarded by feedback that indicates progress toward one's goal can result in wasted effort and resources that might be better directed elsewhere. In fact, overconfidence in one's abilities to change are the heart of what has been referred to as the *false hope syndrome:* "a cycle of failure and renewed effort . . . characterized by unrealistic expectations about the likely speed, amount, ease, and consequences of self-change attempts" (Polivy & Herman, 2002, p. 677). As of yet, however, we have no way of determining when self-efficacy is "too strong" and at what point people should give up trying to achieve their goals. Many successful individuals throughout history have long records of failure and rejection before reaching success through sheer persistence for many years. To pathologize persistence and endurance is to pathologize most of the movers, shakers, and innovators in music, literature, science, politics, and most other fields.

Second, the way in which strong self-efficacy expectancies develop can affect their impact on behavior. Self-efficacy expectancies that are not warranted by past success can lead to complacency and diminished effort and performance over time (Yang, Chuang, & Chiou, 2009), as well as an increased willingness to engage in potentially dangerous behaviors, such as using a cell phone while driving (Schlehofer et al., 2010). Further, people who develop strong self-efficacy expectancies without effort and struggle may set lower goals and may be satisfied with lower quality performance, compared with those who attain strong efficacy expectancies through hard work of progressive mastery, possibly because "[c]omplacent self-assurance creates little incentive to expend the increased effort needed to attain high levels of performance" (Bandura & Jourden, 1991, p. 949).

Third, people may be less likely to seek needed help when self-efficacy is greater than actual abilities. For example, smokers with an inflated sense of self-efficacy to quit smoking are less inclined to enroll in programs to quit smoking and may have less success in quitting smoking (Duffy, Scheumann, Fowler, Darling-Fisher, & Terrell, 2010). This potential disadvantage of unrealistically high self-efficacy and decreased help seeking may apply to other domains, including one's ability to regulate alcohol and other substance use, diet, exercise, and many other behaviors that involve self-regulation. The strategy of mental contrasting noted previously may prevent or ameliorate self-efficacy expectancies that are not in line with abilities by calling attention to and promoting analysis of current obstacles to a goal.

SELF-EFFICACY AND PSYCHOLOGICAL HEALTH AND WELL-BEING

A sense of control over one's behavior, one's environment, and one's own thoughts and feelings is essential for happiness and a sense of well-being. When the world seems predictable and controllable, and when behaviors, thoughts, and emotions seem within their control, people are better able to pursue valued goals, successfully meet life's challenges, build healthy relationships, and achieve personal satisfaction and peace of mind. A weak sense of control is common among people who seek the help of psychotherapists and counselors. Subjective well-being is a broad term that involves how people experience the quality of their lives (Diener, 1984) and includes constructs such as life satisfaction and positive affect. Several studies find that strong self-efficacy expectancies explain how some personality traits (e.g., openness to new experiences) lead to greater subjective well-being. For example, one study found that general self-efficacy mediated the relationship between openness to new experiences and higher levels of subjective well-being (Strobel, Tumasjan, & Spörrle, 2011), perhaps because people who are more open to new experiences are more likely to enter novel situations and explore novel behaviors, which might lead to stronger self-efficacy beliefs and a greater number of success experiences, which then leads to greater well-being.

Expectations of positive and negative future events and states can also influence our sense of well-being in the present. Self-efficacy is an important part of these predictions of future outcomes. Self-efficacy is related to our perceptions of the likelihood of positive future events (i.e., positive future-thinking) and our expectations about positive outcomes from our actions (i.e., optimism).

Positive future-thinking refers to a high perceived likelihood of self-relevant future positive events (MacLeod & Byrne, 1996). Positive future-thinking is positively associated with a variety of beneficial outcomes and negatively associated with a variety of negative outcomes (e.g., suicidal thoughts; Hirsch et al., 2007). Many studies find that stronger self-efficacy expectancies (both general and domain-specific) are associated with stronger expectancies of positive future outcomes in both adolescents and adults (Caprara, Steca, Gerbino, Pacielloi, & Vecchio, 2006; Caprara & Steca, 2006; Epel, Bandura, & Zimbardo, 1999; Kerpelman, Eryigit, & Stephens, 2007).

Although conceptually similar to positive future-thinking, *dispositional optimism*—the tendency to expect positive outcomes from one's actions (Carver, Scheier, & Segerstrom, 2010)—is studied as a distinct construct. Dispositional optimism is consistently linked to positive physical and psychological well-being outcomes (Scheier & Carver, 1993). It is unclear whether having stronger self-efficacy expectancies makes us more optimistic or if being dispositionally more optimistic leads to stronger self-efficacy expectancies. The studies showing a positive relationship between dispositional optimism and self-efficacy (e.g., Waldrop, Lightsey, Ethington, Woemmel, & Coke, 2001) are cross-sectional and do not allow us to determine the temporal causality in the relationship between optimism and self-efficacy. At least one cross-sectional study found that a model in which dispositional optimism mediated the relation between general self-efficacy and life satisfaction fit the data better than a model in which optimism mediated the relation between optimism and life satisfaction (Karademas, 2006). This finding might suggest that self-efficacy precedes optimism, but such inferences can only be verified with longitudinal data.

Theory and research on *hope,* a construct highly similar to optimism, finds that both self-efficacy expectancies (general and domain-specific) and outcome expectancies are important components of hopeful and optimistic thinking about the future (Snyder, 2002).

In addition, individuals with high self-efficacy tend to have more rewarding interpersonal relationships. For example, individuals with greater social self-efficacy (i.e., self-efficacy specific to maintaining interpersonal relationships) experience greater social support and feel less lonely (Wei, Russell, & Zakalik, 2005). This relationship seems to be bidirectional, because other studies find that greater social support from parents and friends leads to greater general self-efficacy (Vieno, Santinello, Pastore, & Perkins, 2007). In addition, the more efficacious spouses (Kaplan & Maddux, 2002) and dating couples (Zapata, 2006) feel about their shared ability to accomplish important shared goals, the more satisfied they are with their relationships. Self-efficacy expectancies also play a major role in a number of common psychological problems and successful psychological interventions. Low self-efficacy expectancies are an important feature of depression (Bandura, Pastorelli, Barbaranelli, & Caprara, 1999; Blazer, 2002; Maddux & Meier, 1995; Riskind, Alloy, & Iacoviello, 2010; Sacco et al., 2005; Wei et al., 2005). People with depression usually believe they are less capable than other people of behaving effectively in many important areas of life. They usually doubt their ability to form and maintain supportive relationships and therefore may avoid potentially supportive people during periods of depression.

Dysfunctional anxiety and avoidant behavior are often the direct result of low self-efficacy expectancies for managing threatening situations (Ahmed & Westra, 2009; Bandura, 1997; Gaudiano & Herbert, 2007; Nicholls, Polman, & Levy, 2010; Preiss, Gayle, & Allen, 2006; Thomasson & Psouni, 2010; Williams, 2016). People who have strong confidence in their abilities to perform and manage potentially difficult situations approach those situations calmly and are not unduly disrupted by difficulties. On the other hand, people who lack confidence in their abilities will either avoid potentially difficult situations or approach them with apprehension, thereby reducing the probability that they will perform effectively. Thus they have fewer success experiences and fewer opportunities to increase their self-efficacy. People with low self-efficacy also respond to difficulties with increased anxiety, which usually disrupts performance, thereby further lowering self-efficacy, and so on. Stressful events often result in physical (e.g., headache) as well as psychological symptoms, and self-efficacy expectancies influence the relationship between stressful events and physical symptoms (Arnstein, Caudill, Mandle, Norris, & Beasley, 1999; Marlowe, 1998). Self-efficacy expectancies also predict effective coping with traumatic life events such as homelessness (Epel et al., 1999), natural disasters, terrorist attacks, and criminal assaults (Benight & Bandura, 2004).

For people with substance abuse problems, self-efficacy for avoiding relapse in high-risk situations and self-efficacy for recovery from relapse predict successful treatment and abstinence (e.g., Kelly, Magill, & Stout, 2009; Van Zundert, Ferguson, Shiffman, & Engels, 2010). The same is true in the successful treatment of people with eating disorders (e.g., Cain, Bardone-Cone, Abramson, Vohs, & Joiner, 2008; Pinto, Guarda, Heinberg, & DiClemente, 2006) and of male sex offenders (e.g., Sawyer & Pettman, 2006; Wheeler, George, & Marlatt, 2006).

Self-efficacy expectancies are also important in psychological interventions and psychotherapy. Most professionally guided interventions, including psychotherapy, are designed to enhance self-regulation because they are concerned with helping people increase a sense of efficacy over important aspects of their lives (Frank & Frank, 1991). Different interventions may be equally effective because they equally enhance self-efficacy for crucial behavioral and cognitive skills (Ahmed & Westra, 2009; Benight & Bandura, 2004; Moos, 2008). Self-efficacy theory emphasizes the importance of arranging a client's experiences in a way that enhances his or her sense of efficacy for specific behaviors in specific problematic and challenging situations. Self-efficacy theory also suggests that formal interventions should provide people with the skills and sense of efficacy for solving problems themselves.

SELF-EFFICACY AND PHYSICAL HEALTH AND WELL-BEING

Most strategies for preventing health problems, enhancing health, and hastening recovery from illness and injury involve changing behavior. In addition, psychology and physiology are tightly intertwined, such that affective and cognitive phenomena are influenced by physiological phenomena and vice versa (e.g., Smith, 2008). Thus expectancies about self-efficacy influence health in two ways—through their influence over the behaviors that influence health and through their direct influence over physiological processes.

First, self-efficacy influences the adoption of healthy behaviors, the cessation of unhealthy behaviors, and the maintenance of behavioral changes in the face of challenge and difficulty. Research on self-efficacy has greatly enhanced our understanding of how and why people adopt healthy and unhealthy behaviors and of how they can most effectively change behaviors that affect health (Bandura, 1997; Maddux, Brawley, & Boykin, 1995; Maddux & Gosselin, 2012). All of the major theories of health behavior—such as protection motivation theory (Maddux & Rogers, 1983), the health belief model (Strecher, Champion, & Rosenstock, 1997), the theory of reasoned action/planned behavior (Ajzen, 1998; Maddux & DuCharme, 1997), the transtheoretical stages-of-change model (Prochaska & Prochaska, 2010), and the health action process model (Schwarzer, Lippke, & Luszczynska, 2011)—include self-efficacy as a key component (see also Maddux, 1993).

In addition, self-efficacy expectancies are crucial to successful change and maintenance of virtually every behavior crucial to health, including exercise, diet, stress management, safe sex (O'Leary, Jemmott, & Jemmott, 2008), smoking cessation, overcoming alcohol abuse, dealing with chronic pain, compliance with treatment and prevention regimens, and detection behaviors such as breast self-examinations (AbuSabha & Achterberg, 1997; Dawson & Brawley, 2000; Holman & Lorig, 1992; Maddux et al., 1995; Reuter et al., 2010).

Self-efficacy expectancies also play a key role in the bridging of the *intention–behavior gap* (Sheeran & Orbell, 2000; Sheeran & Webb, Chapter 25, this volume)—the gap between the intention to engage in a health behavior (based on knowledge of its benefits, for example) and actually doing so. The health action process approach (Schwarzer & Luszczynska, 2008), in broad terms, states that in order to go from intending to engage in a behavior (e.g., intending to lose weight) to actually doing so (e.g., going on a diet), we must plan specific action (e.g., "When I am out to dinner with my friends, and everyone orders a burger, I will order a salad") and coping (e.g. "If I do overeat, I will remind myself that one unhealthy meal does not ruin a diet") behaviors—usually referred to as forming *implementation intentions,* or if–then plans (Gollwitzer, 2014; Hagger et al., 2016). Research shows that self-efficacy affects almost all steps in this process (Maddux & Dawson, 2014). For example, planning is more effective in helping us go from intention to behavior if we also have stronger self-efficacy expectancies for the behavior in question (Koring et al., 2012; Luszczynska, Schwarzer, Lippke, & Mazurkiewicz, 2011).

Second, self-efficacy expectancies influence a number of biological processes that, in turn, influence health and disease (Bandura, 1997). Research suggests that self-efficacy expectancies affect the body's physiological responses to stress, including the immune system (Antoni, 2003; Bandura, 1997; Coussons-Read, Okun, Schmitt, & Giese, 2005; Mausbach et al., 2010; O'Leary & Brown, 1995) and the physiological pathways activated by physical activity (Rudolph & McAuley, 1995). Lack of perceived control over environmental demands can increase susceptibility to infections and hasten the progression of disease (Gomez, Zimmermann, Froehlich, & Knop, 1994). Self-efficacy expectancies affect how the immune system responds to stress (Wiedenfeld et al., 1990). Self-efficacy expectancies also influence the activation of catecholamines, a family of neurotransmitters important to the management of stress and perceived threat, along with the endogenous painkillers referred to as endorphins (Bandura, 1988; Bandura, Barr, Lloyd, Mefford, & Barchas, 1985; Heinrichs et al., 2005; Bandura, 1997; Benight & Bandura, 2004; O'Leary & Brown, 1995; Shenassa, 2001), as well as the production of cortisol under stress (Gaab, Rohleder, Nater, & Ehlert, 2005; Schwerdtfeger, Konermann, & Schönhofen, 2008).

SUMMARY

The very little engine looked up and saw the tears in the dolls' eyes.
And she thought of the good little boys and girls on the other side of
the mountain who would not have any toys or good food unless she
helped. Then she said, "I think I can. I think I can. I think I can."
        —WATTY PIPER, *The Little Engine That Could* (1930/1989)

Some of the most powerful truths also are the simplest—so simple that a child can understand them. The concept of self-efficacy deals with one of these truths—one so simple it can be captured in a children's book of 37 pages (with illustrations), yet so powerful that fully describing its implications has filled thousands of pages in scientific journals and books over the past 30+ years. This truth is that strong expectancies in one's ideas, goals, and capacity for achievement are essential for success. Strong self-efficacy expectancies are important because they lead to effective self-regulation and persistence, which in turn lead to success. Most people see only extraordinary accomplishments of athletes, artists, and others but do not see "the unwavering commitment and countless hours of perseverant effort that produced them" (Bandura, 1997, p. 119; see also Ericsson & Charness, 1994). They then overestimate the role of "talent" in these accomplishments, while underestimating the role of determination and self-regulation.

As individuals contemplate and evaluate themselves and their lives, often the most salient points of reference are their accomplishments, challenges, and failures. In setting goals and trying to attain them, individuals who have faith in their own abilities give themselves an advantage that self-doubters lack. Because self-efficacy is concerned with understanding those factors that people can control, it is the study of human potential and possibilities and of the future.

REFERENCES

Abele, A. E., & Spurk, D. (2009). The longitudinal impact of self-efficacy and career goals on objective and subjective career success. *Journal of Vocational Behavior, 74,* 53–62.

AbuSabha, R., & Achterberg, C. (1997). Review of self-efficacy and locus of control for nutrition- and health-related behavior. *Journal of the American Dietetic Association, 97,* 1122–1133.

Ahmed, M., & Westra, H. A. (2009). Impact of a treatment rationale on expectancy and engagement in cognitive behavioral therapy for social anxiety. *Cognitive Therapy and Research, 33,* 314–322.

Ajzen, I. (1991). The theory of planned behavior. *Organizational Behavior and Human Decision Processes, 50,* 179–211.

Antoni, M. H. (2003). Stress management and psychoneuroimmunology in HIV infection. *CNS Spectrums, 8,* 40–51.

Arnstein, P., Caudill, M., Mandle, C. L., Norris, A., & Beasley, R. (1999). Self-efficacy as a mediator of the relationship between pain intensity, disability and depression in chronic pain patients. *Pain, 80,* 483–491.

Bandura, A. (1977). Self-efficacy: Toward a unifying theory of behavioral change. *Psychological Review, 84,* 191–215.

Bandura, A. (1986). *Social foundations of thought and action.* New York: Prentice-Hall.

Bandura, A. (1988). Self-efficacy conception of anxiety. *Anxiety Research, 1,* 77–98.

Bandura, A. (1992). Social cognitive theory. In R. Vasta (Ed.), *Six theories of child development: Revised formulations and current issues* (pp. 1–60). London: Jessica Kingsley.

Bandura, A. (1997). *Self-efficacy: The exercise of control.* New York: Freeman.

Bandura, A. (1999). A sociocognitive analysis of substance abuse: An agentic perspective. *Psychological Science, 10,* 214–217.

Bandura, A. (2005). The evolution of social cognitive theory. In K. G. Smith & M. A. Hitt (Eds.), *Great minds in management* (pp. 9–35). Oxford, UK: Oxford University Press.

Bandura, A. (2006). Guide for constructing self-efficacy scales. In F. Pajares & T. Urdan (Eds.), *Self-efficacy beliefs of adolescents* (Vol. 5, pp. 307–337). Greenwich, CT: Information Age.

Bandura, A., Barbaranelli, C., Caprara, G. V., & Pastorelli, C. (1996). Multifaceted impact of self-efficacy expectancies on academic functioning. *Child Development, 67,* 1206–1222.

Bandura, A., Barbaranelli, C., Caprara, G. V., & Pastorelli, C. (2001). Self-efficacy beliefs as shapers of children's aspirations and career trajectories. *Child Development, 72,* 187–206.

Bandura, A., Barr, C., Lloyd, S., Mefford, I. N., & Barchas, J. D. (1985). Catecholamine secretion as a function of perceived coping self-efficacy. *Journal of Consulting and Clinical Psychology, 53,* 406–414.

Bandura, A., Caprara, G. V., Barbaranelli, C., Gerbino, M., & Pastorelli, C. (2003). Role of affective self-regulatory efficacy in diverse spheres of psychosocial functioning. *Child Development, 74,* 769–782.

Bandura, A., & Jourden, J. F. (1991). Self-regulatory mechanisms governing the impact of social comparison on complex decision-making. *Journal of Personality and Social Psychology, 60,* 941–951.

Bandura, A., & Locke, E. A. (2003). Negative self-efficacy and goal effects revisited. *Journal of Applied Psychology, 88,* 87–99.

Bandura, A., Pastorelli, C., Barbaranelli, C., & Caprara, G. V. (1999). Self-efficacy pathways to childhood depression. *Journal of Personality and Social Psychology, 76,* 258–269.

Baumeister, R. F., Vohs, K. D., & Tice, D. M. (2007). The strength model of self-control. *Current Directions in Psychological Science, 16,* 351–355.

Bayer, C., & Gollwitzer, P. M. (2007). Boosting scholastic test scores by willpower: The role of implementation intentions. *Self and Identity, 6,* 1–19.

Beattie, S., Woodman, T., Fakehy, M., & Dempsey, C. (2016). The role of performance feedback on the self-efficacy–performance relationship. *Sport, Exercise, and Performance Psychology, 5,* 1–13.

Benight, C. C., & Bandura, A. (2004). Social cognitive theory of posttraumatic recovery: The role of perceived self-efficacy. *Behaviour Research and Therapy, 42,* 1129–1148.

Bennett, K. K., Adams, A. D., & Ricks, J. M. (2012). Pessimistic attributional style and cardiac symptom experiences: Self-efficacy as a mediator. *North American Journal of Psychology, 14,* 293–306.

Berry, J. M., & West, R. L. (1993). Cognitive self-efficacy in relation to personal mastery and goal setting across the life span. *International Journal of Behavioral Development, 16,* 351–379.

Betz, N. E. (2007). Career self-efficacy: Exemplary recent research and emerging directions. *Journal of Career Assessment, 15,* 403–422.

Blazer, D. G. (2002). Self-efficacy and depression in late life: A primary prevention proposal. *Aging and Mental Health, 6,* 315–324.

Boyer, D. A., Zollo, J. S., Thompson, C. M., Vancouver, J. B., Shewring, K., & Sims, E. (2000, June). *A quantitative review of the effects of manipulated self-efficacy on performance.* Poster session presented at the annual meeting of the American Psychological Society, Miami, Florida.

Cain, A. S., Bardone-Cone, A. M., Abramson, L. Y., Vohs, K. D., & Joiner, T. E. (2008). Refining the relationships of perfectionism, self-efficacy, and stress to dieting and binge eating: Examining the appearance, interpersonal, and academic domains. *International Journal of Eating Disorders, 41,* 713–721.

Caprara, G. V., Pastorelli, C., Regalia, C., Scabini, E., & Bandura, A. (2005). Impact of adolescents' filial self-efficacy on quality of family functioning and satisfaction. *Journal of Research on Adolescence, 15,* 71–97.

Caprara, G. V., Scabini, E., Barbaranelli, C., Pastorelli, C., Regalia, C., & Bandura, A. (1998). Impact of adolescents' perceived self-regulatory efficacy on familial communication and antisocial conduct. *European Psychologist, 3,* 125–132.

Caprara, G. V., & Steca, P. (2006). The contribution of self–regulatory efficacy beliefs in managing affect and family relationships to positive thinking and hedonic balance. *Journal of Social and Clinical Psychology, 25,* 603–627.

Caprara, G. V., Steca, P., Gerbino, M., Paciello, M., & Vecchio, G. M. (2006). Looking for adolescents' well-being: Self-efficacy beliefs as determinants of positive thinking and happiness. *Epidemiologia e Psichiatria Sociale, 15,* 30–43.

Carver, C. S., Scheier, M. F., & Segerstrom, S. C. (2010). Optimism. *Clinical Psychology Review, 30,* 879–889.

Cervone, D., Shadel, W. G., Smith, R. E., & Fiori, M. (2006). Self-regulation: Reminders and suggestions from personality science. *Applied Psychology, 55,* 333–385.

Chen, G., Gully, S. M., & Eden, D. (2001). Validation of a new general self-efficacy scale. *Organizational Research Methods, 4,* 62–83.

Ciani, K. D., Easter, M. A., Summers, J. J., & Posada, M. L. (2009). Cognitive biases in the interpretation of autonomic arousal: A test of the construal bias hypothesis. *Contemporary Educational Psychology, 34,* 9–17.

Coussons-Read, M. E., Okun, M. L., Schmitt, M. P., & Giese, S. (2005). Prenatal stress alters cytokine levels in a manner that may endanger human pregnancy. *Psychosomatic Medicine, 67,* 625–631.

Dan, O., Sagi-Schwartz, A., Bar-Haim, Y., & Eshel, Y. (2011). Effects of early relationships on children's perceived control: A longitudinal study. *International Journal of Behavioral Development, 35,* 449–456.

Dawson, K. A., & Brawley, L. R. (2000). Examining the relationship between exercise goals, self-efficacy, and overt behavior with beginning exercisers. *Journal of Applied Social Psychology, 30,* 315–329.

DeBono, A., Shmueli, D., & Muraven, M. (2011). Rude and inappropriate: The role of self-control in following social norms. *Personality and Social Psychology Bulletin, 37,* 136–146.

Diener, E. (1984). Subjective well-being. *Psychological Bulletin, 95,* 542–575.

Doerr, C. E., & Baumeister, R. F. (2010). Self-regulatory strength and psychological adjustment: Implications of the limited resource model of self-regulation. In J. E. Maddux & J. P. Tangney (Eds.), *Social psychological foundations of clinical psychology* (pp. 71–83). New York: Guilford Press.

Duffy, S. A., Scheumann, A. L., Fowler, K. E., Darling-Fisher, C., & Terrell, J. E. (2010). Perceived difficulty quitting predicts enrollment in a smoking-cessation program for patients with head and neck cancer. *Oncology Nursing Forum, 37,* 349–356.

Epel, E. S., Bandura, A., & Zimbardo, P. (1999). Escaping homelessness: The influences of self-efficacy and time perspective on coping with homelessness. *Journal of Applied Social Psychology, 29,* 575–596.

Ericsson, K. A., & Charness, N. (1994). Expert performance: Its structure and acquisition. *American Psychologist, 49,* 725–747.

Fan, W., & Williams, C. M. (2010). The effects of parental involvement on students' academic self-efficacy, engagement and intrinsic motivation. *Educational Psychology, 30,* 53–74.

Ferrari, M. (1996). Observing the observer: Self-regulation in the observational learning of motor skills. *Developmental Review, 16,* 203–240.

Forsyth, A. D., & Carey, M. P. (1998). Measuring self-efficacy in the context of HIV risk reduction: Research challenges and recommendations. *Health Psychology, 17,* 559–568.

Frank, J. D., & Frank, J. B. (1991). *Persuasion and healing: A comparative study of psychotherapy* (3rd ed.). Baltimore: Johns Hopkins University Press.

Gaab, J., Rohleder, N., Nater, U. M., & Ehlert, U. (2005). Psychological determinants of the cortisol stress response: The role of anticipatory cognitive appraisal. *Psychoneuroendocrinology, 30,* 599–610.

Gaudiano, B. A., & Herbert, J. D. (2007). Self-efficacy for social situations in adolescents with generalized social anxiety disorder. *Behavioural and Cognitive Psychotherapy, 35,* 209–223.

Gollwitzer, P. M. (2014). Weakness of the will: Is a quick fix possible? *Motivation and Emotion, 38,* 305–322.

Gomez, V., Zimmermann, G., Froehlich, W., & Knop, J. (1994). Stress, control experience, acute hormonal and immune reactions. *Psychologische Beitrage, 36,* 74–81.

Gross, J. J. (1998). The emerging field of emotion regulation: An integrative review. *Review of General Psychology, 2,* 271–299.

Gully, S. M., Incalcaterra, K. A., Joshi, A., & Beaubien, J. M. (2002). A meta-analysis of team-efficacy, potency, and performance: Interdependence and level of analysis as moderators of observed relationships. *Journal of Applied Psychology, 87*, 819–832.

Hagger, M. S., Luszczynska, A., de Wit, J., Benyamini, Y., Burkert, S., Chamberland, P.-E., . . . Gollwitzer, P. M. (2016). Implementation intention and planning interventions in health psychology: Recommendations from the Synergy Expert Group for research and practice. *Psychology and Health, 31*, 814–839.

Hagger, M. S., Wood, C., Stiff, C., & Chatzisarantis, N. L. D. (2010). Ego depletion and the strength model of self-control: A meta-analysis. *Psychological Bulletin, 136*, 495–525.

Harkin, B., Webb, T. L., Chang, B. P. I., Prestwich, A., Conner, M., Kellar, I., . . . Sheeran, P. (2016). Does monitoring goal progress promote goal attainment?: A meta-analysis of the experimental evidence. *Psychological Bulletin, 142*, 198–229.

Heinrichs, M., Wagner, D., Schoch, W., Soravia, L. M., Hellhammer, D. H., & Ehlert, U. (2005). Predicting posttraumatic stress symptoms from pretraumatic risk factors: A 2-year prospective follow-up study in firefighters. *American Journal of Psychiatry, 162*, 2276–2286.

Hirsch, J. K., Duberstein, P. R., Conner, K. R., Heisel, M. J., Beckman, A., Franus, N., . . . Conwell, Y. (2007). Future orientation moderates the relationship between functional status and suicide ideation in depressed adults. *Depression and Anxiety, 24*, 196–201.

Hirschy, A. J., & Morris, J. R. (2002). Individual differences in attributional style: The relational influence of self-efficacy, self-esteem, and sex role identity. *Personality and Individual Differences, 32*, 183–196.

Hoeppner, B. B., Kahler, C. W., & Gwaltney, C. J. (2014). Relationship between momentary affect states and self-efficacy in adolescent smokers. *Health Psychology, 33*, 1507–1517.

Holden, G. (1991). The relationship of self-efficacy appraisals to subsequent health related outcomes: A meta-analysis. *Social Work in Health Care, 16*, 53–93.

Holden, G., Moncher, M. S., Schinke, S. P., & Barker, K. M. (1990). Self-efficacy of children and adolescents: A meta-analysis. *Psychological Reports, 66*, 1044–1046.

Holman, H. R., & Lorig, K. (1992). Perceived self-efficacy in self-management of chronic disease. In R. Schwarzer (Ed.), *Self-efficacy: Thought control of action* (pp. 305–324). Washington, DC: Hemisphere.

Inzlicht, M., Legault, L., & Teper, R. (2014). Exploring the mechanisms of self-control improvement. *Current Directions in Psychological Science, 23*, 302–307.

Job, V., Walton, G. M., Bernecker, K., & Dweck, C. S. (2015). Implicit theories about willpower predict self-regulation and grades in everyday life. *Journal of Personality and Social Psychology, 108*, 637–647.

Jones, M. V., Mace, R. D., Bray, S. R., MacRae, A. W., & Stockbridge, C. (2002). The impact of motivational imagery on the emotional state and self-efficacy levels of novice climbers. *Journal of Sport Behavior, 25*, 57–73.

Jones, T. L., & Prinz, R. J. (2005). Potential roles of parental self-efficacy in parent and child adjustment: A review. *Clinical Psychology Review, 25*, 341–363.

Judge, T. A., Erez, A., Bono, J. E., & Thoresen, C. J. (2002). Are measures of self-esteem, neuroticism, locus of control, and generalized self-efficacy indicators of a common core construct? *Journal of Personality and Social Psychology, 83*, 693–710.

Junttila, N., Vauras, M., & Laakkonen, E. (2007). The role of parenting self-efficacy in children's social and academic behavior. *European Journal of Psychology of Education, 22*, 41–61.

Kaplan, M., & Maddux, J. E. (2002). Goals and marital satisfaction: Perceived support for personal goals and collective efficacy for collective goals. *Journal of Social and Clinical Psychology, 21*, 157–164.

Kappes, A., Singmann, H., & Oettingen, G. (2012). Mental contrasting instigates goal pursuit by linking obstacles of reality with instrumental behavior. *Journal of Experimental Social Psychology, 48,* 811–818.

Karademas, E. C. (2006). Self-efficacy, social support and well-being. *Personality and Individual Differences, 40,* 1281–1290.

Karoly, P. (2010). Goal systems and self-regulation. In R. Hoyle (Ed.), *Handbook of personality and self-regulation* (pp. 218–242). New York: Wiley-Blackwell.

Kelley, W. M., Wagner, D. D., & Heatherton, T. F. (2015). In search of a human self-regulation system. *Annual Review of Neuroscience, 38,* 389–411.

Kelly, J. F., Magill, M., & Stout, R. L. (2009). How do people recover from alcohol dependence?: A systematic review of the research on mechanisms of behavior change in Alcoholics Anonymous. *Addiction Research and Theory, 17,* 236–259.

Kerpelman, J. L., Eryigit, S., & Stephens, C. J. (2007). African American adolescents' future education orientation: Associations with self-efficacy, ethnic identity, and perceived parental support. *Journal of Youth and Adolescence, 37,* 997–1008.

Kirsch, I. (Ed.). (1999). *How expectancies shape behavior.* Washington, DC: American Psychological Association.

Knudstrup, M., Segrest, S. L., & Hurley, A. E. (2003). The use of mental imagery in the simulated employment interview situation. *Journal of Managerial Psychology, 18,* 573–591.

Koring, M., Richert, J., Parschau, L., Ernsting, A., Lippke, S., & Schwarzer, R. (2012). A combined planning and self-efficacy intervention to promote physical activity: A multiple mediation analysis. *Psychology, Health and Medicine, 17,* 488–498.

Kruglanski, A. W., Chernikova, M., Rosenzweig, E., & Kopetz, C. (2014). On motivational readiness. *Psychological Review, 121,* 367–388.

Larsen, R. J., & Prizmic, Z. (2004). Affect regulation. In R. F. Baumeister & K. D. Vohs (Eds.), *Handbook of self-regulation: Research, theory, and applications* (pp. 40–61). New York: Guilford Press.

Little, T. D., Oettingen, G., Stetsenko, A., & Baltes, P. B. (1995). Children's action-control beliefs about school performance: How do American children compare with German and Russian children? *Journal of Personality and Social Psychology, 69,* 686–700.

Ludwig, K. B., & Pittman, J. F. (1999). Adolescent prosocial values and self-efficacy in relation to delinquency, risky sexual behavior, and drug use. *Youth and Society, 30,* 461–482.

Luszczynska, A., Schwarzer, R., Lippke, S., & Mazurkiewicz, M. (2011). Self-efficacy as a moderator of the planning–behaviour relationship in interventions designed to promote physical activity. *Psychology and Health, 26,* 151–166.

MacLeod, A. K., & Byrne, A. (1996). Anxiety, depression, and the anticipation of future positive and negative experiences. *Journal of Abnormal Psychology, 105,* 286–289.

Maddux, J. E. (1993). Social cognitive models of heath and exercise behavior: An introduction and review of conceptual issues. *Journal of Applied Sport Psychology, 5,* 116–140.

Maddux, J. E. (1999). Expectancies and the social-cognitive perspective: Basic principles, processes, and variables. In I. Kirsch (Ed.), *How expectancies shape behavior* (pp. 17–40). Washington, DC: American Psychological Association.

Maddux, J. E., Brawley, L., & Boykin, A. (1995). Self-efficacy and healthy decision-making: Protection, promotion, and detection. In J. E. Maddux (Ed.), *Self-efficacy, adaptation, and adjustment: Theory, research, and application* (pp. 173–202). New York: Plenum Press.

Maddux, J. E., & Dawson, K. A. (2014). Predicting and changing exercise behavior: Bridging the information-intention-behavior gap. In A. R. Gomes, R. Resende, & A. Albuquerque (Eds.), *Positive human functioning from a multidimensional perspective* (pp. 97–120). New York: Nova Science.

Maddux, J. E., & DuCharme, K. A. (1997). Behavioral intentions in theories of health behavior. In D. Gochman (Ed.), *Handbook of health behavior research: I. Personal and social determinants* (pp. 133–152). New York: Plenum Press.

Maddux, J. E., & Gosselin, J. T. (2012). Self-efficacy. In M. R. Leary & J. P. Tangney (Eds.), *Handbook of self and identity* (2nd ed., pp. 218–238). New York: Guilford Press.

Maddux, J. E., & Meier, L. J. (1995). Self-efficacy and depression. In J. E. Maddux (Ed.), *Self-efficacy, adaptation, and adjustment: Theory, research and application* (pp. 143–169). New York: Plenum Press.

Maddux, J. E., & Rogers, R. W. (1983). Protection motivation and self-efficacy: A revised theory of fear appeals and attitude change. *Journal of Experimental Social Psychology, 19*, 469–479.

Maddux, J. E., & Volkmann, J. R. (2010). Self-efficacy and self-regulation. In R. Hoyle (Ed.), *Handbook of personality and self-regulation* (pp. 315–331). New York: Wiley-Blackwell.

Mandler, J. M. (1992). How to build a baby: II. Conceptual primitives. *Psychological Review, 99*, 587–604.

Marlowe, N. (1998). Self-efficacy moderates the impact of stressful events on headache. *Headache, 38*, 662–667.

Mattanah, J. F., Pratt, M. W., Cowan, P. A., & Cowan, C. P. (2005). Authoritative parenting, parental scaffolding of long-division mathematics, and children's academic competence in fourth grade. *Journal of Applied Developmental Psychology, 26*, 85–106.

Mausbach, B. T., Roepke, S. K., Ziegler, M. G., Milic, M., von Känel, R., Dimsdale, J. E., . . . Grant, I. (2010). Association between chronic caregiving stress and impaired endothelial function in the elderly. *Journal of the American College of Cardiology, 55*, 2599–2606.

McAuley, E. (1993). Self-efficacy and the maintenance of exercise participation in older adults. *Journal of Behavioral Medicine, 16*, 103–113.

McAvay, G., Seeman, T. E., & Rodin, J. (1996). A longitudinal study of change in domain-specific self-efficacy among older adults. *Journals of Gerontology: Series B. Psychological Sciences and Social Sciences, 51*, 243–253.

Mischel, W. (1973). Toward a cognitive social learning reconceptualization of personality. *Psychological Review, 80*, 252–284.

Moos, R. H. (2008). Active ingredients of substance use–focused self-help groups. *Addiction, 103*, 387–396.

Morgenroth, T., Ryan, M. K., & Peters, K. (2015). The motivational theory of role modeling: How role models influence role aspirants' goals. *Review of General Psychology, 19*, 465–483.

Moritz, S. E., Feltz, D. L., Fahrbach, K. R., & Mack, D. E. (2000). The relation of self-efficacy measures to sport performance: A meta-analytic review. *Research Quarterly for Exercise and Sport, 71*, 280–294.

Multon, K. D., Brown, S. D., & Lent, R. W. (1991). Relation of self-efficacy beliefs to academic outcomes: A meta-analytic investigation. *Journal of Counseling Psychology, 38*, 30–38.

Muraven, M., & Baumeister, R. F. (2000). Self-regulation and depletion of limited resources: Does self-control resemble a muscle? *Psychological Bulletin, 126*, 247–259.

Nicholls, A. R., Polman, R., & Levy, A. R. (2010). Coping self-efficacy, pre-competitive anxiety, and subjective performance among athletes. *European Journal of Sport Science, 10*, 97–102.

Nickel, D., & Spink, K. S. (2010). Attributions and self-regulatory efficacy for health-related physical activity. *Journal of Health Psychology, 15*, 53–63.

O'Leary, A., & Brown, S. (1995). Self-efficacy and the physiological stress response. In J. E. Maddux (Ed.), *Self-efficacy, adaptation, and adjustment: Theory, research and application* (pp. 227–248). New York: Plenum Press.

O'Leary, A., Jemmott, L. S., & Jemmott, J. B. (2008). Mediation analysis of an effective sexual risk-reduction intervention for women: The importance of self-efficacy. *Health Psychology, 27*, 180–184.

Oettingen, G. (2012). Future thought and behaviour change. *European Review of Social Psychology, 23,* 1–63.

Oettingen, G. (2014). *Rethinking positive thinking: Inside the new science of motivation.* New York: Penguin Random House.

Oettingen, G., & Gollwitzer, P. M. (Eds.). (2015). *Self-regulation in adolescence.* New York: Cambridge University Press.

Oettingen, G., Little, T. D., Lindenberger, U., & Baltes, P. B. (1994). Causality, agency, and control beliefs in East versus West Berlin children: A natural experiment on the role of context. *Journal of Personality and Social Psychology, 66,* 579–595.

Oettingen, G., Marquardt, M. K., & Gollwitzer, P. M. (2012). Mental contrasting turns positive feedback on creative potential into successful performance. *Journal of Experimental Social Psychology, 48,* 990–996.

Petty, R. E., & Brinol, P. (2010). Attitude change. In R. F. Baumeister & E. J. Finkel (Eds.), *Advanced social psychology: The state of the science* (pp. 217–259). New York: Oxford University Press.

Pinto, A., Guarda, A. S., Heinberg, L. J., & DiClemente, C. C. (2006). Development of the eating disorder recovery self-efficacy questionnaire. *International Journal of Eating Disorders, 39,* 376–384.

Piper, W. (1989). *The little engine that could.* New York: Platt & Monk. (Original work published 1930)

Polivy, J., & Herman, C. P. (2002). If at first you don't succeed: False hopes of self-change. *American Psychologist, 57,* 677–689.

Preiss, R., Gayle, B., & Allen, M. (2006). Test anxiety, academic self-efficacy, and study skills: A meta-analytic assessment. In B. Gayle, R. Preiss, N. Burrell, & M. Allen (Eds.), *Classroom communication and instructional processes: Advances through meta-analysis* (pp. 99–112). Mahwah, NJ: Erlbaum.

Prochaska, J. O., & Prochaska, J. M. (2010). Self-directed change: A transtheoretical model. In J. E. Maddux & J. P. Tangney (Eds.), *Social psychological foundations of clinical psychology* (pp. 431–440). New York: Guilford Press.

Reuter, T., Ziegelmann, J. P., Wiedemann, A. U., Geiser, C., Lippke, S., Schüz, B., . . . Schwarzer, R. (2010). Changes in intentions, planning, and self-efficacy predict changes in behaviors: An application of latent true change modeling. *Journal of Health Psychology, 15,* 935–947.

Riskind, J. H., Alloy, L. B., & Iacoviello, B. M. (2010). Social and cognitive vulnerability to depression and anxiety. In J. E Maddux & J. P. Tangney (Eds.), *Social psychological foundations of clinical psychology* (pp. 272–293). New York: Guilford Press.

Rudolph, D. L., & McAuley, E. (1995). Self-efficacy and salivary cortisol responses to acute exercise in physically active and less active adults. *Journal of Sport and Exercise Psychology, 17,* 206–213.

Russell, J. E. A. (2008). Promoting subjective well-being at work. *Journal of Career Assessment, 16,* 117–131.

Sacco, W. P., Wells, K. J., Vaughan, C. A., Friedman, A., Perez, S., & Matthew, R. (2005). Depression in adults with type 2 diabetes: The role of adherence, body mass index, and self-efficacy. *Health Psychology, 24,* 630–634.

Sadri, G., & Robertson, I. T. (1993). Self-efficacy and work-related behaviour: A review and meta-analysis. *Applied Psychology, 42,* 139–152.

Sawyer, S. P., & Pettman, P. J. (2006). Do clients retain treatment concepts?: An assessment of post treatment adjustment of adult sex offenders. *Sexual Offender Treatment, 1,* 1–14.

Scheier, M. F., & Carver, C. S. (1993). On the power of positive thinking: The benefits of being optimistic. *Current Directions in Psychological Science, 2,* 26–30.

Schlehofer, M. M., Thompson, S. C., Ting, S., Ostermann, S., Nierman, A., & Skenderian, J. (2010). Psychological predictors of college students' cell phone use while driving. *Accident Analysis and Prevention, 42,* 1107–1112.

Schunk, D. H. (1995). Self-efficacy and education and instruction. In J. E. Maddux (Ed.), *Self-efficacy, adaptation, and adjustment: Theory, research, and application* (pp. 281–304). New York: Plenum Press.

Schunk, D. H., & Meece, J. L. (2006). Self-efficacy development in adolescence. In B. Kirshner (Series Ed.) & F. Pajares & T. Urdan (Vol. Eds.), *Adolescence and education: Vol. 5. Self-efficacy beliefs of adolescents* (pp. 71–96). Greenwich, CT: Information Age.

Schwarzer, R., Lippke, S., & Luszczynska, A. (2011). Mechanisms of health behavior change in persons with chronic illness or disability: The Health Action Process Approach (HAPA). *Rehabilitation Psychology, 56,* 161–170.

Schwarzer, R., & Luszczynska, A. (2008). How to overcome health-compromising behaviors. *European Psychologist, 13,* 141–151.

Schwerdtfeger, A., Konermann, L., & Schönhofen, K. (2008). Self-efficacy as a health-protective resource in teachers?: A biopsychological approach. *Health Psychology, 27,* 358–368.

Sevigny, P. R., & Loutzenhiser, L. (2010). Predictors of parenting self-efficacy in mothers and fathers of toddlers. *Child: Care, Health and Development, 36,* 179–189.

Sevincer, A. T., & Oettingen, G. (2013). Spontaneous mental contrasting and selective goal pursuit. *Personality and Social Psychology Bulletin, 39,* 1240–1254.

Sheeran, P., & Orbell, S. (2000). Using implementation intentions to increase attendance for cervical cancer screening. *Health Psychology, 19,* 283–289.

Shenassa, E. D. (2001). Society, physical health and modern epidemiology. *Epidemiology, 12,* 467–470.

Sherer, M., Maddux, J. E., Mercandante, B., Prentice-Dunn, S., Jacobs, B., & Rogers, R. W. (1982). The Self-Efficacy Scale: Construction and validation. *Psychological Reports, 51,* 633–671.

Sherman, N. W. (2002). Motivation, attributions, and self-efficacy in children. *Journal of Physical Education, Recreation, and Dance, 73,* 10–13.

Shields, C. A., Brawley, L. R., & Lindover, T. I. (2006). Self-efficacy as a mediator of the relationship between causal attributions and exercise behavior. *Journal of Applied Social Psychology, 36,* 2785–2802.

Short, S. E., Bruggeman, J. M., Engel, S. G., Marback, T. L., Wang, L. J., . . . Short, M. W. (2002). The effect of imagery function and imagery direction on self-efficacy and performance on a golf-putting task. *Sport Psychologist, 16,* 48–67.

Singer, J. L. (1998). Imaginative play in early childhood: A foundation for adaptive emotional and cognitive development. *International Medical Journal, 5,* 93–100.

Smith, R. F. (2008). Biological bases of psychopathology. In J. E. Maddux & B. W. Winstead (Eds.), *Psychopathology: Foundations for a contemporary understanding* (pp. 67–82). New York: Taylor & Francis.

Snyder, C. R. (2002). Hope theory: Rainbows of the mind. *Psychological Inquiry, 13,* 249–275.

Spink, K. S., & Nickel, D. (2009). Self-regulatory efficacy as a mediator between attributions and intention for health-related physical activity. *Journal of Health Psychology, 15,* 75–84.

Stack, D. M., & Poulin-Dubois, D. (1998). Socioemotional and cognitive competence in infancy: Paradigms, assessment strategies, and implications for intervention. In D. Pushkar, W. M. Bukowski, A. E. Schwartzman, D. M., Stack, & D. R. White (Eds.), *Improving competence across the lifespan: Building interventions based on theory and research* (pp. 37–57). New York: Plenum Press.

Stajkovic, A. D., & Lee, D. S. (2001, August). *A meta-analysis of the relationship between collective efficacy and group performance.* Paper presented at meeting of the National Academy of Management, Washington, DC.

Stajkovic, A. D., & Luthans, F. (1998). Self-efficacy and work-related performance: A meta-analysis. *Psychological Bulletin, 124,* 240–261.

Stajkovic, A. D., & Sommer, S. M. (2000). Self-efficacy and causal attributions: Direct and reciprocal links. *Journal of Applied Social Psychology, 30,* 707–737.

Stipek, D. (2002). *Motivation to learn: Integrating theory and practice* (4th ed.). Needham Heights, MA: Allyn & Bacon.

Strecher, V. J., Champion, V. L., & Rosenstock, I. M. (1997). The health belief model and health behavior. In D. Gochman (Ed.), *Handbook of health behavior research: I. Personal and social determinants* (pp. 71–92). New York: Plenum Press.

Strobel, M., Tumasjan, A., & Spörrle, M. (2011). Be yourself, believe in yourself, and be happy: Self-efficacy as a mediator between personality factors and subjective well-being. *Scandinavian Journal of Psychology, 52,* 43–48.

Tabernero, C., & Wood, R. E. (2009). Interaction between self-efficacy and initial performance in predicting the complexity of task chosen. *Psychological Reports, 105,* 1167–1180.

Taylor, S. E., & Brown, J. D. (1988). Illusion and well-being: A social psychological perspective on mental health. *Psychological Bulletin, 2,* 193–210.

Thomasson, P., & Psouni, E. (2010). Social anxiety and related social impairment are linked to self-efficacy and dysfunctional coping. *Scandinavian Journal of Psychology, 51,* 171–178.

Tolli, A. P., & Schmidt, A. M. (2008). The role of feedback, causal attributions, and self-efficacy in goal revision. *Journal of Applied Psychology, 93,* 692–701.

Urdan, T., & Pajares, F. (Eds.). (2006). *Self-efficacy beliefs of adolescents.* Charlotte, NC: Information Age.

Urdan, T., & Schoenfelder, E. (2006). Classroom effects on student motivation: Goal structures, social relationships, and competence beliefs. *Journal of School Psychology, 44,* 331–349.

Van Zundert, R. M. P., Ferguson, S. G., Shiffman, S., & Engels, R. C. M. E. (2010). Dynamic effects of self-efficacy on smoking lapses and relapse among adolescents. *Health Psychology, 29,* 246–254.

Vancouver, J. B., More, K. M., & Yoder, R. J. (2008). Self-efficacy and resource allocation: Support for a nonmonotonic, discontinuous model. *Journal of Applied Psychology, 93,* 35–47.

Vecchio, G. M., Gerbino, M., Pastorelli, C., Del Bove, G., & Caprara, G. V. (2007). Multifaceted self-efficacy beliefs as predictors of life satisfaction in late adolescence. *Personality and Individual Differences, 43,* 1807–1818.

Vieno, A., Santinello, M., Pastore, M., & Perkins, D. D. (2007). Social support, sense of community in school, and self-efficacy as resources during early adolescence: An integrative model. *American Journal of Community Psychology, 39,* 177–190.

Waldrop, D., Lightsey, O. R., Jr., Ethington, C. A., Woemmel, C. A., & Coke, A. L. (2001). Self-efficacy, optimism, health competence, and recovery from orthopedic surgery. *Journal of Counseling Psychology, 48,* 233–238.

Wei, M., Russell, D. W., & Zakalik, R. A. (2005). Adult attachment, social self-efficacy, self-disclosure, loneliness, and subsequent depression for freshman college students: A longitudinal study. *Journal of Counseling Psychology, 52,* 602–614.

Welch, D. C., & West, R. L. (1995). Self-efficacy and mastery: Its application to issues of environmental control, cognition, and aging. *Developmental Review, 15,* 150–171.

West, R. L., Bagwell, D. K., & Dark-Freudeman, A. (2008). Self-efficacy and memory aging: The impact of a memory intervention based on self-efficacy. *Aging, Neuropsychology, and Cognition, 15,* 302–329.

Wheeler, J. G., George, W. H., & Marlatt, G. A. (2006). Relapse prevention for sexual offend-
    ers: Considerations for the "abstinence violation effect." *Sexual Abuse: A Journal of
    Research and Treatment, 18,* 233–248.
Wieber, F., Odenthal, G., & Gollwitzer, P. (2010). Self-efficacy feelings moderate implemen-
    tation intention effects. *Self and Identity, 9,* 177–194.
Wiedenfeld, S. A., O'Leary, A., Bandura, A., Brown, S., Levine, S., & Raska, K. (1990).
    Impact of perceived self-efficacy in coping with stressors on components of the immune
    system. *Journal of Personality and Social Psychology, 59,* 1082–1094.
Williams, D. M. (2010). Outcome expectancy and self-efficacy: Theoretical implications of
    an unresolved contradiction. *Personality and Social Psychology Review, 14,* 417–425.
Williams, D. M., & Rhodes, R. E. (2014). The confounded self-efficacy construct: Concep-
    tual analysis and recommendations for future research. *Health Psychology Review, 10,*
    1–16.
Williams, S. L. (2016). Anxiety disorders, obsessive–compulsive, and related disorders. In
    J. E. Maddux & B. A. Winstead (Eds.), *Psychopathology: Foundations for a contemporary
    understanding* (4th ed., pp. 141–161). New York: Routledge.
Windle, G., Markland, D. A., & Woods, R. T. (2008). Examination of a theoretical model of
    psychological resilience in older age. *Aging and Mental Health, 12,* 285–292.
Yang, M. L., Chuang, H. H., & Chiou, W. B. (2009). Long-term costs of inflated self-estimate
    on academic performance among adolescent students: A case of second-language
    achievements. *Psychological Reports, 105,* 727–737.
Zapata, S. L. (2006). Goals and collective efficacy: A new and dynamic approach to increase
    relationship satisfaction. Doctoral dissertation, George Mason University, Fairfax, Vir-
    ginia. Available from *www.proquest.com.*
Zhao, H., Seibert, S. E., & Hills, G. E. (2005). The mediating role of self-efficacy in the devel-
    opment of entrepreneurial intentions. *Journal of Applied Psychology, 90,* 1265–1272.
Zimmerman, B. J., & Cleary, T. J. (2006). Adolescents' development of personal agency: The
    role of self-efficacy beliefs and self-regulatory skill. In F. Pajares & T. Urdan (Eds.), *Self-
    efficacy beliefs of adolescents* (pp. 45–69). Charlotte, NC: Information Age.

CHAPTER 10

Positive Future-Thinking, Well-Being, and Mental Health

Andrew K. MacLeod
Rory C. O'Connor

How we think about our own future is intimately bound up with our well-being and mental health. Within the clinical literature, a negative view of the future has long been identified as a central feature of anxiety and depression (e.g., Beck, 1976). Specifying the details of a negative view of the future and how those details might relate to different disorders, though, has not received a great deal of attention. Moreover, positive, as opposed to negative, aspects of a future outlook and their breakdown in emotional disorders have received even less attention. Emerging evidence, however, is beginning to identify how diverse aspects of future-directed thinking, especially positive aspects, relate to different facets of well-being and mental health in variety of ways (see MacLeod, 2017, for a review). For example, expectancies for future positive and negative events relate in different ways to anxiety and depression, and changes to some, but not all, aspects of a person's goals are implicated in depression. The present chapter reviews literature relevant to both these examples to illustrate how different aspects of positive future-thinking are involved in emotional disturbance. By highlighting these specific connections, basic research has the potential to inform interventions, both at the clinical and subclinical levels, through suggesting particular avenues of future-directed thinking that can be the target of therapeutic strategies.

EXPECTANCIES AND GOALS

The expectancies that people have and the goals that they hold for the future are, as already indicated, two main areas in which the links between future-thinking and well-being have been examined. Expectancies and goals are different but overlapping constructs. *Expectancies* describe a broad category of mental representations characterized by varying degrees of belief in what is likely (or unlikely) to happen in the future. A *goal* refers to "the object of a person's ambition or effort" (English Oxford Living Dictionaries, 2016), in other words, mental representations of desired future outcomes that someone is motivated to bring about and is engaged in working toward. Goals and expectancies are distinct from fantasies about future outcomes, which need not have any of the cognitive or motivational elements of working toward the positive outcome that is imagined, or even any belief in its likelihood (Oettingen, 2012). The first part of this chapter reviews evidence on how positive and negative expectancies relate to well-being and mental health, with an emphasis on individuals' own, idiosyncratic, personally relevant expectancies, as well as an emphasis on positive anticipation. The second part of the chapter reviews some particular characteristics of goals and how those characteristics relate to well-being and mental health.

Judged Expectancies of Events

Expectancies, in a broad sense, can be measured through self-reported optimistic and pessimistic attitudes toward the future, for example, endorsing self-report items such as "overall I expect more good things to happen to me than bad" (Scheier, Carver, & Bridges, 1994). Alternatively, expectancy beliefs about specific future events can be measured by presenting people with lists of hypothetical events and asking them to make judgments about the likelihood of those events happening to them (Weinstein, 1980). Expectancies in this latter sense are more the focus of the discussion here. Judgments that desirable future events are likely and undesirable future events unlikely are reliably linked to well-being and mental health. At both clinical and subclinical levels, low expectancies for positive future events are consistently linked to depression, whereas high expectancies for negative events are most often associated with elevated levels of both anxiety and depression (MacLeod, Tata, Kentish, Carroll, & Hunter, 1997; Miranda & Mennin, 2007; Wenze, Gunthert, & German, 2012).

The method of giving people lists of hypothetical future events, such as "you will experience financial difficulties" or "your health and fitness will improve" and asking them to judge the likelihood of those events has the advantage of participants all rating the same items. The disadvantage lies in personal relevance: The listed items might not all be personally relevant or important to an individual making the judgments, and, conversely, some future events that are very important to the person might not be captured by the list. Intuitively, what would seem to matter are the particular, personally relevant events that an individual cares about and actively anticipates. There is also empirical evidence suggesting that likelihood ratings on researcher-provided lists of events differ from individual, self-generated events in their relationships to mood (Bredemeier, Berenbaum, & Spielberg, 2012; Hepburn, Barnhofer, & Williams, 2006).

Measuring Individuals' Own Personal Expectancies

In an attempt to get at the more personally relevant future expectancies that individuals naturally think about and anticipate, MacLeod and colleagues (MacLeod,

Rose, & Williams, 1993) devised the Future-Thinking Task. In this task (see Figure 10.1), people are asked to think spontaneously about things in the future they are looking forward to (positive future-thinking) and not looking forward to (negative future-thinking) in various future time frames. Modeled on verbal fluency tasks (Lezak, Howieson, Bigler, & Tranel, 2012), participants simply have to say aloud as many examples of future expectancies as they can within a time limit, for example, things they are looking forward to over the next year.

The standard measure is the number of responses people are able to think of in each category, but, additionally, people can be re-presented with their responses and asked to make ratings of how likely they think they are to come about and how positive or negative they think they would feel if those outcomes happened (MacLeod et al., 2005). These likelihood and value ratings reflect classic expectancy–value accounts of goal-directed behavior (Eccles & Wigfield, 2002; Oettingen, Pak, & Schnetter, 2001) and can be used to form a composite score (cf., Nagengast et al., 2011). The pattern of findings across studies is essentially the same whether the number of responses or an expectancy–value measure based on participants' ratings of their responses is used, perhaps because both expectancy and value are already inherent in asking people to think of things they are and are not looking forward to. The following subsections review some of the data on the Future-Thinking Task in relation to well-being, mood, and suicidality. The emphasis is on positive future-thinking, although findings are compared with negative future-thinking where data are available.

Well-Being, Depression, and Anxiety

A number of studies have examined the relationship between emotional disturbance (anxiety and depression) and positive and negative future-thinking, as measured by the Future-Thinking Task. In addition, studies have also reported relationships to

---

Participants are given three future time periods (the next week, the next year, the next 5 to 10 years) and asked to try to think of positive things (things they are looking forward to) and negative things (things they are not looking forward to) for each of those time periods.

Standard Instructions

"I'd like to ask you to think about things that might happen to you in the future. I will give you three different time periods in the future, one at a time, and I'd like you to try to think of things that might happen to you in those time periods. I will give you a minute to try to think of as many things as you can. It doesn't matter whether the things are trivial or important, just say what comes to mind. But they should be things that you think will definitely happen or are at least quite likely to happen. If you can't think of anything or if you can't think of many things, that's fine, but just keep trying until the time limit is up."

The order of presentation of negative and positive conditions should be counterbalanced across participants, although within each condition the time periods are always presented in the same order (1 week, 1 year, 5–10 years).

FIGURE 10.1. The Future-Thinking Task. From MacLeod, A. K., Rose, G. S., & Williams, J. M. G. (1993). Components of hopelessness about the future in parasuicide. *Cognitive Therapy and Research, 17,* 441–455. Copyright 1993 by Springer. Reprinted with permission of Springer.

well-being within the general population. Well-being is often conceptualized in a subjective way, such that someone is considered as high in well-being to the extent that he or she typically experiences high levels of positive affect (PA) and low levels of negative affect (NA) and is satisfied with his or her life (Diener, 1984). Within this subjective well-being framework, PA, often represented by high-arousal positive states such as excitement and elation, and NA, reflected in high-arousal negative states such as tension and hostility, are thought to be largely independent of each other (Watson, Clark, & Tellegen, 1988). The first question to ask is whether positive and negative future-thinking correlate with well-being in the general population. More interestingly, do the different aspects of future-directed thinking correlate in varied ways with the different dimensions of well-being?

MacLeod and Conway (2005) found an asymmetry in how positive and negative future-thinking related to affect. In a general community sample, positive future-thinking correlated with PA, but not with NA; NA, in contrast, showed the opposite pattern, correlating only with negative but not positive future-thinking. Life satisfaction, on the other hand, correlated with both (high) positive future-thinking and (low) negative future-thinking, suggesting that there are common as well as distinctive well-being correlates of positive and negative future-thinking. The same distinctive relationships of PA and NA with positive and negative future-thinking, respectively, have also been reported among adolescents (Miles, MacLeod, & Pote, 2004) and in a clinical sample (MacLeod, Tata, Kentish, & Jacobsen, 1997). These differential relationships reinforce the distinctiveness of positive and negative future-thinking and highlight the unique affective correlates of each type of thinking.

Turning to relationships with depression and anxiety, differential relationships have also been found. Rather in the way that lowered likelihood judgments for positive events are linked to depression, groups with depression show reduced positive future-thinking. This is true whether the groups are student samples scoring highly on depression (Kosnes, Whelan, O'Donovan, & McHugh, 2013) or patients with clinical depression (Bjärehed, Sarkohi, & Andersson, 2010; Lavender & Watkins, 2004; MacLeod & Salaminiou, 2001; MacLeod, Tata, Kentish, & Jacobsen, 1997). The reduction in positive future-thinking has also been found in older adults with clinical depression (Conaghan & Davidson, 2002) and in patients with a concurrent physical condition (multiple sclerosis; Moore, MacLeod, Barnes, & Langdon, 2006). Crucially, this reduction in positive anticipation is furnished with greater interest because in these same studies it occurs alongside the *absence* of any increase in negative future-thinking. The lack of effects with negative future-thinking is not attributable simply to lack of sensitivity or some other artifact of the measure, because anxious students (MacLeod & Byrne, 1996) and patients (MacLeod, Tata, Kentish, & Jacobsen, 1997) show elevations in negative future-thinking compared with controls, while showing no reduction in positive future-thinking.

The particular relationship involving reduced positive anticipation may be even more specific than to depression. Inducing a negative mood leads to reductions in positive future-thinking, as would be expected for the preceding findings, but only in those particular individuals who are vulnerable to feelings of hopelessness (i.e., people who report that they usually experience high levels of hopelessness when in a negative mood). Williams, Van der Does, Barnhofer, Crane, and Segal (2008) had participants complete the Leiden Index of Depression Sensitivity (LEIDS; Van der Does, 2002), which assesses the particular sorts of experiences people say they have while they are in a negative mood state. After a negative mood induction, the high scorers on the hopelessness subscale showed the greatest reduction in positive future-thinking, an effect that was independent of depression. As would be expected from the already-reported findings, there was no relationship between LEIDS hopelessness scores and changes in negative future-thinking. O'Connor and Williams (2014) found similar vulnerability effects in people who had previously reported frequent feelings of entrapment (specific beliefs about not being able to escape from painful thoughts or external circumstances), a construct closely related to hopelessness. Again, this effect was independent of depressive symptoms. Hopelessness about the future has been identified as the key component of depression for suicidal behavior (Salter & Platt, 1990). These findings suggest, therefore, that a lack of positive future-thinking might be especially salient in those who are high in hopelessness and who are suicidal, something that has indeed been found to be the case.

Suicidality

As noted above, the lack of positive anticipation may play an important role in the etiology and course of suicidal ideation and behavior. Indeed, in a series of studies, MacLeod and colleagues have demonstrated precisely this—time and again, suicidality was associated with the absence of positive future-thinking rather than with the presence of negative future-thinking (MacLeod, Pankhania, Lee, & Mitchell, 1997; MacLeod et al., 1998; MacLeod et al., 2005). Clinically, these findings are important, as they highlight that the valence of specific future thoughts is crucial to understanding suicide risk and that the presence of negative future-thinking is not functionally equivalent to the absence of positive future-thinking (MacLeod et al., 1998; MacLeod et al., 1993).

This suicidal versus nonsuicidal group difference effect (i.e., lower levels of positive future-thinking being found in suicidal vs. nonsuicidal groups) has also been replicated in clinical and nonclinical populations (Conaghan & Davidson, 2002; Hunter & O'Connor, 2003; O'Connor, O'Connor, O'Connor, Smallwood, & Miles, 2004; Sidley, Calam, Wells, Hughes, & Whitaker, 1999). The deleterious effect of the absence of positive future-thinking has also been shown to interact with high levels of stress to further increase the risk of hopelessness and suicidal ideation (O'Connor et al., 2004). In a sample of college students, levels of hopelessness and suicidal ideation were elevated among students who reported low levels of positive future thinking together with high levels of stress (O'Connor et al., 2014).

Low levels of positive future-thinking may also strengthen the relationship between high entrapment (see the earlier discussion) and suicide risk. This finding is particularly important because entrapment is posited to be the proximal psychological risk factor that leads to suicide ideation (O'Connor, 2011; Rasmussen et al., 2010; Williams, 2001). Moreover, an absence of positive future thoughts during an acute suicidal crisis may also impede recovery in the short term. In one study, low levels of positive future thoughts, when assessed within 24 hours of a suicide attempt, predicted poorer recovery (in terms of high levels of suicidal ideation) in the 2–3 months following an index episode after controlling for baseline depression, anxiety, and even self-reported hopelessness (O'Connor, Fraser, Whyte, MacHale, & Masterton, 2008). Indeed, in this study of 144 patients who had attempted suicide, low positive future-thinking and high levels of baseline suicidal ideation were the only significant predictors of suicidal ideation at follow-up when all predictors were considered together in a multivariate model.

Although there is considerable evidence that the absence of positive future-thinking is implicated in the etiology and course of a suicidal crisis, a recent longer term follow-up study points to a more complex relationship between positive future-thinking and suicide risk than was originally thought. In a 15-month prospective study, O'Connor and colleagues investigated, for the first time, whether positive future thoughts were always protective and whether they predicted suicide risk in the medium term (O'Connor, Smyth, & Williams, 2015). To address the former question, they adapted an existing coding frame for future-thinking (Godley, Tchanturia, MacLeod, & Schmidt, 2001) and classified the content of positive future thoughts into categories. Guided by suicide theory, they reasoned that not all types of future-thinking (content) would be protective. Specifically, they hypothesized that future thoughts that focused on changing a personal attribute—something specific to the individual (e.g., being happy, labeled intrapersonal positive future-thinking)—may not be protective if it becomes impossible to realize this hoped-for change over time. The findings were consistent with this conjecture. In univariate analyses, although low levels of other types of positive future-thinking (namely, achievement- and financial-related future thoughts) were associated with suicidal behavior (consistent with all of the earlier research), *high* levels of intrapersonal future-thinking were also positively associated with further suicidal behavior. Moreover, in the multivariate analyses, intrapersonal positive future-thinking was the only significant future-thinking predictor of suicidal behavior, suggesting that not all positive future-thinking is beneficial over time.

More recent research on positive fantasies (defined as fantasies about an idealized future) also supports the seemingly counterintuitive intrapersonal positive future-thinking effect (Oettingen, Mayer, & Portnow, 2016). Across a series of studies, Oettingen and colleagues (2016) found that although positive fantasies seemed to protect against depressive symptoms concurrently, the reverse was true longitudinally, with positive fantasies predicting depressive symptoms longitudinally. The mechanism(s) to explain the positive fantasies and the intrapersonal positive future-thinking effects (described earlier) are unclear. For example, future research should further investigate the extent to which low effort (as proposed by Oettingen et al., 2016) or the realization that some future thoughts are not achievable (as proposed by O'Connor et al., 2015) explain these findings. Nonetheless, taking these findings together with the broader research literature, it is clear that the absence of positive future-thinking is associated with a suicidal crisis. However, future research should focus on the content of the positive future thoughts, as some positive future thoughts may not be protective.

Employing a different method of assessment, Sargalska, Miranda, and Marroquin (2011) investigated the extent to which being "as certain as one can be" that positive events will not happen in the future predicted concurrent suicidal ideation. In this study of college students, certainty that positive events will not happen and uncertainty that negative events will occur were associated with suicidal ideation, and these relationships were partially accounted for by hopelessness. Moreover, the relationship between certainty about the absence of positive future expectancies and concurrent suicidal ideation remained significant even after controlling for hopelessness and depression. These findings highlight the utility of employing different methods of assessing positive future-thinking. Whereas a lot of research focuses on valence only (e.g., O'Connor et al., 2007), the Sargalska et al. (2011) findings suggest that another charteristic of positive future-thinking (namely, certainty) is important to consider when assessing risk of suicidal ideation.

The theoretical work on positive anticipation has also contributed to the development of a treatment intervention designed specifically to target future-oriented cognitions for suicidal patients. In the Netherlands, van Beek, Kerkhof, and Beekman (2009) have developed a program of "future-oriented group training" for suicidal patients that consists of 10 weekly group training sessions, including discussion, exercises, and future goal formulation, guided by a workbook to promote more realistic thinking and future goal setting. The results of this trial offer promise; although intention-to-treat analyses yielded a nonsignificant effect in the reduction of suicidal ideation at 12 months, the per-protocol analysis (on those who adhered to the intervention) suggests a significant reduction in suicidal ideation (van Beek, 2013).

Section Summary

There is clear evidence that anticipating positive and negative future experiences, as indicated by likelihood judgments and elicited thoughts about what one is looking forward to or not looking forward to, are linked to states of emotional well-being. Low anticipation of positive events is linked to elevated depression and lowered positive affect, as well as to suicidality. In contrast, an increase in anticipated negative events is associated with high negative affect and elevated anxiety. Furthermore, the particular content of what it is that people are anticipating looks to be important and is an area for future research.

Goals

The second main way in which a person's positive thoughts about the future are manifested is in his or her goals. There is a substantial literature on goals and well-being, and it is beyond the scope of this chapter to review these findings. Other chapters in this volume (see Part III) address some aspects of the goals literature. The particular focus in this section is on how people relate to their goals, and two main areas are discussed. The first area relates to the process of disengaging, or failing to disengage, from goals when they are proving to be difficult to attain, as well as the related process of establishing and engaging with new goals. The second, and linked, area to be discussed is how goals can be overvalued, to the point at which they are seen as essential for future happiness and fulfilment.

Disengagement–Reengagement

Each of us is driven by the pursuit of goals; indeed, "goals give meaning to people's lives, [that] understanding the person means understanding the person's goals" (Carver, 2004). As noted previously, their importance is reflected in the substantial literature on self-regulation that highlights the central role of goal attainment as a determinant of well-being (Carver & Scheier, 1998; Heckhausen, Wrosch, & Schulz, 2010; Wrosch, Scheier, Carver, & Schulz, 2003; Wrosch, Scheier, Miller, Schulz, & Carver, 2003). However, in this section, we focus on what happens when a goal proves unattainable. As limited-capacity information processers, at some stage, we have to decide when enough is enough and the costs of continuing to pursue a goal outweigh the benefits. To investigate this process of goal regulation when confronted with unattainable goals, Wrosch and colleagues developed the Goal Adjustment Scale, which comprises two subscales (Wrosch, Scheier, Miller, et al., 2003). The first subscale, Goal Disengagement, taps the ease with which respondents are able to reduce effort in the pursuit of a goal and relinquish commitment toward its attainment (e.g., "It's easy for me to reduce my effort toward the goal"; Wrosch, Scheier, Miller, at al., 2003). Goal Reengagement, the second subscale, assesses the extent to which respondents are able to generate new goals that are attainable (e.g., "I convince myself that I have other meaningful goals to pursue").

Research from different populations across the lifespan highlights the potentially pernicious and protective effects of the regulation of unattainable goals on subjective well-being, depression, and suicidality (O'Connor, Fraser, Whyte, MacHale, & Masterton, 2009; O'Connor, O'Carroll, Ryan, & Smyth, 2012; Wrosch & Scheier, 2003; Wrosch, Scheier, Miller, et al., 2003). For example, high levels of disengagement have been shown to be independently associated with high levels of mastery, low stress, low intrusive thoughts, low depressive symptoms, and positive subjective well-being (Heckhausen, Wrosch, & Fleeson, 2001; Wrosch & Heckhausen, 1999; Wrosch, Scheier, Miller, et al., 2003). The potentially protective effects of goal reengagement are also considerable, with evidence that high levels of goal reengagement predict subjective well-being beyond the effect of goal disengagement (Wrosch, Scheier, Miller, et al., 2003).

The ability to disengage from old goals and reengage with new ones may be particularly important in populations in which attainment of existing goals becomes more difficult. In a 6-year follow-up study of older adults, there was clear evidence that disengaging in unattainable goals may be protective (Dunne, Wrosch, & Miller, 2011). As depressive symptoms increased over time, those who had poor goal disengagement capacities experienced more depressive symptoms. Moreover, among those who experienced increases in disability, the greater their capacity to disengage was, the less they showed an increase in depressive symptoms. Goal disengagement and reengagement have also been shown to predict well-being following advanced breast cancer diagnosis up to 12 months postdiagnosis (Lam et al., 2016). In a study of 193 women, high goal disengagement and low reengagement were associated with lower baseline anxiety, while high goal disengagement predicted a slower rate of change in anxiety. In addition, those who reported being able to disengage and reengage with new goals showed lower baseline depression (Lam et al., 2016).

There is some evidence that goal disengagement and reengagement can combine to predict risk of suicidal behavior. Across two studies, O'Connor and colleagues demonstrated that high levels of goal reengagement linked to lower suicidal ideation and attempts over time in patients who had attempted suicide (O'Connor et al., 2009; O'Connor et al., 2012). However, in another study of 237 patients admitted to hospital following a suicide attempt, the relationship between goal disengagement, reengagement, and subsequent suicide risk (or another episode of hospital-treated self-harm) varied as a function of age (O'Connor et al., 2012). Specifically, among younger adults, risk of self-harm was elevated if, at baseline, they reported low levels of disengagement and low levels of reengagement. Conversely, self-harm was significantly more likely among those older adults who reported high levels of disengagement and low levels of reengagement at baseline. For the older adults, the authors posited that the findings yielded evidence for complete disengagement, as they had no reasons for living and therefore were at increased risk of suicide. In contrast, they reasoned that the young people who had not disengaged and had not generated new goals were at elevated risk because they were engaged in painful goal pursuit akin to MacLeod and Conway's concept of *painful engagement* (MacLeod & Conway, 2007), discussed in the following section. Given the importance of goal disengagement and reengagement, future research should focus on exploring the extent to which self-regulatory processes—such as implementation intentions (the formation of if–then plans) and mental contrasting (mentally considering one's desired future, thinking about potential obstacles and how to overcome such obstacles; Fritzsche, Schlier, Oettingen, & Lincoln, 2016; Henderson, Gollwitzer, & Oettingen, 2007; Oettingen, 2012)—facilitate goal pursuit in suicidal individuals.

Although we have focused on goal disengagement and reengagement as the key processes here, other authors have suggested overlapping constructs such as tenacious goal pursuit and flexible goal pursuit adjustment, which have also been shown to be related to positive emotional well-being (Coffey, Gallagher, Desmond, & Ryall, 2014). Irrespective of method of assessment, though, the findings are unambiguous: How people respond to unattainable goals is strongly linked to their well-being.

Painful Engagement

Perhaps surprisingly, those who are depressed, even those who are suicidal, are able to describe personal goals: When asked to generate goals, they do not differ from control participants in the number of personal goals they are able to think of (Dickson, Moberly, & Kinderman, 2011; Vincent, Boddana, & MacLeod, 2004). What does appear to distinguish them clearly from their nondepressed or nonsuicidal counterparts is that they judge those goals as relatively unlikely to be realized. One question that can be asked is why some people believe their goals are unlikely to be realized. Undoubtedly, there are numerous contributors, ranging from social and economic circumstances through to psychological factors such as poor planning ability (Vincent et al., 2004). A second question links to the findings reviewed in the previous section about why people who have mood disturbances have difficulty disengaging from goals that they see as being relatively unlikely to be realized. Some people appear to get stuck in a state of painful engagement. Painful engagement describes a state in which an individual does have personal goals for the future, believes those goals are relatively unlikely to be realized, yet is unable to let go of them. In this situation, why would someone not disengage from their low-likelihood goals and go on to engage with new, different goals? Restricted opportunities, lack of skills to identify new goals and pursue them, and impaired motivation are likely contributors. But the answer may also lie in a "pull" toward their current goals which is difficult to overcome.

Conditional Goal Setting

Engaging with new goals is unlikely to happen unless someone disengages from persistently unattainable goals, and one candidate for the pull toward current goals and the failure to disengage from them is the overvaluation of those current goals. In fact, the person might see attainment of his or her goals as the only way that he or she will ever experience happiness in the future. Goal theories suggest that goals are organized hierarchically, in which higher order goals, such as to be happy or fulfilled, are linked to subgoals, whose attainment will contribute to the achievement of that higher order goal (Carver & Scheier, 1990). The system works well when there is this coherent linkage, but it is also possible for the links to be in place too strongly and inflexibly. In such cases, the goals at the different levels become overly identified with each other. Street (2002) labels this phenomenon *conditional goal setting*. For example, if someone believes that the only way of being happy in the future is to spend the rest of her life with her husband, who has left her, then, at one level, it would never make sense to let go of that goal, because however unlikely it is seen as, there is no alternative. Given such beliefs toward their important goals, it is perhaps not surprising that people find it difficult to disengage from those goals when they are failing and to move on to new, different goals.

Conditional goal setting has been measured by identifying people's goals and assessing to what degree they endorse statements such as "I can only be happy if . . ." in relation to their important goals. High levels of conditional goal setting are related to depression (Crane, Barnhofer, Hargus, Amarasinghe, & Winder, 2010; Street, 2002). They are also related specifically to levels of hopelessness in individuals with depression (Hadley & MacLeod, 2010), as well as being elevated in those who have recently exhibited suicidal behavior (Danchin, MacLeod, & Tata, 2010). Danchin et al. (2010) compared their suicidal group not only to a standard mood control group but also to a group of psychiatric patients with comparably high levels of depression who were not suicidal; the suicidal group showed significantly higher levels of conditional goal setting than both of the other two groups (the group with depression also scored higher than the standard-mood controls). Consistent with the findings reported by Hadley and MacLeod (2010), the suicidal group, although equivalent in depression to the psychiatric controls, did have significantly higher levels of hopelessness about the future, suggesting that hopelessness and suicidality have specific links with conditional goal setting.

It is perhaps not surprising that those who are suicidal and are high in levels of hopelessness would endorse items about only being able to be happy in the future if certain important future events happened. What would be more interesting, perhaps, would be to show that goals are not only seen as *necessary* but are also seen as *sufficient* for future happiness. Danchin et al. (2010) reversed the conditional goal-setting statements, this time asking participants how happy and fulfilled people thought they *would* be *if* the goal *was* achieved. The suicidal patients showed stronger endorsement of these positive statements than did either the psychiatric or general population control groups; that is, they anticipated experiencing higher levels of happiness upon achievement of their goals than did either of the other two groups. Coughlan, Tata, and MacLeod (2016) examined this issue more directly by first asking participants to rate their levels of subjective and psychological well-being. Participants then spent some time envisaging and imagining their most important goal being achieved. Finally, they completed the same well-being measures again, this time under instructions to provide ratings about how they anticipated they would feel with their most important goal achieved. Despite being significantly lower on the various measures of well-being at the outset, after the envisaging phase, suicidal participants gave *anticipated* well-being ratings that were equivalent to those of the controls.

Interestingly, the findings on conditional goal setting connect to the work of Oettingen and colleagues (e.g., Oettingen, 2012) showing that people are able to derive emotional benefit in the present through simply entertaining fantasies about the future. This form of future-thought can get in the way of taking the sometimes difficult steps toward achieving goals because of the immediate emotional benefits such thoughts provide. It remains an interesting question whether those with serious mood disturbance do show this form of future-thinking about their goals, and, if so, whether it can be changed through contrasting the present with the future fantasy, an approach that has been found to be an effective goal-regulation strategy in other circumstances, even in those with depression (Fritzsche et al., 2016). Clearly, mental contrasting would need to be handled carefully in those who have severe depression or are suicidal, but moving people away from their fantasy thinking about goals to a more realistic appraisal in which they either start to engage with the steps needed to move toward the goals or disengage and engage with new goals is an important therapeutic aim.

SUMMARY AND CONCLUSION

How people think about their own futures is fundamental to their mental health and well-being. In this chapter, we have focused on two aspects of positive future-thinking—expectancies, especially in the active sense of anticipating what positive and negative experiences one might have in the future, and goals. It has become clear that problems with positive future-thinking are central to the difficulties experienced by many of those who have depression, and particularly those who are suicidal. A lack of positive thoughts about the future, in the absence of increased negative thoughts, is reliably associated with depression and suicidality, including future risk of further suicidal behavior. Furthermore, the nature of those thoughts appears to be important, in that a focus on one's own feeling states is associated with worse outcomes. Well-being is also associated with goals. In this chapter, we have focused on how people respond to their goals—how they respond when their goals are proving to be unattainable and whether they can then engage with and pursue new goals. People with mood disturbance have difficulty with both of these aspects of relating to goals, possibly because of the degree of valuing of, and investment in, the goals that they currently hold, leading them to a position of painful engagement. Understanding more about how lack of positive future-thinking is related to low well-being, including extreme states of low well-being, offers opportunities to intervene and help those experiencing such states of distress, including those at elevated risk of suicide.

REFERENCES

Beck, A. T. (1976). *Cognitive therapy and the emotional disorders*. Madison, CT: International Universities Press.

Bjärehed, J., Sarkohi, A., & Andersson, G. (2010). Less positive or more negative?: Future-directed thinking in mild to moderate depression. *Cognitive Behaviour Therapy, 39,* 37–45.

Bredemeier, K., Berenbaum, H., & Spielberg, J. M. (2012). Worry and perceived threat of proximal and distal undesirable outcomes. *Journal of Anxiety Disorders, 26,* 425–429.

Carver, C. S. (2004). Self-regulation of action and affect. In R. F. V. Baumeister & K. D. Vohs (Eds.), *Handbook of self-regulation: Research, theory and applications* (pp. 13–39). New York: Guilford Press.

Carver, C. S., & Scheier, M. F. (1990). Origins and functions of positive and negative affect: A control-process view. *Psychological Review, 97,* 19–35.

Carver, C. S., & Scheier, M. F. (1998). *On the self-regulation of behaviour*. New York: Cambridge University Press.

Coffey, L., Gallagher, P., Desmond, D., & Ryall, N. (2014). Goal pursuit, goal adjustment, and affective well-being following lower limb amputation. *British Journal of Health Psychology, 19,* 409–424.

Conaghan, S., & Davidson, K. M. (2002). Hopelessness and the anticipation of positive and negative future experiences in older parasuicidal adults. *British Journal of Clinical Psychology, 41,* 233–242.

Coughlan, K., Tata, P., & MacLeod, A. K. (2016). Personal goals, well-being and deliberate self-harm. *Cognitive Therapy and Research, 41*(3), 434–443.

Crane, C., Barnhofer, T., Hargus, E., Amarasinghe, M., & Winder, R. (2010). The relationship between dispositional mindfulness and conditional goal setting in depressed patients. *British Journal of Clinical Psychology, 49,* 281–290.

Danchin, C. L., MacLeod, A. K., & Tata, P. (2010). Painful engagement in deliberate self-harm: The role of conditional goal setting. *Behaviour Research and Therapy, 48,* 915–920.

Dickson, J. M., Moberly, N. J., & Kinderman, P. (2011). Depressed people are not less motivated by personal goals but are more pessimistic about attaining them. *Journal of Abnormal Psychology, 120,* 975–980.

Diener, E. (1984). Subjective well-being. *Psychological Bulletin, 95,* 542–575.

Dunne, E., Wrosch, C., & Miller, G. E. (2011). Goal disengagement, functional disability, and depressive symptoms in old age. *Health Psychology, 30,* 763–770.

Eccles, J. S., & Wigfield, A. (2002). Motivational beliefs, values, and goals. *Annual Review of Psychology, 53,* 109–132.

English Oxford Living Dictionaries. (2016). Retrieved from *https://en.oxforddictionaries.com/definition/goal*.

Fritzsche, A., Schlier, B., Oettingen, G., & Lincoln, T. M. (2016). Mental contrasting with implementation intentions increases goal-attainment in individuals with mild to moderate depression. *Cognitive Therapy and Research, 40,* 557–564.

Godley, J., Tchanturia, K., MacLeod, A., & Schmidt, U. (2001). Future-directed thinking in eating disorders. *British Journal of Clinical Psychology, 40,* 281–295.

Hadley, S. A., & MacLeod, A. K. (2010). Conditional goal-setting, personal goals and hopelessness about the future. *Cognition and Emotion, 24,* 1191–1198.

Heckhausen, J., Wrosch, C., & Fleeson, W. (2001). Developmental regulation before and after a developmental deadline: The sample case of "biological clock" for childbearing. *Psychology and Aging, 16,* 400–413.

Heckhausen, J., Wrosch, C., & Schulz, R. (2010). A motivational theory of life-span development. *Psychological Review, 117,* 32–60.

Henderson, M. D., Gollwitzer, P. M., & Oettingen, G. (2007). Implementation intentions and disengagement from a failing course of action. *Journal of Behavioural Decision Making, 20,* 81–102.

Hepburn, S. R., Barnhofer, T., & Williams, J. M. G. (2006). Effects of mood on how future events are generated and perceived. *Personality and Individual Differences, 41,* 801–811.

Hunter, E. C., & O'Connor, R. C. (2003). Hopelessness and future thinking in parasuicide: The role of perfectionism. *British Journal of Clinical Psychology, 42,* 355–365.

Kosnes, L., Whelan, R., O'Donovan, A., & McHugh, L. A. (2013). Implicit measurement of positive and negative future thinking as a predictor of depressive symptoms and hopelessness. *Consciousness and Cognition, 22,* 898–912.

Lam, W. W. T., Yeo, W., Suen, J., Ho, W. M., Tsang, J., Soong, I., . . . Fielding, R. (2016). Goal adjustment influence on psychological well-being following advanced breast cancer diagnosis. *Psycho-Oncology, 25,* 58–65.

Lavender, A., & Watkins, E. (2004). Rumination and future thinking in depression. *British Journal of Clinical Psychology, 43,* 129–142.

Lezak, M. D., Howieson, D. B., Bigler, E. D., & Tranel, D. (2012). *Neuropsychological assessment* (5th ed.). New York: Oxford University Press.

MacLeod, A. K. (2017). *Prospection, well-being and mental health.* New York: Oxford University Press.

MacLeod, A. K., & Byrne, A. (1996). Anxiety, depression, and the anticipation of future positive and negative experiences. *Journal of Abnormal Psychology, 105,* 286–289.

MacLeod, A. K., & Conway, C. (2005). Well-being and the anticipation of future positive experiences: The role of income, social networks, and planning ability. *Cognition and Emotion, 19,* 357–374.

MacLeod, A. K., & Conway, C. (2007). Well-being and positive future thinking for the self versus others. *Cognition and Emotion, 21,* 1114–1124.

MacLeod, A. K., Pankhania, B., Lee, M., & Mitchell, D. (1997). Parasuicide, depression and the anticipation of positive and negative future experiences. *Psychological Medicine, 27,* 973–977.

MacLeod, A. K., Rose, G. S., & Williams, J. M. G. (1993). Components of hopelessness about the future in parasuicide. *Cognitive Therapy and Research, 17,* 441–455.

MacLeod, A. K., & Salaminiou, E. (2001). Reduced positive future-thinking in depression: Cognitive and affective factors. *Cognition and Emotion, 15,* 99–107.

MacLeod, A. K., Tata, P., Evans, K., Tyrer, P., Schmidt, U., Davidson, K., . . . Catalan, J. (1998). Recovery of positive future thinking within a high-risk parasuicide group: Results from a pilot randomized controlled trial. *British Journal of Clinical Psychology, 37,* 371–379.

MacLeod, A. K., Tata, P., Kentish, J., Carroll, F., & Hunter, E. (1997). Anxiety, depression, and explanation-based pessimism for future positive and negative events. *Clinical Psychology and Psychotherapy, 4,* 15–24.

MacLeod, A. K., Tata, P., Kentish, J., & Jacobsen, H. (1997). Retrospective and prospective cognitions in anxiety and depression. *Cognition and Emotion, 11,* 467–479.

MacLeod, A. K., Tata, P., Tyrer, P., Schmidt, U., Davidson, K., & Thompson, S. (2005). Hopelessness and positive and negative future thinking in parasuicide. *British Journal of Clinical Psychology, 44,* 495–504.

Miles, H., MacLeod, A. K., & Pote, H. (2004). Retrospective and prospective cognitions in adolescents: Anxiety, depression, and positive and negative affect. *Journal of Adolescence, 27,* 691–701.

Miranda, R., & Mennin, D. S. (2007). Depression, generalized anxiety disorder, and certainty in pessimistic predictions about the future. *Cognitive Therapy and Research, 31,* 71–82.

Moore, A. C., MacLeod, A. K., Barnes, D., & Langdon, D. W. (2006). Future-directed thinking and depression in relapsing-remitting multiple sclerosis. *British Journal of Health Psychology, 11,* 663–675.

Nagengast, B., Marsh, H. W., Scalas, L. F., Xu, M. K., Hau, K.-T., & Trautwein, U. (2011). Who took the 'x' out of expectancy-value theory?: A psychological mystery, a substantive-methodological synergy, and a cross-national generalization. *Psychological Science, 22,* 1058–1066.

O'Connor, R. C. (2011). Towards an integrated motivational–volitional model of suicidal behavior. In R. O'Connor, S. Platt, & J. Gordon (Eds.), *International handbook of suicide prevention: Research, policy and practice* (pp. 181–198). Malden, MA: Wiley-Blackwell.

O'Connor, R. C., Fraser, L., Whyte, M.-C., MacHale, S., & Masterton, G. (2008). A comparison of specific positive future expectancies and global hopelessness as predictors of suicidal ideation in a prospective study of repeat self-harmers. *Journal of Affective Disorders, 110,* 207–214.

O'Connor, R. C., Fraser, L., Whyte, M.-C., MacHale, S., & Masterton, G. (2009). Self-regulation of unattainable goals in suicide attempters: The relationship between goal disengagement, goal reengagement and suicidal ideation. *Behaviour Research and Therapy, 47,* 164–169.

O'Connor, R. C., O'Carroll, R. E., Ryan, C., & Smyth, R. (2012). Self-regulation of unattainable goals in suicide attempters: A two year prospective study. *Journal of Affective Disorders, 142,* 248–255.

O'Connor, R. C., O'Connor, D. B., O'Connor, S. M., Smallwood, J., & Miles, J. (2004). Hopelessness, stress, and perfectionism: The moderating effects of future thinking. *Cognition and Emotion, 18,* 1099–1120.

O'Connor, R. C., Smyth, R., & Williams, J. M. G. (2015). Intrapersonal positive future thinking predicts repeat suicide attempts in hospital-treated suicide attempters. *Journal of Consulting and Clinical Psychology, 83,* 169–176.

O'Connor, R. C., Whyte, M.-C., Fraser, L., Masterton, G., Miles, J., & MacHale, S. (2007). Predicting short-term outcome in well-being following suicidal behaviour: The conjoint effects of social perfectionism and positive future thinking. *Behaviour Research and Therapy, 45,* 1543–1555.

O'Connor, R. C., & Williams, J. M. G. (2014). The relationship between positive future thinking, brooding, defeat and entrapment. *Personality and Individual Differences, 70,* 29–34.

Oettingen, G. (2012). Future thought and behaviour change. *European Review of Social Psychology, 23,* 1–63.

Oettingen, G., Mayer, D., & Portnow, S. (2016). Pleasure now, pain later: Positive fantasies about the future predict symptoms of depression. *Psychological Science, 27,* 345–353.

Oettingen, G., Pak, H., & Schnetter, K. (2001). Self-regulation of goal-setting: Turning free fantasies about the future into binding goals. *Journal of Personality and Social Psychology, 80,* 736–753.

Rasmussen, S. A., Fraser, L., Gotz, M., MacHale, S., Mackie, R., Masterton, G., . . . O'Connor, R. C. (2010). Elaborating the cry of pain model of suicidality: Testing a psychological model in a sample of first-time and repeat self-harm patients. *British Journal of Clinical Psychology, 49,* 15–30.

Salter, D., & Platt, S. (1990). Suicidal intent, hopelessness and depression in a parasuicide population: The influence of social desirability and elapsed time. *British Journal of Clinical Psychology, 29,* 361–371.

Sargalska, J., Miranda, R., & Marroquin, B. (2011). Being certain about an absence of the positive: Specificity in relation to hopelessness and suicidal ideation. *International Journal of Cognitive Therapy, 4,* 104–116.

Scheier, M. F., Carver, C. S., & Bridges, M. W. (1994). Distinguishing optimism from neuroticism (and trait anxiety, self-mastery, and self-esteem): A reevaluation of the Life Orientation Test. *Journal of Personality and Social Psychology, 67,* 1063–1078.

Sidley, G. L., Calam, R., Wells, A., Hughes, T., & Whitaker, K. (1999). The prediction of parasuicide repetition in a high-risk group. *British Journal of Clinical Psychology, 38,* 375–386.

Street, H. (2002). Exploring relationships between goal setting, goal pursuit and depression: A review. *The Australian Psychologist, 37,* 95–103.

Van Beek, W. (2013). *Future-thinking in suicidal patients: Development and evaluation of a future oriented group training in a randomized controlled trial.* Doctoral dissertation, Vrije University, Amsterdam, The Netherlands.

Van Beek, W., Kerkhof, A., & Beekman, A. (2009). Future oriented group training for suicidal patients: A randomized clinical trial. *BMC Psychiatry, 9,* 7.

Van der Does, W. (2002). Cognitive reactivity to sad mood: Structure and validity of a new measure. *Behaviour Research and Therapy, 40,* 105–120.

Vincent, P. J., Boddana, P., & MacLeod, A. K. (2004). Positive life goals and plans in parasuicide. *Clinical Psychology and Psychotherapy, 11,* 90–99.

Watson, D., Clark, L. A., & Tellegen, A. (1988). Development and validation of brief measures of positive and negative affect: The PANAS scales. *Journal of Personality and Social Psychology, 54,* 1063–1070.

Weinstein, N. D. (1980). Unrealistic optimism about future life events. *Journal of Personality and Social Psychology, 39,* 806–820.

Wenze, S. J., Gunthert, K. C., & German, R. E. (2012). Biases in affective forecasting and recall in individuals with depression and anxiety symptoms. *Personality and Social Psychology Bulletin, 38,* 895–906.

Williams, J. M. G. (2001). *The cry of pain.* London: Penguin.

Williams, J. M. G., Van der Does, A. J. W., Barnhofer, T., Crane, C., & Segal, Z. S. (2008). Cognitive reactivity, suicidal ideation and future fluency: Preliminary investigation of a differential activation theory of hopelessness/suicidality. *Cognitive Therapy and Research, 32,* 83–104.

Wrosch, C., & Heckhausen, J. (1999). Control processes before and after passing a developmental deadline: Activation and deactivation of intimate relationship goals. *Journal of Personality and Social Psychology, 77,* 415–427.

Wrosch, C., & Scheier, M. F. (2003). Personality and quality of life: The importance of optimism and goal adjustment. *Quality of Life Research, 12,* 59–72.

Wrosch, C., Scheier, M. F., Carver, C. S., & Schulz, R. (2003). The importance of goal disengagement in adaptive self-regulation: When giving up is beneficial. *Self and Identity, 2,* 1–20.

Wrosch, C., Scheier, M. F., Miller, G. E., Schulz, R., & Carver, C. S. (2003). Adaptive self-regulation of unattainable goals: Goal disengagement, goal reengagement, and subjective well-being. *Personality and Social Psychology Bulletin, 29,* 1494–1508.

CHAPTER 11

Generalized Optimism

Charles S. Carver
Michael F. Scheier

Optimists are people who expect things to work out well for them; pessimists are people who expect things to work out badly for them. Optimism is a personality trait: a continuously varying dimension of generalized expectancies about one's own future. As a construct, it is intrinsically future-oriented, although it draws upon experiences from the past to suggest what that future will be like.

The optimism construct is related to several other constructs discussed in this book, and yet it is different from them. Optimism is not really about imagining a particular future (as others discuss in Part I of this volume), but differences in optimism clearly reflect variations in how people orient themselves to the future. Optimism definitely represents positive thinking, but it does not consist of positive fantasies and daydreams (cf. Oettingen, 2012, 2014). Optimism is not really about goals and plans per se (as others discuss in Part III of this volume), but it very likely has a large influence on the ways in which people go about pursuing their goals and plans and the success with which they do so. Optimism as we discuss it here is generalized, an expectation for one's broad future, rather than being focused on a particular domain of life (as other discuss in some of the other chapters in Part II). Furthermore, it is a property that seems not to entail any particular comparison with other people (which is an element discussed in some other chapters of the volume).

OPTIMISM AND PESSIMISM

Optimism as a concept has roots in centuries of folk psychology, and it has been studied as a scientific topic for at least 30 years. Because it is based on expectancies for the future, the scientific conception of optimism also has roots in a long history of expectancy–value models of motivation (Eccles & Wigfield, 2002). Expectancy-value theories assume that behavior reflects pursuit of goals: desired states or activities. The more important a goal is, the greater its *value* (Austin & Vancouver, 1996; Carver & Scheier, 1998; Higgins, 2006). The other element is *expectancy*—the degree of confidence that the goal can be reached. People who doubt they can reach a goal withdraw their effort. They may stop trying prematurely, or they may never really start. People who are confident about reaching a goal persevere, even in the face of adversity.

Expectancies exist at many levels of inclusiveness. Confidence and doubt can pertain to very narrow contexts (e.g., the ability to raise and place one's foot 16 inches forward), to somewhat broader contexts (e.g., the ability to cross a street unaided), to even broader ones (e.g., the ability to navigate an unfamiliar city with a map), and to some contexts that are quite broad indeed (e.g., the ability to travel throughout the world). Optimism, as conceptualized here, is a generalized sense of confidence: confidence pertaining to life, rather than to just a specific context (Scheier & Carver, 1992). This breadth means that the expectancy it reflects should apply in many different contexts (without denying that narrower expectancies in those same contexts are also relevant—cf. Scheier et al., 1989). Optimists should generally tend to be more confident and persistent, whereas pessimists should tend to be more doubtful and hesitant.

Measurement

Research has taken two pathways to assessing optimism. One is to ask people directly whether they expect outcomes in their lives to be good or bad (Scheier & Carver, 1992). This approach underlies the Life Orientation Test (LOT) and its revision the LOT-R (Scheier, Carver, & Bridges, 1994). People indicate their degree of agreement or disagreement with statements about the future (e.g., "I'm always optimistic about my future," and "I rarely count on good things happening to me" [reverse coded]).

Another approach follows from the idea that expectancies for the future stem from causal interpretations of the past (Peterson & Seligman, 1984). If past failures are seen as having stable causes, then one should expect failure in the future because the cause is likely to remain in place. If past failures have unstable causes, however, one might expect a potentially brighter future because the cause may not be present any longer. Rather than measuring optimism and pessimism directly, this approach measures attributions about the causes of events, focusing on the idea that some attributions foster more optimistic expectations than others (Peterson & Seligman, 1984).

It turns out, however, that attributions for negative events correlate only modestly with direct measures of generalized expectancies (Ahrens & Haaga, 1993; Peterson & Vaidya, 2001). Thus, despite the fact that there is conceptual similarity underlying the two approaches, the two are not interchangeable. In part because the attributional style measure is more difficult to administer, researchers have come to rely more and more on assessing expectancies directly.

Whichever approach is used, assessment in any typical group yields a continuous distribution of scores. We commonly refer to optimists and pessimists here as though they were distinct classes, but in fact people range from very optimistic to very pessimistic, with most being somewhere between. Most people actually are on the optimistic side of neutral, but to differing degrees. Far fewer people actually disagree with optimistic items and agree with pessimistic items (Segerstrom, 2006a). Therefore, some of the differences attributed to optimism versus pessimism might be more accurately attributed to greater versus lesser degrees of optimism.

Before we continue, we should mention one more issue about assessment— which also links to a conceptual issue. Some items of the LOT-R refer to good outcomes, others refer to bad outcomes. This was because the intent behind the scale was to assess both confidence that good outcomes would occur and confidence that bad outcomes would fail to occur. We had no reason to believe that people who were optimistic about one class of outcome would be pessimistic about the other. However, responses to the two sets of items do not correlate as strongly as expected. This raises a question as to whether the imperfect association derives from method (the fact that people semantically process good and bad items differently) or from substance (there are two distinct traits, one pertaining to good outcomes, the other pertaining to bad outcomes).

The answer is not entirely clear. In some studies, the item subsets have differentially predicted outcomes (e.g., Marshall, Wortman, Kusulas, Hervig, & Vickers, 1992; Robinson-Whelen, Kim, MacCallum, & Kiecolt-Glaser, 1997), but in many other studies they have not. A statistical issue has also been raised: that the loss of reliability associated with reducing the scale length (by splitting it into two sets of 3 items) might yield spurious differences between the two subscales (Segerstrom, Evans, & Eisenlohr-Moul, 2011). There remains disagreement on this question. Some people take a unidimensional view (Rauch, Schweizer, & Moosbrugger, 2007; Segerstrom et al., 2011); others prefer a two-dimensional view (Herzberg, Glaesmer, & Hoyer, 2006). For descriptive simplicity, we treat optimism–pessimism here as one dimension.

Finally, we reiterate that optimism is a trait. Your level of optimism is part of your personality. As is true of all research on personality, research on optimism entails measuring variations in the trait across a group of people and relating the trait to some other variable. By definition, this research is correlational. This makes it exceedingly difficult to be certain that the predictor (in this case, optimism) is the cause of variation in the other variable. This difficulty is dealt with in some instances by including measures of other potential causes to see whether they account for the associations found for optimism. However, fundamentally this uncertainty is an occupational hazard for personality psychologists. There simply is no way other than this to study variations in personality (Carver & Scheier, 2012).

Origins of Optimism

If a person's degree of optimism is a trait, where does this trait come from? As with most traits, there is evidence for both genetic and environmental contributions to optimism. One study estimated the heritability of LOT scores at approximately 25% (Plomin et al., 1992). This is a lower heritability than many traits display, but still a substantial genetic contribution. On the other hand, childhood environment, in the form of parental warmth, financial security, and parental socioeconomic status (SES), has also predicted adult optimism (Heinonen, Räikkönen, & Keltikangas-Järvinen, 2005; Heinonen et al., 2006).

In adulthood, there is evidence of both stability and change, again consistent with other traits. Test–retest correlations have been relatively high over periods of a few weeks to 3 years, ranging from .58 to .79 (Atienza, Stephens, & Townsend, 2004; Lucas, Diener, & Suh, 1996; Scheier & Carver, 1985; Scheier et al., 1994). However, correlations over 10 years are more mixed, with one study finding a correlation of .35 in young adulthood (Segerstrom, 2007), and another finding a correlation of .71 in middle age (Matthews, Räikkönen, Sutton-Tyrrell, & Kuller, 2004). Thus it seems that optimism continues to evolve even in adulthood, as is true of most traits (Roberts, Walton, & Viechtbauer, 2006).

What might prompt such changes in optimism in adulthood? One possibility is that resources in adulthood continue to influence later optimism, just as childhood resources did. Consistent with this view, optimism displays a strong socioeconomic gradient among adults, particularly with occupational class and income (Boehm, Chen, Williams, Ryff, & Kubzansky, 2015). Increases in social resources in adulthood (e.g., friendship networks) may also foster greater optimism. In a 10-year follow-up of first-year law students, increases in social resources correlated with increases in optimism (Segerstrom, 2007).

Although more research is needed on how optimism evolves across the lifespan, it appears that positive expectations for the future are fostered by the very resources that help people who have positive expectations to attain better outcomes. Therefore, change in optimism over time may reflect an upward spiral of optimism and resources, in which resources promote optimism, and optimism in turn promotes resource growth (e.g., college graduation, social network development).

BEHAVIORAL MANIFESTATIONS OF OPTIMISM

The optimism dimension has been studied in a fairly wide range of contexts. Some of them follow fairly directly from the motivational underpinnings of the construct. Others range more widely.

Motivational Phenomena

One obvious area in which optimism should play a role in behavior is in active goal pursuit. As we said early on, expectancy–value models assume that greater confidence should promote greater engagement in goal-directed efforts. Optimists' approach orientation to goals is evident in their greater persistence at goals assigned to them in laboratory experiments (e.g., solving anagrams; Solberg Nes, Segerstrom, & Sephton, 2005). It is also evident in their daily lives. One study found that highly optimistic college freshmen were only half as likely to drop out of school before their sophomore year as were more pessimistic ones (Solberg Nes, Evans, & Segerstrom, 2009). Another study found that optimistic law students had higher income 10 years later than those less optimistic (Segerstrom, 2007), suggesting stronger goal pursuit in their professional careers.

In another study of goal pursuit across an academic semester, optimistic students were found to be more committed to their goals and to make more progress toward those goals across the semester (Segerstrom & Solberg Nes, 2006). On the other hand, optimistic students also had more goal conflict, which occurs when pursuing one goal interferes with pursuit of another. Two kinds of conflict were assessed in this study. *Resource* conflict arises when goals compete for resources such as time and energy (e.g., "go to more parties" competes with "study harder"). *Inherent* conflict arises when progress toward one goal inherently undermines progress toward another (e.g., "be outgoing" competes with "do not draw attention to myself"). Optimism was related to greater resource conflict, but not to inherent conflict.

Optimists in this study also did better at balancing expectancy and value against the costs associated with goal conflict (Segerstrom & Solberg Nes, 2006). Specifically, the optimistic students were more guided by goal importance: The more important the goal, the more effort they dedicated to it, and the more likely they were to achieve it. The more pessimistic students did not pursue (or achieve) highly valued goals to a greater degree than less valued ones. Thus optimism seems to predispose people to more efficient and effective pursuit of valued goals (for further evidence on this, see Geers, Wellman, & Lassiter, 2009).

Greater persistence at goal striving among optimists has also been shown in studies of people facing health challenges. One study found that optimistic women with fibromyalgia persisted at health and social goals in the face of pain and fatigue to a greater extent than did less optimistic women (Affleck et al., 2001). Another study found that more optimistic breast cancer patients were less likely to let social activities be disrupted by their disease and its treatment (Carver, Lehman, & Antoni, 2003).

A particular challenge arises when goals become unattainable. In that case, it is often better to disengage from them and set new ones that are more attainable (Wrosch, Scheier, Carver, & Schulz, 2003). Optimists and pessimists do not differ in their reports that they find it easy to disengage from unattainable goals, but optimists do report finding it easier to take up new goals. Optimistic older adults have also been found to be more likely to replace activities lost to illness and to have higher well-being 1 year later as a consequence (Duke, Leventhal, Brownlee, & Leventhal, 2002; Rasmussen, Wrosch, Scheier, & Carver, 2006).

Optimism has been related to both tenacious and flexible goal pursuit (for a review of how these properties are interwoven in effective goal pursuit, see Gollwitzer, Parks-Stamm, Jaudas, & Sheeran, 2008). Perhaps suprisingly, given the connection between confidence and tenacity, one study has found that flexibility in goal pursuit accounted for more of optimists' better subjective well-being than did tenacity (Hanssen et al., 2015). It is important to be able to let go and shift to something else (flexibility), and it appears that optimists are able to navigate that issue well.

There is evidence that engaging in mental contrasting of one's desired end and one's current situation plays an important role both in effective goal pursuit and in the disengagement from unattainable goals (e.g., Kappes & Oettingen, 2014; Oettingen, 2012). Given the evidence reviewed above about the motivational correlates of optimism, it would seem a reasonable idea that optimists are more likely to make such mental contrasts than pessimists. Though there exists a valid tool to assess the spontaneous use of mental contrasting (Sevincer & Oettingen, 2013), this is a hypothesis that, to the best of our knowledge, has not been tested.

Social Correlates of Optimism

Although it may be most intuitive to point to the principle of goal engagement with respect to such domains as academics and achievement, goal engagement also seems implicated in other beneficial effects of optimism. Optimism fosters the building of social resources, which are very important in life. Social resources can lessen the impact of negative events (e.g., via social support) or promote positive events (e.g., being invited to parties). Optimistic college freshmen have been found to have larger increases in their social networks over their first semester than less optimistic ones (Brissette, Scheier, & Carver, 2002).

How does optimism build social resources? There likely are several contributors. One contributor is certainly that other people perceive optimists as being desirable social partners. People who espouse a positive outlook are socially accepted more than those who express a negative outlook (Carver, Kus, & Scheier, 1994; Helweg-Larsen, Sadeghian, & Webb, 2002). Actual interactions with optimists are also more positive in their emotional tone (Räikkönen, Matthews, Flory, Owens, & Gump, 1999), whereas pessimists sometimes make others feel burdened (Ruiz, Matthews, Scheier, & Schulz, 2006).

Another contributor to the difference in social outcomes is that optimists perceive their partners as being supportive to a greater extent than do less optimistic people (Srivastava, McGonigal, Richards, Butler, & Gross, 2006). Consistent with this, optimists also perceive that they have more social support in general than do pessimists (e.g., Abend & Williamson, 2002; Trunzo & Pinto, 2003).

Finally, optimists work harder, or perhaps work more effectively, at their relationships, even under stress. In one study of married couples across a 2-year span, optimism was initially related to better relationship quality, fewer negative interactions, and more cooperative problem solving during a discussion. At follow-up, optimism was related to better relationship quality and greater likelihood of the relationship's having survived (Assad, Donnellan, & Conger, 2007).

EMOTIONAL WELL-BEING

Another aspect of life in which optimism has been studied is subjective well-being. A very simple but pervasive effect of optimism and pessimism occurs on how people feel when they encounter problems. When life gets difficult, emotions range from enthusiasm and eagerness to anger, anxiety, and depression. Degree of optimism relates to the balance among these feelings. Because optimists expect good outcomes, even when things are hard, the result is a more positive mix of feelings. Pessimists, expecting bad outcomes, have more negative feelings—anxiety, anger, sadness—even despair (Carver & Scheier, 1998; Scheier & Carver, 1992).

This is a simple point, but it has been studied extensively. Optimism and distress have been examined in contexts that include students starting college (Aspinwall & Taylor, 1992; Brissette et. al., 2002); survivors of missile attacks (Zeidner & Hammer, 1992); cancer caregivers (Given et al., 1993); Alzheimer's caregivers (Hooker, Monahan, Shifren, & Hutchinson, 1992; Shifren & Hooker, 1995); and people dealing with stresses of childbirth (Carver & Gaines, 1987), coronary artery bypass surgery (Fitzgerald, Tennen, Affleck, & Pransky, 1993; Scheier et al., 1989), failed attempts at in vitro fertilization (Litt, Tennen, Affleck, & Klock, 1992), bone marrow transplantation (Curbow, Somerfield, Baker, Wingard, & Legro, 1993), cancer (Carver et al., 1993; Friedman et al., 1992), and the progression of AIDS (Taylor et al., 1992).

These studies vary in complexity and thus in what they are able to show. Many of them are cross-sectional, relating optimism to distress in one or another difficult situation. What those studies do *not* show is whether optimistic people were less distressed even prior to adversity. Studies that assess distress at multiple time points give a better picture of how distress changes over time and circumstances and allow control for prior distress. As an example, in one study, pregnant women completed the LOT and a depression scale in their last trimester. They completed the depression scale again 3 weeks after delivery. Optimism was related to lower depression symptoms both during pregnancy and in the postpartum period after controlling for symptoms during pregnancy. Thus optimism appeared to confer resistance to postpartum depressive symptoms (Carver & Gaines, 1987).

Much of the longitudinal research on optimism and subjective well-being focuses on people coping with health stressors, including cardiovascular disease and cancer. Here are a few representative results. Controlling for presurgical life satisfaction, optimists had higher life satisfaction 8 months after coronary artery bypass graft (CABG) surgery, an effect occurring through specific optimism about their surgery (Fitzgerald et al., 1993). Optimists in another study retained higher quality of life even up to 5 years after CABG (Scheier et al., 1989). In the context of treatment for ischemic heart disease, lower optimism related to more symptoms of depression both after hospitalization and at a 1-year follow-up after controlling for symptoms of depression at hospitalization (Shnek, Irvine, Stewart, & Abbey, 2001).

Another important health challenge is cancer. In one study, women diagnosed with breast cancer were interviewed at diagnosis, on the day before surgery, a few days afterward, and 3, 6, and 12 months later. Optimism predicted decreases in distress over time, conferring resilience during the full year (Carver et al., 1993). In another study, head and neck cancer patients showed similar results (Allison, Guichard, & Gilain, 2000).

Patients are not the only ones affected by health conditions: Caregiving for patients is also stressful; sometimes the well-being of caregivers is affected even more than that of patients (Roach, Averill, Segerstrom, & Kasarskis, 2009). Higher optimism among cancer caregivers has predicted less depression and less adverse impact of caregiving on their physical health (Given et al., 1993). Similar results have been found for caregivers of spouses with Alzheimer's disease (Hooker et al., 1992; Shifren & Hooker, 1995).

Optimism is important across the full range of stress, both severe stressors such as health threats and less severe stressors such as life transitions. For example, students starting college or law school, assessed when arriving on campus and later in the semester, had less distress if they were more optimistic (Aspinwall & Taylor, 1992; Brissette et al., 2002; Segerstrom, Taylor, Kemeny, & Fahey, 1998). At the other end of the adult lifespan, the simple process of aging brings challenges such as loss of mobility, minor and major illness, and bereavement. In elderly men, optimism has predicted significantly lower cumulative incidence of depression symptoms across a 15-year follow-up (Giltay, Zitman, & Kromhout, 2006). Optimism's inverse relation to depressive symptoms appears to diminish somewhat, however, as people approach very old age (Wrosch, Jobin, & Scheier, 2017).

Mechanisms of Emotional Well-Being

Why do optimists have higher emotional well-being? One potential path to differences in well-being concerns how one copes with stress. There are many ways to cope (Compas, Connor-Smith, Saltzman, Thomsen, & Wadsworth, 2001; Folkman & Moskowitz, 2004; Skinner, Edge, Altman, & Sherwood, 2003) and many ways to categorize coping (Carver & Connor-Smith, 2010; Skinner et al., 2003). A distinction that was made early in the analysis of coping divided problem-focused coping—doing something about the stressor to blunt its impact—from emotion-focused coping—soothing distress (Lazarus & Folkman, 1984). Another distinction is made between engagement or approach coping—dealing with the stressor or emotions stemming from it—and disengagement or avoidance coping—escaping the stressor or emotions stemming from it (e.g., Roth & Cohen, 1986; Skinner et al., 2003).

Early studies of situational coping responses and general coping styles (e.g., Scheier, Carver, & Bridges, 2001) found that optimists were approach copers and pessimists were avoidant copers. Conceptually similar results have followed. A meta-analysis of optimism and coping crossed the two distinctions described above, fitting coping responses into the four resulting categories (Solberg Nes & Segerstrom, 2006). Optimism was positively associated with both problem-focused and emotion-focused subsets of engagement coping. Optimists also were responsive to the kind of stressor being confronted. They used more problem-focused coping for controllable stressors (e.g., academic demands) and more emotion-focused coping for uncontrollable ones (e.g., trauma). Thus optimism predicted active attempts to change stressful circumstances and also to accommodate to those circumstances in ways that reflect flexible engagement.

Some studies described just earlier with respect to emotional well-being also examined coping processes. Before CABG surgery, optimists reported planning for their futures and setting goals for recovery and focused less on negative aspects of the experience, such as distress and symptoms. After surgery, optimists reported seeking out information about what they would be required to do in the months ahead, and they were less likely to say they were suppressing thoughts about their symptoms (Scheier et al., 1989).

In the context of cancer, pessimistic women used more cognitive avoidance in coping with an upcoming biopsy than optimists, and cognitive avoidance before the biopsy predicted greater distress afterward (Stanton & Snider, 1993). More optimistic breast cancer patients in the first year after diagnosis were more likely to accept the situation's reality, place it in as positive a light as possible, use humor, and decrease efforts to push the reality of the situation away and to give up. Optimism correlated with lower distress, largely through coping (Carver et al., 1993). Finally, in another study of women under treatment for breast cancer, more optimistic women endorsed more fighting spirit (confronting and trying to beat cancer) and less of a sense of giving up. Again, coping accounted for the some of the relationship between higher optimism before diagnosis and quality of life a year afterward (Schou, Ekeberg, & Ruland, 2005).

In sum, optimists differ from pessimists in how they cope with stress. Particularly noteworthy may be a contrast between acceptance, an optimistic strategy, and overt denial, a pessimistic strategy. Acceptance does not mean giving up, but rather a restructuring of one's perceptions and goals. Indeed, acceptance may actually serve the purpose of keeping the person goal engaged and "life engaged" (Scheier & Carver, 2001). In contrast, overt denial (refusing to accept the reality of the situation) is trying to maintain a worldview that no longer applies.

OPTIMISM AND PHYSICAL HEALTH

The preceding section on emotional well-being included frequent mention of physical health. This reflects the fact that much of the research on optimism has been conducted in the field of health psychology. Aside from subjective well-being, optimism has also been linked to physical well-being.

Several examples of the relationship of optimism to physical health come from work on cardiovascular health (for broader treatment, see Mens, Scheier, & Carver, in press; Rasmussen, Scheier, & Greenhouse, 2009). Carotid intima thickness, a physical marker of the development of heart disease, was measured in middle-aged women. Pessimists had increases over 3 years in intima thickness, but optimists had almost no increase (Matthews et al., 2004). Another project examined patterns of rehospitalization after CABG, which is quite common (Scheier et al., 1999). Optimism predicted significantly less likelihood of rehospitalization and a longer time before its occurrence, independent of self-esteem, depression, and neuroticism (see also Tindle et al., 2012).

Perhaps the most compelling evidence linking optimism to cardiovascular health comes from large epidemiological studies. A large sample of participants in the Women's Health Initiative (a sample of over 95,000), all of whom were free of cancer and cardiovascular disease at study entry, were followed for 8 years. Optimists were less likely than pessimists to develop coronary heart disease (CHD), were less likely to die from CHD, and had lower total mortality (Tindle et al., 2009). Men and women age 50 and older in the Health and Retirement Survey ($N = 6,808$) were followed for 4 years; each quartile elevation in optimism was associated with 32% lower odds of heart failure after controlling for age and sex. After controlling for demographic, behavioral, and biological factors, higher optimism was still associated with 22% lower odds of heart failure (Kim, Smith, & Kubzansky, 2014).

Healing and immunity may also be affected by optimism. In one study men were classified after a skin biopsy as "slow healers" and "fast healers." Fast healers were more optimistic than slow healers (Ebrecht et al., 2004). Another study found that optimism predicted better immune response to the influenza vaccine among older adults (Kohut, Cooper, Nickolaus, Russell, & Cunnick, 2002). Immune responses are tricky to interpret, though, because they are sometimes suppressed when there are other behavioral demands, so as to conserve energy (Segerstrom, 2010). Under very high challenge, optimism has been related to lower, rather than higher, immune responses. This has been interpreted as suggesting a pattern of greater engagement with demanding goals, resulting in suppression of immune responses (Segerstrom, 2005, 2006b).

Mechanisms of Physical Health

Why do optimists have better health outcomes than pessimists? Two possibilities stand out (and they are by no means mutually exclusive). One possibility follows from the better profile of emotional responses to adversity that optimists display (less distress and more positive emotions). This pattern of emotional experiences, which follows in part from the pattern of coping reactions that optimists use (as described earlier in the chapter), doubtlessly results in lower physiological strain over time, resulting in better health (e.g., Wrosch, Scheier, & Miller, 2013).

The other possibility is motivational and behavioral. Part of remaining healthy is doing the right things and avoiding the wrong things. One way in which optimism might promote well-being and health is by seeking knowledge about potential risks. Consistent with this reasoning, in one study adults higher in optimism knew more about risk factors for heart attack than those who were less optimistic (Radcliffe & Klein, 2002).

Optimists not only know more about risks, they also act to decrease them. Among patients in cardiac rehabilitation, optimists were more successful in lowering saturated fat, body fat, and an index of overall coronary risk and in increasing exercise (Shepperd, Maroto, & Pbert, 1996). Five years after surgery, more optimistic cardiac bypass patients were more likely to be taking vitamins, to be eating low-fat foods, and to be enrolled in cardiac rehabilitation (Scheier & Carver, 1992).

Another important health challenge is avoidance of contact with the human immunodeficiency virus (HIV). Management of risk of infection with HIV also provides a context for proactive health-related behaviors. By avoiding certain sexual practices, people can reduce risk of infection. Among HIV-negative gay men, optimists reported fewer anonymous sexual partners than pessimists, suggesting efforts to safeguard their health (Taylor et al., 1992).

In contrast, the tendency to give up among pessimists can manifest as health-defeating behaviors. For example, excessive alcohol use is often seen as an escape from problems. Among women with a family history of alcoholism, more pessimistic women were more likely than optimists to report drinking problems (Ohannessian, Hesselbrock, Tennen, & Affleck, 1993). In another study, pessimists who had been treated for alcohol abuse were more likely to drop out of aftercare and return to drinking than optimists (Strack, Carver, & Blaney, 1987). In yet another study, pessimistic women were more likely than optimistic women to engage in substance abuse during their pregnancies (Park, Moore, Turner, & Adler, 1997).

In sum, optimists do not stick their heads in the metaphorical sand. Rather, they attend to health risks and take action to minimize them. They selectively focus on risks that relate to potentially serious health problems that apply to them personally (Aspinwall & Brunhart, 1996). For example, optimists were more likely to want to learn the results of genetic testing when they felt they were at high risk, whereas pessimists were less likely (Tabor et al., 2015).

Because optimism predisposes people to engage with rather than disengage from their goals, and because engagement results in better long-term outcomes than disengagement, experience presumably teaches optimists that their own efforts play an important part in the positive futures that they expect. For that reason, they are quicker to engage those efforts and to monitor a need for them. Conversely, pessimism can lead people into self-defeating patterns. The result can be less persistence, more avoidance coping, and various kinds of health-damaging behavior. Without confidence about the future, it is harder to remain engaged in life.

Does Optimism Have Drawbacks?

Thus far, the evidence reviewed suggests that optimists have happy and fulfilling lives. Compared with pessimists, they are less distressed when they encounter adversity. They deal with difficulty by coping in better ways: using problem-focused coping when there is something to do and accommodative coping when there is not. They accomplish their goals to a greater degree and acquire more resources in so doing. These properties all sound quite adaptive.

Are there contexts in which optimism can lead to problems? Maybe. Consider gambling. Gibson and Sanbonmatsu (2004) reasoned that gambling is a context in which confidence and persistence can be counterproductive, because in the long run gambling is always a losing proposition. In a survey, optimists reported more confidence in their ability to win at gambling than did less optimistic people, but despite that greater confidence, they did not report more frequent gambling or a greater tendency to gamble longer than intended. In the lab, pessimists were more likely than optimists to display the so-called gambler's fallacy: betting more after a win and betting less after a loss. So it is not entirely clear that optimism creates problem tendencies even in the gambling context. More research on this question is clearly needed.

Others have asked whether the persistence displayed by optimists can create problems because they fail to recognize what they cannot accomplish. Certainly people sometimes have to recognize that goals are lost and that the adaptive course is to give up on them (Wrosch et al., 2003). Does optimism prevent disengagement? As we already pointed out, some studies have found that optimists did not find it easier to disengage from life goals than pessimists, but they did not find it harder either, and they were more flexible than pessimists in managing their goals (Hanssen et al., 2015; Rasmussen et al., 2006).

Another laboratory study provided experimental control over goals, examining people's willingness to quit tasks on which they were failing. Some engaged in a difficult (actually impossible) task for which there was no alternative task to turn to; for others, there was an alternative. With no alternative, everyone persisted at the impossible task. Given another task, however, optimists gave up on a task they could not master in order to turn to a similar task that they *could* perhaps master. Indeed, when they had been led to think the other task measured a somewhat different skill, they outperformed the less optimistic people on it (Aspinwall & Richter, 1999). Therefore, the available evidence does not suggest that optimists are worse than pessimists at disengaging when disengaging is appropriate.

Finally, it has been suggested that optimism might set people up for disappointment when the expected positive future fails to manifest itself (Schwarzer, 1994; Tennen & Affleck, 1987). A few studies have explicitly assessed optimism and distress before and after bad news, including failure at in vitro fertilization, breast cancer diagnosis, and cardiovascular disease relapse. People who were more optimistic before receiving bad news were not more emotionally vulnerable, and in some cases they were protected (Litt et al., 1992; Helgeson, 2003; Stanton & Snider, 1993). One possible mechanism is that, after potential disappointment, optimists are more disposed to think about how things could have been worse (Barnett & Martinez, 2015).

Optimists do not look at the world through rose-colored glasses. As described previously, they cope with acceptance rather than denial and seek information about risk more than do pessimists. However, there do appear to be very specific cases in which optimism may have drawbacks. It is not clear how rare these cases are, or whether other variables limit the range of any potential problems. The overall body of evidence suggests that the benefits of optimism far outweigh the drawbacks, but this question certainly will remain a topic for future work.

Concluding Comment

There is a great deal of evidence showing that people with positive expectations for the future respond to difficulty and adversity more adaptively than those with negative expectations. Indeed, optimism seems to confer benefits in both intrapersonal and interpersonal domains, and in the absence and presence of stress. Expectancies predict how people approach both threats and opportunities, and they relate to the success and well-being that results.

References

Abend, T. A., & Williamson, G. M. (2002). Feeling attractive in the wake of breast cancer: Optimism matters, and so do interpersonal relationships. *Personality and Social Psychology Bulletin, 28*, 427–436.

Affleck, G., Tennen, H., Zautra, A., Urrows, S., Abeles, M., & Karoly, P. (2001). Women's pursuit of personal goals in daily life with fibromyalgia: A value–expectancy analysis. *Journal of Consulting and Clinical Psychology, 69*, 587–596.

Ahrens, A. H., & Haaga, D. A. F. (1993). The specificity of attributional style and expectations to positive and negative affectivity, depression, and anxiety. *Cognitive Therapy and Research, 17*, 83–98.

Allison, P. J., Guichard, C., & Gilain, L. (2000). A prospective investigation of dispositional optimism as a predictor of health-related quality of life in head and neck cancer patients. *Quality of Life Research, 9*, 951–960.

Aspinwall, L. G., & Brunhart, S. N. (1996). Distinguishing optimism from denial: Optimistic beliefs predict attention to health threats. *Personality and Social Psychology Bulletin, 22*, 993–1003.

Aspinwall, L. G., & Richter, L. (1999). Optimism and self-mastery predict more rapid disengagement from unsolvable tasks in the presence of alternatives. *Motivation and Emotion, 23*, 221–245.

Aspinwall, L. G., & Taylor, S. E. (1992). Modeling cognitive adaptation: A longitudinal investigation of the impact of individual differences and coping on college adjustment and performance. *Journal of Personality and Social Psychology, 61*, 755–765.

Assad, K. K., Donnellan, M. B., & Conger, R. D. (2007). Optimism: An enduring resource for romantic relationships. *Journal of Personality and Social Psychology, 93*, 285–297.

Atienza, A. A., Stephens, M. A. P., & Townsend, A. L. (2004). Role stressors as predictors of changes in women's optimistic expectations. *Personality and Individual Differences, 37*, 471–484.

Austin, J. T., & Vancouver, J. B. (1996). Goal constructs in psychology: Structure, process, and content. *Psychological Bulletin, 120*, 338–375.

Barnett, M. D., & Martinez, B. (2015). Optimists: It could have been worse; Pessimists: It could have been better: Dispositional optimism and pessimism and counterfactual thinking. *Personality and Individual Differences, 86,* 122–125.

Boehm, J. K., Chen, Y., Williams, D. R., Ryff, C., & Kubzansky, L. D. (2015). Unequally distributed psychological assets: Are there social disparities in optimism, life satisfaction, and positive affect? *PLOS ONE, 10*(2), e0118066.

Brissette, I., Scheier, M. F., & Carver, C. S. (2002). The role of optimism in social network development, coping, and psychological adjustment during a life transition. *Journal of Personality and Social Psychology, 82,* 102–111.

Carver, C. S., & Connor-Smith, J. (2010). Personality and coping. *Annual Review of Psychology, 61,* 679–704.

Carver, C. S., & Gaines, J. G. (1987). Optimism, pessimism, and postpartum depression. *Cognitive Therapy and Research, 11,* 449–462.

Carver, C. S., Kus, L. A., & Scheier, M. F. (1994). Effects of good versus bad mood and optimistic versus pessimistic outlook on social acceptance versus rejection. *Journal of Social and Clinical Psychology, 13,* 138–151.

Carver, C. S., Lehman, J. M., & Antoni, M. H. (2003). Dispositional pessimism predicts illness-related disruption of social and recreational activities among breast cancer patients. *Journal of Personality and Social Psychology, 84,* 813–821.

Carver, C. S., Pozo, C., Harris, S. D., Noriega, V., Scheier, M. F., Robinson, D. S., . . . Clark, K. C. (1993). How coping mediates the effect of optimism on distress: A study of women with early stage breast cancer. *Journal of Personality and Social Psychology, 65,* 375–390.

Carver, C. S., & Scheier, M. F. (1998). *On the self-regulation of behavior.* New York: Cambridge University Press.

Carver, C. S., & Scheier, M. F. (2012). *Perspectives on personality* (7th ed.). Upper Saddle River, NJ: Pearson Education.

Compas, B. E., Connor-Smith, J. K., Saltzman, H., Thomsen, A. H., & Wadsworth, M. E. (2001). Coping with stress during childhood and adolescence: Problems, progress, and potential in theory and research. *Psychological Bulletin, 127,* 87–127.

Curbow, B., Somerfield, M. R., Baker, F., Wingard, J. R., & Legro, M. W. (1993). Personal changes, dispositional optimism, and psychological adjustment to bone marrow transplantation. *Journal of Behavioral Medicine, 16,* 423–443.

Duke, J., Leventhal, H., Brownlee, S., & Leventhal, E. A. (2002). Giving up and replacing activities in response to illness. *Journal of Gerontology: Psychological Sciences, 57B,* 367–376.

Ebrecht, M., Hextall, J., Kirtley, L.-G., Taylor, A. M., Dyson, M., & Weinman, J. (2004). Perceived stress and cortisol levels predict speed of wound healing in healthy male adults. *Psychoneuroendrocrinology, 29,* 798–809.

Eccles, J. S., & Wigfield, A. (2002). Motivational beliefs, values, and goals. *Annual Review of Psychology, 53,* 109–132.

Fitzgerald, T. E., Tennen, H., Affleck, G., & Pransky, G. S. (1993). The relative importance of dispositional optimism and control appraisals in quality of life after coronary artery bypass surgery. *Journal of Behavioral Medicine, 16,* 25–43.

Folkman, S., & Moskowitz, J. T. (2004). Coping: Pitfalls and promise. *Annual Review of Psychology, 55,* 745–774.

Friedman, L. C., Nelson, D. V., Baer, P. E., Lane, M., Smith, F. E., & Dworkin, R. J. (1992). The relationship of dispositional optimism, daily life stress, and domestic environment to coping methods used by cancer patients. *Journal of Behavioral Medicine, 15,* 127–141.

Geers, A. L., Wellman, J. A., & Lassiter, G. D. (2009). Dispositional optimism and engagement: The moderating influence of goal prioritization. *Journal of Personality and Social Psychology, 96,* 913–932.

Gibson, B., & Sanbonmatsu, D. M. (2004). Optimism, pessimism, and gambling: The downside of optimism. *Personality and Social Psychology Bulletin, 30,* 149–160.

Giltay, E. J., Zitman, F. G., & Kromhout, D. (2006). Dispositional optimism and the risk of depressive symptoms during 15 years of follow-up: The Zutphen Elderly Study. *Journal of Affective Disorders, 91,* 45–52.

Given, C. W., Stommel, M., Given, B., Osuch, J., Kurtz, M. E., & Kurtz, J. C. (1993). The influence of cancer patients' symptoms and functional states on patients' depression and family caregivers' reaction and depression. *Health Psychology, 12,* 277–285.

Gollwitzer, P. M., Parks-Stamm, E. J., Jaudas, A., & Sheeran, P. (2008). Flexible tenacity in goal pursuit. In J. Y. Shah & W. L. Gardner (Eds.), *Handbook of motivation science* (pp. 325–341). New York: Guilford Press.

Hanssen, M. M., Vancleef, L. M. G., Vlaeyen, J. W. S., Hayes, A. F., Schouten, E. G. W., & Peters, M. L. (2015). Optimism, motivational coping, and well-being: Evidence supporting the importance of flexible goal adjustment. *Journal of Happiness Studies, 16,* 1525–1537.

Heinonen, K., Räikkönen, K., & Keltikangas-Järvinen, L. (2005). Dispositional optimism: Development over 21 years from the perspectives of perceived temperament and mothering. *Personality and Individual Differences, 38,* 425–435.

Heinonen, K., Räikkönen, K., Matthews, K. A., Scheier, M. F., Raitakari, O. T., Pulkki, L., . . . Keltikangas-Järvinen, L. (2006). Socioeconomic status in childhood and adulthood: Associations with dispositional optimism and pessimism over a 21-year follow-up. *Journal of Personality, 74,* 1111–1126.

Helgeson, V. S. (2003). Cognitive adaptation, psychological adjustment, and disease progression among angioplasty patents: 4 years later. *Health Psychology, 22,* 30–38.

Helweg-Larsen, M., Sadeghian, P., & Webb, M. S. (2002). The stigma of being pessimistically biased. *Journal of Social and Clinical Psychology, 21,* 92–107.

Herzberg, P. Y., Glaesmer, H., & Hoyer, J. (2006). Separating optimism and pessimism: A robust psychometric analysis of the revised Life Orientation Test (LOT–R). *Psychological Assessment, 18,* 433–438.

Higgins, E. T. (2006). Value from hedonic experience *and* engagement. *Psychological Review, 113,* 439–460.

Hooker, K., Monahan, D., Shifren, K., & Hutchinson, C. (1992). Mental and physical health of spouse caregivers: The role of personality. *Psychology and Aging, 7,* 367–375.

Kappes, A., & Oettingen, G. (2014). The emergence of goal pursuit: Mental contrasting connects future and reality. *Journal of Experimental Social Psychology, 54,* 25–39.

Kim, E. S., Smith, J., & Kubzansky, L. D. (2014). Prospective study of the association between dispositional optimism and incident heart failure. *Circulation: Heart Failure, 7,* 394–400.

Kohut, M. L., Cooper, M. M., Nickolaus, M. S., Russell, D. R., & Cunnick, J. E. (2002). Exercise and psychosocial factors modulate immunity to influenza vaccine in elderly individuals. *Journals of Gerontology: Series A: Biological Sciences and Medical Sciences, 57A,* 557–562.

Lazarus, R. S., & Folkman, S. (1984). *Stress, appraisal, and coping.* New York: Springer.

Litt, M. D., Tennen, H., Affleck, G., & Klock, S. (1992). Coping and cognitive factors in adaptation to *in vitro* fertilization failure. *Journal of Behavioral Medicine, 15,* 171–187.

Lucas, R. E., Diener, E., & Suh, E. (1996). Discriminant validity of well-being measures. *Journal of Personality and Social Psychology, 71,* 616–628.

Marshall, G. N., Wortman, C. B., Kusulas, J. W., Hervig, L. K., & Vickers, R. R., Jr. (1992). Distinguishing optimism from pessimism: Relations to fundamental dimensions of mood and personality. *Journal of Personality and Social Psychology, 62,* 1067–1074.

Matthews, K. A., Räikkönen, K., Sutton-Tyrrell, K., & Kuller, L. H. (2004). Optimistic attitudes protect against progression of carotid atherosclerosis in healthy middle-aged women. *Psychosomatic Medicine, 66,* 640–644.

Mens, M. G., Scheier, M. F., & Carver, C. S. (in press). Optimism and physical health. In K. Sweeny & M. L. Robbins (Eds.), *Wiley encyclopedia of health psychology.* New York: Wiley.

Oettingen, G. (2012). Future thought and behavior change. *European Review of Social Psychology, 23,* 1–63.

Oettingen, G. (2014). *Rethinking positive thinking: Inside the new science of motivation.* New York: Penguin Random House.

Ohannessian, C. M., Hesselbrock, V. M., Tennen, H., & Affleck, G. (1993). Hassles and uplifts and generalized outcome expectancies as moderators on the relation between a family history of alcoholism and drinking behaviors. *Journal of Studies on Alcohol, 55,* 754–763.

Park, C. L., Moore, P. J., Turner, R. A., & Adler, N. E. (1997). The roles of constructive thinking and optimism in psychological and behavioral adjustment during pregnancy. *Journal of Personality and Social Psychology, 73,* 584–592.

Peterson, C., & Seligman, M. E. P. (1984). Causal explanations as a risk factor for depression: Theory and evidence. *Psychological Review, 91,* 347–374.

Peterson, C., & Vaidya, R. S. (2001). Explanatory style, expectations, and depressive symptoms. *Personality and Individual Differences, 31,* 1217–1223.

Plomin, R., Scheier, M. F., Bergeman, C. S., Pedersen, N. L., Nesselroade, J. R., & McClearn, G. E. (1992). Optimism, pessimism, and mental health: A twin/adoption analysis. *Personality and Individual Differences, 13,* 921–930.

Radcliffe, N. M., & Klein, W. M. P. (2002). Dispositional, unrealistic, and comparative optimism: Differential relations with the knowledge and processing of risk information and beliefs about personal risk. *Personality and Social Psychology Bulletin, 28,* 836–846.

Räikkönen, K., Matthews, K. A., Flory, J. D., Owens, J. F., & Gump, B. B. (1999). Effects of optimism, pessimism, and trait anxiety on ambulatory blood pressure and mood during everyday life. *Journal of Personality and Social Psychology, 76,* 104–113.

Rasmussen, H. N., Scheier, M. F., & Greenhouse, J. B. (2009). Optimism and physical health: A meta-analytic review. *Annals of Behavioral Medicine, 37,* 239–256.

Rasmussen, H. N., Wrosch, C., Scheier, M. F., & Carver, C. S. (2006). Self-regulation processes and health: The importance of optimism and goal adjustment. *Journal of Personality, 74,* 1721–1747.

Rauch, W. A., Schweizer, K., & Moosbrugger, H. (2007). Method effects due to social desirability as a parsimonious explanation of the deviation from unidimensionality in LOT-R scores. *Personality and Individual Differences, 42,* 1597–1607.

Roach, A. R., Averill, A. J., Segerstrom, S. C., & Kasarskis, E. J. (2009). The dynamics of quality of life in ALS patients and caregivers. *Annals of Behavioral Medicine, 37,* 197–206.

Roberts, B. W., Walton, K. E., & Viechtbauer, W. (2006). Patterns of mean-level change in personality traits across the life course: A meta-analysis of longitudinal studies. *Psychological Bulletin, 132,* 1–25.

Robinson-Whelen, S., Kim, C., MacCallum, R. C., & Kiecolt-Glaser, J. K. (1997). Distinguishing optimism from pessimism in older adults: Is it more important to be optimistic or not to be pessimistic? *Journal of Personality and Social Psychology, 73,* 1345–1353.

Roth, S., & Cohen, L. J. (1986). Approach, avoidance, and coping with stress. *American Psychologist, 41,* 813–819.

Ruiz, J. M., Matthews, K. A., Scheier, M. F., & Schulz, R. (2006). Does who you marry matter for your health?: Influence of patients' and spouses' personality on their partners' psychological well-being following coronary artery bypass surgery. *Journal of Personality and Social Psychology, 91,* 255–267.

Scheier, M. F., & Carver, C. S. (1985). Optimism, coping, and health: Assessment and implication of generalized outcome expectancies. *Health Psychology, 4,* 219–247.

Scheier, M. F., & Carver, C. S. (1992). Effects of optimism on psychological and physical well-being: Theoretical overview and empirical update. *Cognitive Therapy and Research, 16,* 201–228.

Scheier, M. F., & Carver, C. S. (2001). Adapting to cancer: The importance of hope and purpose. In A. Baum & B. L. Andersen (Eds.), *Psychosocial interventions for cancer* (pp. 15–36). Washington, DC: American Psychological Association.

Scheier, M. F., Carver, C. S., & Bridges, M. W. (1994). Distinguishing optimism from neuroticism (and trait anxiety, self-mastery, and self-esteem): A reevaluation of the Life Orientation Test. *Journal of Personality and Social Psychology, 67,* 1063–1078.

Scheier, M. F., Carver, C. S., & Bridges, M. W. (2001). Optimism, pessimism, and psychological well-being. In E. C. Chang (Ed.), *Optimism and pessimism: Implications for theory, research, and practice* (pp. 189–216). Washington, DC: American Psychological Association.

Scheier, M. F., Matthews, K. A., Owens, J. F., Magovern, G. J., Lefebvre, R. C., Abbott, R. A., . . . Carver, C. S. (1989). Dispositional optimism and recovery from coronary artery bypass surgery: The beneficial effects on physical and psychological well-being. *Journal of Personality and Social Psychology, 57,* 1024–1040.

Scheier, M. F., Matthews, K. A., Owens, J. F., Schulz, R., Bridges, M. W., Magovern, G. J., Sr., . . . Carver, C. S. (1999). Optimism and rehospitalization following coronary artery bypass graft surgery. *Archives of Internal Medicine, 159,* 829–835.

Schou, I., Ekeberg, O., & Ruland, C. M. (2005). The mediating role of appraisal and coping in the relationship between optimism–pessimism and quality of life. *Psycho-Oncology, 14,* 718–727.

Schwarzer, R. (1994). Optimism, vulnerability, and self-beliefs as health-related cognitions: A systematic overview. *Psychology and Health, 9,* 161–180.

Segerstrom, S. C. (2005). Optimism and immunity: Do positive thoughts always lead to positive effects? *Brain, Behavior, and Immunity, 19,* 195–200.

Segerstrom, S. C. (2006a). *Breaking Murphy's law.* New York: Guilford Press.

Segerstrom, S. C. (2006b). How does optimism suppress immunity?: Evaluation of three affective pathways. *Health Psychology, 25,* 653–657.

Segerstrom, S. C. (2007). Optimism and resources: Effects on each other and on health over 10 years. *Journal of Research in Personality, 41,* 772–786.

Segerstrom, S. C. (2010). Resources, stress, and immunity: An ecological perspective on human psychoneuroimmunology. *Annals of Behavioral Medicine, 40,* 114–125.

Segerstrom, S. C., Evans, D. R., & Eisenlohr-Moul, T. A. (2011). Optimism and pessimism dimensions in the Life Orientation Test–Revised: Method and meaning. *Journal of Research in Personality, 45,* 126–129.

Segerstrom, S. C., & Solberg Nes, L. (2006). When goals conflict but people prosper: The case of dispositional optimism. *Journal of Research in Personality, 40,* 675–693.

Segerstrom, S. C., Taylor, S. E., Kemeny, M. E., & Fahey, J. L. (1998). Optimism is associated with mood, coping, and immune change in response to stress. *Journal of Personality and Social Psychology, 74,* 1646–1655.

Sevincer, A. T., & Oettingen, G. (2013). Spontaneous mental contrasting and selective goal pursuit. *Personality and Social Psychology Bulletin, 39,* 1240–1254.

Sheppard, J. A., Maroto, J. J., & Pbert, L. A. (1996). Dispositional optimism as a predictor of health changes among cardiac patients. *Journal of Research in Personality, 30,* 517–534.

Shifren, K., & Hooker, K. (1995). Stability and change in optimism: A study among spouse caregivers. *Experimental Aging Research, 21,* 59–76.

Shnek, Z. M., Irvine, J., Stewart, D., & Abbey, S. (2001). Psychological factors and depressive symptoms in ischemic heart disease. *Health Psychology, 20,* 141–145.

Skinner, E. A., Edge, K., Altman, J., & Sherwood, H. (2003). Searching for the structure of coping: A review and critique of category systems for classifying ways of coping. *Psychological Bulletin, 129,* 216–269.

Solberg Nes, L., Evans, D. R., & Segerstrom, S. C. (2009). Optimism and college retention: Mediation by motivation, performance, and adjustment. *Journal of Applied Social Psychology, 39,* 1887–1912.

Solberg Nes, L., & Segerstrom, S. C. (2006). Dispositional optimism and coping: A meta-analytic review. *Personality and Social Psychology Review, 10,* 235–251.

Solberg Nes, L., Segerstrom, S. C., & Sephton, S. E. (2005). Engagement and arousal: Optimism's effects during a brief stressor. *Personality and Social Psychology Bulletin, 31,* 111–120.

Srivastava, S., McGonigal, K. M., Richards, J. M., Butler, E. A., & Gross, J. J. (2006). Optimism in close relationships: How seeing things in a positive light makes them so. *Journal of Personality and Social Psychology, 91,* 143–153.

Stanton, A. L., & Snider, P. R. (1993). Coping with breast cancer diagnosis: A prospective study. *Health Psychology, 12,* 16–23.

Strack, S., Carver, C. S., & Blaney, P. H. (1987). Predicting successful completion of an aftercare program following treatment for alcoholism: The role of dispositional optimism. *Journal of Personality and Social Psychology, 53,* 579–584.

Tabor, J. M., Klein, W. M. P., Ferrer, R. A., Lewis, K. L., Biesecker, L. G., & Biesecker, B. B. (2015). Dispositional optimism and perceived risk interact to predict intentions to learn genome sequencing results. *Health Psychology, 34,* 718–728.

Taylor, S. E., Kemeny, M. E., Aspinwall, L. G., Schneider, S. G., Rodriguez, R., & Herbert, M. (1992). Optimism, coping, psychological distress, and high-risk sexual behavior among men at risk for acquired immunodeficiency syndrome (AIDS). *Journal of Personality and Social Psychology, 63,* 460–473.

Tennen, H., & Affleck, G. (1987). The costs and benefits of optimistic explanations and dispositional optimism. *Journal of Personality, 55,* 377–393.

Tindle, H. A., Belnap, B. H., Houck, P. R., Mazumdar, S., Scheier, M. F., Matthews, K. A., . . . Rollman, B. L. (2012). Optimism, response to treatment of depression, and rehospitalization after coronary artery bypass graft surgery. *Psychosomatic Medicine, 74,* 200–207.

Tindle, H. A., Chang, Y., Kuller, L. H., Manson, J. E., Robinson, J. G., Rosal, M. C., . . . Matthews, K. A. (2009). Optimism, cynical hostility, and incident coronary heart disease and mortality in the Women's Health Initiative. *Circulation, 120,* 656–662.

Trunzo, J. J., & Pinto, B. M. (2003). Social support as a mediator of optimism and distress in breast cancer survivors. *Journal of Consulting and Clinical Psychology, 4,* 805–811.

Wrosch, C., Jobin, J., & Scheier, M. F. (2017). Do the emotional benefits of optimism vary across older adulthood?: A life span perspective. *Journal of Personality, 85,* 388–397.

Wrosch, C., Scheier, M. F., Carver, C. S., & Schulz, R. (2003). The importance of goal disengagement in adaptive self-regulation: When giving up is beneficial. *Self and Identity, 2,* 1–20.

Wrosch, C., Scheier, M. F., & Miller, G. E. (2013). Goal adjustment capacities, subjective well-being, and physical health. *Social and Personality Psychology Compass, 7,* 847–860.

Zeidner, M., & Hammer, A. L. (1992). Coping with missile attack: Resources, strategies, and outcomes. *Journal of Personality, 60,* 709–746.

CHAPTER 12

Fluctuations in Future Outlooks
Unrealistic Optimism and Pessimism in Outcome Predictions

James A. Shepperd
Angelica Falkenstein
Kate Sweeny

Part of what makes humans distinct from other animals is their ability to contemplate the future (Gilbert & Wilson, 2007). Humans can imagine what is likely to occur and then prepare accordingly. Presumably, it would serve people's interests to be accurate in their forecasts—to know when undesired outcomes lie ahead and when they do not. However, four decades of research show that predictions about the future are often remarkably optimistic. The number of incoming college freshmen who declare that they are pre-med compared with the number who graduate pre-med illustrates the enormous optimism people can hold about the future. Yet people can also be remarkably pessimistic in their predictions. We discuss research on people's outlooks about the future. We first address the general tendency for people to display unrealistic optimism in predictions. We also review why people are optimistic, as well as the boundary conditions on unrealistic optimism. Next, we discuss evidence that people sometimes abandon their optimistic outlook in favor of a more realistic or even pessimistic outlook as the future moves to the present. We review why people shift from optimism, as well as factors that influence these shifts.

Our discussion focuses on outlooks or predictions that are unrealistically optimistic or unrealistically pessimistic. By *optimistic* we mean high expectations of favorable outcomes and low expectations of unfavorable outcomes; by *pessimistic* we mean low expectations of favorable outcomes and high expectations of unfavorable outcomes. By *unrealistic*, we mean an unjustifiable expectation that personal outcomes will differ from the outcomes of one's peers (e.g., "I am less likely to experience smoking-related illnesses than are other smokers who smoke a similar amount") or from the outcomes suggested by some quantitative, objective standard ("I believe my risk of lung cancer is below average even though epidemiological data suggest that my risk is average or above average").

UNREALISTIC OPTIMISM

Unrealistic optimism refers to expectations about what will happen in the future that deviate from objective indicators of one's likely outcomes. For example, people believe they are less likely than their peers to experience unfavorable outcomes such as car accidents (McKenna, 1993), smoking-related illnesses (Myers, 2014), sexual violence (Chapin & Coleman, 2012), infringement of online computer privacy (Baek, Kim, & Bae, 2014), virus infections (Cho, Lee, & Lee, 2013), and contracting a variety of diseases (for a review, see Shepperd, Klein, Waters, & Weinstein, 2013). Conversely, people believe they are more likely than their peers to experience favorable outcomes such as graduating from college, getting married, maintaining a healthy lifestyle, and quitting smoking (Borrelli, Hayes, Dunsiger, & Fava, 2009; Chock, 2011; Weinstein, 1980). People also display unrealistic optimism in estimates of how long it will take to complete tasks, a phenomenon that researchers call the *planning fallacy* (Kahneman & Tversky, 1982). For example, people underestimate how long it will take to complete one's tax return (Buehler & Griffin, Chapter 27, this volume; Buehler, Griffin, & MacDonald, 1997, Study 1), solve puzzles (Buehler & Griffin, Chapter 27, this volume; Buehler et al., 1997, Study 2), write a report (Koole & Spijker, 2000), and assemble a computer stand (Byram, 1997).

A review of the literature reveals that investigators use the term *unrealistic optimism* to refer to two distinct beliefs (Shepperd et al., 2013). The first, *unrealistic comparative optimism,* refers to the erroneous belief that one's personal outcomes will be more favorable than the outcomes of one's peers. The logic underlying this form of unrealistic optimism is that the risk estimates for a group of people should be average; that is, the estimates of people who report below-average risk should balance out the estimates of people who report above-average risk. A group displays unrealistic optimism when the mean of their estimates is below average for undesirable outcomes or above average for desirable outcomes (Shepperd, Waters, Weinstein, & Klein, 2015). The second form of unrealistic optimism—*unrealistic absolute optimism*—refers to the erroneous belief that personal outcomes will be more favorable than the outcomes suggested by some objective standard, such as the population base rate, past experience, or the judgments of experts. For example, although 38% of all marriages in the United States end in divorce, research participants often report that their personal chance of divorce is much less, around 20% in one study (Rothman, Klein, & Weinstein, 1996).

Both forms of unrealistic optimism share overlap with dispositional optimism in that they represent positive expectations about the future. Not surprisingly, studies find that unrealistic optimism and dispositional optimism are correlated, with correlations typically ranging from .10 to .30 (Davidson & Prkachin, 1997; Fowler & Geers, 2015). However, unrealistic optimism and dispositional optimism are distinct. Dispositional optimism represents a general, trait-like tendency to expect positive outcomes, and these expectations may or may not be unrealistic. In contrast, unrealistic optimism represents unrealistic personal predictions about specific events and not merely positive expectations in general.

Unrealistic optimism has also been theoretically and empirically differentiated from fantasies about the future (Oettingen, 2012, 2014; Oettingen & Mayer, 2002). Unrealistic optimism represents an expectation of what will happen in the future and typically is at least somewhat grounded in past behavior, in intentions to act, or in actuarial data. By contrast, fantasies represent streams of thought similar to daydreams in that they are embellished desires about future outcomes. Moreover, fantasies are typically unrelated—or perhaps even inversely related—to activities that might bring the desired outcome about (Oettingen & Mayer, 2002). Finally, unrealistic optimism is distinct from mental simulations (Taylor, Pham, Rivkin, & Armor, 1998) such as simulating moving toward a goal (process simulation) and simulating obtaining a goal (outcome simulation). With the various forms of simulation, people imagine proceeding through the steps required to achieve a goal or what would happen if one did or did not achieve a goal. Although mental simulations may contribute to unrealistic optimism, unrealistic optimism is distinct in that it represents expectations about what will transpire.

CAUSES OF UNREALISTIC OPTIMISM

Although theorists have proposed a variety of explanations for unrealistic optimism, all of the explanations fall within three broad categories: motivation, use of available information, and biased information processing (for a review, see Shepperd, Carroll, Grace, & Terry, 2002).

Motivation

The first category of explanations addresses the observation that people wish to believe (or wish others to believe) that unwanted events are unlikely to happen to them, or at least are less likely to happen to them than to other people. Research on this first category of explanations has found support for two sources of motivations for unrealistic optimism: self-enhancement and self-presentation. Regarding self-enhancement, it feels good to believe that favorable outcomes are likely and unfavorable outcomes are unlikely to happen in one's future. People are able to sustain self-enhancing beliefs by focusing not on what might or will happen, but on what they would like to happen (Krizan & Windschitl, 2007; Sherman, 1980; Stuart, Windschitl, Smith, & Scherer, 2017), and people's judgment of the likelihood of an disease increase in step with their ratings of the desirability of the event (Biner, Angle, Park, Mellinger, & Barber, 1995). For example, the more important or consequential research participants rate a disease, the less likely they are to report that the disease will happen to them compared with others (Kirscht, Haefner, Kegeles, & Rosenstock, 1966). Likewise, the more college students rate divorce as stressful and unpleasant, the less likely they are to report that their eventual marriage will end in divorce (Perloff, 1987).

The second motivation is grounded in research on self-presentation and involves conveying a desired image to others, an image that may include the assertion that one's risk for unfavorable outcomes is low, or at least lower than the risk of other people. Importantly, the presentation of low risk for unfavorable outcomes may not be deliberative or even conscious (Schlenker, 1985). Several studies provide evidence that self-presentational concerns may motivate unrealistic optimism. For instance, research participants in one study displayed less social acceptance toward targets who expressed comparative pessimism in their risk judgments (i.e., predicted that they were at greater risk than other people for unfavorable outcomes) because they assumed that the targets were hopeless, sad, and depressed (Helweg-Larsen, Sadeghian, & Webb, 2002). The realization that social acceptance is linked to appearing optimistic may lead people to conclude that they should be unrealistically optimistic in their personal predictions if they wish to be liked (Armor, Massey, & Sackett, 2008). Other research finds that people sometimes are strategic in their displays of unrealistic optimism. Specifically, people are less inclined to claim that their risk for unfavorable outcomes is less than that of their peers if they believe they might be held accountable for their overly optimistic predictions (Tyler & Rosier, 2009).

Available Information

The second category of explanations suggests that unrealistic optimism arises naturally from the kind of information people have at their disposal when making risk judgments. People typically have a great deal of information about themselves when making personal judgments (Kruger, 1999). They know their personal history, the efforts they take to avoid or lower their risk for unwanted outcomes and to achieve desired outcomes, and their plans and intentions regarding future events, and people rely heavily on this information when calculating their risk or predicting what will transpire. For example, when young smokers estimate their comparative risk for smoking-related illnesses such as cancer and emphysema, they consider how frequently they smoke, their willpower, their level of addiction, and the likelihood that they will still be smoking 10 years later (Weinstein, Slovic, & Gibson, 2004). However, they lack or fail to use similar information about the average person.

Several studies illustrate how the disparity in information about oneself versus comparison targets can lead to unrealistic optimism in personal risk estimates. One study found that actors rely on their intentions when making personal estimates, whereas observers, who lack access to the actors' intentions, do not (Kruger & Gilovich, 2004). Specifically, when reporting how charitable they are, actors consider their intentions to engage in charitable actions. In contrast, observers—who have no access to the actors' intentions—consider only whether the actor did or did not engage in charitable actions. Other studies find that providing people with population base rate information diminished unrealistic optimism in personal predictions for unfavorable events (Weinstein, 1983; Weinstein & Lachendro, 1982). Finally, research shows that encouraging people to think about the control that other people have over a future outcome can reduce unrealistic optimism (Hoorens & Smits, 2001).

Even when it is available, people may fail to use information about the average person when making risk judgments because the "average person" is rather abstract. Research on the person-positivity bias has demonstrated that the more an entity resembles a specific, visualizable human being, the more favorably observers regard that entity (Sears, 1983). The "average person" is an amorphous exemplar or prototype rather than a specific person. And as an amorphous prototype, the average person is viewed as less human—and thus less favorably—than the self. Accordingly, people tend to rate an amorphous, less human-like target as more likely to experience unfavorable outcomes. In line with this argument, when instructed to rate their risk for unfavorable outcomes relative to a specific target rather than the amorphous average person, people display less unrealistic optimism (Alicke, Klotz, Breitenbecher, Yurak, & Vredenburg, 1995; Hoorens & Buunk, 1993).

Much of the research described in this second category of explanations for unrealistic optimism is pertinent to unrealistic comparative optimism. Yet evidence suggests that information disparity can contribute to unrealistic absolute optimism as well, such that providing people with base rate information can diminish unrealistic absolute optimism (Weinstein, 1983; Weinstein & Lachendro, 1982).

Information Processing

Researchers have identified a variety of heuristics and biases that characterize the way people process information, two of which—the representativeness heuristic and egocentric thinking—are particularly relevant to unrealistic optimism. The representativeness heuristic (Tversky, 1977) is an information-processing shortcut whereby, when applied to risk estimates, people judge the likelihood of an event happening to them based on how similar they are to the typical person who experiences the event (Weinstein, 1980). For example, if asked to estimate the likelihood that they will become HIV infected, people might imagine the stereotypical person who is HIV positive—someone who is gay, promiscuous, or uses intravenous drugs—and base their personal risk judgment on their similarity to this image.

Evidence for the role of the representativeness heuristic in unrealistic optimism comes from a clever study in which researchers asked participants to estimate their risk for various unfavorable events (e.g., car accident, heart attack) relative to that of a friend. Not surprisingly, participants displayed unrealistic optimism in their estimates, rating their risk as lower than that of their friend. More telling was that participants reported selecting different friends for each event. For car accidents, participants typically selected a friend who was a reckless driver. For heart attacks, participants typically selected a friend with a high number of risk factors (Perloff & Fetzer, 1986). Apparently, each event evoked thoughts of the stereotypical person who was at high risk for the event, which in turn prompted participants to select from their various friends one who matched the stereotype. Participants then judged their risk relative to this high-risk friend.

Beyond the representativeness heuristic, research finds that people are quite egocentric when making comparative judgments (Chambers, Windschitl, & Suls, 2003). When asked to evaluate their risk relative to that of the average person, people appear not to rationally weigh their risk factors against the risk factors of the average person. Rather, they merely consider their personal risk factors and infer their comparative risk accordingly. If they believe that their risk is high, they conclude that their risk is higher than average. If they believe that their risk is low, they conclude that their risk is lower than average. As such, comparative judgments sometimes are not comparative at all; they instead are simply self-judgments (Eiser, Pahl, & Prins, 2001).

Several studies illustrate this egocentric bias in risk judgments. For example, researchers often assess comparative judgments with a single item, such as, "How likely are you to experience _____ relative to the average person?" (*1 = much less likely than the average person; 5 = much more likely than the average person*). Importantly, researchers sometimes include measures of personal and target risk estimates by asking, "How likely are you to experience _____?" and "How likely is the average person to experience _____?" (*1 = not at all likely; 5 = very likely*). Consistent with the argument that comparative judgments are really self-judgments, comparative judgments typically correlate strongly with personal estimates but are uncorrelated with target estimates (Eiser et al., 2001; Klar & Giladi, 1999).

Other studies have demonstrated the egocentric nature of comparative judgments by creating subtle variations in item framing to shift attention away from personal risk toward the risk of the average person. For example, participants in one study (Eiser et al., 2001) supplied likelihood estimates for 12 events. In the *self-focus* condition, participants estimated how likely it was that the event would happen to them compared with others. In the *other-focus* condition, participants estimated how likely it was that the event would happen to others compared with them. The findings were consistent with the egocentric explanation for unrealistic optimism: Although participants showed unrealistic optimism for all 12 events, their optimism was greater in the self-focus condition than in the other-focus condition. In addition, in the self-focus condition, comparative judgments correlated strongly ($r = .75$) with participants' personal ratings. Participants who reported that the outcome was unlikely to happen to them also reported that the event was less likely to happen to them than to the average person. In contrast, comparative judgments were uncorrelated with participants' target ratings ($r = .01$). This latter finding suggests that participants did not consider the average person's risk when making their comparative judgments (Eiser et al., 2001).

In the other-focus condition, the comparative judgment again correlated strongly ($r = .72$) with participants' personal ratings. This finding once again highlights the overlap between personal and comparative judgments. In addition, comparative judgments also correlated with participants' target rating ($r = -.35$; Eiser et al., 2001). The negative correlation indicates that participants who reported that the unfavorable outcome was likely to happen to the average person also reported that the unfavorable outcome was less likely to happen to them than to the average person. Moreover, the finding that comparative and target estimates were correlated suggests that participants did consider the average person's risk when making their comparative judgments.

Summary

The three categories of explanations we have discussed undoubtedly overlap. However, none by itself can sufficiently account for unrealistic optimism, as evident by the fact that manipulations designed to address any one of the three causes rarely eliminates unrealistic optimism entirely. Moreover, as we note elsewhere (Shepperd et al., 2002), the motivations and processes that elicit unrealistic optimism can become quite automatic, so much so that unrealistic optimism for many events may acquire an almost heuristic quality that allows people to draw the speedy conclusion that they are less at risk for unfavorable events than are others (Alicke et al., 1995). Finally, it is noteworthy that most of the research we discussed on the causes of unrealistic optimism pertained to unrealistic comparative optimism, primarily because researchers have conducted far fewer studies on unrealistic absolute optimism. The first two categories of causes (motivation and available information) are almost certainly equally relevant to both unrealistic comparative and unrealistic absolute optimism. It remains unknown the extent to which information processing—particularly the representativeness heuristic and egocentric thinking—contribute to unrealistic absolute optimism. Thus, understanding the causes of unrealistic absolute optimism remains a viable topic for future research.

Boundary Conditions on Unrealistic Optimism

We noted in the prior section that changes in the context or in the framing of items can decrease or even eliminate unrealistic optimism. Beyond these moderators, a number of studies reveal that people can be selective in their expression of unrealistic optimism (for a more extensive review, see Helweg-Larsen & Shepperd, 2001). We discuss three boundary conditions on unrealistic optimism that have received considerable attention: perceived control, prior experience, and outcome frequency. All of the boundary conditions reflect constraints on people's predictions of what awaits in the future.

Perceived Control

Among the most replicated findings in the literature on unrealistic optimism is the finding that people display less unrealistic optimism for uncontrollable outcomes than for controllable outcomes (for reviews, see Harris, 1996; Klein & Helweg-Larsen, 2002). When outcomes are controllable, people can take action to avoid outcomes that are undesirable and take action to ensure the occurrence of desirable outcomes. When outcomes are uncontrollable, people are in a weak position to defend their optimistic outlook. Perhaps nowhere is the role of perceived control more evident than in a study of automobile accidents, in which research participants predicted that they were less likely to experience an automobile accident if they were the drivers rather than the passengers (McKenna, 1993). Other research has examined trait-like perceptions of control and found that a greater sense of personal control corresponds with greater unrealistic optimism (Hoorens & Buunk, 1993).

Although much of the research on unrealistic optimism and control examines unrealistic comparative optimism, this literature consistently finds that greater control corresponds with lower personal risk judgments but is uncorrelated with target risk judgments. Because unrealistic absolute optimism is defined by how a personal judgment compares with some objective criterion, perceived control should moderate the expression of unrealistic absolute optimism as well. Research on the planning fallacy supports this proposition (Buehler et al., 1997; Buehler & Griffin, Chapter 27, this volume).

Prior Experience

Both theory and research suggest that expectations for the future flow from past experience (Bandura, 1977; Caprara et al., 2008; Mischel, Cantor, & Feldman, 1996; Olson, Roese, & Zanna, 1996; Pajares & Johnson, 1996). Accordingly, a number of studies find that people display less unrealistic optimism about unfavorable outcomes with which they have prior experience (Helweg-Larsen & Shepperd, 2001). By prior experience, we mean at least one incident of the target event occurring in a person's life. For example, people display less unrealistic optimism about earthquakes and hurricanes following personal experience with these events (Helweg-Larsen, 1999; Trumbo, Lueck, Marlatt, & Peek, 2011), less unrealistic optimism about contracting a sexually transmitted infection if they have had an infection in the previous 4 months (Van der Velde, Hooykaas, & Van Der Pligt, 1992), and less unrealistic optimism about avoiding negative Internet events (e.g., having personal information stolen, getting a computer virus) if they had experienced such events in the past (Campbell, Greenauer, Macaluso, & End, 2007).

Prior experience with an unfavorable outcome may influence unrealistic optimism through several routes (Helweg-Larsen & Shepperd, 2001). First, prior experience may diminish people's sense of personal control over the outcome, leading them to believe that they cannot avoid it or are no more likely than others to avoid the event. Second, prior experience may increase the accessibility of the unfavorable outcome, keeping it at the front of one's mind where it can influence later risk judgments. Third, prior experience with an unfavorable outcome may color one's sense of what can happen in the future, forcing people to acknowledge that they are at some degree of risk.

As with perceived control, personal experience influences personal risk judgments rather than judgments made on behalf of targets. Thus, although much of the research on prior experience examined its effect on unrealistic comparative optimism, the findings will likely hold for unrealistic absolute optimism, such that prior experience with an unfavorable outcome is likely to decrease unrealistic absolute optimism for that outcome.

Outcome Frequency

A number of studies demonstrate that people show greater unrealistic comparative optimism for rare unfavorable outcomes than for common unfavorable outcomes. Conversely, people show greater unrealistic comparative optimism for common favorable outcomes than for uncommon favorable outcomes (Chambers et al., 2003). How do we account for this asymmetry in judgments? One explanation is egocentric thinking. As noted earlier, when making comparative judgments, people consider their personal information yet neglect information about others. People show unrealistic comparative optimism for rare unfavorable outcomes because they reason that if the outcomes are unlikely to happen to them, then they are less likely to happen to them than to other people. In a similar vein, people show unrealistic comparative optimism for common favorable outcomes because they reason that if the outcomes are likely to happen to them, then they are more likely to happen to them than to other people. People fail to consider that rare unfavorable outcomes are also unlikely to happen to others and that common favorable outcomes are also likely to happen to others.

It is noteworthy that research shows an opposite pattern for unrealistic absolute optimism. People tend to show greater unrealistic absolute optimism for common unfavorable outcomes than for rare unfavorable outcomes, yet they show greater unrealistic absolute pessimism for rare favorable outcomes than for common favorable outcomes (Chambers et al., 2003; Kruger & Burrus, 2004; Price, Pentecost, & Voth, 2002). The asymmetry here likely arises from ignorance of the base rate (Fischhoff, 1981; Slovic, 1987). Specifically, people likely underestimate the rarity of low-prevalence outcomes. Put simply, people understand that rare events are rare, yet fail to understand how rare they are. This failure leads people to overestimate the prevalence—and thus their likelihood of experiencing—rare events, whether favorable or unfavorable. For favorable events, the overestimation translates into unrealistic absolute optimism; for unfavorable events, the overestimation translates into unrealistic absolute pessimism. Evidence supporting the argument that ignorance of the base rate accounts for these departures from unrealistic absolute optimism comes from several studies that provide people with base rate information. These studies consistently find that people show less unrealistic absolute optimism (as well as less unrealistic comparative optimism) when they receive base rate information than when they do not (Rothman et al., 1996; Sweeny & Shepperd, 2007; Weinstein & Lyon, 1999).

Summary

People are not always unrealistically optimistic. They do not show unrealistic optimism for uncontrollable events or when perceived control is low, and when they have prior experience with the unwanted outcome. They also show less unrealistic comparative optimism for rare favorable events and for common unfavorable events. Conversely, they show less unrealistic absolute optimism for common favorable events and for rare unfavorable events.

Importantly, our list of boundary conditions omits one important moderator of unrealistic optimism. In the past two decades, numerous studies have shown that people will shelve their optimism in favor of a more realistic or even pessimistic outlook if they anticipate that their optimistic outlook might be challenged. The next section discusses how and when people abandon their optimism in predictions about the future.

TEMPORAL FLUCTUATIONS IN UNREALISTIC OPTIMISM

Nearness in time to performance or to the arrival of important news serves as a reality check for the unrealistically optimistic. A robust literature demonstrates how sobering the temporal proximity of a performance or feedback can be when envisioning future outcomes, such as starting salaries (Shepperd, Ouellette, & Fernandez, 1996), performance on tests of personal ability (Gilovich, Kerr, & Medvec, 1993), success of public presentations (Kettle & Häubl, 2010), and grades on academic exams (Jiga-Boy, 2008; Shepperd et al., 1996). People tend to become more pessimistic in their outcome predictions as they approach the event in question (Sweeny & Krizan, 2013).

In a classic demonstration of this shift from optimism, students in one study predicted their scores on a midterm exam at four points in time: at the start of the semester, just after taking the exam, 1 hour before learning their grades, and immediately before learning their grades (Shepperd et al., 1996). At the start of the semester, students were unrealistically optimistic, presumably because they had every intention of attending lectures and office hours, keeping up with the reading, and getting an early start on studying. Following the exam, students' predictions were quite realistic, grounded in the knowledge of how much they actually studied and how their preparations aligned with the exam itself. Perhaps most interesting, however, were students' predictions in the final moments before learning their grades: Students abandoned all pretense of optimism, displaying unrealistically pessimistic predictions at the moment of truth.

Reasons for Shifts from Optimism at the Moment of Truth

Dozens of studies have replicated and expanded this seminal study, and a recent meta-analysis (Sweeny & Krizan, 2013) concluded that the tendency to shift away from unrealistic optimism as objective feedback draws near is quite robust (average $d = .40$). This literature has identified two broad explanations for these shifts: responding to changing information and emotion regulation.

Information-Based Shifts

Why does the proximity of an event temper unrealistic optimism? One reason is that as people approach an event, they encounter new information that prompts them to reappraise the likelihood of various outcomes. Using a midterm exam for illustration, students may acquire new information about the population base rate (e.g., performance of students in past semesters) or about the demands of the task itself (e.g., the difficulty of the material) as they prepare, or they may gain new information about themselves based on their experiences in other classes (Kappes, Oettingen, & Mayer, 2012). This information constrains unrealistic optimism (Carroll, Sweeny, & Shepperd, 2006). Additionally, the very act of preparing provides information about the demands of performance, the perseverance and skill required to obtain a good outcome, and how well one's personal abilities match up to the task at hand (Gilovich et al., 1993). Similarly, people form expectations based in part on their plans and intentions. The passage of time often reveals that these plans are unrealistic, thus demanding an adjustment in one's predictions to account for the plans that remain unexecuted (Carroll et al., 2006). Finally, people's emotional states can provide information (albeit unreliable information) about their likely outcomes. According to the mood-as-information hypothesis, feelings of anxiety point to the possibility that future events may not turn out as hoped (Schwarz, 2011). Consistent with this possibility, one study demonstrated that rising anxiety in anticipation of feedback plays a key role in shifting people away from unrealistic optimism (Shepperd, Grace, Cole, & Klein, 2005).

Even when no new information is available, shifts away from unrealistic optimism can occur in response to a deeper analysis of existing information (Sweeny & Krizan, 2013). Construal-level theory suggests that people view temporally distant events in a high-level, abstract fashion, with greater attention to desires and motivations than to context or details (Liberman, Trope, & Wakslak, 2007). This abstract perspective allows considerable space to embrace an unrealistically optimistic outlook. However, as an event draws near, construal of the event becomes more concrete and detail oriented, and these newly apparent details often constrain predictions (Nussbaum, Liberman, & Trope, 2006). For example, as the day of a midterm exam approaches, students may begin to consider their particular skill at multiple-choice exams or the likelihood that they will forgo a party to get a good night's sleep prior to the exam. Even after the exam is over, shifts in construal level may account for a further slide toward pessimism as people increasingly focus on details of their potential outcomes. In conjunction with rising anxiety, the potential for negative consequences (e.g., failing the exam) may be especially salient as the moment of truth draws near (Trope & Liberman, 2003).

Another reason people reconsider existing information in the face of impending feedback is the increasing awareness that their expectations may be disconfirmed (Lerner & Tetlock, 1999). People could look foolishly overconfident if they maintain unrealistic optimism. As such, even simple awareness of one's own expectations tends to prompt a downward revision away from unrealistic optimism (Armor & Sackett, 2006). When faced with increasing accountability pressures, people scrutinize existing information and turn to self-criticism, which diminishes the biased processing that maintains unrealistic optimism (Lerner & Tetlock, 1999).

Finally, proximity to an uncertain outcome might prompt mental contrasting, a process that entails imagining a desired future outcome while also identifying present-moment obstacles to reaching that outcome (Oettingen, 2012, 2014). When people engage in mental contrasting, they consider the effort that it would take to overcome obstacles standing in the way of a desired outcome, and they exert the necessary effort only if they believe they are likely to achieve the outcome. Put another way, people embrace a more realistic outlook when they engage in mental contrasting. Initial evidence suggests that people are more likely to engage in mental contrasting when a desired outcome is more immediate and salient (Sevincer, Schlier, & Oettingen, 2015, Study 2), which points to mental contrasting as another route by which people abandon unrealistic optimism at the moment of truth.

Bracing for the Worst

Although people sometimes shift away from optimism in response to changing information, at other times the shift serves an emotion regulation function. Optimism generally feels good, even if that optimism is unfounded. However, unrealistic optimism has a cost: shattering disappointment in the face of disconfirming evidence (Shepperd & McNulty, 2002; Sweeny & Shepperd, 2010). In fact, considerable evidence finds that the more optimistic people are about a particular outcome, the greater is their risk for disappointment (Zeelenberg, Van Dijk, Manstead, & der Pligt, 1998).

Given this tradeoff, people are often strategic in their departures from optimism, making outcome predictions based on a risk–benefit ratio between optimism and pessimism (Armor & Sackett, 2006). Optimism puts people in a frame of mind to take advantage of opportunities, whereas pessimism prepares people to deal with setbacks, including the blow of disappointment that would accompany bad news (Carroll et al., 2006). To the extent that the potential consequences of bad news become more salient as the moment of truth draws near, the need to prepare for setbacks intensifies, and unrealistic optimism may fade.

On the other hand, pessimism can also serve a motivating function for some people. Some highly capable people, in anticipation of performance, make excessively pessimistic predictions about the outcome. The pessimistic predictions produce anxiety that these *defensive pessimists* use to prepare for the performance and ensure that the unwanted outcome does not transpire (Norem & Cantor, 1986). In this case, shifts away from unrealistic optimism serve a seemingly undesirable emotion regulation function by fostering anxiety, yet this anxiety motivates success for defensive pessimists. In contrast, strategic optimists are at the opposite end of the spectrum, garnering motivation from upbeat, even unrealistically optimistic thinking (Norem & Cantor, 1986). Interestingly, recent research found that across nearly two dozen studies, defensive pessimists were just as likely as strategic optimists to lower their expectations as a moment of truth drew near (Sweeny & Falkenstein, 2016), suggesting that both individual and contextual factors motivate the strategic management of expectations.

Summary

When anticipating the future, people depart from unrealistically optimistic predictions for a variety of reasons. Most intuitively, people may gain information along the way that constrains their otherwise unmitigated optimism. Prior to a performance, efforts to prepare shed new light on the demands of performance and how well one's skills and abilities match up with those demands. As time passes, people begin to view the event and perhaps the implications of that event in a more concrete and detailed fashion, which may reveal considerations that were invisible from a distant and abstract point of view. Impending feedback also underscores accountability concerns, and when these concerns are coupled with rising anxiety, people may weigh more heavily the possibility that their expectations could exceed their ultimate outcomes. Furthermore, as the ability to prepare for an outcome diminishes with time, people realize they may be unable to implement the plans that would guarantee a desired outcome.

Information about performance and potential outcomes are not the only source of shifts from unrealistic optimism. People strategically lower their expectations to regulate their emotional states. People may hedge their predictions to avoid crippling disappointment if their outcomes fall short of their hopes, and some people may even embrace pessimism in an effort to motivate preparative efforts and ultimately secure success. For all of these reasons, people show a robust tendency to abandon unrealistic optimism as they approach objective feedback; however, certain conditions limit this tendency.

BOUNDARY CONDITIONS ON FLUCTUATIONS IN OPTIMISM

Although a variety of circumstances can prompt people to shift away from unrealistic optimism over time, evidence suggests that people are particular likely to shift under three conditions: when the feared outcome is (1) severe, (2) personally relevant, and (3) relatively rare. First, people are more likely to brace for the worst when the worst-case scenario is particularly fearsome. For example, participants in one study more readily abandoned optimism about their likelihood of having a disease with severe consequences compared with a disease with relatively benign consequences (Taylor & Shepperd, 1998). Importantly, the effects of outcome severity on outcome predictions can be quite subtle, reflecting the cognitive or semantic framing of an outcome as a missed opportunity (i.e., a failure to gain something) versus a loss. When faced with the possibility of either a financial windfall or a financial setback, students in one study persisted in their unrealistic optimism about the windfall but braced for the worst when it came to the setback. In this study, university students learned of a university billing error. Some students read that 25% of students were underbilled by the university and would soon receive a bill in the mail (a loss). Other students learned that 25% of students were overbilled by the university and would soon receive a check (a gain). All students then estimated the likelihood that they were one of the affected students. Whereas the estimates of students in the gain condition were realistic, hovering close to the 25% base rate, the estimates of students in the loss condition were pessimistic. This effect was particularly strong for students high in financial need, for whom an unexpected bill would represent a serious setback (Shepperd, Findley-Klein, Kwavnick, Walker, & Perez, 2000).

Second, people are more likely to brace for outcomes that are personally relevant than for outcomes that are not personally relevant. That is, people are disinclined to brace for outcomes that pertain solely or primarily to another person, even a close a friend (Sweeny, Shepperd, & Carroll, 2009). Many of the motivations to brace that we discussed earlier are moot in the face of others' impending outcomes: People may have little insight into others' preparatory efforts, they cannot directly experience others' rising anxiety, they will not be held accountable if outcomes deviate from expectations, and they have little need to manage their emotions over others' outcomes. In fact, people experience little disappointment when others' outcomes turn out worse than expected (Carroll, Shepperd, Sweeny, Carlson, & Benigno, 2007).

Consistent with this reasoning are the findings from a series of experiments in which pairs of friends were assigned the role of applicant or interviewer in a mock job interview. The interviews were videotaped, and an external evaluator would ostensibly judge whether the "applicant" did or did not get the job. Immediately after the interview, interviewers were far more optimistic than applicants about the applicant's chance of being "hired." Moreover, as the announcement of the hiring decision drew near, applicants became less confident that they would be hired, whereas their friends remained unchanged in their optimistic predictions. A follow-up experiment revealed that people braced for their friends only when they personally had a stake in the game; that is, when they personally would benefit or suffer based on their friends' outcome (Sweeny et al., 2009).

Third, people brace more for rare events than for relatively common events (Sweeny & Shepperd, 2007). This difference is likely due in part to the fact that rare events, by their nature, are less expected. Research shows that unwelcome outcomes produce more disappointment when they are unexpected than when they are expected (Shepperd & McNulty, 2002). People may also brace more for rare outcomes because they perceive them as more severe. Specifically, people view rare negative events as more severe than common negative events (Jemmott, Ditto, & Croyle, 1986).

We noted earlier that unrealistic optimism is greater for rare negative events than for rare positive events, which would seem inconsistent with the finding of a shift to pessimism for rare events as the moment of truth draws near. The inconsistency, however, is more apparent than real and highlights the importance of anticipating a possible challenge to personal predictions. When making predictions about a rare event that may or may not happen in the distant future, people have considerable room for optimism. Moreover, the rarity of the event particularly lends itself to unrealistic comparative optimism because of egocentric thinking (Chambers et al., 2003; Eiser et al., 2001). People think the event is unlikely to happen to them and thus that it is less likely to happen to them than to others. By contrast, when making predictions about a rare event that may occur in the near future, people no longer have the luxury of being optimistic but instead face the possibility, no matter how remote, that an unwanted event may happen in the immediate future. Because rare events are unexpected and thus more likely to produce disappointment, people are particularly inclined to brace for rare events than for common events.

In sum, people do not always shift their predictions downward when facing impending feedback. Research finds that people are most inclined to shift their predictions toward pessimism when the outcome is more serious, when the outcome is personally consequential rather than pertaining only to others, and when the outcome is rare.

SUMMARY

Unrealistic optimism is a pervasive phenomenon in social judgment (Shepperd et al., 2013). It occurs in part because people are motivated to believe, or have others believe, that they are unlikely to experience unfavorable events, or at least less likely than others to experience such events. It also can arise from differences in the amount of information people have about themselves versus the comparison standard—either some objective standard such as the population base rate or a comparison target such as the average person. Finally, unrealistic optimism can be a natural consequence of the way people process information, particularly the tendency for people to use the representativeness heuristic in making judgments and to be egocentric when evaluating their risk.

Although unrealistic optimism is commonplace, it does not occur for all outcomes. Egocentric thinking prompts unrealistic comparative optimism for rare unfavorable outcomes and for common favorable outcomes. Conversely, it prompts unrealistic absolute optimism for common unfavorable outcomes and for rare favorable outcomes. Finally, people display greater unrealistic optimism when their predictions are less constrained. Accordingly, people show relatively little unrealistic optimism when outcomes are uncontrollable, when they have base rate information, and when they have personal experience with the unfavorable event.

Unrealistic optimism typically disappears, and sometimes is replaced by unrealistic pessimism, when the moment of truth draws near and people face the possibility that their optimistic predictions might be disconfirmed. In such instances, people often gain information that leads them to temper their optimistic expectations. They also come to realize that their outcomes may fall short of their expectations, producing disappointment should they remain optimistic. The shift from optimism in outcome predictions occurs most readily for outcomes that are rare, serious, and personally relevant.

We opened this chapter with the suggestion that it would serve people's interests to be accurate in their forecasts—to know when undesired outcomes lie ahead and when they do not. Research on unrealistic optimism, as well as departures from unrealistic optimism, suggest that people are often remarkably inaccurate in their forecasts. As we have explained, these unrealistic predictions are quite sensible given the conditions under which people make predictions about their future outcomes. Moreover, unrealistic optimism and the shift to unrealistic pessimism may serve people well. Unrealistic optimism feels good in the moment (Sweeny & Shepperd, 2010), has interpersonal benefits (Helweg-Larsen et al., 2002), and may even facilitate goal-directed behavior, persistence, and postive affect (Armor & Taylor, 1998). As the moment of truth draws near, the shift from optimism offers its own benefits, including less disappointment when outcomes turn out poorly (Shepperd & McNulty, 2002; Sweeny & Shepperd, 2010) and, for some, anxiety that they can harness toward actions that ensure that their gloom-and-doom predictions are not realized (Norem & Cantor, 1986). Thus inaccurate forecasts can also serve people's interests.

REFERENCES

Alicke, M. D., Klotz, M. L., Breitenbecher, D. L., Yurak, T. J., & Vredenburg, D. S. (1995). Personal contact, individuation, and the better-than-average effect. *Journal of Personality and Social Psychology, 68*, 804–825.

Armor, D. A., Massey, C., & Sackett, A. M. (2008). Prescribed optimism: Is it right to be wrong about the future? *Psychological Science, 19*, 329–331.

Armor, D. A., & Sackett, A. M. (2006). Accuracy, error, and bias in predictions for real versus hypothetical events. *Journal of Personality and Social Psychology, 91*, 583–600.

Armor, D. A., & Taylor, S. E. (1998). Situated optimism: Specific outcome expectancies and self-regulation. In M. P. Zanna (Ed.), *Advances in experimental social psychology* (Vol. 30, pp. 309–379). New York: Academic Press

Baek, Y. M., Kim, E., & Bae, Y. (2014). My privacy is okay, but theirs is endangered: Why comparative optimism matters in online privacy concerns. *Computers in Human Behavior, 31*, 48–56.

Bandura, A. (1997). *Self-efficacy: The exercise of control.* New York: Freeman.

Biner, P. M., Angle, S. T., Park, J. H., Mellinger, A. E., & Barber, B. C. (1995). Need state and the illusion of control. *Personality and Social Psychology Bulletin, 21*, 899–907.

Borrelli, B., Hayes, R. B., Dunsiger, S., & Fava, J. L. (2009). Risk perception and smoking behavior in medically ill smokers: A prospective study. *Addiction, 105*, 1100–1108.

Buehler, R., Griffin, D., & MacDonald, H. (1997). The role of motivated reasoning in optimistic time predictions. *Personality and Social Psychology Bulletin, 23,* 238–247.

Byram, S. J. (1997). Cognitive and motivational factors influencing time prediction. *Journal of Experimental Psychology: Applied, 3,* 216–239.

Campbell, J., Greenauer, N., Macaluso, K., & End, C. (2007). Unrealistic optimism in Internet events. *Computers in Human Behavior, 23,* 1273–1284.

Caprara, G. V., Fida, R., Vecchione, M., Del Bove, G., Vecchio, G. M., Barbaranelli, C., . . . Bandura, A. (2008). Longitudinal analysis of the role of perceived self-efficacy for self-regulated learning in academic continuance and achievement. *Journal of Educational Psychology, 100,* 525–534.

Carroll, P. J., Shepperd, J. A., Sweeny, K., Carlson, E., & Benigno, J. P. (2007). Disappointment for others. *Cognition and Emotion, 21,* 1565–1576.

Carroll, P. J., Sweeny, K., & Shepperd, J. A. (2006). Forsaking optimism. *Review of General Psychology, 10,* 56–73.

Chambers, J. R., Windschitl, P. D., & Suls, J. (2003). Egocentrism, event frequency, and comparative optimism: When what happens frequently is "more likely to happen to me." *Personality and Social Psychology Bulletin, 29,* 1343–1356.

Chapin, J. R., & Coleman, G. (2012). Optimistic bias about dating/relationship violence among teens. *Journal of Youth Studies, 15,* 645–655.

Cho, H., Lee, J., & Lee, J. (2013). Optimistic bias about H1N1 flu: Testing the links between risk communication, optimistic bias, and self-protection behavior. *Health Communication, 28,* 146–158.

Chock, T. M. (2011). The influence of body mass index, sex, and race on college students' optimistic bias for lifestyle healthfulness. *Journal of Nutrition Education and Behavior, 43,* 331–338.

Davidson, K., & Prkachin, K. (1997). Optimism and unrealistic optimism have an interacting impact on health-promoting behavior and knowledge changes. *Personality and Social Psychology Bulletin, 23,* 617–625.

Eiser, J. R., Pahl, S., & Prins, Y. R. A. (2001). Optimism, pessimism, and the direction of self-other comparisons. *Journal of Experimental Social Psychology, 37,* 77–84.

Fischhoff, B. (1981). When do base rates affect predictions? *Journal of Personality and Social Psychology, 41,* 671–680.

Fowler, S. L., & Geers, A. L. (2015). Dispositional and comparative optimism interact to predict avoidance of a looming health threat. *Psychology and Health, 30,* 456–474.

Gilbert, D. T., & Wilson, T. D. (2007). Prospection: Experiencing the future. *Science, 317,* 1351–1354.

Gilovich, T., Kerr, M., & Medvec, V. H. (1993). Effect of temporal perspective on subjective confidence. *Journal of Personality and Social Psychology, 64,* 552–560.

Harris, P. (1996). Sufficient grounds for optimism? The relationship between perceived controllability and optimistic bias. *Journal of Social and Clinical Psychology, 15,* 9–52.

Helweg-Larsen, M. (1999). (The lack of) optimistic biases in response to the Northridge earthquake: The role of personal experience. *Basic and Applied Social Psychology, 21,* 119–129.

Helweg-Larsen, M., Sadeghian, P., & Webb, M. A. (2002). The stigma of being pessimistically biased. *Journal of Social and Clinical Psychology, 21,* 92–107.

Helweg-Larsen, M., & Shepperd, J. A. (2001). Do moderators of the optimistic bias affect personal or target risk estimates?: A review of the literature. *Personality and Social Psychology Review, 5,* 74–95.

Hoorens, V., & Buunk, B. P. (1993). Social comparison of health risks: Locus of control, the person-positivity bias, and unrealistic optimism. *Journal of Applied Social Psychology, 23,* 291–302.

Hoorens, V., & Smits, T. (2001). Why do controllable events elicit stronger comparative optimism than uncontrollable events? *Revue International de Psychologie Sociale, 14,* 11–44.

Jemmott, J. B., Ditto, P. H., & Croyle, R. T. (1986). Judging health status: Effects of perceived prevalence and personal relevance. *Journal of Personality and Social Psychology, 50,* 899–905.

Jiga-Boy, G. M. (2008). *Adaptive thinking about the future: Temporal construal, health-related behaviour, and perceived temporal distance.* Unpublished doctoral dissertation, University of Grenoble II, Grenoble, France.

Kahneman, D., & Tversky, A. (1982). Intuitive prediction: Biases and corrective procedures. In D. Kahneman, P. Slovic, & A. Tversky (Eds.), *Judgment under uncertainty: Heuristics and biases* (pp. 414–421). Cambridge, UK: Cambridge University Press.

Kappes, H. B., Oettingen, G., & Mayer, D. (2012). Positive fantasies predict low academic achievement in disadvantaged students. *European Journal of Social Psychology, 42,* 53–64.

Kettle, K. L., & Häubl, G. (2010). Motivation by anticipation: Expecting rapid feedback enhances performance. *Psychological Science, 21,* 545–547.

Kirscht, J. F., Haefner, D. P., Kegeles, S. S., & Rosenstock, I. M. (1966). A national study of health beliefs. *Journal of Health and Human Behavior, 7,* 248–254.

Klar, Y., & Giladi, E. E. (1999). Are most people happier than their peers, or are they just happy? *Personality and Social Psychology Bulletin, 25,* 585–594.

Klein, C. T. F., & Helweg-Larsen, M. (2002). Perceived control and the optimistic bias: A meta-analytic review. *Psychology and Health, 17,* 437–446.

Koole, S., & Spijker, M. (2000). Overcoming the planning fallacy through willpower: Effects of implementation intentions on actual and predicted task-completion times. *European Journal of Social Psychology, 30,* 873–888.

Krizan, Z., & Windschitl, P. D. (2007). The influence of outcome desirability on optimism. *Psychological Bulletin, 133,* 95–121.

Kruger, J. (1999). Lake Wobegon be gone!: The "below-average effect" and the egocentric nature of comparative ability judgments. *Journal of Personality and Social Psychology, 77,* 221–232.

Kruger, J., & Burrus, J. (2004). Egocentrism and focalism in unrealistic optimism (and pessimism). *Journal of Experimental Social Psychology, 40,* 332–340.

Kruger, J., & Gilovich, T. (2004). Actions, intentions, and self-assessment: The road to self-enhancement is paved with good intentions. *Personality and Social Psychology Bulletin, 30,* 328–339.

Lerner, J. S., & Tetlock, P. E. (1999). Accounting for the effects of accountability. *Psychological Bulletin, 125,* 255–275.

Liberman, N., Trope, Y., & Wakslak, C. (2007). Construal level theory and consumer behavior. *Journal of Consumer Psychology, 17,* 113–117.

McKenna, F. P. (1993). It won't happen to me: Unrealistic optimism or illusion of control? *British Journal of Psychology, 84,* 39–50.

Mischel, W., Cantor, N., & Feldman, S. (1996). Principles of self-regulation: The nature of will power and self-control. In E. T. Higgins & A. W. Kruglanski (Eds.), *Social psychology: Handbook of basic principles* (pp. 329–360). New York: Guilford Press.

Myers, L. B. (2014). Changing smokers' risk perceptions—for better or worse? *Journal of Health Psychology, 19,* 325–332.

Norem, J. K., & Cantor, N. (1986). Defensive pessimism: Harnessing anxiety as motivation. *Journal of Personality and Social Psychology, 51,* 1208–1217.

Nussbaum, S., Liberman, N., & Trope, Y. (2006). Predicting the near and distant future. *Journal of Experimental Psychology: General, 135,* 152–161.

Oettingen, G. (2012). Future thought and behaviour change. *European Review of Social Psychology, 23,* 1–63.

Oettingen, G. (2014). *Rethinking positive thinking: Inside the new science of motivation*. New York: Penguin Random House.

Oettingen, G., & Mayer, D. (2002). The motivating function of thinking about the future: Expectations versus fantasies. *Journal of Personality and Social Psychology, 83,* 1198–1212.

Olson, J. M., Roese, N. J., & Zanna, M. P. (1996). Expectancies. In E. T. Higgins & A. W. Kruglanski (Eds.), *Social psychology: Handbook of basic principles* (pp. 211–238). New York: Guilford Press.

Pajares, F., & Johnson, M. J. (1996). Self-efficacy beliefs and the writing performance of entering high school students. *Psychology in the Schools, 33,* 163–175.

Perloff, L. S. (1987). Social comparison and illusions of invulnerability to negative life events. In C. R. Snyder & C. Ford (Eds.), *Coping with negative life events: Clinical and social psychological perspectives on negative life events* (pp. 217–242). New York: Plenum Press.

Perloff, L. S., & Fetzer, B. K. (1986). Self–other judgments and perceived vulnerability to victimization. *Journal of Personality and Social Psychology, 50,* 502–510.

Price, P. C., Pentecost, H. C., & Voth, R. D. (2002). Perceived event frequency and the optimistic bias: Evidence for a two–process model of personal risk judgments. *Journal of Experimental Social Psychology, 38,* 242–252.

Rothman, A. J., Klein, W. M., & Weinstein, N. D. (1996). Absolute and relative biases in estimations of personal risk. *Journal of Applied Social Psychology, 26,* 1213–1236.

Schlenker, B. R. (1985). Identity and self-identification. In B. R. Schlenker (Ed.), *The self and social life* (pp. 65–99). New York: McGraw-Hill.

Schwarz, N. (2011). Feelings-as-information theory. In P. Van Lange, A. W. Kruglanski, & E. T. Higgins (Eds.), *Handbook of theories of social psychology* (pp. 289–308). Thousand Oaks, CA: SAGE.

Sears, D. O. (1983). The person-positivity bias. *Journal of Personality and Social Psychology, 44,* 233–250.

Sevincer, A. T., Schlier, B., & Oettingen, G. (2015). Ego depletion and the use of mental contrasting. *Motivation and Emotion, 39,* 876–891.

Shepperd, J. A., Carroll, P. J., Grace, J., & Terry, M. (2002). Exploring the causes of comparative optimism. *Psychologica Belgica, 42,* 65–98.

Shepperd, J. A., Findley-Klein, C., Kwavnick, K. D., Walker, D., & Perez, S. (2000). Bracing for loss. *Journal of Personality and Social Psychology, 78,* 620–634.

Shepperd, J. A., Grace, J., Cole, L. J., & Klein, C. (2005). Anxiety and outcome predictions. *Personality and Social Psychology Bulletin, 31,* 267–275.

Shepperd, J. A., Klein, W. M. P., Waters, E. A., & Weinstein, N. D. (2013). Taking stock of unrealistic optimism. *Perspectives on Psychological Science, 8,* 395–411.

Shepperd, J. A., & McNulty, J. K. (2002). The affective consequences of expected and unexpected outcomes. *Psychological Science, 13,* 85–88.

Shepperd, J. A., Ouellette, J. A., & Fernandez, J. K. (1996). Abandoning unrealistic optimism: Performance estimates and the temporal proximity of self-relevant feedback. *Journal of Personality and Social Psychology, 70,* 844–855.

Shepperd, J. A., Waters, E. A., Weinstein, N. D., & Klein, W. M. P. (2015). A primer on unrealistic optimism. *Current Directions in Psychological Science, 24,* 232–237.

Sherman, S. J. (1980). On the self-erasing nature of errors in prediction. *Journal of Personality and Social Psychology, 39,* 211–221.

Slovic, P. (1987). Perception of risk. *Science, 236,* 280–285.

Stuart, J. O., Windschitl, P. D., Smith, A. R., & Scherer, A. M. (2017). Behaving optimistically: How the (un)desirability of an outcome can bias people's preparations for it. *Journal of Behavioral Decision Making, 30,* 54–69.

Sweeny, K., & Falkenstein, A. (2016). *Even optimists get the blues: Inter-individual consistency in the tendency to brace for the worst.* Unpublished manuscript, University of California, Riverside, CA.

Sweeny, K., & Krizan, Z. (2013). Sobering up: A quantitative review of temporal declines in expectations. *Psychological Bulletin, 139,* 702–724.

Sweeny, K., & Shepperd, J. A. (2007). Do people brace sensibly?: Risk judgments and event likelihood. *Personality and Social Psychology Bulletin, 33,* 1064–1075.

Sweeny, K., & Shepperd, J. A. (2010). The costs of optimism and the benefits of pessimism. *Emotion, 10,* 750–753.

Sweeny, K., Shepperd, J. A., & Carroll, P. J. (2009). Expectations for others' outcomes: Do people display compassionate bracing? *Personality and Social Psychology Bulletin, 35,* 160–171.

Taylor, K. M., & Shepperd, J. A. (1998). Bracing for the worst: Severity, testing, and feedback timing as moderators of the optimistic bias. *Personality and Social Psychology Bulletin, 24,* 915–926.

Taylor, S. E., Pham, L. B., Rivkin, I. D., & Armor, D. A. (1998). Harnessing the imagination: Mental simulation, self-regulation, and coping. *American Psychologist, 53,* 429–439.

Trope, Y., & Liberman, N. (2003). Temporal construal. *Psychological Review, 110,* 403–421.

Trumbo, C., Lueck, M., Marlatt, H., & Peek, L. (2011). The effect of proximity to Hurricanes Katrina and Rita on subsequent hurricane outlook and optimistic bias. *Risk Analysis, 31,* 1907–1918.

Tversky, A. (1977). Features of similarity. *Psychological Review, 84,* 327–352.

Tyler, J. M., & Rosier, J. G. (2009). Examining self-presentation as a motivational explanation for comparative optimism. *Journal of Personality and Social Psychology, 97,* 716–727.

Van der Velde, F. W., Hooykaas, C., & Van Der Pligt, J. (1992). Risk perception and behavior: Pessimism, realism, and optimism about AIDS-related health behavior. *Psychology and Health, 6,* 23–38.

Weinstein, N. D. (1980). Unrealistic optimism about future life events. *Journal of Personality and Social Psychology, 39,* 806–820.

Weinstein, N. D. (1983). Reducing unrealistic optimism about illness susceptibility. *Health Psychology, 2,* 11–20.

Weinstein, N. D., & Lachendro, E. (1982). Egocentrism as a source of unrealistic optimism. *Personality and Social Psychology Bulletin, 8,* 195–200.

Weinstein, N. D., & Lyon, J. E. (1999). Mindset, optimistic bias about personal risk and health-protective behaviour. *British Journal of Health Psychology, 4,* 289–300.

Weinstein, N. D., Slovic, P., & Gibson, G. (2004). Accuracy and optimism in smokers' beliefs about quitting. *Nicotine and Tobacco Research, 6,* 375–380.

Zeelenberg, M., Van Dijk, W. W., Manstead, A. S. R., & der Pligt, J. (1998). The experience of regret and disappointment. *Cognition and Emotion, 12,* 221–230.

CHAPTER 13

A Neuroeconomist's Perspective on Thinking about the Future

Anna B. Konova
Paul W. Glimcher

WHAT WOULD A NEUROECONOMIST DO?: OVERVIEW AND GOALS OF THIS CHAPTER

Toward the end of the 1990s, a group of scientists from the disciplines of neuroscience, economics, and psychology came together, recognizing that they had a common goal: to understand how humans and other animals make decisions, express preferences, and trade off outcomes. Each discipline brings its unique contribution to this common goal. Speaking a bit too broadly, economics provides the theoretical framework for understanding choice, psychology the experimental tools for the study of choice behavior and constructs for capturing mental life, and neuroscience the measurement tools for elucidating the choice machinery at a reduced and mechanistic level. The hybrid approach that emerged from the conglomeration of each of these disciplines' contributions to the study of decision making is now known as *neuroeconomics*.

In this chapter, we describe how scientists who employ this neuroeconomic approach typically think about decisions that involve tradeoffs between outcomes that occur at different points in time (in the future vs. today, for example), also known as *intertemporal choices*. Our primary goal is to provide the reader with the context within which neuroeconomists think about this particular class of decision problems. To do this, we provide an introduction to more traditional (neoclassical) economic theories of choice as they influenced the development of neuroeconomics. We first review the history of modern notions of "utility" or "subjective value"—a subject-specific quantity associated with how valuable a given outcome is to a given individual—before turning our attention to a more detailed discussion of the intertemporal choice models commonly used to capture how time specifically influences subjective notions of value in *reduced-form* (mathematical–economic) theories. We then describe how these models are combined with neuroscientific tools by neuro-economists to understand what happens in the brain as a person makes intertemporal choices. What happens in the brain, neuroeconomists typically argue, can in turn help us narrow down the set of plausible models of choice (be those models psychological or economic in origin), by excluding those which cannot be plausibly mapped to a neural hardware for implementation or inspire new models linked to biological constraints or features. We then summarize key empirical findings that show people *discount* (value less) outcomes set to occur in the future in highly predictable, albeit idiosyncratic, ways. We highlight a core set of brain regions whose coordinated activity is thought to underlie this behavior. We conclude by taking drug addiction as a case study of how a psychological pathology might reflect these brain and behavior interactions under conditions of ill health.

NEUROECONOMIC TOOLS

In the most general sense, a neuroeconomist: (1) observes people's *behavior*; (2) thinks about theory and tests which *models or classes of models of choice* explain this behavior (at various reductive levels of analysis); and (3) identifies what the *neurobiological processes* are that enable this behavior by linking the "best-fitting" model of choice to brain data. In this section, we review the central tools most neuroeconomists use to accomplish these goals before focusing on intertemporal choice as a representative area in which much progress has been made using the neuroeconomic approach.

Economic Models of Choice

Early Notions of Utility and What a "Neuroeconomic" Theory of Choice Might Look Like

To traditional economists, all of human behavior can be described as having the ultimate goal of maximizing a theoretical quantity called *utility*. Von Neumann and Morgenstern (1944) and Savage (1954) defined utility as the *implicit* value to a specific individual of any object or event in the outside world, be it the utility derived from wealth, love, social status, or another source. But it is important to remember that economists see this as a subjective experience. To make that clear, consider one of the earliest puzzles of the classical economic revolution of the 18th and 19th centuries: the *diamond–water paradox*. Water is essential for survival, and diamonds have limited use-value, but despite this fact, people are willing to pay far more for diamonds than for water. Why is the subjective value, or utility, of diamonds so high and the subjective value of water so low? The philosopher Adam Smith argued that this apparent contradiction stems from a person's subjective utility being fundamentally tied to scarcity. Because we are wealthy in water, Smith argued, we place very little value on a small increment in that "water-wealth," but the opposite is true of diamonds. The idea that the utility you experience from a single diamond or a single liter of water diminishes as you possess more and more (formally a *diminishing marginal utility*) was revolutionary and spurred what became known as the *marginal revolution*. Formal assumptions of the marginal revolution were that (1) people maximize utility as evidenced by their choices; (2) people experience utility from owning or consuming goods, and it is the behavior of those people which defines value (not the economist); and (3) the amount of utility experienced per unit of most goods follows a function that "diminishes at the margin," or slowly bends downward in slope (a curve relating happiness/satisfaction/utility—and hence price—to quantity; see Figure 13.1).

Interestingly, in some ways the paradox at the center of the marginal revolution echoed ideas from choice theory pioneered almost a century earlier by the probability theorist Blaise Pascal, who was working to understand people's decisions when gambling. He came to the notion of *expected value,* a quantity that is the product of the magnitude of a potential outcome (e.g., amount of money that could be won from a gamble) and the probability of that outcome occurring (e.g., the winning probability). Pascal argued that what one should do to maximize one's welfare (or net wealth) is to aim to maximize expected value. He proposed that, given two options, a chooser should compute each option's expected value and simply select the one with the higher of the two. But Pascal ignored a critical empirical observation that was important to the economists of the marginal revolution: There are significant individual differences in starting welfare (or "wealth"), which have implications for what one should do. What one should do depends on where one is on the curve—rich or poor in any particular quantity.

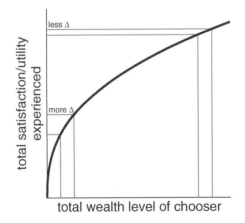

FIGURE 13.1. Diminishing marginal utility. During the marginal revolution, scholars working to develop a formal theory of choice realized that the "utility" a person experiences by owning things or by monetary gains depends both on the intrinsic value of those objects (which is itself very complex) and how much of them the person possesses. The function mapping objective value (or quantity) to utility is often assumed to be a power function with an exponent referred to as "alpha." Alpha captures individual differences in the rate of diminishing utility experienced for a given object by different people. Here we show such a function for money for an individual whose alpha takes on a value below 1. As the total number of dollars this chooser possesses increases, the amount of utility he or she experiences with each additional dollar increase diminishes. When he or she only has a couple of dollars, an additional dollar results in a greater increase in utility than when he or she has many dollars, as illustrated by the distance between the two sets of horizontal lines.

For a psychologist, reconciling the marginal revolution's idea of diminishing marginal utility with Pascal's expected value requires understanding the work of the mathematician Daniel Bernoulli, who suggested that, rather than maximizing expected value, choosers should be seen as maximizing instead a more subjective quantity: expected utility (a transformation of expected value). Expected utility differs critically from expected value because, unlike expected value, it is a more psychological and subjective, rather than an objective, measure. Bernoulli argued that the satisfaction or utility derived from a given unit of a good x is a nonlinear function of how much that unit of good x increases a chooser's total welfare, as determined by $u(x)$. For a chooser, which course of action offers higher utility (e.g., taking \$7,000 for sure or a 50% chance of \$20,000) depends on (1) what that chooser's $u(x)$ function looks like and (2) his or her total wealth. Bernoulli assumed that $u(x)$ was a logarithmic function for everyone, but it is now accepted that the form of $u(x)$ is more complicated and can be represented in many ways. For our purposes, we employ in this discussion a power function with an exponent (typically referred to as "alpha") that differs across individuals and determines the rate of diminishing utility for good x. That is, for Pascal:

$$\text{Utility} = \text{Expected Value and } (0.5 \times \$20{,}000) > (1 \times \$7{,}000).$$

The chooser should go for the gamble.

But for Bernoulli and modern utility theorists, for whom utility follows a nonlinear monotonic function,

$$\text{Utility} = \log(\$) \text{ or } \$^{\text{alpha}} \text{ and } [0.5 \times \log(\$20{,}000)] < [1 \times \log(\$7{,}000)]$$
$$\text{or } (0.5 \times \$20{,}000^{0.5}) < (1 \times \$7{,}000^{0.5}).$$

The chooser should go for the safe bet.

Notice that for Bernoulli all of the subjectivity of a chooser is embedded in the utility function. He assumed that there was no subjectivity in the perception of *probability*. It was not until the work of the economist Leonard Savage in the 1950s that the notion of "subjective probability" was introduced, a point that we return to later.

Revealed Preference

The end of the 19th century brought on a new revolution in economics—the ordinal revolution—which was spearheaded by the Italian economist Vilfredo Pareto. Although Bernoulli's and the marginal revolution's notions of utility significantly advanced our understanding of what a theory of choice might look like, both critically assumed that utility can be *measured* as a specific numerical function that allowed one to identify, for example, that one option was exactly twice as good as another. Pareto argued that such precise quantitative comparisons could not be made based on data about simple choice but, rather, argued that only statements about one option being better than another (not better by a certain fraction) could be made based on observations about what people prefer. He showed, through a famous mathematical proof, that asking people which of two options they preferred could only reveal a *rank order* for goods in terms of utility, never a numerical (or metric) distance. Take, for example, a chooser who prefers apples to oranges and oranges to grapes. Pareto showed that, for this chooser, one could represent her utilities as u(apples) = 3, u(oranges) = 2, and u(grapes) = 1, or that the utilities she assigned to these fruit could be any other ordered set of numbers that preserved this ranking and thus predicted the observed choice ordering! Pareto's demonstration that a unique value for utility could not be derived from simple choice experiments led to one of the most important tenets of early 20th-century economics: that utility must be considered a mathematically *ordinal* (just rank ordered) and not a cardinal (a truly numerical) quantity.

Recognizing the problem with measuring utility directly, the American economist Paul Samuelson proposed an advance to Pareto's approach that preserved most of its features while providing new tools for thinking about choice. The question Samuelson sought to answer was whether the choices we might observe in a given experiment could be proven to be inconsistent with all possible utility functions—whether there is a pattern of choice which fundamentally disproves utility theory. He sought to develop a simple way of describing patterns of choices that were fundamentally incompatible with the idea that the chooser assigned even simple rank-order utilities to options such as apples and oranges. To accomplish this, he developed a formal test for this kind of consistency, the weak axiom of revealed preference (WARP; now often confusingly called *rationality* [Samuelson, 1938]), a condition that must be satisfied by any pattern of choice that is consistent with maximizing utility—for any possible utility function (though with some minor restrictions on the craziness of the function). Simply put, Samuelson showed that, for WARP to be satisfied, the following must be true: (1) if A is chosen when both A and B are available, then A is said to be preferred to B ($A \succ B$, strict preference) or is at least as good as B ($A \succsim B$, weak preference); but (2) it cannot be the case that B is clearly preferred to A ($B \succ A$). This may seem trivial, but with just this assumption and a bit of math, Samuelson (1938) was able to prove that an individual who chooses apples over oranges and oranges over pears cannot also *prefer* pears over apples—if she or he has a stable underlying utility representation. It is worth noting that, although we can say that an individual obeying WARP in his or her choices shows behavior consistent with maximization of some utility function, because of WARP's ordinal nature, we cannot say anything about the shape of that utility function.

Extending Samuelson's (1938) approach further, Hendrik Houthakker (1950) developed what is now known as the generalized axiom of revealed preference (GARP). Whereas obeying WARP is a *necessary* condition for maximizing and representing utility, Houthakker sought to identify what might be a *necessary* and *sufficient* condition for a utility representation—the kind of choice behavior that indicates unambiguously that the individual was behaving *as if* she or he really did have a utility representation of some kind. What Houthakker did with GARP was to consider how an individual's choices order when several options are available with a subtle assumption about how increasing the quantity of a desirable good increased the utility of that good—a test to determine whether an individual's choices necessarily and sufficiently obey *transitivity* (Figure 13.2). A chooser who obeys GARP is one who is transitive and, roughly speaking, monotonic (he or she obeys the general rule: more is better, or at least not worse) in his or her preferences. Obeying GARP, in turn, means that there exists a monotonic utility function (or, more accurately, a family of such functions) that this chooser behaves as if he or she is maximizing. We *still* do not know from this test what that function(s) looks like, though now we do know that there is *at least one* function-shape that can account for the individual's choices and hence that the individual can, in principle, be viewed as a utility maximizer under the conditions being studied.

A chooser who violates GARP is said to be "irrational"—he or she has inconsistent preferences, and the claim that he or she is acting as if he or she is maximizing a monotonic utility function is falsified. To put that another way, a chooser who violates GARP cannot be described as having a stable internal representation of value guiding his or her choice, and when we can make this observation, we know this for sure. The notion of rationality causes a lot of confusion in the cross-talk between economists and other scholars. Rationality in the economic sense only means that a person's preferences are internally consistent—that they are transitive. That a person prefers a bag of chips over a lifetime supply of caviar is not irrational in the economic sense regardless of whether it seems crazy to a caviar-lover.

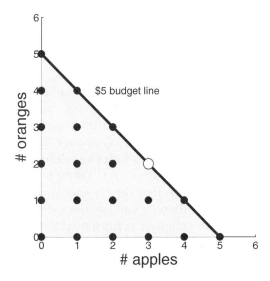

FIGURE 13.2. Economic rationality and a test of transitivity. Rationality in the economic sense means that a person's choices obey transitivity—that they are internally consistent. In the formal test of transitivity, using a budget set choice problem, choosers are asked to allocate a fixed amount of money to purchasing two goods. In this example, the chooser has a budget of $5 to spend on apples and oranges, which cost $1 apiece. Each point on the graph depicts a possible combination of apples and oranges the chooser can afford. Assuming the chooser must spend all of his or her money, he or she can choose any point (bundle) that lies on the $5 budget line, and in this example, the chooser selected the circled point as the preferred option (three apples and two oranges). What this tells us is that for this chooser the white circled point is *at least as good* as every other point on the budget line (because he or she selected it). It also tells us that every point in the shaded area below the line is *strictly worse* than at least one point on the line. Given this reasoning, we can conclude that anyone who also selects a point in the shaded area cannot be described as having a monotonic utility function that he or she is acting to maximize.

What is so important about revealed preference and rationality is that, with these tools in hand, a choice experiment reveals what an individual prefers. If Mary chose a cookie over an apple when she had the choice of both, then in that moment Mary must have preferred the cookie. That Mary feels regret that she went for the cookie instead of the apple has no bearing on what her preferences are, from an economist's perspective. That is, *unless her expressed regret has consequences for her behavior* (e.g., when faced with the choice between a cookie and an apple a second time, under equal circumstances, she chooses the apple), then—based on her behavior—an economist from the 1950s would conclude that Mary had made a mistake.

Expected Utility Theory

The groundwork reviewed above contributed to the origin of what is now known as expected utility (EU) theory (Savage, 1954; Von Neumann & Morgenstern, 1944). EU theory uses the neoclassical approach to describe choices under uncertainty developed by Samuelson (1938) but adds one new idea: that probabilistic outcomes can be used as a way to measure precisely the metrical shape of the utility representation (if it exists). To accomplish this, EU theory added additional axioms to the transitivity axiom (the axiom that requires a person's choices be internally consistent, as tested with GARP) that took advantage of *probability* as a ruler to determine the relationship in utility space between different choice options. These additional axioms are *completeness, continuity,* and *independence,* and their due attention is beyond the scope of this chapter. Very broadly speaking, completeness assumes that people have well-defined preferences, continuity implies that the utility function maximized is continuous, and independence guards against preference shifts in the presence of irrelevant choice alternatives (for a complete and accessible explanation of these axioms for this audience, see Glimcher, 2010). Critically, the objects of choice in EU theory are referred to as lotteries—defined by a probability and a prize (e.g., 25% chance of winning 100 pears). Taken together, if a chooser obeys GARP, there exists a utility function that the chooser is maximizing. If the chooser also obeys the other EU axioms, then we can further say that the expected utility of any option (the lottery) that the chooser is presented with is equal to the utility of the prize multiplied by the probability of receiving the prize.

RISK ATTITUDES

A critical insight here is that the curvature of the utility function tells us something about a person's risk attitude in the EU model—indeed, the curvature of the utility function fully specifies risk attitude for a consistent chooser (when one exists). In EU, a concave utility function over prize x (i.e., when the curvature of the utility function for x takes on a value below 1 and the function bends downward, as shown in Figure 13.1) is synonymous with saying that a person is risk averse in choices involving prize x. This person will, for example, prefer $50 for sure to a 50% chance of $100 because receiving $50 carries a utility that is more than half the utility of receiving $100—*consistent with diminishing marginal utility over total wealth.* The opposite is said for a person whose utility function is convex (i.e., when the curvature of the utility function for x takes on a value above 1 and the function bends upward). This person is said to be risk seeking (or risk loving) and will prefer a 50% chance of $100 to $50 for sure as demonstrated by the same rationale.

Risky Choices as Captured by Prospect Theory

Economic models such as EU theory are built on logical statements about choice. Their strength is in their falsifiability. But this may also be their greatest weakness: Under many conditions we can show that people do not obey the EU axioms, and therefore their choices are inconsistent with EU theory. A series of observations made by experimental psychologists indeed highlighted this flaw, showing that the neoclassical theories did not capture many kinds of human choice behavior and may thus be insufficient as a basis for our understanding of choice. When faced with probabilities that are very small or very large, for example, people consistently behave as if they violate the independence axiom, as most famously demonstrated in the Allais paradox (Allais, 1953). In the Allais paradox experiments, people are asked to decide between two lotteries, A and B, and then between two other lotteries, C and D. In a typical example, A is a 100% chance of $1 million, and B is an 89% chance of $1 million, a 1% chance of nothing, and a 10% chance of $5 million. In the second pair, C is an 89% chance of nothing and an 11% chance of $1 million, and D is a 90% chance of nothing and a 10% chance of $5 million. In reality, after removing any implied "common consequence" components of the lotteries (89% of $1 million for A and B, and 89% of nothing for C and D), the two pairs of lotteries can be reduced to the same choice (11% chance of $1 million vs. 10% chance of $5 million). But despite this formal equivalence, most people choose A from the first pair and D from the second pair, which would imply that they both prefer an 11% chance of $1 million over a 10% chance of $5 million *and* a 10% chance of $5 million over an 11% chance of $1 million, violating the independence axiom. One implication of these findings is that any unified theory of choice needs to recognize that there are certain *constraints* (be it biological or other) that make us inconsistent and that influence our decision process and that perhaps these behavioral patterns should not be ignored but rather used to inform theory.

Aiming to allow choice prediction even when choosers were being inconsistent, when it could be proven that no fixed internal representation of value existed, Kahneman and Tversky (1979) suggested an alternative to EU theory, known as prospect theory. This made prospect theory fundamentally different from EU theory because it was, in essence, a fittable predictive model rather than a logical theory in the economic sense. Prospect theory permits fitted solutions that approximate behavior even when one can prove that the kind of representation prospect theory employs cannot, fundamentally, be correct in the economic sense. Prospect theory achieved this by modifying EU theory with three classes of "parameterizations." The first was the idea that, in addition to the transformation of prizes in the computation of utility, there was a transformation of probabilities as well that related objective probabilities to *subjective probabilities,* an extension of an idea first introduced by Savage (1954). A second change had to do with how utilities were defined. Instead of being referenced to a chooser's total wealth (the original notion of diminishing marginal utility), Kahneman and Tversky (1979) argued for the presence of a moving *reference point* against which utilities are compared (how much the chooser is set to gain or lose relative to his or her reference point). The third change stemmed from the reference point idea and allowed "losses" to be considered as distinct from "gains" (a notion not present in EU theory) with their own mapping from prize (objective value) space to utility space. This is also referred to as *loss aversion*–the idea that people behave as if the shape of their utility function for losses is different (steeper) than that for gains (Figure 13.3).

A critical distinction between EU theory and prospect theory and, more broadly, a difference in the way economists and psychologists think about theories of choice is that, whereas the former describes how people *should* behave (in the sense that it describes consistent logical behavior), the latter makes it possible to basically describe with a utility-like model how people *do* behave, even when their behavior can be proven mathematically not to be describable with a utility-like functional representation. Put another way, EU theory is a *prescriptive* (or normative) theory of choice (and thus does a good job when people are being logical), whereas prospect theory is a *descriptive* theory of choice that can be used under nonlogical conditions.

To help illustrate this difference between EU theory and prospect theory more concretely, we return to the notion of risk attitudes. The specific formulation of utility in prospect theory is made with the forethought of *accommodating* empirical observations about how people behave in situations involving fully known (and hence explicitly stated) risk. These observations are: (1) people are risk averse for

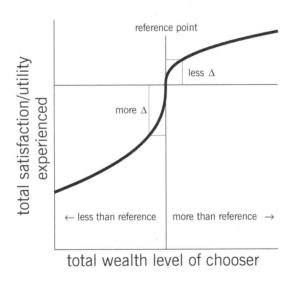

FIGURE 13.3. Shape of the "value" function according to prospect theory. The value function (Kahneman & Tversky [1979] never called it a utility function because they wanted the function to be used even when choice behavior proved that no utility representation was formally possible for a particular chooser) in prospect theory is centered on a subjective "reference point." The amount of gain or total wealth of a chooser is determined as a deviation from this reference point. The difference in the curvature of the utility function on the left versus the right side of the reference point accounts for the empirical observation that people are risk averse for gains (or relative gains) and risk seeking for losses (or relative losses). This effect, also referred to as loss aversion, is thought to occur because a given amount of gain produces smaller increases in satisfaction than the same magnitude of loss decreases satisfaction.

high-probability gains (they tend to *underweight* the likelihood of positive outcomes when the probability with which they are expected to occur is fairly *high,* for example, preferring option *A* over option *B* in our Allais paradox example); (2) risk averse for low-probability losses (they tend to *overweight* the likelihood of negative outcomes when the probability with which they are expected to occur is fairly *low,* such as when purchasing insurance); (3) risk seeking for low-probability gains (they tend to *overweight* the likelihood of positive outcomes when the probability with which they are expected to occur is fairly *low,* such as when going to a casino or purchasing lottery tickets); and (4) risk seeking for high-probability losses (they tend to *underweight* the likelihood of negative outcomes when the probability with which they are expected to occur is fairly *high,* preferring to avoid a sure loss at almost any cost). In prospect theory, risk attitudes are captured (though not in a unique way—many possible combinations of these parameters can capture each risk attitude) by (1) the curvature of the positive and negative value functions, (2) the magnitude of the loss aversion coefficient, and (3) the curvature of the subjective "probability weighting function."

Models of Temporal Discounting and How They Differ

Another factor (in addition to wealth and risk) that is consequential to how human choosers behave is how they weigh the present relative to the future, also known as *intertemporal choice.* Here we briefly review theoretical models of intertemporal choice before discussing the behavioral and neuroimaging evidence for this particular class of decision problems in the second part of this chapter.

It is no surprise that what we do today bears consequences for how much better or worse off we will be in the future. This is captured, for example, by our choice today of what we eat (e.g., high-fat foods), drink (e.g., massive amounts of alcohol), or choose more generally to do (e.g., exercise, smoke cigarettes). See Figure 13.4 for Walter Mischel's famous "marshmallow test," in which he showed that the ability of young children to delay gratification (waiting to get a better treat) was predictive of how financially and academically successful they became later in life and how likely they were to avoid going to jail or using drugs. See Mischel and Metzner (1962) for a description of the original studies and Mischel et al. (2011) for a complete survey of this work.

A consistent finding across all species tested with approaches like the marshmallow test is that choosers of all ages place less weight on outcomes the further in the future they are set to occur. This is the same (for an economist) as saying that there is a decrease in the utility of the delayed outcome as a function of time. For a given chooser, the rate at which the utility (or idiosyncratic subjective value) of an outcome decreases with time is referred to as this chooser's *discount rate,* a factor that shows considerable individual differences. The steepness of the discount rate describes a chooser's patience (with steeper discounting indicating more impatience). The discount rate, like most quantities stemming from economics, is estimated by observing people's choices, for example, when faced with sooner smaller and later larger outcomes ($50 today vs. $100 in 365 days).

The specific *shape of the discounting function,* however, is a point of ongoing debate that mirrors the tension between EU theory and prospect theory. The

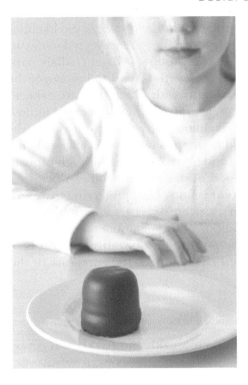

FIGURE 13.4. The marshmallow test. In a famous series of studies in the 1960s conducted by then Stanford University psychologist Walter Mischel, kids were given a choice between having one marshmallow as soon as they wanted and waiting several minutes alone with the tempting single marshmallow until an experimenter returned to the room, at which point they would get two marshmallows. How willing kids were to wait (i.e., to delay gratification) was predictive of how successful they became later in life in multiple domains, including academics and financial stability. See Mischel and Metzner (1962) for a description of the original studies and Mischel et al. (2011) for a complete survey of this work. Photo by Kai Schwabe/Food Collection/Getty Images.

neoclassical economists Fishburn and Rubinstein (1982) and Strotz (1956) theorized that decision makers *should* (in order to be logically consistent) employ exponential discounting such that the utility of a given outcome (say monetary amount) should decrease at a fixed rate for each unit of time it is pushed into the future (Figure 13.5), given by:

$$\text{Discounted Utility } (A, t) = A \times e^{-\delta t}$$

Smaller values of the discount factor δ indicate shallower discounting. They were led to this conclusion when it became clear that any other shape of the discount function could lead to logically inconsistent choice behavior (Strotz, 1956). This is a critically important point that is often unclear. If a human chooser weighted the value of an outcome using anything other than an exponential function, then he or she would be *intransitive in time,* just as a person who prefers apples to oranges to pears but prefers pears to apples is intransitive now. And, of course, this would mean that no temporal-utility representation could account for his or her behavior.

Fishburn and Rubinstein (1982) completed what is now considered the standard proof of this fact using a modified form of the EU theory axioms with the addition of axioms about *impatience* and *stationarity*. Impatience refers to a preference for positive outcomes to occur sooner and negative outcomes to occur later. Stationarity refers to a consistency of behavior in time such that if a chooser is willing to wait 1 more day for a reward that could have been received in 364 days, he or she should also be willing to wait 1 more day for a reward that could have been received today.

Substantial empirical work, however, again shows that people violate the Fishburn and Rubinstein axioms under many conditions;[1] they do not have consistent preferences over time. Instead, most people's choices suggest that having to wait 1 day to receive a reward that could have been received today decreases the utility of that reward to a greater extent than having to wait 365 days to receive a reward that could have been received 364 days from today (Figure 13.5).

Mazur (1987) showed in seminal work that the discounting behavior of pigeons could best be explained by an alternative, hyperbolic or hyperbolic-like function, a form of discounting that has since received vast support across species, including in humans. This functional form assumes that choosers treat the near and distant future differently: the rate at which the utility of a reward decreases with time to its delivery is *faster* for the more proximal than the more distant future. Here, the

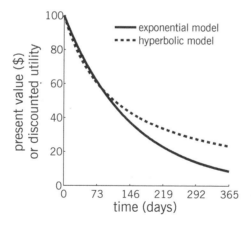

FIGURE 13.5. How the present value (or discounted utility) of $100 diminishes with time according to exponential discounting and hyperbolic discounting. The graph shows that having to wait 1 year to receive $100, for this moderately patient individual, is worth about the same as getting $8 today, according to exponential discounting, and $23 today, according to hyperbolic discounting. The rate of decrease in utility of the $100 is constant through time in the exponential model but is faster for the near future and slower for the distant future in the hyperbolic model. This difference in the rate of change through time in the hyperbolic model results in inconsistent preferences over time: having to wait 1 day from today to receive the $100 reduces its value by about $1, but having to wait 365 days instead of 364 days reduces its value by only $0.05.

---

[1] There is debate about whether they violate the stationarity axiom (Laibson, 1997) or the ordering axiom (Kable & Glimcher, 2010).

discount rate κ determines the rate of decrease, and smaller values of κ indicate shallower discounting:

$$\text{Discounted Utility } (A, t) = \frac{A}{1 + kt}$$

An unsatisfying aspect of hyperbolic discounting for economists is that hyperbolic discounting implies that choosers are necessarily inconsistent in their preferences with respect to time. To account for the empirically observed departures from exponential discounting while preserving stationarity, Phelps and Pollak (1968), and later Laibson (1997), popularized the use of the quasi-hyperbolic discounting model. In this form of discounting, rewards are discounted exponentially (by a constant rate δ over time), but the utility of delayed rewards (i.e., when $t > 0$) is additionally reduced relative to immediate rewards by a second constant "bias" term β:

$$\text{Discounted Utility } (A, t) = \beta \times (A \times e^{-\delta t})$$

For economists, quasi-hyperbolic discounting is preferred to hyperbolic discounting, even if it may also not be very predictive under some conditions (e.g., Laibson, 1997), because it does not require a complete departure from exponential discounting, as the exponent is preserved and all of the inconsistency emerges uniquely from a "present bias." When the bias term β is 1, that is, when delayed rewards are not treated in some special way compared with immediate rewards, this functional form reduces to exponential discounting. When β approaches 0, delayed rewards are given less weight and immediate rewards prevail. The β parameter is thus an intuitive way to assess how far a chooser departs from normative, exponential discounting. Its usage has been central to mapping temporal discounting onto *dual process theories* of decision making in which there is a perceived battle between the hot–cool (Metcalfe & Mischel, 1999) or affective–deliberative (Bernheim & Rangel, 2004; Loewenstein & O'Donoghue, 2004) self. The distinctions among exponential, hyperbolic, and quasi-hyperbolic models make interesting predictions about what we might observe at the neural, implementation, level of intertemporal choice decision making. We come back to this point later, after we review the tools neuroeconomists use to get at these underlying mechanisms.

Before we do that, however, it is worth pausing for a moment to point out that, as the careful reader might have noticed, in the three prominent models of temporal discounting discussed, the delayed reward, A appears without an exponent in the equations. That is, these models assume an embedded *linear* utility function consistent with risk neutrality, such that there is no subjective transformation of the objective value of A. Yet we know that most people do not have linear utility functions; instead, most people behave as though they have nonlinear utility functions (usually concave, consistent with risk aversion). This assumption of linear utility might importantly affect the estimation of an individual's idiosyncratic discount rate, which is invariably influenced by that individual's idiosyncratic utility curvature. This issue has recently come to the forefront of research in temporal discounting, although there is still much work to be done. Nevertheless, it seems clear now, as Andreoni and Sprenger (2012) showed, that the presence versus absence of certainty can bias people's time preferences and that jointly eliciting risk and time preferences can improve the accuracy of discount rate estimates (Andersen, Harrison, Lau, & Rutstrom, 2008). More recent work has focused on how to best capture these interdependencies in the experimental setting (Andreoni, Kuhn, & Sprenger, 2015).

EXPERIMENTAL TOOLS FROM PSYCHOLOGY AND NEUROSCIENCE USED IN NEUROECONOMICS

In this section, we review the basic tools that neuroeconomists use to study decision making in human choosers. We specifically focus on how these tools (mostly stemming from experimental psychology and neuroscience) can help researchers test some of the core predictions of the theoretical models (mostly stemming from economics) that we have reviewed in the preceding sections. We first describe the key features of a decision-making experiment and how researchers use the choice data generated to "fit" these models. We then describe how these experiments can be performed using functional brain imaging techniques, and how the neural data generated with those techniques can be combined with a study participant's choice data and the theoretical model under study.

The Notion of Incentive Compatibility

We can estimate a decision maker's risk preference and discount rate by asking him or her to participate in a laboratory experiment. In a typical neuroeconomic laboratory experiment, participants are asked to make a series of choices about goods (e.g., snacks) or money that they can *actually* receive with some probability or at a given delay. That participants make choices with real consequences (as compared with hypothetical choices with no direct consequences to them), referred to as *incentive compatibility,* is thought by many to be extremely important for eliciting an individual's "true preferences." Economic journals as a rule do not publish studies that lack real incentives (e.g., choosing a delayed reward of $100 in 365 days and actually getting the $100 in 365 days). This practice has been argued to contribute to the relatively high replication rates seen in experimental and behavioral economics studies relative to other fields, in which the use of hypothetical decisions and incentives is more common (Camerer et al., 2016).

Because in a typical experiment more than one choice needs to be made by participants and because paying according to each choice can become costly if meaningful incentives are used, task earnings are usually determined by a random draw of one or several of the series of choices the participant made. Paying from a subset of randomly determined choices after the experiment is complete also helps reduce strategy use—for example, stockpiling earnings to then gamble more in a later part of the experiment. Participants are instructed, without deception, that they should treat each of their choices as independent and important because only one or a subset of these choices will determine their earnings, and they do not know which at the time of choice.

Once enough choice observations are made, the experimenter typically picks a model (e.g., hyperbolic discounting) and, using minimization algorithms, tries to find the parameters of that model that best capture a participant's choices (e.g., her or his discount rate). This analytical approach is referred to as a "model-based" or "parametric" analysis. How good the model is at capturing a participant's preferences depends not only on the assumptions of the model but also on the quality of the experiment (e.g., if a sufficiently probative "choice set" was used and if enough observations were made).

Human Neuroscience Tools

The unique contribution neuroscience brings to neuroeconomics is the direct measurement of *subjective value* in the brain. Subjective values are related to utilities and value functions with the difference being that subjective values are directly observable (for a detailed discussion of this topic, see Glimcher, 2010, Section 3). Using a variety of neuroscientific tools, it is now possible to measure directly, or to infer quite precisely, the activity levels of neurons or populations of neurons encoding the subjective values of options in single-choice sets actually being presented experimentally to laboratory participants.

Measurement Techniques

The most widely used measurement tool by neuroeconomists to study how the brain represents utility or subjective value in humans is functional magnetic resonance imaging (fMRI). Although other measurement tools are also available to study human decision making—including scalp and intracranial electroencephalography (EEG), magnetoencephalography (MEG), and positron emission tomography (PET), fMRI is by far the most common. This is likely because fMRI is a noninvasive and fairly flexible technique with a good balance between spatial and temporal resolution. fMRI takes advantage of the fact that blood oxygen levels increase in areas of the brain where there is more metabolic activity due to neuronal activity. These increases in oxygenated blood—measured with the blood-oxygen-level-dependent (BOLD) contrast—can be used as an indirect readout of the amount of neuronal activity in the area of increase. For a comprehensive description of how fMRI and the BOLD signal work, the interested reader is referred to Huettel, Song, and McCarthy (2009).

In a typical neuroeconomic fMRI study, participants make choices on economic tasks such as the ones we described in the section above while fMRI data are collected. However, these tasks need to be adapted for use during fMRI, keeping a couple of limitations of the BOLD response in mind—mainly those pertaining to its "delay to peak," the observation that the BOLD signal is a sluggish representation of underlying brain activity (on the order of 5–15 seconds), and its troublingly low signal-to-noise ratio. These constraints require adequate temporal separation of the events of interest (in this case, the choices a participant is asked to make) and repetition to enhance detection power. To capture how the brain computes or represents utility and implements choice, data analysis typically focuses on the time window during which participants consider their options and prepare a response. A neuroeconomics experiment aims to correlate brain activity during this time window with economic model parameters or with a participant's choices or both.

Model-Based fMRI

In a typical model-based fMRI study (see Figure 13.6), a time series of values is derived from a computational model of a specific cognitive process (e.g., the discounted utility of the option offered on each trial of an intertemporal choice task as determined by a given participant's κ value) and then correlated against the fMRI data from that participant performing the task to determine which brain regions show a response profile consistent with the model. The goal is to map model-derived parameters onto their specific underlying brain circuits, to determine not only what regions are potentially responsible for generating this particular cognitive process but *how* this process is implemented in these brain regions. This is the key advantage of the model-based approach over more conventional analytical approaches to neuroimaging data (O'Doherty, Hampton, & Kim, 2007).

A special form of model-based fMRI is called a *neurometric* analysis (as opposed to a psychometric analysis, in which a model is fit to behavior or ratings provided by the participant). In a neurometric analysis, the model is fit directly to neural responses. This is difficult to do in associative brain areas (such as the prefrontal cortex) but is now common practice in the vision and audition sciences that focus on the sensory cortices in which signals are more closely tied to experimental inputs (visual stimuli or sounds as they evoke responses in visual or auditory cortices).

THE CASE OF INTERTEMPORAL CHOICE: PUTTING IT ALL TOGETHER

In this section, we focus on how neuroeconomists have worked to better understand why people often choose immediate rewards over rewards to be received in the future, even if the future rewards are bigger.

Quasi-hyperbolic (dual-system-style) discounting would predict the engagement of two neural systems in the decision to take the larger, later reward, an account we discussed earlier as having to do with the competition between two "selves." One system would push behavior toward less patience (i.e., toward the immediate reward as demonstrated by a lower beta term) and the other system would push behavior toward more patience. Initial evidence using fMRI in human participants indeed seemed to suggest, based on a fairly complex inference, that one set of brain regions, the ventromedial prefrontal cortex (VMPFC), ventral striatum, and posterior cingulate cortex (PCC), was more active when participants chose the immediate relative to the delayed options in an intertemporal choice experiment (McClure, Laibson, Loewenstein, & Cohen, 2004). Also another set of regions, the dorsolateral prefrontal cortex and posterior parietal cortex, was active when the participant made a more difficult choice compared with an easier choice. These two groups of regions could be construed as mapping onto beta and delta regions, respectively, because in the first case (when participants chose the immediate rewards) there was more activity in beta regions relative to delta regions, and vice versa when participants chose the delayed reward.

But putting this early evidence aside for a moment, it is, of course, also logically possible that a single hyperbolically discounting system is used to evaluate all rewards, with each reward's utility determined by how far away in time it is to be

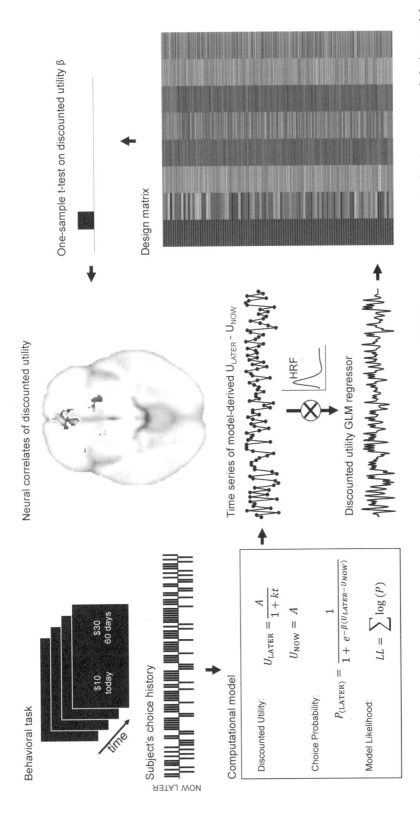

FIGURE 13.6. Steps involved in conducting a model-based functional magnetic resonance (fMRI) study. In this example of an intertemporal choice model-based fMRI study, participants first make binary choices between some amount of money to be delivered without delay (NOW) and a larger amount of money to be delivered with some delay (LATER). Based on the series of choices the participant makes, the experimenter estimates a discount rate parameter that minimizes the difference between the model predictions and the observed behavior. The best-fitting parameters are then used to generate a time series, for example, of discounted utility or difference in utility of the NOW versus LATER options seen on each trial of the experiment. This time series is then convolved with a basis function such as a canonical hemodynamic function (or HRF) to account for the lag in the BOLD response. This convolved time series of discounted utility can then be used as a predictor variable, along with other predictors, in a regression analysis against the simultaneously collected fMRI data. The experimenter can then visualize in which regions of the brain BOLD activity correlates with discounted utility. Adapted from O'Doherty, Hampton, and Kim (2007) and Glascher and O'Doherty (2010).

received by a simple hyperbolic calculation. Pitting these two competing accounts against each other (and avoiding some of the complex structural inference of the earlier McClure et al., 2004, study), Kable and Glimcher (2007) estimated what individual participants' discount rates were based on the choices they made in a long and detailed intertemporal choice experiment. The authors then used this estimate to construct what the discounted utility of each option on a given trial of the experiment would be for a given participant based on that participant's own discount rate. Using the model-based fMRI analysis approach we discussed in the previous sections, this study revealed that activity in a small set of brain regions, all part of the proposed beta regions, that is, the VMPFC, ventral striatum, and PCC, increased hyperbolically exactly as the utility of the offer increased (Figure 13.7)—a study now widely seen to demonstrate a single system for hyperbolically representing discounted value. In a follow-up study, Kable and Glimcher (2010) showed that this was also true in the context of deciding about two delayed rewards (in which there could be no "present bias") rather than about a delayed and an immediate reward. In this study, participants anchored their discounting behavior to the soonest possible reward, not simply to the present, and the magnitude of activation in the VMPFC, striatum, and PCC was not higher when an immediate reward could be chosen relative to when only a delayed reward could be chosen. Instead, activity in these regions encoded the subjective value of immediate and delayed rewards. Together, these two studies provided what is now typically seen as unequivocal evidence that the VMPFC, striatum, and PCC track discounted utility, or discounted subjective value, and not immediacy, impulsivity, or some "hot" response to a reward. Moreover, the shape of the discounting function that maximized the correspondence between the brain and behavioral data in both studies was hyperbolic, providing further evidence that human participants do not decide according to exponential discounting.

Although both perspectives have since found empirical support, the latter (unified system) view provides a more parsimonious account (from a neurobiological perspective) about how we might decide about the future. Further work continues to show that the VMPFC, striatum, and PCC are not active exclusively or disproportionately more for immediate rewards. Instead, these regions are now thought to form what is referred to as the brain's valuation system, a set of brain regions that track the value of choice options across a variety of decision contexts and reward types (Bartra, McGuire, & Kable, 2013).

Is Temporal Discounting a Loss of Self-Control?

An outstanding question pertains to whether steeper discounting reflects a loss of self-control, as the quasi-hyperbolic discounting model would predict. Many studies have linked steeper discount rates to maladaptive behaviors presumed to result from poor self-control and/or lack of forethought, including gambling, obesity, low achievement, and credit card debt (Story, Vlaev, Seymour, Darzi, & Dolan, 2014). Excessive discounting is also a feature of many psychiatric disorders that are characterized by problems with self-control, most notably impulse control disorders (American Psychiatric Association, 2013) and drug addiction (Baler & Volkow, 2006). Although these findings are highly suggestive of a link between self-control

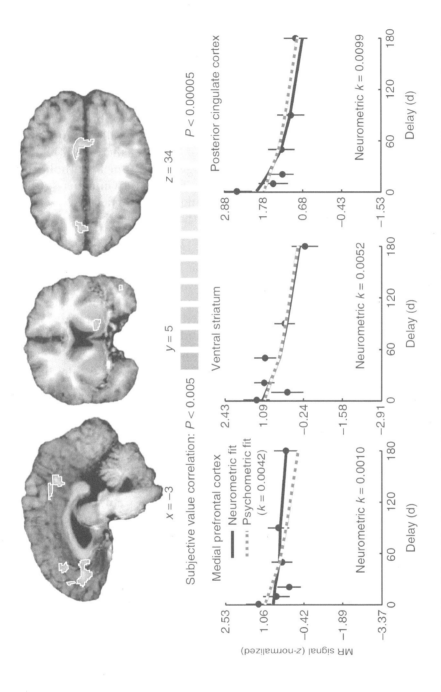

FIGURE 13.7. Brain areas that track individual discounted utilities. The top panel shows which regions' BOLD activity correlated with discounted utility for each individual based on his or her own discount rate parameter κ. These regions are the ventromedial prefrontal cortex (VMPFC), ventral striatum, and posterior cingulate cortex, which, based on meta-analytic data, are thought to form a unified system of valuation for all types of rewards and decision contexts. The bottom panel shows, for an example participant, a close match between the predicted response in each region as a function of delay given that participant's behaviorally derived discount rate and the brain's response to each delay (the neural discount rate). Together, these data show that these three regions are directly involved in the valuation of delayed outcomes to guide choice for those outcomes. Reprinted by permission of Macmillan Publishers from Kable, J. W., & Glimcher, P. W. (2007). The neural correlates of subjective value during intertemporal choice. *Nature Neuroscience, 10,* 1625–1633.

and temporal discounting, based on this evidence alone one might draw the conclusion that self-control as indexed by temporal discounting is a between-subjects phenomenon—a stable interindividual difference—rather than a capacity or resource that can be depleted or "lost."

However, there is also compelling evidence that temporal discounting is not (or at least is not only) a stable interindividual difference or trait. It can be affected, within an individual, by his or her current physiological needs or emotional state and by external, contextual influences (e.g., how the decision problem is framed; Lempert & Phelps, 2016). More recent work also shows that cognitively taxing activities (6 hours of working-memory and set-switching tasks) can make laboratory participants less patient, presumably by interfering with the neural structures that support self-control, such as the dorsolateral prefrontal cortex (Blain, Hollard, & Pessiglione, 2016). The problem here, though, is in the interpretation of an increase in discounting as self-control failure. There are many reasons why individuals should discount delayed rewards at different rates. One reason is that these delayed rewards might fail to materialize or come too late to satisfy the organism's *current* needs. There is an opportunity cost that comes with waiting (Story, Moutoussis, & Dolan, 2015), and certain states or external contexts might shift this cost. We return to this point in the next section, in which we describe how a neuroeconomist might think about excessive discounting behavior, such as that seen in drug addiction. Furthermore, without consideration for an individual's beliefs about the experimental paradigm, it is difficult to know whether these changes in the discount rate reflect a change in the certainty about receiving the prospective reward, a change in time perception, or a change in the rate at which future rewards are discounted.

Temporal Discounting and Psychopathology: The Case of Drug Addiction

Addiction is a chronic, relapsing disease characterized by continued drug taking despite many harmful health and social consequences (American Psychiatric Association, 2013). The addicted individual becomes preoccupied with the addictive substance (e.g., alcohol or heroin), despite efforts to stop or cut down drug taking, even when the positive experiences derived from the drug are markedly reduced. Addiction is considered a brain disease because drugs change the brain's chemistry, particularly in regions that form the brain's valuation system. At the core of this system are dopamine fibers that originate in the ventral tegmental area and terminate in the ventral striatum and in other regions, including the VMPFC. Although different drugs of abuse have different mechanisms of action, they have all been shown to produce a surge of dopamine in the ventral striatum in exerting their reinforcing effects (e.g., the feelings of "high" and "euphoria"; see Chen, Hopf, & Bonci, 2010; Laruelle et al., 1995; Sulzer, 2011; Volkow, Fowler, Wang, Ding, & Gatley, 2002; Volkow et al., 1997).

A large body of literature indicates that steeper discount rates are a hallmark feature of drug addiction (MacKillop et al., 2011). This is not surprising given that the brain circuits affected by addiction are primarily those that support intertemporal choice that we reviewed in the preceding sections (Volkow & Baler, 2015). The steepness of an individual's temporal discounting has even been proposed as a candidate behavioral marker for addiction (Bickel, 2015; Bickel, Koffarnus, Moody, & Wilson, 2014). Many have argued that impulsivity as captured by higher discount rates is a risk factor for drug addiction—something that precedes drug use that puts a person at risk for developing addiction, along with other disorders of impulse control (Bickel, Jarmolowicz, Mueller, Koffarnus, & Gatchalian, 2012). However, laboratory animal work, as well as a handful of studies in humans, show that various drugs of abuse and those that act on dopamine have a direct impact on discounting behavior (de Wit, 2009; Setlow, Mendez, Mitchell, & Simon, 2009), although it is not clear where in the brain dopamine has its effects, which result in changes in discounting. In one fMRI study, for example, the dopamine precursor L-DOPA increased discounting via its effects on value representations in the striatum (Pine, Shiner, Seymour, & Dolan, 2010). In another study, modafinil (a wakefulness-promoting drug used as a cognitive enhancer) reduced discounting, presumably by its effects in the VMPFC and via modulation of functional connectivity or cross-talk between the superior frontal gyrus (which contains the dorsolateral prefrontal cortex, a presumed "delta" region) and the striatum (Schmaal et al., 2014). These studies suggest that the relationship between excessive discounting and drug use is not clear-cut and might be determined by certain symptoms or stages of the disease.

Whereas most psychologists and clinicians think about the relatively steeper discount rates seen in addicted individuals as reflecting a general lack of self-control, some economists have taken a different perspective. In their classic paper, Becker and Murphy (1988) argued that people have knowledge of what will happen to them in the future if they use drugs and "rationally" (consistently) decide to do so, knowing the consequences. The choice to engage in drug taking is "rational" (in the economic sense) because, for the addicted individual, the present holds greater value than the future. This is because past drug consumption has raised the marginal utility of current consumption (known as the reinforcement effect), whereas the prospect of future tolerance, or the need for higher doses of the drug to achieve the same level of reinforcement, decreases the value of the future. Another theory used to explain excessive temporal discounting in addiction as a rational process is the melioration theory (Herrnstein & Prelec, 1991; Heyman, 1996). The melioration theory considers individuals who are addicted to drugs as more myopic—they are unable to see or appreciate the future consequences of their actions. Instead, an individual faced with two options (e.g., to take the drug or not) will choose the one that gives him or her the higher payoff in utility at the time of choosing. Melioration theory explains addiction as a series of seemingly rational choices that eventually lead to an irrational outcome, which the individual would have seen had he or she been forward looking.

CAN WE CHANGE OUR TENDENCY TO DISCOUNT POSITIVE FUTURE OUTCOMES?

Given that steeper discount rates have been linked to numerous maladaptive health and social outcomes and are considered a core aspect of addiction psychopathology, some researchers have asked whether there are effective strategies people can use to self-regulate their discount rate, particularly in situations in which the more appealing immediate course of action is in conflict with one's long-term goals (e.g., smoking after having recently quit). One promising approach may be the use of mental contrasting (Oettingen, 2000, 2012; Oettingen, Pak, & Schnetter, 2001; Oettingen & Schwörer, 2013)—a process by which an individual compares his or her long-term goals (maintaining abstinence and overall good health) with the obstacles of current reality (relieving the stress of a work day with a cigarette) as a way to explicate tangible steps to overcome that reality and to meet his or her respective goal. Mental contrasting has also been combined with implementation intentions. These are if–then plans (Gollwitzer, 1999, 2014) that link goal-directed responses to specified situational cues. Mental contrasting with implementation intentions (MCII) turns out to be a particularly effective self-regulation tool to change behavior in multiple life domains (health, social, occupational; Oettingen & Schwörer, 2013). Even in laboratory studies of economic decision making, both MCII (e.g., involving social fairness; Bieleke, Gollwitzer, Oettingen, & Fischbacher, 2016) and implementation intentions (e.g., involving unknown or not fully known probabilistic outcomes; Doerflinger, Martiny-Huenger, & Gollwitzer, 2017) were effective self-regulation tools.

Mental contrasting and implementation intentions could thus also help to reduce the rate of temporal discounting. One psychological mechanism by which this strategy could work is by making the future seem more *concrete* and *certain*. Indeed, people consistently exhibit shallower discounting behavior when delayed outcomes are described in terms of a calendar date or event (e.g., December 25th, or Christmas) rather than in terms of a more abstract passage of time (e.g., 65 days from today), presumably because this framing manipulation helps one concretize his or her future (Read, Frederick, Orsel, & Rahman, 2005). In addition, a related process, episodic future-thinking, in which a person mentally simulates future experiences (what it would feel like to get $100 on Christmas), has been shown to reduce individual discount rates in laboratory studies (Peters & Buchel, 2010). Engaging in episodic future-thinking (and possibly mental contrasting) is likely inherent to choosing to wait for delayed rewards, as individuals with frontotemporal dementia, whose memory and imagination systems are atrophied, discount future outcomes *to a greater extent* than their neurotypical counterparts (Bertoux, de Souza, Zamith, Dubois, & Bourgeois-Gironde, 2015; Chiong et al., 2016; Lebreton et al., 2013).

Finally, strategies that focus on the choice process itself might also have some efficacy in biasing choice toward that consistent with one's long-term goals. For example, directing attention toward specific attributes of the choice options (the magnitude of reward vs. the delay to reward) can differentially promote immediate versus delayed choices (Lempert & Phelps, 2016). Other strategies include elaborating on the possible outcomes of a decision before making a choice (by first generating arguments favoring delayed consumption followed by arguments favoring immediate consumption; Weber et al., 2007) and focusing on choice options in the "explicit zero" format (as in a choice between $10 today and nothing in the future rather than simply $10 today; Magen, Dweck, & Gross, 2008; Magen, Kim, Dweck, Gross, & McClure, 2014).

The Future of Thinking about the Future

Much progress has been made in the past decade using the neuroeconomic approach to understand how people incorporate information about time into their value-based decisions and what the neural substrates of these types of decisions are. This research suggests that most people behave as if they are hyperbolic discounters, weighing the near future more heavily than the distant future. The discounted utility of future rewards is represented in brain regions thought to form a unified valuation system, including the VMPFC and striatum, suggesting that time (or delay) to reward is another factor that modulates subjective value (utility), similar to uncertainty, cost, or effort. Several outstanding questions remain, however. What is the relationship between these other factors (e.g., uncertainty) and time? Is steep discounting an adaptive reflection of an individual's environment and beliefs, or is it related to self-control failure? What is the neurobiological foundation of an individual's discount rate? As research aiming to address these questions intensifies, we look forward to achieving a deeper understanding of temporal discounting.

Acknowledgments

We would like to thank Silvia Lopez-Guzman for helpful discussions. Anna B. Konova is supported by a Ruth R. Kirschstein National Research Service Award (1F32DA03964-01).

References

Allais, M. (1953). Behavior of the rational man before risk: Criticism of American school postulates and axioms. *Econometrica, 21,* 503–546.

American Psychiatric Association. (2013). *Diagnostic and statistical manual of mental disorders* (5th ed.). Arlington, VA: Author.

Andersen, S., Harrison, G. W., Lau, M. I., & Rutstrom, E. E. (2008). Eliciting risk and time preferences. *Econometrica, 76,* 583–618.

Andreoni, J., Kuhn, M. A., & Sprenger, C. (2015). Measuring time preferences: A comparison of experimental methods. *Journal of Economic Behavior and Organization, 116,* 451–464.

Andreoni, J., & Sprenger, C. (2012). Risk preferences are not time preferences. *American Economic Review, 102,* 3357–3376.

Baler, R. D., & Volkow, N. D. (2006). Drug addiction: The neurobiology of disrupted self-control. *Trends in Molecular Medicine, 12,* 559–566.

Bartra, O., McGuire, J. T., & Kable, J. W. (2013). The valuation system: A coordinate-based meta-analysis of BOLD fMRI experiments examining neural correlates of subjective value. *NeuroImage, 76,* 412–427.

Becker, G. S., & Murphy, K. M. (1988). A theory of rational addiction. *Journal of Political Economy, 96,* 675–700.

Bernheim, B. D., & Rangel, A. (2004). Addiction and cue-triggered decision processes. *American Economic Review, 94,* 1558–1590.

Bertoux, M., de Souza, L. C., Zamith, P., Dubois, B., & Bourgeois-Gironde, S. (2015). Discounting of future rewards in behavioural variant frontotemporal dementia and Alzheimer's disease. *Neuropsychology, 29,* 933–939.

Bickel, W. K. (2015). Discounting of delayed rewards as an endophenotype. *Biological Psychiatry, 77,* 846–847.

Bickel, W. K., Jarmolowicz, D. P., Mueller, E. T., Koffarnus, M. N., & Gatchalian, K. M. (2012). Excessive discounting of delayed reinforcers as a trans-disease process contributing to addiction and other disease-related vulnerabilities: Emerging evidence. *Pharmacology and Therapeutics, 134,* 287–297.

Bickel, W. K., Koffarnus, M. N., Moody, L., & Wilson, A. G. (2014). The behavioral- and neuro-economic process of temporal discounting: A candidate behavioral marker of addiction. *Neuropharmacology, 76*(Part B), 518–527.

Bieleke, M., Gollwitzer, P. M., Oettingen, G., & Fischbacher, U. (2016). Social value orientation moderates the effects of intuition versus reflection on responses to unfair ultimatum offers. *Journal of Behavioral Decision Making, 30*(2), 569–581.

Blain, B., Hollard, G., & Pessiglione, M. (2016). Neural mechanisms underlying the impact of daylong cognitive work on economic decisions. *Proceedings of the National Academy of Sciences of the USA, 113,* 6967–6972.

Camerer, C. F., Dreber, A., Forsell, E., Ho, T. H., Huber, J., Johannesson, M., . . . Wu, H. (2016). Evaluating replicability of laboratory experiments in economics. *Science, 351,* 1433–1436

Chen, B. T., Hopf, F. W., & Bonci, A. (2010). Synaptic plasticity in the mesolimbic system: Therapeutic implications for substance abuse. *Annals of the New York Academy of Sciences, 1187,* 129–139.

Chiong, W., Wood, K. A., Beagle, A. J., Hsu, M., Kayser, A. S., Miller, B. L., . . . Kramer, J. H. (2016). Neuroeconomic dissociation of semantic dementia and behavioural variant frontotemporal dementia. *Brain, 139,* 578–587.

de Wit, H. (2009). Impulsivity as a determinant and consequence of drug use: A review of underlying processes. *Addiction Biology, 14,* 22–31.

Doerflinger, J. T., Martiny-Huenger, T., & Gollwitzer, P. M. (2017). Planning to deliberate thoroughly: If–then planned deliberation increases the adjustment of decisions to newly available information. *Journal of Experimental Social Psychology, 69,* 1–12.

Fishburn, P. C., & Rubinstein, A. (1982). Time preference. *International Economic Review, 23,* 677–694.

Glascher, J. P., & O'Doherty, J. P. (2010). Model-based approaches to neuroimaging: Combining reinforcement learning theory with fMRI data. *Wiley Interdisciplinary Reviews: Cognitive Science, 1,* 501–510.

Glimcher, P. W. (2010). *Foundations of neuroeconomic analysis.* New York: Oxford University Press.

Gollwitzer, P. M. (1999). Implementation intentions: Strong effects of simple plans. *American Psychologist, 54,* 493–503.

Gollwitzer, P. M. (2014). Weakness of the will: Is a quick fix possible? *Motivation and Emotion, 38,* 305–322.

Herrnstein, R. J., & Prelec, D. (1991). Melioration: A theory of distributed choice. *Journal of Economic Perspectives, 5,* 137–156.

Heyman, G. M. (1996). Resolving the contradictions of addiction. *Behavioral and Brain Sciences, 19,* 561–610.

Houthakker, H. S. (1950). Revealed preference and the utility function. *Economica–New Series, 17,* 159–174.

Huettel, S. A., Song, A. W., & McCarthy, G. (2009). *Functional magnetic resonance imaging* (2nd ed.). Sunderland, MA: Sinauer Associates.

Kable, J. W., & Glimcher, P. W. (2007). The neural correlates of subjective value during intertemporal choice. *Nature Neuroscience, 10,* 1625–1633.

Kable, J. W., & Glimcher, P. W. (2010). An "as soon as possible" effect in human intertemporal decision making: Behavioral evidence and neural mechanisms. *Journal of Neurophysiology, 103,* 2513–2531.

Kahneman, D., & Tversky, A. (1979). Prospect theory: Analysis of decision under risk. *Econometrica, 47,* 263–291.

Laibson, D. (1997). Golden eggs and hyperbolic discounting. *Quarterly Journal of Economics, 112,* 443–477.

Laruelle, M., Abi-Dargham, A., van Dyck, C. H., Rosenblatt, W., Zea-Ponce, Y., . . . Innis, R. B. (1995). SPECT imaging of striatal dopamine release after amphetamine challenge. *Journal of Nuclear Medicine, 36,* 1182–1190.

Lebreton, M., Bertoux, M., Boutet, C., Lehericy, S., Dubois, B., Fossati, P., & Pessiglione, M. (2013). A critical role for the hippocampus in the valuation of imagined outcomes. *PLOS Biology, 11,* e1001684.

Lempert, K. M., & Phelps, E. A. (2016). The malleability of intertemporal choice. *Trends in Cognitive Sciences, 20,* 64–74.

Loewenstein, G., & O'Donoghue, T. (2004). *Animal spirits: Affective and deliberative processes in economic behavior.* Ithaca, NY: Cornell University Press.

MacKillop, J., Amlung, M. T., Few, L. R., Ray, L. A., Sweet, L. H., & Munafo, M. R. (2011). Delayed reward discounting and addictive behavior: A meta-analysis. *Psychopharmacology (Berlin), 216,* 305–321.

Magen, E., Dweck, C. S., & Gross, J. J. (2008). The hidden-zero effect: Representing a single choice as an extended sequence reduces impulsive choice. *Psychological Science, 19,* 648–649.

Magen, E., Kim, B., Dweck, C. S., Gross, J. J., & McClure, S. M. (2014). Behavioral and neural correlates of increased self-control in the absence of increased willpower. *Proceedings of the National Academy of Sciences of the USA, 111,* 9786–9791.

Mazur, J. E. (1987). An adjusting procedure for studying delayed reinforcement. In M. L. Commons, J. E. Mazur, J. A. Nevin, & H. C. Rachlin (Eds.), *Quantitative analyses of behavior: Vol. 5. The effect of delay and of intervening events on reinforcement value* (pp. 55–73). Hillsdale, NJ: Erlbaum.

McClure, S. M., Laibson, D. I., Loewenstein, G., & Cohen, J. D. (2004). Separate neural systems value immediate and delayed monetary rewards. *Science, 306,* 503–507.

Metcalfe, J., & Mischel, W. (1999). A hot/cool-system analysis of delay of gratification: Dynamics of willpower. *Psychological Review, 106,* 3–19.

Mischel, W., Ayduk, O., Berman, M. G., Casey, B. J., Gotlib, I. H., Jonides, J., . . . Shoda, Y. (2011). "Willpower" over the life span: Decomposing self-regulation. *Social Cognitive and Affective Neuroscience, 6,* 252–256.

Mischel, W., & Metzner, R. (1962). Preference for delayed reward as a function of age, intelligence, and length of delay interval. *Journal of Abnormal Psychology, 64,* 425–431.

O'Doherty, J. P., Hampton, A., & Kim, H. (2007). Model-based fMRI and its application to reward learning and decision making. *Annals of the New York Academy of Sciences, 1104,* 35–53.

Oettingen, G. (2000). Expectancy effects on behavior depend on self-regulatory thought. *Social Cognition, 18,* 101–129.

Oettingen, G. (2012). Future thought and behaviour change. *European Review of Social Psychology, 23,* 1–63.

Oettingen, G., Pak, H., & Schnetter, K. (2001). Self-regulation of goal setting: Turning free fantasies about the future into binding goals. *Journal of Personality and Social Psychology, 80,* 736–753.

Oettingen, G., & Schwörer, B. (2013). Mind wandering via mental contrasting as a tool for behavior change. *Frontiers in Psychology, 4,* 562.

Peters, J., & Buchel, C. (2010). Episodic future thinking reduces reward delay discounting through an enhancement of prefrontal–mediotemporal interactions. *Neuron, 66,* 138–148.

Phelps, E. S., & Pollak, R. A. (1968). On second-best national saving and game-equilibrium growth. *Review of Economic Studies, 35,* 185–199.

Pine, A., Shiner, T., Seymour, B., & Dolan, R. J. (2010). Dopamine, time, and impulsivity in humans. *Journal of Neuroscience, 30,* 8888–8896.

Read, D., Frederick, S., Orsel, B., & Rahman, J. (2005). Four score and seven years from now: The date/delay effect in temporal discounting. *Management Science, 51,* 1326–1335.

Samuelson, P. A. (1938). A note on the pure theory of consumer's behaviour. *Economica–New Series, 5,* 61–71.

Savage, L. J. (1954). *Foundations of statistics.* New York: Wiley.

Schmaal, L., Goudriaan, A. E., Joos, L., Dom, G., Pattij, T., van den Brink, W., . . . Veltman, D. J. (2014). Neural substrates of impulsive decision making modulated by modafinil in alcohol-dependent patients. *Psychological Medicine, 44,* 2787–2798.

Setlow, B., Mendez, I. A., Mitchell, M. R., & Simon, N. W. (2009). Effects of chronic administration of drugs of abuse on impulsive choice (delay discounting) in animal models. *Behavioural Pharmacology, 20,* 380–389.

Story, G. W., Moutoussis, M., & Dolan, R. J. (2015). A computational analysis of aberrant delay discounting in psychiatric disorders. *Frontiers in Psychology, 6,* 1948.

Story, G. W., Vlaev, I., Seymour, B., Darzi, A., & Dolan, R. J. (2014). Does temporal discounting explain unhealthy behavior?: A systematic review and reinforcement learning perspective. *Frontiers in Behavioral Neuroscience, 8,* 76.

Strotz, R. H. (1956). Myopia and inconsistency in dynamic utility maximization. *Review of Economic Studies, 23,* 165–180.

Sulzer, D. (2011). How addictive drugs disrupt presynaptic dopamine neurotransmission. *Neuron, 69,* 628–649.

Volkow, N. D., & Baler, R. D. (2015). NOW vs LATER brain circuits: Implications for obesity and addiction. *Trends in Neurosciences, 38,* 345–352.

Volkow, N. D., Fowler, J. S., Wang, G. J., Ding, Y. S., & Gatley, S. J. (2002). Role of dopamine in the therapeutic and reinforcing effects of methylphenidate in humans: Results from imaging studies. *European Neuropsychopharmacology, 12,* 557–566.

Volkow, N. D., Wang, G. J., Fischman, M. W., Foltin, R. W., Fowler, J. S., Abumrad, N. N., . . . Shea, C. E. (1997). Relationship between subjective effects of cocaine and dopamine transporter occupancy. *Nature, 386,* 827–830.

Von Neumann, J., & Morgenstern, O. (1944). *Theory of games and economic behavior.* Princeton, NJ: Princeton University Press.

Weber, E. U., Johnson, E. J., Milch, K. F., Chang, H., Brodscholl, J. C., & Goldstein, D. G. (2007). Asymmetric discounting in intertemporal choice: A query-theory account. *Psychological Science, 18,* 516–523.

CHAPTER 14

Anticipated Regret

A Prospective Emotion about the Future Past

Marcel Zeelenberg

Regret is the emotion experienced when looking back at decisions that went awry. It is typically associated with feeling responsible for the bad outcome and kicking oneself over the mistake made. No book about the psychology of thinking about the future would be complete without a chapter on regret. That might seem surprising, since regret is a backward-looking emotion. But regret is also forward looking, in the sense that decision makers can anticipate regret happening in the future. People's decisions are sometimes influenced by these anticipations, in such a way that they choose in order to avoid future regret. In this chapter, I first describe what regret is. Next I turn to anticipated regret and discuss economic and psychological theories about this forward-looking type of regret. I also briefly review some empirical research on the effects of anticipated regret. Then I turn to the questions, "Is anticipated regret an emotion?" and "How does it differ from the more prototypical retrospective regret?" In order to answer those two questions, I describe hitherto unpublished research comparing the experiential qualities of anticipated regret and retrospective regret. I end with a discussion of the strategies that decision makers may use to regulate their anticipated regrets. Let us start with examining what regret is.

Regret is a painful emotion, not only because one is confronted with a bad decision outcome, but even more so because it points to one's own role in causing that bad outcome. Put differently, we feel regret over bad decision outcomes that were produced by our own choices; it was our fault. Hence it may come as no surprise that Saffrey, Roese, and Summerville (2008) found that regret was the most intense of a series of negative emotions.

Regret is a universal experience in the sense that it is experienced all over the globe and that it seems to feel the same in different countries or cultures. We recently studied the experiential qualities of regret (and disappointment and guilt as benchmark emotions) in the United States, Israel, Taiwan, and the Netherlands (Breugelmans, Zeelenberg, Gilovich, Huang, & Shani, 2014). We found that in all four countries, regret is a distinct emotion that differs systematically from disappointment and guilt. In that study, we adopted a procedure developed by Roseman, Wiest, and Swartz (1994) in which emotions are conceptualized as multicomponent phenomena that may differ on a number of dimensions. Roseman et al. (1994) asked participants to recall one particular emotion and further asked them to rate the extent to which they experienced certain feelings, thoughts, action tendencies (what you are inclined to do at that moment), emotivations[1] (what you want to achieve), and engaged in certain actions. Roseman et al. (1994) included 10 negative emotions in their study and found that "discrete emotions have distinctive goals and action tendencies, as well as thoughts and feelings" (p. 206). In our study we found that regret, guilt, and disappointment were associated with specific feelings, thoughts, action tendencies, and emotivations, and that this pattern was stable across the four cultures. This procedure also revealed that regret can be assessed with five items measuring the specific components that make up this emotion, as expressed in this statement: "I felt *regret*. I felt *angry* with myself. I thought that I was *responsible* for the situation. I thought that I had made a *mistake*. I wanted to *correct* my mistake." These items were found to be indicative of regret across cultures and could be used as a reliable scale to measure experiences of regret (Cronbach's alpha ranged between .80 and .86 in the four countries). We also found that guilt and disappointment were associated with specific items (for details, see Breugelmans et al., 2014). In other words, there seems to be structural equivalence of regret over cultures. This is not only interesting but also important for theories of regret. This structural equivalence makes it more likely that these theories are globally applicable.

In addition to being painful and universal, regret is also frequent. Susan Shimanoff, a communication researcher, studied verbal expressions of emotions in everyday communication. In a first study with audiotaped conversations of 30 students and written transcripts of 30-minute conversations of 20 married couples, she found that regret was the most frequently named negative emotion (and the only emotion being mentioned more often was the positive emotion of love; Shimanoff, 1984). In another study, in which she audiotaped the everyday conversations of 26 dyads, she found that regret was the most frequently used emotion word (Shimanoff, 1985). This prevalence of regret is also evident in Barry Cadish's 2001 book *Damn!: Reflections on Life's Biggest Regrets*. Cadish asked thousands of people, from different countries and different walks of life, via his website *RegretsOnly. com* to report their most intense regret. Cadish writes that "regrets are universal; nearly everyone has them. Regrets transcend age, gender, race, culture, nationality,

---

[1] Roseman (1984) introduced the term *emotivations,* or *emotivational goals,* to refer to the distinctive motives or goals that accompany discrete emotions. They are called emotivations to distinguish them from the traditional motivations, such as hunger and need for achievement. Roseman et al. (1994, p. 207) provide the following examples of emotivations "in fear, wanting to avoid danger; in anger, wanting to hurt someone; and in sadness, wanting to recover from loss."

religion, language, social status, and geographic location" (p. 2). The earlier cited Saffrey et al. (2008) also investigated the frequency of different positive and negative emotions, in addition to their intensity. The negative emotions in their study were anger, anxiety, boredom, disappointment, fear, guilt, jealousy, regret, and sadness. Regret was rated as being the most intense of these negative emotions and second most frequent (anxiety was rated as the most frequent negative emotion).

Carmon and Ariely (2000) might provide some insight into why regret is frequent. These scholars studied how people set selling and buying prices in transactions and found that sellers tend to focus on the benefits of possessing an item, whereas buyers tend to focus on salient reference prices. Put differently, people have a natural tendency to focus on the forgone instead of on what can be obtained. Such a focus is clearly conducive to regret. Similarly, Carmon, Wertenbroch, and Zeelenberg (2003) examined the role of deliberation in consumer decisions. They found that when decision makers closely consider different choice options, choosing one of them produces a sense of immediate postdecisional regret over losing the others, because it felt as if they already owned them.

Feeling regret is thus universal, painful, and frequent, and I believe that these three features may be the key to understanding why we feel regret and what regret does. Regret is a functional emotion, improving future decision making (e.g., Bourgeois-Gironde, 2010; Roese, 2005; Zeelenberg, 1999, 2018). The experience of regret has many cognitive and behavioral correlates and can motivate people to undo their decisions. Regret can also help people to learn from the mistakes made and to prevent such mistakes in the future. It is precisely because regret is so painful that it is so functional. That is why we do not easily forget our mistakes (Wagenaar, 1986, 1992) and why we try to right our wrongs (Zeelenberg, Van der Pligt, & Manstead, 1998).

Research has also documented that our current judgments and decisions may be driven by the regret that we experience over previous decisions that went awry. Inman, Dyer, and Jia (1997) had participants make eight choices between lottery pairs (sets of gambles) and afterward provided them with the outcomes of the chosen and unchosen gambles. After this information, they asked the participants, for each decision, how happy or unhappy they were with that decision. This measure of postchoice valuation was influenced not only by the outcome of the decision but also by the outcome of the unchosen gamble (a proxy for regret). The more regret there was (i.e., the better the outcome of the unchosen gamble), the less happy they were with their choice. Thus postdecisional evaluations of a choice were influenced by the regret that was associated with that choice.

Inman and Zeelenberg (2002) studied regret following switch versus repeat purchases. They found that justifiability of decisions may attenuate regret following bad outcomes. And this effect carried over to subsequent decisions. Zeelenberg and Pieters (1999, 2004a) surveyed consumers who were dissatisfied with the delivery of a service and assessed how dissatisfied they were, how disappointed they were, and how much regret they felt. They also assessed whether the consumers complained, switched, and engaged in negative word-of-mouth. They found that both these emotions had a direct effect on behavior over and above the effects of (dis)satisfaction. Regret was associated with switching behavior, whereas disappointment was associated with negative word-of-mouth. Of course, these are only a few examples of research showing that the experience of regret can influence behavior.

ANTICIPATED REGRET

One of the interesting things about regret is that we do not have to wait passively for regret to happen to us. We can sort of feel it beforehand, before a decision is made. At this point in time, before the decision, we may contemplate what to choose and think about what can go wrong. And we can envision how we would respond emotionally to these wrong decisions, and hence try to prevent these bad outcomes from happening. This is intuitive ("if something is bad for you, you may want to avoid it") and has been long known. The statistician Leonard Savage proposed already in 1951 that people can make decisions using a strategy or decision rule that he called "minimax regret." In this strategy, regret is defined as the difference in value between the actual outcome of the chosen option and the highest possible outcome of the rejected options. The strategy implies that one tries to minimize the maximum regret. Put differently, you compute the possible regret for each option, and then choose the one for which the maximum regret is lowest. This rule is useful when one has no knowledge about the probabilities of the possible outcomes (see also Acker, 1997; Zeelenberg, 2015), as it ignores the likelihood with which an event occurs and incorporates only how the outcomes compare. Sometimes ignoring probabilities makes sense. But, in many cases, probabilities are known. Even when they are not known, one is often able to rank-order the states of the world in terms of their likelihood. Such rank ordering should help in determining the importance of the associated outcomes in the final decision. In these cases, minimax regret is not a good strategy, and one might turn to approaches that take the rank order into account and arrive at decisions that are closer to utility maximizing (Kmietowicz & Pearman, 1981).

The economists Bell (1982), Loomes and Sugden (1982), and Sage and White (1983) took the minimax regret idea one step further, integrated it with standard utility theory, and formalized it in regret theory. Even though these authors proposed slightly different theories, I use the term *regret theory* as a generic name for all these theories. Regret theory also takes into account the opposite of regret: rejoicing (sometimes called elation), the emotion felt when the outcome of the chosen option compares favorably with the outcomes of the unchosen options. In addition, regret theory takes into account the probability of regret and rejoicing, such that they weight heavier when they are more likely. In short, regret theory is a modified version of expected utility (EU) theory. In EU theory, the attractiveness of choice option, its expected utility, is the weighed average of the utility ($\approx$ value) of all possible outcomes, where the weights are the likelihood of that outcome occurring. Regret theory assumes that the EU of an option depends not only on the likelihood and value of the outcomes but also on the regret or rejoicing one may feel over the choice. More about regret theory later.

Psychologists also realized that anticipated regret might be a force to be reckoned with in decision making. Kahneman and Tversky (1979) thought about the role of regret when working on their prospect theory, but "eventually abandoned this approach because it did not elegantly accommodate the patter of results that we labeled 'reflection'" (Kahneman, 2000, p. x).[2] It is telling that Kahneman (2011, p. 286–287) recently referred to regret and disappointment as the two obvious blind spots in prospect theory. He wrote, "The emotions regret and disappointment are real, and decision makers surely anticipate these emotions when making their choices" (p. 288).

A few years before prospect theory and regret theory were published, the psychologists Janis and Mann (1977) wrote extensively about the psychological processes that occur when people make important decisions. They expressed elegantly how decision makers' fear of future regret influences their behavioral decisions and how these are made. Moreover, they believed that anticipating future regret may help us to make better decisions, because this anticipation causes us to think more elaborately before making the decision. In their own words:

> Before undertaking any enterprise "of great pith and moment," we usually delay action and think about what might happen that could cause regret. . . . Anticipatory regret is a convenient generic term to refer to the main psychological effects of the various worries that beset a decision maker before any losses actually materialize. . . . Such worries, which include anticipatory guilt and shame, provoke hesitation and doubt, making salient the realization that even the most attractive of the available choices might turn out badly. (p. 222)

Thus, roughly at the same time that both psychologists and economists increase their research attention with respect to decision processes in both fields, they discover that emotional influences such as regret may be important. The economists, though, had a colder and more rational process in mind when talking about the impact of anticipated regret, as the following description of regret theory makes clear.

Regret theory is based on a number of simple assumptions. The first, and least controversial, is that we can feel emotions as the result of a choice when we compare the outcomes obtained to the outcomes that would have been if we had chosen differently. There is now ample evidence for this assumption (e.g., Boles & Messick, 1995). The second assumption is that these emotions influence or color the experience of the outcomes. Negative emotions reduce the experienced utility of a decision outcome, and positive emotions increase the utility. Support for this assumption is found in Inman et al. (1997), Taylor (1997), and Mellers, Schwartz, and Ritov (1999). The third assumption, already a bit more controversial, is that we can predict these feelings beforehand. This is controversial because extensive research on affective forecasting (Wilson & Gilbert, 2003) shows that we are not always accurate in predicting our future feelings. We tend to overshoot in our predictions such that we expect our emotions to be more intense and to last longer than they actually do (but see Mellers et al., 1999, for accurate predictions of regret; and Fernandez-Duque, & Landers, 2008, for underpredictions of regret). But one might argue that

---

[2]Kahneman and Tversky (1982a, 1982b) wrote about the psychology of regret and the differential regrets for action and inaction in their work on the simulation heuristic and counterfactual thinking, but they never formalized their ideas on regret in decision making.

it does not matter for regret theory how accurately we predict the intensity of our regrets; the fact that we predict them is what matters for regret theory. The fourth and most important assumption, and also the one that was most provocative at the time, is that we take these predicted emotions into account when choosing and that we choose in such a way that we avoid regret and strive for rejoicing. In other words, we are regret averse. There is now quite some support for the ideas that we take regret into account when making decisions. Next I present a very selective review, highlighting some of the ways in which anticipated regret has an influence on behavioral decisions. Bleichrodt and Wakker (2015) provide a detailed review of the research on regret theory in economics. Zeelenberg and Pieters (2007) review the research from the fields of psychology and consumer research.

EMPIRICAL DEMONSTRATIONS OF THE IMPACT OF ANTICIPATED REGRET ON DECISION MAKING

Richard and Van der Pligt (1991) were, to my best knowledge, the first who studied the effects of anticipated regret (and related emotions) in a more generalized attitude–behavior framework (Ajzen, 1991). They asked more than 800 adolescents about their sexual behaviors: more specifically, they asked about their attitudes, subjective norms, self-efficacy, habits, and anticipated affective reactions (including regret, worry, and discontent). Richard and Van der Pligt found that anticipated regret predicted condom use, independent of other predictors such as attitudes and habits. They replicated these findings in many other studies on health behavior (for a review, see Van der Pligt, Zeelenberg, van Dijk, de Vries, & Richard, 1998).

It seems reasonable to assume that anticipated regret can strengthen people's commitment to their intentions, no matter whether these intentions pertain to reaching set goals (intentions that specify desired outcomes, such as losing weight, or desired behaviors, such as eating healthy food) or to the implementation of how one wants to reach these set goals (so-called if–then plans that specify when, where, and how one wants to strive for the set goal; Gollwitzer, Wieber, Myers, & McCrea, 2010). In the process of setting goals and making plans, people may run mental simulations (Kahneman & Tversky, 1982a, 1982b; Taylor, Pham, Rivkin, & Armor, 1998) that have the by-product of making clear when regret may be the result. Abraham and Sheeran (2003) argued that anticipation of regret "binds people to their intentions by associating failure to act with aversive affect" (p. 496). When people are strongly committed to their goal intentions and implementation intentions, the likelihood that people will act on these intentions is enhanced, and thus the rate of goal attainment increases (Gollwitzer & Sheeran, 2006).

Two recent meta-analyses, one of 25 studies coming from 20 articles (Sandberg & Conner, 2008) and the other of 81 studies from 79 articles (Brewer, DeFrank, & Gilkey, 2016) documented a strong link between anticipated regret and behavioral intentions and a moderate relation between anticipated regret, intentions, and health behaviors. A narrative literature review by Koch (2014) supports these findings. Interestingly, before this empirical work on health behaviors of ordinary people, Tymstra (1989) already indicated the "imperative" character of anticipated regret in medical testing. He reasoned that the moment medical technology allows for new screening procedures, anticipated regret over not using these new technologies pushes doctors (and most likely also patients) toward overusage of tests that may be less than informative and also very expensive. These ideas about how anticipated regret influences the prescriptive decisions of doctors were later elaborated upon and formalized by Hozo and Djulbegovic (2008).

Findings of anticipated regret influencing behavioral decision making have also been found in the domain of consumer behavior. Simonson (1992) was one of the first to apply the ideas of anticipatory regret to consumer decision making. He asked people to think about the regret they would feel after having made a wrong choice of products. This induction of anticipated regret made people more likely to purchase items that would shield them from potential postchoice regret. In this case, these regret-minimizing choices were choices for higher priced, well-known brands over a potentially better but less expensive lesser known brand that is thus riskier. Inman and McAlister (1994) found that anticipations of regret might explain why people often use coupons just before the expiration date.

Anticipated regret can also influence lottery play. Wolfson and Briggs (2002; see also Van de Ven & Zeelenberg, 2011) studied the behavior of players in the British National Lottery in 1997, when they introduced a second weekly drawing (a Wednesday drawing in addition to the traditional Saturday drawing). Wolfson and Briggs (2002) found that those playing with a fixed set of numbers in the Saturday drawing were more likely to also participate in the Wednesday drawing. Wolfson and Briggs did not assess anticipated regret, but the idea was that these players were "locked in" because they anticipated the regret they would feel upon finding out that "their numbers" had won on Wednesday and that they had not played. Thus the lottery players had to play Wednesday as well to avoid regret. Similarly, Zeelenberg and Pieters (2004b) studied the decisions of lottery players in the Netherlands and found that the anticipation of regret can explain the behavioral decisions of players in the postcode lottery, but not in the state lottery. This is the case because, in the postcode lottery, the postcode is the lottery ticket, and if one does not play, one could still find out that one would have won had one played. Thus, again, people play the lottery in order to prevent the regret from not playing.

Finally, Croy, Gerrans, and Speelman (2015) found that anticipated regret might help people to save for retirement. It is well known that when people are themselves responsible for their pension planning, this often results in saving too little. Combining this finding with the persuasive attempts of the lotteries described above suggests that inviting people to think about the regret they feel when retiring with too little money may be a fruitful intervention.

This selective review of the literature shows only a few of the instances in which it was found that the anticipation of regret can influence the decisions and choices that people make. It does demonstrate, I hope, the wide range of behaviors in which anticipated regret may influence choice. Now that we know that anticipated regret can be so influential across domains, it may be relevant to understand a bit better what anticipated regret actually is. As described earlier, in regret theory, anticipated regret is simply the expected reaction to the value difference between the outcome of the chosen option and that of the unchosen option. It is not clear whether anticipated regret qualifies as an emotion. There has been discussion of whether regret (the retrospective form) is an emotion (see Landman, 1993), but it is now commonly accepted that it is. But when it comes to anticipated regret, there may be some disagreement.

IS ANTICIPATED REGRET AN EMOTION?

The fact that anticipated regret has such an effect on behavioral choice shows that regret aversion is a clear motivator. That lends some support to the idea that anticipated regret is an emotional experience. But note that there has been some discussion about whether this is the case. The exact definition of *emotion* has been a matter of dispute among many (Kleinginna & Kleinginna, 1981). However, there is agreement on several aspects. Emotions are acute, relatively momentary, object-based experiences of goal relevance. This definition helps us to conceive of what an emotion is but does not really help us to decide whether anticipated regret is an emotion. The question is, of course, hard to answer, but it may be instructive to see what different people have written about this.

Frijda (2007) refers to anticipated emotions as *virtual emotions*. Virtual emotions are "representations of the emotion one would have under certain circumstances, including virtual readiness for particular types of action and posture" (p. 41). I interpret this as anticipated emotions not being full-blown emotions but having important emotional and motivational qualities. Let us also see how we can answer the question concerning the emotionality of anticipated regret by looking at regret theory and related research efforts.

In regret theory, regret (and rejoicing) are conceptualized in a rather cognitive, cold, and calculative way. According to this theory, we compare decision outcomes and "compute" the associated regret and related emotions, and then we compute the rational choice, given the potential of regret and elation. Thus regret is conceived as an outcome of a decision that one can weigh and take into account. The emotional qualities of regret are not central in this reasoning, other than that regret is an aversive state that decision makers would like to avoid.

This stands in contrast with how Janis and Mann (1977) wrote about anticipated regret. In their words, anticipated regret may be felt when contemplating a decision, and it goes together with worries, feelings of guilt, and hypervigilance. It is an emotion that does not (or not only) change how we evaluate the outcomes, but even more so an emotion that changes the way in which we approach the decision and finally make it. Reb (2008) found support for the ideas of Janis and Mann (1977) that anticipated regret leads to more careful and better decisions. In a series of five studies, he found that making regret salient to decision makers induced them to use more time to reach a decision and to collect more information before making the final choice.

A thing to note is that Janis and Mann (1977) refer to *anticipatory* regret instead of *anticipated* regret, the term that is used in regret theory. Loewenstein, Weber, Hsee, and Welch (2001) elaborated on a potential distinction between anticipated and anticipatory emotions in judgment and decision making (J/DM) research. They write:

> Anticipatory emotions are immediate visceral reactions (e.g., fear, anxiety, dread) to risks and uncertainties. Anticipated emotions are typically not experienced in the

immediate present but are expected to be experienced in the future. To the extent that J/DM research has addressed emotions, the emotions that have been taken into account are anticipated emotions. . . . These anticipated emotions are a component of the expected consequences of the decision; they are emotions that are expected to occur when outcomes are experienced, rather than emotions that are experienced at the time of decision. (pp. 267–268)

This distinction between anticipated and anticipatory regret makes sense conceptually, but I think this distinction is hard to make in many everyday situations. For example, when thinking about the feelings of regret one might experience when having unprotected sex, the regret is likely to be both anticipated and anticipatory in nature. And the same applies to the regret one might feel when one is about to buy a house or an expensive car or when thinking about vaccinating one's child and the associated risks. In all these cases, the anticipated regret refers to both a prospective outcome and a clear immediate emotional experience. Many researchers have been using the terms *anticipated* and *anticipatory regret* in different ways or interchangeably (cf. Koch, 2014). Thus I opt for the pragmatic solution provided by Koch (p. 398) and "use the term 'anticipated regret' to denote a prospective, aversive, and cognitive emotion (i.e., an emotion that requires thinking) that influences decision making."

Janis and Mann's (1977) words on anticipated regret bring forward another issue. I read them as meaning that anticipated regret is something related to, but at the same time different from, retrospective regret. As yet, it is unclear how this anticipated sense of regret may differ from the retrospective one, which intuitively seems more prototypical. Anticipated regret, by definition, is more forward-looking and probably more proactive than its retrospective cousin. But do these two emotional states differ only in these respects, or are there other aspects that distinguish between them? This is the question addressed next.

ARE ANTICIPATED REGRET AND RETROSPECTIVE REGRET DIFFERENT EMOTIONS?

In what follows, I describe an unpublished study (Zeelenberg, Van Dijk, & Manstead, 2003) that we conducted to investigate the extent to which these two types of regret experiences (anticipated and retrospective) differ and to which they are similar. The importance of the question concerning the experience of these two emotional states lies in the fact that research has demonstrated that both states affect behavioral decisions, as reviewed earlier in this chapter. And, if we would like to understand how that influence takes place, it is insightful to understand the experiential qualities of these emotions (Zeelenberg, Nelissen, Breugelmans, & Pieters, 2008). If we believe that emotions exist for the sake of behavioral guidance, we need to understand what the experience and anticipation of regret entails and which behaviors these experiences motivate. Only then can we shed light on how anticipated and retrospective regret can shape subsequent decision making.

Because we wanted to compare the two emotional states, we turned to traditional emotion research, in which the expertise in comparing and disentangling different emotional states can be found. We chose to adopt the methodology of

Frijda, Kuipers, and Ter Schure (1989). Their approach is similar to that of Rose-man et al. (1994), discussed earlier, but in some ways more comprehensive. Frijda et al. (1989) asked participants to remember instances of 32 emotional states. They also asked them to rate their experiences on appraisal dimensions and modes of action readiness. Appraisals are interpretations of the situation that link what happens to a person's goals, concerns, and well-being. An important appraisal dimension is agency (whether one is responsible for an event, or someone else, or circumstances). People may differ in the specific appraisals that are elicited by a particular event, but the same patterns of appraisals always give rise to the same emotions. If one accepts responsibility for a bad decision outcome, regret is typically felt. But, if that same bad outcome is appraised as caused by someone else, or by circumstances, disappointment is typically felt (Van Dijk & Zeelenberg, 2002). An understanding of appraisals helps to understand why specific emotions arise from precipitating events—that is, what the antecedents of specific emotions are. Appraisal theory is a well-accepted theory of emotion causation, and different appraisal patterns are related with different emotional experiences (for a review, see Scherer, Schorr, & Johnstone, 2001). Emotions can be furthermore distinguished by patterns of action readiness (also referred to as *action tendencies*) that accompany the emotion. Patterns of action readiness refer to the motivational states that are part of the emotional experience. These patterns involve focusing of attention, experienced arousal, muscular preparation, goal priority, or felt readiness. Action readiness has control precedence, implying that it overrules other goals. Many emotions can be differentiated in terms of action readiness, as shown by Frijda et al. (1989). For example, when one is fearful, running away has priority. But when angry, moving toward the source of the anger may be prioritized (Bougie, Pieters, & Zeelenberg, 2003). Next I explain how we used Frijda et al.'s method to study the differences and similarities between anticipated and retrospective regret.

We asked 70 Tilburg University students to recall a concrete memory about a purchase decision over which they experienced substantial regret in retrospect (*retrospective regret condition*) or to recall a purchase decision over which they experienced substantial anticipatory regret before the decision (*anticipated regret condition*). We asked for purchase decisions because they are frequent and easy to recall. Moreover, using such mundane decisions makes it more likely that we find comparable decisions in both conditions. In order to make clear what we wanted them to remember, they were provided with the definition of regret or anticipated regret taken from Reber (1986). Because the instruction was in Dutch, the definition was taken from the Dutch translation of Reber's original English edition, published in 1986. After they provided information about the purchase situation, we asked them about the emotions, appraisals, and states of action readiness that they experienced in that situation (closely based on the study by Frijda et al., 1989; the exact items are shown in Tables 14.1, 14.2 and 14.3).

The average *emotion ratings* for both regret conditions are shown in Table 14.1. The events reported in both conditions were associated with equal amounts of experienced regret, which is desirable because differences on the other dimensions cannot be attributed to the intensity of regret. Interestingly, the anticipatory emotions that we included (worry, fear, and concern) received higher ratings in the anticipated regret condition, whereas the three retrospective emotions included (disappointment, dissatisfaction, and frustration) received higher ratings in the retrospective regret condition. This pattern of results was as expected and thus provided first support for the idea that both regret experiences may differ on some important dimensions.

Next we turn to the *appraisal ratings*. The average ratings for both regret conditions are shown in Table 14.2. Here we found that the two conditions did not differ significantly for most appraisal dimensions. Only 3 out of 11 dimensions differed significantly. There were differences for Pleasantness. Although, as one would expect, both experiences were appraised as unpleasant (i.e., below the neutral midpoint), retrospective regret experiences are clearly less pleasant (or, better, more unpleasant). This makes sense if one realizes that in the case of retrospective regret the bad decision has already happened and that, in cases of anticipated regret, the bad decision may still be prevented. Anticipated regret also scores higher on Expectedness, perhaps reflecting the fact that decision makers, in these situations, already brace for the worst. It could reflect that we might anticipate regret for many decisions and only experience regret for a subset of those. This would indicate that we more often anticipate regret than actually experience it, making anticipations of regret more prevalent and more expected. The final difference was found for the appraisal dimension of Modifiability: whether the situation's outcome was immutable or whether it could still be changed. Anticipatory regret scored higher and above the midpoint, which is likely to reflect the functionality of this emotion in protecting the self from faulty decisions. Experienced or retrospective regret scored below the midpoint, suggesting that little can be done about the outcome. This is interesting, because the tendency or willingness to undo regretted outcomes is an important element of the regret experience (Breugelmans et al., 2014). Thus people realize it is hard to modify the regretted outcomes but still wish they had been different. In sum, we found that the appraisal pattern for both types of regret were similar, with a few differences that seem to make sense.

TABLE 14.1. Mean Emotion Ratings per Regret Condition

	Anticipated Regret			Retrospective Regret			
	M	SD		M	SD	F(1, 69)	p
Regret	4.66	1.30	=	4.94	1.24	0.89	.35
Worry	3.68	1.63	>	2.23	1.42	15.57	<.001
Disappointment	2.86	1.93	<	4.43	1.31	42.57	<.001
Fear	2.46	1.52	>	1.63	0.96	7.37	.008
Dissatisfaction	4.09	1.79	<	5.40	1.50	11.10	<.001
Concerned	3.71	1.66	>	1.91	1.25	25.79	<.001
Frustrated	3.57	1.85	<	4.51	1.74	4.82	.031

Note. Entries are mean responses and standard deviations. Participants were asked the following: "It is of course possible that you experienced multiple emotions and feelings during this event. Could you indicate how intense the following emotions were felt during the event?." Ratings were made on 7-point scales, with endpoints labeled *not intense* (1) and *very intense* (7). Items adapted from Frijda et al. (1989).

TABLE 14.2. Appraisal Variables and Items and Ratings per Regret Condition

Variable	Items (and scale anchors)	Anticipated M (SD)		Retrospective M (SD)	F(1,69)	p
Pleasantness	Was it a pleasant or unpleasant situation? (1 = unpleasant, 7 = pleasant)	3.46 (0.95)	>	2.57 (1.12)	12.74	< .001
Outcome	Did you know how the situation would end? (1 = did not know, 7 = did know)	3.00 (1.78)	=	3.29 (2.11)	0.38	.542
Suddenness	Was it a situation that had already lasted for some time, or one that had developed all of a sudden? (1 = already lasted for some time, 7 = developed all of a sudden)	4.69 (1.89)	=	4.49 (2.05)	0.18	.673
Expectedness	Was it an unexpected or an expected situation? (1 = very unexpected, 7 = very expected)	4.03 (1.71)	>	3.14 (1.61)	4.99	.029
Importance	Was the situation unimportant or important to you? (1 = very unimportant, 7 = very important)	3.86 (1.48)	=	3.66 (1.49)	0.32	.575
Modifiability	Was the situation's outcome immutable, or could someone or something still change it in some way? (1 = situation was immutable, 7 = could still be changed)	5.06 (1.78)	>	2.94 (2.06)	21.13	< .001
Self responsible	Were you responsible for what happened or had happened? (1 = not at all responsible, 7 = very responsible)	5.91 (1.40)	=	5.29 (1.90)	2.48	.12
Other responsible	Was someone else responsible for what happened or had happened? (1 = not at all responsible, 7 = very responsible)	3.43 (2.23)	=	3.14 (1.99)	0.32	.573
Circumstances	Was what happened or had happened attributable to circumstances? (1 = not at all, 7 = completely)	3.91 (1.85)	=	3.11 (1.81)	3.34	.072
Familiarity	Had you experienced the situation before, or was it new to you? (1 = experienced before, 7 = new)	4.14 (2.22)	=	4.49 (2.15)	0.43	.514
Time of event	Was your emotion elicited by something that had occurred in the past, occurred now, or was to occur in the future? (1 = in the past, 4 = now, 7 = in the future)	4.23 (1.72)	=	3.91 (1.01)	0.87	.354

Note. Entries are mean responses and standard deviations for items assessing the appraisal of the emotion-eliciting situation (adopted from Frijda et al., 1989). The scales on which the items could be answered ranged from 1 to 7; 4 was the neutral point. Items adapted from Frijda et al. (1989).

TABLE 14.3. Mean Action Readiness Variables and Items Ratings per Regret Condition

Variable	Item	Anticipated M (SD)		Retrospective M (SD)	$F(1,69)$	p
Option knowledge	I wanted to know everything about the different options I considered during the purchase.	4.54 (1.70)	>	3.40 (1.68)	7.97	.006
Comparison	I had the urge to compare all the products with each other.	4.43 (1.82)	>	3.37 (1.80)	5.97	.017
Protection	I wanted to protect myself from someone or something.	4.63 (1.75)	=	3.83 (1.85)	3.44	.068
Rejection	I did not want to have anything to do with someone or something.	2.43 (1.56)	=	2.94 (1.63)	1.83	.181
Understanding	I wanted to pay close attention to understand the situation better.	3.89 (1.78)	=	3.89 (1.68)	0.00	1.000
Don't want	I did not want to be like this, I did not want to exist.	2.09 (1.52)	=	1.97 (1.47)	0.10	.75
Inhibition	I felt inhibited, paralyzed.	2.20 (1.37)	=	2.20 (1.73)	0.00	1.000
Disappear from view	I wanted to disappear, to dissolve into nothingness.	1.71 (1.10)	=	1.74 (1.31)	0.01	.922
Undo	I had the strong urge to do something to undo the situation.	3.83 (1.93)	<	5.43 (1.50)	14.97	< .001
Focus	I wanted to focus all my attention to what happened.	4.29 (1.74)	=	3.60 (1.63)	2.89	.094
Kicking oneself	I felt the urge to kick myself.	3.09 (1.96)	<	4.89 (1.76)	16.32	< .001
Other control	I had the urge to leave things to others regarding what had to be done.	3.74 (2.01)	>	2.14 (1.54)	14.04	< .001
In command	I felt I was in command, I held the ropes.	4.60 (1.54)	=	4.40 (1.68)	0.27	.606
Apathy	I had absolutely no motivation or interest anymore.	2.49 (1.54)	=	2.91 (1.63)	1.28	.263
Do the best	I had the urge to do the best I could do in order to achieve my goals in a better way.	4.51 (1.87)	=	3.83 (1.74)	2.52	.117

Note. Entries are mean responses and standard deviations. Participants indicated the applicability of the action readiness items on 7-point scales, with endpoints labeled *not applicable* (1) and *very much applicable* (7). They were adapted from Frijda et al. (1989).

Let us finally turn to the *action readiness items*. These items reflect the motivational experiences that accompany the emotion. The specific items, and the average ratings for both regret conditions, are shown in Table 14.3. Interestingly, the action readiness items revealed a few more differences than the appraisal items, which might reveal some of the functions of these two states. Here 5 out of the 15 items showed significant differences. Anticipated regret participants reported higher scores on the item tapping Option Knowledge ("I wanted to know everything about the different options I considered during the purchase") and on the item tapping Comparison ("I had the urge to compare all products with each other"). Both items assess a need for information search (cf. Reb, 2008). The participants in the anticipated regret condition also scored higher on the item Other Control ("I had the urge to leave things to others regarding to what had to be done"). Together, these items show an increased readiness to act in order to prevent a bad decision from happening or to ensure that one will not regret the decision by increasing its justifiability. Experienced regret participants reported higher scores on the items tapping Undo ("I had the strong urge to undo the situation") and Kicking Oneself ("I felt the urge to kick myself"), reflecting a stronger focus on what happened, one's causal role in this, and how to deal with it (cf. Breugelmans et al., 2014).

Taken together, this study found some interesting similarities and differences between anticipated and retrospective regret. We found that anticipated regret goes together with other prospective emotions, such as fear, worry and concern, whereas retrospective regret goes together with backward-looking emotions, such as disappointment, dissatisfaction, and frustration. Both experiences have similar appraisal patterns, with understandable differences on pleasantness, expectedness, and modifiability. The associated patterns of action readiness also show a number of similarities. Anticipated and retrospective regret both are experiences that activate and that seem to promote a problem-solving state of mind. It is telling that in both the anticipated regret and retrospective regret conditions, the action readiness items that assess withdrawal or apathy are low, whereas those related to understanding what happened and taking control are relatively high. This clearly shows the pragmatic character of regret. Anticipated and retrospective regret differ with respect to a few items. Undoing and kicking oneself were more strongly associated with retrospective regret, revealing that this emotion stimulates focusing on the forgone and most likely learning from mistakes. Information search and delegating the decision to others was more apparent in anticipated regret, illustrating the fearing-the-future part of this emotion, and the tendencies to cope with that.

REGULATION OF ANTICIPATED REGRET

The study described above was important input for our theory of regret regulation (Pieters & Zeelenberg, 2007; Zeelenberg & Pieters, 2006, 2007, 2008). The core idea in this theory is that decision makers are regret averse. Hence they try to regulate their regrets: Decision makers are motivated to avoid regret, and when it happens despite these attempts, they engage in ameliorative behaviors or manage, deny, or suppress their experience of regret. Our theory is pragmatic; it assumes that "feeling is for doing" (cf. Zeelenberg et al., 2008), and it stresses how emotions exist for the sake of behavioral guidance. Because of that pragmatic approach, we needed to understand what the experience of regret (anticipated and retrospective) entails, which behaviors it motivates, and how it can shape subsequent decision making. That is where the reported study came in handy.

Our regret regulation theory acknowledges that regret bridges the past and the future in the present and incorporates both anticipated and retrospective regret. The different ways in which anticipated and retrospective regret are related to self-regulation might be linked to the work on mental contrasting future and reality (e.g., Oettingen, Pak, & Schnetter, 2001; Oettingen, 2012). Oettingen and colleagues identify various modes of self-regulation. I think that the regulation of anticipated regret is most close to their expectancy-based route to self-regulation. Here, decision makers set and pursue goals by engaging in mental contrasting of fantasies and obstacles in reality. In such contrasting, the question is how to overcome obstacles in the current reality to attain the desired future. When generating these thoughts and fantasies, the first step is to simulate the future, and hence one is also likely to generate futures that incorporate regret. As we found in the section on empirical demonstrations of the impact of anticipated regret on decision making, such anticipations of regret facilitate the outcome that people stick to their intentions and are more successful in self-regulation. Successful self-regulation should equally ensue after people mentally contrast a desired future that is void of regret (e.g., having done everything one can to get a good grade) with obstacles that may stand in the way of achieving this regret-free future (e.g., feeling too shy to ask for help). Such mental contrasting should guarantee both satisfactory decision making (e.g., deciding to approach the professor for help) and the successful prevention of regret.

We have described different regulation strategies that decision makers can engage in to regulate their regrets. The main strategic options for regulation are the same for anticipated and experienced regret, although the specific mechanics differ (see Pieters & Zeelenberg, 2007). We differentiate goal-focused, decision-focused, alternative-focused and feeling-focused regulation strategies.

Goal-focused strategies deal with goal setting and the critical reference value of an outcome (below which one becomes unsatisfied). The strategy to prevent regret is to decrease your goal level, so that regret is less likely. This is consistent with the *bracing for loss* literature (Shepperd, Findley-Klein, Kwavnick, Walker, & Perez, 2000). Bracing refers to decision makers' modifying their expectations about their decision outcomes in order to regulate the negative feelings about those undesired outcomes. Carroll, Sweeny, and Sheppard (2006) apply this to regret and argue that "People may also brace to avoid regret in case their action (or inaction) fails to produce a desired consequence" (p. 63). "With avoiding disappointment or regret, people prepare for the anticipated emotional consequences of an undesired outcome. For example, bracing to avoid disappointment prepares people for the impact of bad news by taking away the element of surprise" (p. 66). Thus regret can be prevented by psychologically preparing for a negative decision outcome via lowering one's goal level.

Decision-focused strategies aim at the decision process and outcome at hand. The strategies in this category focus on the decision process in order to increase decision quality (gathering more information, thinking better, etc.) and decision justifiability (making sure you have good reasons for your decision, sticking to defaults, picking normative choices), to transfer decision responsibility (letting other, more qualified people make the decision), and, finally, to delay or avoid decisions (making no decisions means no regret).

Alternative-focused strategies deal with the rejected alternatives. The strategies in this category focus on the alternatives that are not chosen. Because regret stems from comparing what is to what might have been, these play an important role. The strategies are ensuring decision reversibility (so that you can undo the regret later on, if it happens) and avoiding feedback about forgone alternatives (if you do not know what you miss out on, there is no regret).

Finally, *feeling-focused strategies* cope with the experience of regret directly rather than indirectly, as in the previous ones. Sometimes expecting the worst can, by means of a contrast effect, make the regret feel less intense. This particular strategy might be most helpful after the decision is made and before the outcomes are known. If one trivializes all regrets beforehand, there will be no need anymore to avoid them. This may cause reckless behavior and the associated bad decisions.

These strategies for the regulation of anticipated regret are aimed at preventing regret from happening or at minimizing its potential intensity when it happens. When we first described these strategies (Zeelenberg & Pieters, 2006), we thought they would play an important role in coping with anticipated regret and preventing future regret, but we had not studied these strategies in full. We did not expect that all regulation strategies would be equally successful or equally prevalent. It could even be the case that some of these strategies would actually increase long-term regret (delegating the decision, for example, could result in more self-recrimination if the decision turns out badly).

Bjälkebring and colleagues studied the usage of the different strategies in various samples and found support for the ideas in regret regulation theory (Bjälkebring, Västfjäll, Svenson, & Slovic, 2015; Bjälkebring, Västfjäll, & Boo, 2013; Västfjäll, Peters, & Bjälkebring, 2010). Bjälkebring et al. (2013) studied the regrets and regulation of regrets by younger and older adults and found that older people generally report fewer regrets, both anticipated and retrospectively. Their research indicates that older people delay decisions when they expect regret and that these older adults also expect regret to happen, which dampens it when it actually does. Bjälkebring et al. (2015) reports an 8-day Web-based diary method in which they asked participants about retrospective regrets and anticipated regrets (they refer to these as *experienced* and *forecasted* regrets). They also asked them to indicate to what extent they used different strategies to prevent or regulate regret. They found that participants regretted 30% of their past decisions and forecasted regret in 70% of future decisions. This corresponds to our findings reported earlier, that anticipated regret is more expected and more prevalent. Bjälkebring and colleagues found support for the usage of the different strategies, and they also found that information search and expecting to feel regret are the most efficient strategies for regulating anticipated regret. Overall, these results are promising, and they reveal that regulation and prevention of regret are important strategies in many decisions. But clearly more research is needed to ascertain when which strategy is used and how successful they are.

CODA

It has been long known that anticipated regret can influence the choices that we make. Formal models have been developed to describe how this takes place, and over the last decades there have been ample empirical demonstrations of the effects of anticipated regret. In this chapter I have briefly reviewed this work and presented hitherto unpublished research that shows how anticipated regret is both similar to and different from retrospective regret. This research was input for our integrative theory of regret regulation. Regret is the prototypical decision-related emotion, and anticipated regret draws heavily on our ability to mentally simulate the future. I hope that a better understanding of the psychological processes underlying the anticipation of regret will result in an improved understanding of how we make decisions and how we cope with the uncertain future.

REFERENCES

Abraham, C., & Sheeran, P. (2003). Acting on intentions: The role of anticipated regret. *British Journal of Social Psychology, 42,* 495–511.
Acker, M. A. (1997). Tempered regrets under total ignorance. *Theory and Decision, 42,* 207–213.
Ajzen, I. (1991). The theory of planned behavior. *Organizational Behavior and Human Decision Processes, 50,* 179–211.
Bell, D. E. (1982). Regret in decision making under uncertainty. *Operations Research, 30,* 961–981.
Bjälkebring, P., Västfjäll, D., & Boo, J. (2013). Regulation of experienced and anticipated regret for daily decisions in younger and older adults in a Swedish one-week diary study. *Journal of Gerontopsychology and Geriatric Psychiatry, 26,* 233–241.
Bjälkebring, P., Västfjäll, D., Svenson, O., & Slovic, P. (2015). Regulation of experienced and anticipated regret in daily decision making. *Emotion, 16,* 381–386.
Bleichrodt, H., & Wakker, P. P. (2015). Regret theory: A bold alternative to the alternatives. *Economic Journal, 125,* 493–532.
Boles, T. L., & Messick, D. M. (1995). A reverse outcome bias: The influence of multiple reference points on the evaluation of outcomes and decisions. *Organizational Behavior and Human Decision Processes, 61,* 262–275.
Bougie, R., Pieters, R., & Zeelenberg, M. (2003). Angry customers don't come back, they get back: The experience and behavioral implications of anger and dissatisfaction in services. *Journal of the Academy of Marketing Sciences, 31,* 377–391.
Bourgeois-Gironde, S. (2010). Regret and the rationality of choices. *Philosophical Transactions of the Royal Society B: Biological Sciences, 365,* 249–257.
Breugelmans, S. M., Zeelenberg, M., Gilovich, T., Huang, W.-H., & Shani, Y. (2014). Generality and cultural variation in the experience of regret. *Emotion, 14,* 1037–1048.
Brewer, N. T., DeFrank, J. T., & Gilkey, M. B. (2016). Anticipated regret and health behavior: A meta-analysis. *Health Psychology, 35,* 1264–1275.
Cadish, B. (2001). *Damn!: Reflections on life's biggest regrets.* Kansas City, MO: Andrews McMeel.
Carmon, Z., & Ariely, D. (2000). Focusing on the forgone: Why value can appear so different to buyers and sellers. *Journal of Consumer Research, 2,* 360–370.
Carmon, Z., Wertenbroch, K., & Zeelenberg, M. (2003). Option attachment: When deliberating makes choosing feel like losing. *Journal of Consumer Research, 30,* 15–29.

Carroll, P., Sweeny, K., & Shepperd, J. A. (2006). Forsaking optimism. *Review of General Psychology, 10,* 56–73.

Croy, G., Gerrans, P., & Speelman, C. P. (2015). A mediating role for anticipated regret in predicting retirement savings intention between groups with (without) past behaviour. *Australian Journal of Psychology, 67,* 87–96.

Fernandez-Duque, D., & Landers, J. (2008). "Feeling more regret than I would have imagined": Self-report and behavioral evidence. *Judgment and Decision Making, 3,* 449–456.

Frijda, N. H. (2007). *The laws of emotion.* New York: Erlbaum.

Frijda, N. H., Kuipers, P., & Ter Schure, E. (1989). Relations among emotion, appraisal, and emotional action readiness. *Journal of Personality and Social Psychology, 57,* 212–228.

Gollwitzer, P. M., & Sheeran, P. (2006). Implementation intentions and goal achievement: A meta-analysis of effects and processes. *Advances in Experimental Social Psychology, 38,* 69–119.

Gollwitzer, P. M., Wieber, F., Meyers, A. L., & McCrea, S. M. (2010). How to maximize implementation intention effects. In C. R. Agnew, D. E. Carlston, W. G. Graziano, & J. R. Kelly (Eds.), *Then a miracle occurs: Focusing on behavior in social psychological theory and research* (pp. 137–161). New York: Oxford University Press.

Hozo, I., & Djulbegovic, B. (2008). When is diagnostic testing inappropriate or irrational?: Acceptable regret approach. *Medical Decision Making, 28,* 540–553.

Inman, J. J., Dyer, J. S., & Jia, J. (1997). A generalized utility model of disappointment and regret effects on post-choice valuation. *Marketing Science, 16,* 97–111.

Inman, J. J., & McAlister, L. (1994). Do coupon expiration dates affect consumer behavior? *Journal of Marketing Research, 16,* 423–428.

Inman, J. J., & Zeelenberg, M., (2002). Regret in repeat purchase versus switching decisions: The attenuating role of decision justifiability. *Journal of Consumer Research, 29,* 116–128.

Janis, I. L., & Mann, L. (1977). *Decision making.* New York: Free Press.

Kahneman, D. (2000). Preface. In D. Kahneman & A. Tversky (Eds.), *Choices, values and frames* (pp. ix–xvii). New York: Cambridge University Press.

Kahneman, D. (2011). *Thinking, fast and slow.* New York: Farrar, Strauss, & Giroux.

Kahneman, D., & Tversky, A. (1979). Prospect theory: An analysis of decision under risk. *Econometrica, 47,* 263–292.

Kahneman, D., & Tversky, A. (1982a). The psychology of preferences. *Scientific American, 246,* 160–173.

Kahneman, D., & Tversky, A. (1982b). The simulation heuristic. In D. Kahneman, P. Slovic, & A. Tversky (Eds.), *Judgment under uncertainty: Heuristics and biases* (pp. 201–208). New York: Cambridge University Press.

Kleinginna, P. R., & Kleinginna, A. M. (1981). A categorized list of emotion definitions, with suggestions for a consensual definition. *Motivation and Emotion, 5,* 345–379.

Kmietowicz, Z. W., & Pearman, A. D. (1981). *Decision theory and incomplete knowledge.* Aldershot, UK: Gower.

Koch, E. J. (2014). How does anticipated regret influence health and safety decisions?: A literature review. *Basic and Applied Social Psychology, 36,* 397–412.

Landman, J. (1993). *Regret: The persistence of the possible.* New York: Oxford University Press.

Loewenstein, G. F., Weber, E. U., Hsee, C. K., & Welch, N. (2001). Risk as feelings. *Psychological Bulletin, 127,* 267–286.

Loomes, G., & Sugden, R. (1982). Regret theory: An alternative theory of rational choice under uncertainty. *Economic Journal, 92,* 805–824.

Mellers, B. A., Schwartz, A., & Ritov, I. (1999). Emotion-based choice. *Journal of Experimental Psychology: General, 128,* 1–14.

Oettingen, G. (2012). Future thought and behaviour change. *European Review of Social Psychology, 23,* 1–63.

Oettingen, G., Pak, H., & Schnetter, K. (2001). Self-regulation of goal setting: Turning free fantasies about the future into binding goals. *Journal of Personality and Social Psychology, 80,* 736–753.

Pieters, R., & Zeelenberg, M. (2007). A theory of regret regulation 1.1. *Journal of Consumer Psychology, 17,* 29–35.

Reb, J. (2008). Regret aversion and decision process quality: Effects of regret salience on decision process carefulness. *Organizational Behavior and Human Decision Processes, 105,* 169–182.

Reber, A. S. (1986). *Dictionary of psychology.* London: Penguin/Viking.

Richard, R., & van der Pligt, J. (1991). Factors affecting condom use among adolescents *Journal of Community and Applied Social Psychology, 1,* 105–116.

Roese, N. J. (2005). *If only: How to turn regret into opportunity.* New York: Broadway Books.

Roseman, I. J. (1984). Cognitive determinants of emotions: A structural theory. In P. Shaver (Ed.), *Review of personality and social psychology* (Vol. 5, pp. 11–36). Berkeley, CA: SAGE.

Roseman, I. J., Wiest, C., & Swartz, T. S. (1994). Phenomenology, behaviors, and goals differentiate discrete emotions. *Journal of Personality and Social Psychology, 67,* 206–211.

Saffrey, C., Roese, N., & Summerville, A. (2008). Praise for regret: People value regret above other negative emotions. *Motivation and Emotion, 32,* 46–54.

Sage, A. P., & White, E. B. (1983). Decision and information structures in regret models of judgment and choice. *IEEE Transactions on Systems, Man, and Cybernetics, 13,* 136–145.

Sandberg, T., & Conner, M. (2008). Anticipated regret as an additional predictor in the theory of planned behaviour: A meta-analysis. *British Journal of Social Psychology, 47,* 589–606.

Savage, L. J. (1951). The theory of statistical decision. *Journal of the American Statistical Association, 46,* 55–67.

Scherer, K. R., Schorr, A., & Johnstone, T. (Eds.). (2001). *Appraisal processes in emotion: Theory, methods, research.* New York: Oxford University Press.

Shepperd, J. A., Findley-Klein, C., Kwavnick, K. D., Walker, D., & Perez, S. (2000). Bracing for loss. *Journal of Personality and Social Psychology, 78,* 620–634.

Shimanoff, S. B. (1984). Commonly named emotions in everyday conversations. *Perceptual and Motor Skills, 58,* 514.

Shimanoff, S. B. (1985). Expressing emotions in words: Verbal patterns of interaction. *Journal of Communication, 35,* 16–31.

Simonson, I. (1992). The influence of anticipating regret and responsibility on purchase decisions. *Journal of Consumer Research, 19,* 105–118.

Taylor, K. A. (1997). A regret theory approach to assessing consumer satisfaction. *Marketing Letters, 8,* 229–238.

Taylor, S. E., Pham, L. B., Rivkin, I. D., & Armor, D. A. (1998). Harnessing the imagination: Mental simulation, self-regulation, and coping. *American Psychologist, 53,* 429–439.

Tymstra, T. (1989). The imperative character of medical technology and the meaning of "anticipated decision regret." *International Journal of Technology Assessment in Health Care, 5,* 207–213.

Van de Ven, N., & Zeelenberg, M. (2011). Regret aversion and the reluctance to exchange lottery tickets. *Journal of Economic Psychology, 32,* 194–200.

Van der Pligt, J., Zeelenberg, M., van Dijk, W. W., de Vries, N. K., & Richard, R. (1998). Affect, attitudes and decisions: Let's be more specific. *European Review of Social Psychology, 8,* 33–66.

Van Dijk, W. W., & Zeelenberg, M. (2002). Investigating the appraisal patterns of regret and disappointment. *Motivation and Emotion, 26,* 321–331.

Västfjäll, D., Peters, E., & Bjälkebring, P. (2010). The experience and regulation of regret across the adult life span. In I. Nyklicek, A. Vingerhoets, & M. Zeelenberg (Eds.), *Emotion regulation and well-being* (pp. 165–181). New York: Springer.

Wagenaar, W. A, (1986). My memory: A study of autobiographical memory over six years. *Cognitive Psychology, 18,* 225–252.

Wagenaar, W. A. (1992). Remembering my worst sins: How autobiographical memory serves the updating of the conceptual self. In M. A. Conway, D. C. Rubin, H. Spinnler, & W. A. Wagenaar (Eds.), *Theoretical perspectives on autobiographical memory* (pp. 263–274). Amsterdam, The Netherlands: Kluwer.

Wilson, T. D., & Gilbert, D. T. (2003). Affective forecasting. In M. Zanna (Ed.), *Advances in experimental social psychology* (Vol. 35, pp. 345–411). New York: Elsevier.

Wolfson, S., & Briggs, P. (2002). Locked into gambling: Anticipatory regret as a motivator for playing the National Lottery. *Journal of Gambling Studies, 18,* 1–17.

Zeelenberg, M. (1999). The use of crying over spilled milk: A note on the rationality and functionality of regret. *Philosophical Psychology, 13,* 326–340.

Zeelenberg, M. (2015). Robust satisficing via regret minimizing. *Journal of Marketing Behavior, 1,* 157–166.

Zeelenberg, M. (2018). Anticipated regret. In R. Parrott (Ed.), *Oxford encyclopedia of health and risk message design and processing.* New York: Oxford University Press.

Zeelenberg, M., Nelissen, R. M. A., Breugelmans, S. M., & Pieters, R. (2008). On emotion specificity in decision making: Why feeling is for doing. *Judgment and Decision Making, 3,* 18–27.

Zeelenberg, M., & Pieters, R. (1999). Comparing service delivery to what might have been: Behavioral responses to regret and disappointment. *Journal of Service Research, 2,* 86–97.

Zeelenberg, M., & Pieters, R. (2004a). Beyond valence in customer dissatisfaction: A review and new findings on behavioral responses to regret and disappointment in failed services. *Journal of Business Research, 57,* 445–455.

Zeelenberg, M., & Pieters, R. (2004b). Consequences of regret aversion in real life: The case of the Dutch postcode lottery. *Organizational Behavior and Human Decision Processes, 93,* 155–168.

Zeelenberg, M., & Pieters, R. (2006). Looking backward with an eye on the future: Propositions toward a theory of regret regulation. In L. J. Sanna & E. C. Chang (Eds.), *Judgments over time: The interplay of thoughts, feelings, and behaviors* (pp. 210–229). New York: Oxford University Press.

Zeelenberg, M., & Pieters, R. (2007). A theory of regret regulation 1.0. *Journal of Consumer Psychology, 17,* 3–18.

Zeelenberg, M., & Pieters, R. (2008). On the consequences of mentally simulating future forgone outcomes: A regret regulation perspective. In K. D. Markman, W. M. P. Klein, & J. A. Suhr (Eds.), *The handbook of imagination and mental simulation* (pp. 417–428). New York: Psychology Press.

Zeelenberg, M., Van der Pligt, J., & Manstead, A. S. R. (1998). Undoing regret on Dutch television: Apologizing for interpersonal regrets involving actions and inactions. *Personality and Social Psychology Bulletin, 24,* 1113–1119.

Zeelenberg, M., Van Dijk, W. W., & Manstead, A. S. R. (2003, August). Fearing the future vs. focusing on the forgone: Investigating anticipatory and retrospective regrets. In T. Gärling (Chair), *Anticipatory and anticipated emotions in decision making.* Symposium conducted at the SPUDM-19 Conference, Zurich, Switzerland.

CHAPTER 15

Thinking about the Future
A Construal Level Theory Perspective

Michael Gilead
Yaacov Trope
Nira Liberman

After millions of years of gradual upgrades, humans now come fully equipped with biological machinery that allows them to identify all sorts of events that occur in their environment. This ability is very useful, because humans also come with machinery that efficiently uses the knowledge that was extracted from their surroundings in order to guide behavior. For example, without much ingenuity and effort on their part, they have a sense of smell that can detect the existence of nearby pizza and a control of limbs that allow them to approach and consume it. And yet, although this machinery provides access to plenty of valuable information, there is much more going on in the world than these built-in features currently detect.

A *Homo erectus* would have had a much better chance to survive and reproduce if one day she would awake knowing that behind the hill, a place she has never visited, there is an orchard with tasty fruit; that she should not trust this knowledge to her friend, because she will tell everyone else and deplete the orchard; that next year, there is a 50% chance that a tornado will destroy the orchard, so she should exploit it as fast as she can. Such knowledge, however, is out of reach, mainly because it is not part of direct experience. Within construal level theory (CLT; Trope & Liberman, 2010; Liberman & Trope, 2008, 2014), the above-mentioned epistemic obstacles are called *dimensions of psychological distance*. Liberman and Trope argued that much of the ignorance that humans face in their daily lives is due to *spatial distance, temporal distance, hypotheticality* (uncertainty about the ontological status of things), or *social distance*.

Several theories of prospective cognition (e.g., Bar, 2009; Schacter, Addis, & Buckner, 2007; Suddendorf & Corballis, 2007; Gilbert & Wilson, 2007) have stressed that the ability to predict the future is what led to proto-humans' evolutionary success. In short, the person who was about to enter a grizzly bear's cave but suddenly gained a glimpse into the unfortunate result of such an action would have survived his future-myopic friend. As such, these theories argue that the ultimate function of cognition is to predict the future (see Bar, 2011). CLT is consistent with these theories. It suggests, however, that the future is just one of a number of sources of ignorance that humans must cope with. As indicated above, other dimensions of psychological distance (i.e., spatial distance, social distance, hypotheticality) also generate ignorance. Therefore, according to the conceptualization of CLT, cognition is best understood as an attempt to overcome the unknown, rather than an attempt to predict the future. We refer to the process whereby individuals try to traverse the various dimensions of psychological distance as *mental travel*.

Mental travel encompasses traversing the future (which has been addressed in literatures on prospection, e.g., Gilbert & Wilson, 2007; Schacter et al., 2007), traversing of social perspectives (which has been addressed in literatures on perspective taking and theory of mind; for example, Premack & Woodruff, 1978; Epley, Keysar, Van Boven, & Gilovich, 2004; Wimmer & Perner, 1983), and counterfactual reasoning (which has been addressed in literatures on reasoning, problem solving and decision making; e.g., Byrne, 2002; Roese, 1997).

In the current chapter, we describe how this process of mental travel is treated within the framework of CLT. We begin by describing the widespread idea according to which mental travel is accomplished by relying on a process of episodic simulation that includes concrete contextual details; we describe the possible limitations of mental simulation and highlight the alternative to this view, namely, that mental travel often relies on more abstract, decontextualized mental representations. We explicate the tradeoff associated with relying on more abstract and more concrete mental representations during mental travel—a tradeoff which is at the basis of the predictions of CLT. We then review some recent evidence that support the key predictions of CLT, describe how this line of research may inform our understanding of the neural bases of mental travel, and conclude by highlighting how this research informs our understanding of important behavioral phenomena.

HOW DO WE MENTALLY TRAVEL?

Much research in recent years has attempted to delineate the process whereby individuals try to predict future events. It is often assumed that our memories of specific episodes are the critical reservoir of information on which we rely to predict future events (e.g., Schacter et al., 2007; Suddendorf & Corballis, 2007). A central principle in many theories is that mental time travel is done by using our episodic memories to "simulate" future events. For example, when John is considering whether he should call or text Dana, with whom he went on a date yesterday, he could "run a simulation" of the conversation: "The phone is ringing, no one is picking up. I am ending the call. Now I don't know whether she's busy or whether she's not interested. This is very stressful." Having simulated this occurrence, John might decide that his best course of action is to send a text message on Facebook so that he can see whether she read the message or not.

When a simulation is vivid and detailed enough so that it bears resemblance to reality, many cognitive processes that respond to occurrences in the real world will "go online." The simulation may activate within us mechanisms that generate affective and motivational states, it may activate behavioral schemas and scripts that are associated with the event we are simulating, and it may give rise to various cognitions that typically emerge in such events. Once these processes have occurred, we just need to self-reflect on our affect, behavior, and cognition, and we can assess whether this simulated scenario is in line with our goals or not. In other words, by "running a simulation," the person performing it can generate new knowledge about the future situation.

For example, in order to decide whether I would like to have a business meeting at the neighborhood café, I might build on episodic memories of past experiences there to simulate entering it, hearing the familiar noise and smelling the bakery, meeting friends and neighbors and feeling embarrassed by their gaze. I might simulate ordering my usual coffee and croissant and, while enjoying my beloved drink, also dealing with the many crumbs the croissant leaves on the business papers. Upon considering all these, I might decide to look for a better place.

SIMULATION CAN BE PROBLEMATIC

Although mental simulation can be an effective way of mental travel, it has some underappreciated caveats. When I imagine being chased by a tiger, or when I read about a person running away from a tiger, I should not confuse these thoughts with the presence of an actual tiger, as the appropriate and adaptive reaction is quite different depending on whether one is dealing with a real or imagined predator. However, research on simulation processes (see Barsalou, 2008, for a review) tells us that these different reactions share some similarities such that simulating events activate the perceptual and motor networks that typically become activated when we encounter a real tiger. For example, research has shown that merely reading the word *tiger* activates an actual avoidance response (Chen & Bargh, 1999) and that language comprehension recruits brain regions that process sensorimotor experience (e.g., Hauk, Johnsrude, & Pulvermüller, 2004). Thus it could have been easy to confuse representations with reality.

Although individuals who do not suffer from psychosis do not typically confuse real experiences with imagined ones, there are cases in which such confusions do occur. Evidence within reality monitoring theory (Johnson & Raye, 1981) suggests that more concrete, vivid representations are more readily confused with reality (and thus are more likely to create false memories) than more abstract representations. For example, the more people imagine an event in vivid and concrete details, including time and place, sensory details (sound and touch), and motor actions, the more they are likely to confuse this imaginary event with an event that really happened (e.g., Goff & Roediger, 1998). Similarly, neuroimaging evidence from individuals with schizophrenia reveals that their auditory hallucinations are caused by the reactivation of early auditory cortex regions that subserve hearing actual real-world voices (Dierks et al., 1999).

Gilead, Liberman, and Maril (2012, 2013) suggested that a critical function of abstract (vs. more concrete, vivid) mental representations is that they enable a separation of reality from imagination. According to this view, the strength of abstract representations is their possible low correlation with their referents. For example, the concept *animal* might refer to many instances of real-world experiences with animals. Thus, when one activates this concept in mind, this activation will diffuse across innumerable specific experiences with cats, dogs, birds, and so on, supplying each of them with a small amount of activation. Activating the concept *Danny's dog when he was a puppy* will excite a more limited set of representations, supposedly allowing a more vivid mental image that would be more readily confused with actually seeing the dog.

Indeed, functional magnetic resonance imaging (fMRI) evidence (Van Dam, Rueschemeyer, & Bekkering, 2010) suggests that the abstractness of described motor sentences (i.e., "Clean the table"—which is an activity that can be performed in any number of ways—vs. "Wipe the table") modulates the degree to which imagery-related motor-cortex activity is recorded. Thus, the generality and lack of specificity inherent to abstraction might serve to attenuate activation of specific experiential instances, and doing so creates a much needed buffer between reality and its representation.

Supporting this notion, research found that when people strategically encode a counterfactual (vs. factual) scenario for a future memory test, they tend to omit the perceptual details of the event (Gilead et al., 2012; Wakslak, Trope, Liberman, & Alony, 2006). Furthermore, evidence from neuroimaging studies (Tettamanti et al., 2008; Gilead et al., 2013) shows that activation within sensorimotor cortical regions is diminished whenever people contemplate counterfactual (vs. factual) scenarios.

THERE ARE ALTERNATIVES TO MENTAL SIMULATION

Despite a strong emphasis in the recent literature on the importance of simulation in prospection (e.g., Moulton & Kosslyn, 2009; Barsalou, 2009; Schacter et al., 2007; Gilbert & Wilson, 2007), it is clearly not the only way by which mental travel occurs. Rather, people can mentally travel by using inference processes such as thinking by analogy (e.g., Gentner & Medina, 1998) and logical deduction (e.g., Goodwin & Johnson-Laird, 2013; Evans, 2003).

For example, consider the case of a prime minister facing a crisis of increasing military tension with a foreign country. The prime minister tries to predict which action would reduce the risk of war. One possibility is to remain unyielding, hopefully deterring opponent countries from further provocation; a second possibility is to offer concessions, hoping that they would alleviate the tensions. The prime minister may begin by considering a series of propositions: "My opponent cares about staying in power"; "A military strike will hurt rather than help his ability to stay in power"; therefore, "He is likely bluffing; if I stand my ground there's a good possibility that the situation will be resolved." Clearly, the prime minister can also simulate the scenarios (i.e., "I am giving a speech on TV, I am sitting in my office, drinking a glass of water . . . I am nervous"); however, such a simulation is not mandatory.

The distinction between logical inference and simulation has been the subject of much discussion in the literature on mentalizing/theory of mind reasoning (Flavell, 1999; Gordon, 1986; Gallese & Goldman, 1998; Gilead et al., 2016), which, in the terminology of CLT, can be seen as the attempt to mentally travel across the barrier of social distance. However, this discussion has been relatively neglected in the literature on humans' capacity to reason about future events, which highlights the simulation process, but not theory-based inference processes (but see Szpunar, Spreng, & Schacter, 2014, for a notable exception).

Whereas the type of mental travel that occurs via simulation is believed to necessarily rely on contextualized, detailed, and vivid mental representations that resemble reality (i.e., on "episodic memory"), inference-based processes are more flexible in that they can rely on more abstract, decontextualized mental representations (i.e., on "semantic" memory). As we now discuss, the degree to which the mental traveler utilizes concrete (vs. abstract) mental representations could be highly consequential.

The Tradeoff between Accuracy and Detail

Astrologers have long noticed that it can be very easy to predict the future. For example, it can be predicted with near certainty that "sometimes in the next week you will experience an affective state, you will attempt to achieve some goal, and you will consume nutrients." These predictions are likely to be accurate, because they are so general that they pertain to innumerable different instances. However, such predictions will not provide you with much useful information to guide your behavior.

In contrast, consider a prediction according to which "next Tuesday you will sit on the train next to a 52-year-old Latvian orthodontist; he will sneeze in your direction, which will result in you catching the flu virus." If this prediction is accurate, it is very useful—it will mean that you should be watchful on your Tuesday train ride. However, the specificity of such a prediction renders it very unlikely to be accurate (unless it turns out that you have specific intelligence regarding a conspiracy by Latvian orthodontists to infect train passengers on Tuesday).

Thus, a central challenge in the attempt to deal with the unknowability of life is generating a mental representation that is both general enough so that it pertains to a variety of possible events and specific enough so that it produces actionable recommendations to guide behavior. Thus the mental traveler needs to optimize a tradeoff between accuracy and detail (or in the terminology of Goldsmith, Koriat, & Weinberg-Eliezer, 2002, the tradeoff between accuracy and the grain size; see also Rosch, Mervis, Gray, Johnson, & Boyesbraem, 1976).

How can a mental traveler set the optimal goal for level of accuracy and detail? One important clue that he or she can use is the level of information currently at hand. For example, if I know that you are a white male from Ohio who always voted for the Republican candidate, I can predict with reasonable certainty that you will vote for the Republican nominee again, although it will be difficult for me to know whether you oppose same-sex marriage or not. If I also know that you are very religious and oppose gun legislation, I can venture and predict that you oppose same-sex marriage. Thus the mental traveler should always evaluate the degree of knowledge she or he currently has before venturing to make highly specific bets.

Based on this rationale, CLT suggests that when people think about objects that are psychologically distant—and, therefore, likely to be more unknowable—the optimum in terms of the tradeoff between level of accuracy and detail will shift toward a lower emphasis on the latter. For example, if the temperature right now is 80 degrees, I can generate a relatively specific prediction for the next hour (e.g., it's going to be between 75 and 85 degrees). However, the temperature in the more distant future (e.g., a week from now) is much less knowable; therefore, if I try to generate a specific prediction, I am much more likely to err. Generating a more general prediction seems to be a better strategy in that situation (Kruger, Fiedler, Koch, & Alves, 2014).

To further exemplify the rationale behind CLT, imagine that you live in a city where pickpockets focus on stealing and selling cellular phones. If you are now traveling to a neighboring city, you might be advised to pay attention to your phone. However, if you are traveling to a different continent altogether, it is possible that in this distant place pickpockets are more interested in stealing wallets, cameras, or jewelry. In light of this, it is advisable for you to expect the unexpected and to be watchful of your *belongings,* rather than being watchful of your *cell phone.* These more abstract and general representations are referred to within CLT as "high-level construals" and are contrasted with more concrete and detailed "low-level construals" (see Shapira, Liberman, Trope, & Rim, 2012, for further discussion of the notion of level of construal).

The central prediction of CLT is that the behavior of individuals will be consistent with this normative prescription for prediction and mental travel. Namely, that mental travelers will be sensitive to the degree of psychological distance they wish to traverse, such that as psychological distance increases, they will tend to construe psychologically distant entities in a more general and abstract manner.

EVIDENCE FOR THE RELATION BETWEEN PSYCHOLOGICAL DISTANCE AND LEVEL OF CONSTRUAL

Ever since the first publication on CLT (Liberman & Trope, 1998), much research has examined its empirical predictions. A meta-analysis published in 2014 identified 106 published papers and 267 studies that focused on investigating the relation between level of construal and psychological distance (Soderberg, Callahan, Kochersberger, Amit, & Ledgerwood, 2015). This research shows that increasing the psychological distance that individuals try to traverse results in a higher level of construal. Although a comprehensive review of this research is beyond the scope of this chapter (for such reviews, see Soderberg et al., 2015; Liberman & Trope, 2008, 2014; Trope & Liberman, 2003, 2010), we now briefly describe a few recent examples of empirical research into the predictions of CLT.

Two recent studies (i.e., Snefjella & Kuperman, 2015; Bhatia & Walasek, 2016) have sought to examine the predictions of CLT by using publicly accessible "big data" corpora of natural language use. In Snefjella and Kuperman (2015), the authors used a dataset that included millions of messages posted on online social network sites (e.g., "tweets" posted on the social network Twitter). Relying on concreteness norms of 40,000 English words (Brysbaert, Warriner, & Kuperman, 2014), the authors automatically assessed the linguistic concreteness of each of the messages. Next, the authors used automated text analysis to investigate how the psychological distance from the referents described in the messages relates to linguistic concreteness.

In the domain of temporal distance, the authors compared the level of concreteness in messages that contained the terms *minutes from now, hours from now, months from now,* and so forth; similarly, they compared the concreteness of message that contained terms such as *yesterday, last week, last month,* and so forth. In the domain of spatial distance, the authors examined the distance between the Global Positioning System (GPS) coordinate from which a tweet was sent and the GPS coordinate of a location referred to in the message. In the domain of social distance, the authors compared the concreteness of messages that referred to family members (e.g., husband, wife, spouse), friends (e.g., friend, ally), coworkers, and so forth.

Across the temporal, spatial, and social distance, the results showed that references to more distal objects decreased linguistic concreteness; more specifically, linguistic concreteness seems to be a curvilinear function of the logarithm of psychological distance. Replicating these results, a study by Bhatia and Walasek (2016) that relied on an automated analysis of additional big datasets (e.g., texts in news articles) also concluded that concreteness is a curvilinear function of distance and may be specifically best described as an exponential function.

Both the studies of Snefjella and Kuperman (2015) and Bhatia and Walasek, (2016) examined the context wherein individuals think and write *about* psychologically distant entities. Another interesting context wherein recent research has investigated the predictions of CLT examines the context wherein individuals communicate *with* psychologically distant recipients.

For example, in an experiment by Joshi, Wakslak, Raj, and Trope (2016, Study 2), students were asked to describe a day in their lives to incoming students who would be joining their school. In the proximal condition, the incoming student was from their own state, and in the distal condition, the student was from a geographically distant state. The authors analyzed the level of concreteness of the descriptions provided by the students using a validated coding scheme (the linguistic categorization model; Coenen, Hedebouw, & Semin, 2006). As predicted, the results showed that when participants wrote a message to a student residing in a faraway state, they used more abstract descriptions.

Similarly, in an experiment by Amit, Wakslak, and Trope (2013, Experiment 4), participants were asked to describe themselves to a fellow participant in the experiment, who would read their message either in a few minutes or in 3 months' time. They were to introduce themselves by selecting various symbols of objects that they liked and that represented who they were (e.g., bikes, books). Half of the objects were presented in a concrete medium—by presenting the visual image of the object (e.g., a picture of a book)—and half of the object symbols were presented in a more abstract medium—by using a verbal category label (e.g., the word "books"). The results showed that when participants believed that their message would be read in the distant future, they preferred to use the more abstract medium (i.e., verbal labels), and when they believed their message would be read in the near future, they preferred to use the more concrete medium (i.e., visual symbols).

Importantly, the effects of psychological distance on construal level are not limited to communicative–interpersonal contexts but primarily reflect intrapersonal cognitive processes (Soderberg et al., 2015). A demonstration of this comes from a series of experiments by Kruger et al. (2014). In these studies, participants were asked to generate assessments of various magnitudes by giving a sort of "confidence interval" (i.e., giving an assessment of the minimal and maximal magnitudes). The findings revealed that when the quantities that were to be assessed were described as physically distant (e.g., the length of bridges that were described to American participants as being in France or in the United States; the number of food items in a bowl that were described as an American or a French cuisine), participants gave less specific estimates of magnitudes (i.e., broader confidence intervals). Participants also provided less specific estimates when psychological distance was manipulated on the dimension of hypotheticality (e.g., whether a drawing of a bridge mentioned that it already existed, or that it was only currently a blueprint).

THE NEURAL MECHANISMS OF MENTAL TRAVEL AND THEIR RELATION TO REPRESENTATIONAL ABSTRACTNESS

Considerable research has investigated the neural bases of various types of mental travel across different dimensions of psychological distance, such as thinking about the future (e.g., Addis, Wong, & Schacter, 2007), imagining hypothetical scenarios (e.g., Hassabis, Kumaran, & Maguire, 2007), and taking the perspective of others (e.g., Mitchell, Banaji, & Macrae, 2005). This research suggests that, indeed, it seems appropriate to consider different types of mental travel as sharing an important common denominator. Across these different lines of research, the neural activity associated with mental travel seemed to focus in regions of the so-called default-mode network (Raichle et al., 2001), and especially in the medial prefrontal cortex, posterior cingulate cortex, and the temporoparietal junction (see Gilead et al., 2013; Spreng, Mar, & Kim, 2009, for meta-analyses).

Early research on the default network has suggested that activation in this network is higher when participants are resting idly in the scanner. This led researchers to believe that activity in this network may reflect the baseline state of the brain, whenever it is not interrupted by demanding cognitive functioning (Raichle et al., 2001). Later research gradually acknowledged that our cognition is never really idle and suggested that default network activity is related to cognitive processes that are engaged when participants' minds wander (Mason et al., 2007), such as episodic memory retrieval (Buckner & Carroll, 2007). In light of this, much of the literature on prospective mind has taken the involvement of the default network as evidence that mental travel occurs via a process of "episodic simulation" of the type described in earlier sections.

And yet, more recent evidence suggests that the default network also subserves the processing of more decontextualized and abstract mental representation (i.e., semantic rather than episodic memory). A comprehensive meta-analysis of functional neuroimaging studies of semantic processing (Binder, Desai, Graves, & Conant, 2009) concluded that semantic processing occurs within a distributed network of regions, which includes the posterior inferior parietal lobe, the middle temporal gyrus, the fusiform and parahippocampal gyri in the medial temporal lobe, the dorsomedial prefrontal cortex, the inferior frontal gyrus, the ventromedial prefrontal cortex, and the posterior cingulate gyrus. This network broadly overlaps with the default network—however, the default network also typically includes the hippocampus (e.g., Buckner, Andrews-Hanna, & Schacter, 2008).

Attempts at finer-grained analysis of the default network suggested that it may encompass a distinct subsystem (i.e., the medial temporal lobe subsystem), which includes the hippocampus, parahippocampal cortex, the retrosplenial cortex, and the posterior inferior parietal lobule (e.g., Yeo et al., 2011)—and also, possibly, the ventral aspects of the medial prefrontal cortex (Andrews-Hanna, Reidler, Sepulcre, Poulin, & Buckner, 2010). Further supporting the possible functional importance of this subsystem, neuroimaging research on episodic memory (e.g., Kim, 2016) suggests that, although both semantic and episodic memory rely on the default network, accessing episodic memories relies to a greater extent on the medial–temporal lobe subsystems.

Based on this evidence, it appears likely that the best available description of default network functionality pertains to the representational capacities it affords (e.g., Binder et al., 2009) and that these capacities subserve its involvement in mental travel. Whenever we see that the medial–temporal subsystem of the default network is involved in mental travel, this may reflect the involvement of detailed episodic simulation processes. However, whenever this medial–temporal activity is not present, this might mean that mental travel occurred via an inferential process that relies on more abstract mental representations.

Based on CLT, we could predict that whenever individuals think about more proximal individuals, times, and places or of events that are less hypothetical, we should see greater involvement of the medial–temporal lobe subnetwork of the default network. Partly supporting this prediction, Tamir and Mitchell (2011) have found that thinking of psychologically proximal events across all different distance dimensions (temporal, social, spatial, and hypotheticality) recruit parts of the medial–temporal subsystem (the retrosplenial cortex and the ventral medial prefrontal cortex).

Furthermore, the medial temporal subsystem was shown to be active when reading sentences that describe psychologically proximal (vs. distal) events (Gilead et al., 2013) and is reliably implicated in processing concrete (vs. abstract) language (see the meta-analysis of concrete language processing by Wang, Conder, Blitzer, & Shinkareva, 2010). Thus evidence converges to highlight that mental travel can rely on more concrete, episodic, and detailed representations, but that such information may be omitted when considering psychologically distant events.

CONSEQUENCES OF THE RELATION BETWEEN PSYCHOLOGICAL DISTANCE AND LEVEL OF CONSTRUAL

So far we have discussed the cognitive and neural bases of mental travel, focusing on the assertions of CLT concerning the relation between psychological distance and representational abstractness. In the last section of the chapter, we discuss some of the behavioral consequences associated with increased psychological distance and with higher level of construal.

Consider an example of two analysts at an investment firm, trying to decide whether to recommend investing in coal or in green energy. The elections are coming up soon, and the Democratic candidate promised to support the green energy industry, whereas the Republican candidate promised to support the coal industry.

In light of this, the two analysts are trying to build a model to predict the outcome of the election. Both of them know that in previous elections, polling data (which now favor the Democratic candidate) and job growth data (which now favor the Republican candidate) were predictive of election outcomes. Analyst A decides to generate the most detailed model possible and incorporate both job growth data and polling data into the model. Analyst B prefers a parsimonious model and decides to omit job growth data from the model. In such a situation, despite the fact that both analysts had the same data, Analyst A may recommend investing in coal, and Analyst B may recommend investing in green energy. (It's worthwhile to note that both of their decisions are justifiable; sometimes a model that incorporates more predictors will be more successful in predicting future outcomes, whereas at other times such models can run the risk of being overfitted to historical data).

Just like these analysts, the degree to which individuals' mental construals are detailed and rich in information can have different consequences for people's behavior. When we generate construals that are less detailed, we must decide which information to leave out of the picture. To the extent that certain types of information are more readily omitted, this could have important and predictable effects on behavior.

One important regularity is that more abstract construals often retain the features that are considered as being central or defining of the object or event in question. For example, if you ask people "What is a party?", they might tell you that a party is "a fun social gathering with food and drinks." If you continue probing them to generate a more detailed answer, they might get to more incidental/peripheral features, such as "a party is also something that takes a lot of time to organize, entails doing dishes and spending money." Thus, in this case, the more abstract construal is described as a positive event, but the more detailed representation also contains negative features. Such a pattern will entail that when individuals consider the possibility of organizing a party a year from now, they will generate a more abstract construal of the event, which will make it seem like a great idea. When they consider throwing a party 1 week from now, they will generate a more concrete and detailed construal of the event, which now includes the idea of doing dishes. Supporting this intuition, much research on construal level theory has documented how such distant-dependent changes in mental construal can predictably alter individuals' choices across innumerable behavioral contexts (e.g., Trope, Liberman, & Wakslak, 2007; Liberman, Trope, & Wakslak, 2007).

Another way to know what information will be retained as construals become more abstract is to ask what features people consider to be stable and invariant across different contexts. For example, personality traits (e.g., being helpful) could be manifested differently in different contexts (e.g., giving money to charity, helping people who got stuck by the side of the road). Therefore, if you see John giving money to charity, construing this behavior more abstractly will mean retaining a stable trait description (i.e., "John is helpful"). Assuming that you live in New York and you hear that John crossed the bridge to nearby New Jersey and gave money to a beggar there, you might construe John's behavior relatively concretely and predict that he will not help you if you ever got stuck by the side of the road. If, however, you hear that John's charitable behavior occurred in a more distant place (e.g., San Diego), you might conclude that he is just a generally helpful guy and will probably assist you whenever you're in need.

Throughout the years, research within CLT has documented many important behavioral consequences associated with construing events more abstractly or more concretely—in such diverse domains as consumer research (e.g., Trope, Liberman, & Wakslak, 2007), self-regulation (Eyal, Sagristano, Trope, Liberman, & Chaiken, 2009; Fujita, Trope, Liberman, & Levin-Sagi, 2006), person perception (e.g., Rim, Uleman, & Trope, 2009; Eyal & Epley, 2010), and negotiations (De Dreu, Giacomantonio, Shalvi, & Sligte, 2009; Henderson, Trope, & Carnevale, 2006). (For a comprehensive review of this literature we refer the readers to Soderberg et al., 2015; Trope & Liberman, 2003, 2010; Liberman & Trope, 2008, 2014).

SUMMARY

In the current chapter we have outlined construal level theory's perspective on future-oriented cognition. We argued that in order to be able to think about future events, people rely on mental processes that are similar to those involved in traversing other dimensions of psychological distance (e.g., hypotheticality, social distance, spatial distance) and that, despite the importance of episodic simulation processes, mental travel also occurs by relying on inference processes that can utilize relatively abstract and decontextualized mental representation. We described how increasing psychological distance entails relying on mental representations that are increasingly abstract, and we surveyed the behavioral and neural evidence that supports this assertion. Clearly, much more work is needed in order to further understand the higher order cognitive processes that allow us to think about the future. However, based on the past research reviewed herein, there is good reason to predict that future research into future-oriented cognition will continue to bring about exciting ideas and novel discoveries.

ACKNOWLEDGMENT

The work reported in this chapter was supported by Grants No. 2011080 to Nira Liberman and Yaacov Trope, BSF Grant No. 2015258 to Michael Gilead, BSF Grant No. 2016090 to Nira Liberman and Yaacov Trope, and NSF Grant No. BCS 1349067 to Yaacov Trope.

REFERENCES

Addis, D. R., Wong, A. T., & Schacter, D. L. (2007). Remembering the past and imagining the future: Common and distinct neural substrates during event construction and elaboration. *Neuropsychologia, 45*, 1363–1377.

Amit, E., Wakslak, C., & Trope, Y. (2013). The use of visual and verbal means of communication across psychological distance. *Personality and Social Psychology Bulletin, 39*, 43–56.

Andrews-Hanna, J. R., Reidler, J. S., Sepulcre, J., Poulin, R., & Buckner, R. L. (2010). Functional-anatomic fractionation of the brain's default network. *Neuron, 65*, 550–562.

Bar, M. (2009). The proactive brain: Memory for predictions. *Philosophical Transactions of the Royal Society B: Biological Sciences, 364*, 1235–1243.

Bar, M. (Ed.). (2011). *Predictions in the brain: Using our past to generate a future*. New York: Oxford University Press.

Barsalou, L. W. (2008). Grounded cognition. *Annual Review of Psychology, 59,* 617–645.

Barsalou, L. W. (2009). Simulation, situated conceptualization, and prediction. *Philosophical Transactions of the Royal Society B: Biological Sciences, 364,* 1281–1289.

Bhatia, S., & Walasek, L. (2016). Event construal and temporal distance in natural language. *Cognition, 152,* 1–8.

Binder, J. R., Desai, R. H., Graves, W. W., & Conant, L. L. (2009). Where is the semantic system?: A critical review and meta-analysis of 120 functional neuroimaging studies. *Cerebral Cortex, 19,* 2767–2796.

Brysbaert, M., Warriner, A. B., & Kuperman, V. (2014). Concreteness ratings for 40 thousand generally known English word lemmas. *Behavior Research Methods, 46*(3), 904–911.

Buckner, R. L., Andrews-Hanna, J. R., & Schacter, D. L. (2008). The brain's default network: Anatomy, function, and relevance to disease. In A. Kingstone & M. B. Miller (Eds.), *Year in cognitive neuroscience 2008* (Vol. 1124, pp. 1–38). Malden, MA: Wiley-Blackwell.

Buckner, R. L., & Carroll, D. C. (2007). Self-projection and the brain. *Trends in Cognitive Sciences, 11,* 49–57.

Byrne, R. M. J. (2002). Mental models and counterfactual thoughts about what might have been. *Trends in Cognitive Sciences, 6,* 426–431.

Chen, M., & Bargh, J. A. (1999). Consequences of automatic evaluation: Immediate behavioral predispositions to approach or avoid the stimulus. *Personality and Social Psychology Bulletin, 25,* 215–224.

Coenen, L. H. M., Hedebouw, L., & Semin, G. R. (2006). *The linguistic category model (LCM) manual.* Unpublished manuscript.

De Dreu, C. K. W., Giacomantonio, M., Shalvi, S., & Sligte, D. (2009). Getting stuck or stepping back: Effects of obstacles and construal level in the negotiation of creative solutions. *Journal of Experimental Social Psychology, 45,* 542–548.

Dierks, T., Linden, D. E., Jandl, M., Formisano, E., Goebel, R., Lanfermann, H., . . . Singer, W. (1999). Activation of Heschl's gyrus during auditory hallucinations. *Neuron, 22,* 615–621.

Epley, N., Keysar, B., Van Boven, L., & Gilovich, T. (2004). Perspective taking as egocentric anchoring and adjustment. *Journal of Personality and Social Psychology, 87,* 327–339.

Evans, J. S. T. (2003). In two minds: Dual-process accounts of reasoning. *Trends in Cognitive Sciences, 7,* 454–459.

Eyal, T., & Epley, N. (2010). How to seem telepathic: Enabling mind reading by matching construal. *Psychological Science, 21,* 700–705.

Eyal, T., Sagristano, M. D., Trope, Y., Liberman, N., & Chaiken, S. (2009). When values matter: Expressing values in behavioral intentions for the near vs. distant future. *Journal of Experimental Social Psychology, 45,* 35–43.

Flavell, J. H. (1999). Cognitive development: Children's knowledge about the mind. *Annual Review of Psychology, 50,* 21–45.

Fujita, K., Trope, Y., Liberman, N., & Levin-Sagi, M. (2006). Construal levels and self-control. *Journal of Personality and Social Psychology, 90,* 351–367.

Gallese, V., & Goldman, A. (1998). Mirror neurons and the simulation theory of mind-reading. *Trends in Cognitive Sciences, 2,* 493–501.

Gentner, D., & Medina, J. (1998). Similarity and the development of rules. *Cognition, 65,* 263–297.

Gilbert, D. T., & Wilson, T. D. (2007). Prospection: Experiencing the future. *Science, 317,* 1351–1354.

Gilead, M., Boccagno, C., Silverman, M., Hassin, R. R., Weber, J., & Ochsner, K. N. (2016). Self-regulation via neural simulation. *Proceedings of the National Academy of Sciences of the USA, 113,* 10037–10042.

Gilead, M., Liberman, N., & Maril, A. (2012). Construing counterfactual worlds: The role of abstraction. *European Journal of Social Psychology, 42,* 391–397.

Gilead, M., Liberman, N., & Maril, A. (2013). The language of future-thought: An fMRI study of embodiment and tense processing. *NeuroImage, 65,* 267–279.

Goff, L. M., & Roediger, H. L. (1998). Imagination inflation for action events: Repeated imaginings lead to illusory recollections. *Memory and Cognition, 26,* 20–33.

Goldsmith, M., Koriat, A., & Weinberg-Eliezer, A. (2002). Strategic regulation of grain size in memory reporting. *Journal of Experimental Psychology–General, 131,* 73–95.

Goodwin, G. P., & Johnson-Laird, P. N. (2013). The acquisition of Boolean concepts. *Trends in Cognitive Sciences, 17,* 128–133.

Gordon, R. (1986). Folk psychology as simulation. *Mind and Language, 1,* 158–171.

Hassabis, D., Kumaran, D., & Maguire, E. A. (2007). Using imagination to understand the neural basis of episodic memory. *Journal of Neuroscience, 27,* 14365–14374.

Hauk, O., Johnsrude, I., & Pulvermüller, F. (2004). Somatotopic representation of action words in human motor and premotor cortex. *Neuron, 41,* 301–307.

Henderson, M. D., Trope, Y., & Carnevale, P. J. (2006). Negotiation from a near and distant time perspective. *Journal of Personality and Social Psychology, 91,* 712–729.

Johnson, M. K., & Raye, C. L. (1981). Reality monitoring. *Psychological Review, 88,* 67–85.

Joshi, P. D., Wakslak, C. J., Raj, M., & Trope, Y. (2016). Communicating with distant others: The functional use of abstraction. *Social Psychological and Personality Science, 7,* 37–44.

Kim, H. (2016). Default network activation during episodic and semantic memory retrieval: A selective meta-analytic comparison. *Neuropsychologia, 80,* 35–46.

Kruger, T., Fiedler, K., Koch, A. S., & Alves, H. (2014). Response category width as a psychophysical manifestation of construal level and distance. *Personality and Social Psychology Bulletin, 40,* 501–512.

Liberman, N., & Trope, Y. (1998). The role of feasibility and desirability considerations in near and distant future decisions: A test of temporal construal theory. *Journal of Personality and Social Psychology, 75,* 5–18.

Liberman, N., & Trope, Y. (2008). The psychology of transcending the here and now. *Science, 322,* 1201–1205.

Liberman, N., & Trope, Y. (2014). Traversing psychological distance. *Trends in Cognitive Sciences, 18,* 364–369.

Liberman, N., Trope, Y., & Wakslak, C. (2007). Construal level theory and consumer behavior. *Journal of Consumer Psychology, 17,* 113–117.

Mason, M. F., Norton, M. I., Van Horn, J. D., Wegner, D. M., Grafton, S. T., & Macrae, C. N. (2007). Wandering minds: The default network and stimulus-independent thought. *Science, 315,* 393–395.

Mitchell, J. P., Banaji, M. R., & Macrae, C. N. (2005). The link between social cognition and self-referential thought in the medial prefrontal cortex. *Journal of Cognitive Neuroscience, 17,* 1306–1315.

Moulton, S. T., & Kosslyn, S. M. (2009). Imagining predictions: Mental imagery as mental emulation. *Philosophical Transactions of the Royal Society B: Biological Sciences, 364,* 1273–1280.

Premack, D., & Woodruff, G. (1978). Does the chimpanzee have a theory of mind? *Behavioral and Brain Sciences, 1,* 515–526.

Raichle, M. E., MacLeod, A. M., Snyder, A. Z., Powers, W. J., Gusnard, D. A., & Shulman, G. L. (2001). A default mode of brain function. *Proceedings of the National Academy of Sciences of the USA, 98,* 676–682.

Rim, S., Uleman, J. S., & Trope, Y. (2009). Spontaneous trait inference and construal level theory: Psychological distance increases nonconscious trait thinking. *Journal of Experimental Social Psychology, 45,* 1088–1097.

Roese, N. J. (1997). Counterfactual thinking. *Psychological Bulletin, 121,* 133–148.

Rosch, E., Mervis, C. B., Gray, W. D., Johnson, D. M., & Boyesbraem, P. (1976). Basic objects in natural categories. *Cognitive Psychology, 8,* 382–439.

Schacter, D. L., Addis, D. R., & Buckner, R. L. (2007). Remembering the past to imagine the future: The prospective brain. *Nature Reviews Neuroscience, 8,* 657–661.

Shapira, O., Liberman, N., Trope, Y., & Rim, S. (2012). Levels of mental construal. In S. T. Fiske & C. N. Macrae, *SAGE handbook of social cognition* (pp. 229–250). London: SAGE.

Snefjella, B., & Kuperman, V. (2015). Concreteness and psychological distance in natural language use. *Psychological Science, 26,* 1449–1460.

Soderberg, C. K., Callahan, S. P., Kochersberger, A. O., Amit, E., & Ledgerwood, A. (2015). The effects of psychological distance on abstraction: Two meta-analyses. *Psychological Bulletin, 141,* 525–548.

Spreng, R. N., Mar, R. A., & Kim, A. S. (2009). The common neural basis of autobiographical memory, prospection, navigation, theory of mind, and the default mode: A quantitative meta-analysis. *Journal of Cognitive Neuroscience, 21,* 489–510.

Suddendorf, T., & Corballis, M. C. (2007). The evolution of foresight: What is mental time travel, and is it unique to humans? *Behavioral and Brain Sciences, 30,* 299–313.

Szpunar, K. K., Spreng, R. N., & Schacter, D. L. (2014). A taxonomy of prospection: Introducing an organizational framework for future-oriented cognition. *Proceedings of the National Academy of Sciences of the USA, 111,* 18414–18421.

Tamir, D. I., & Mitchell, J. P. (2011). The default network distinguishes construals of proximal versus distal events. *Journal of Cognitive Neuroscience, 23,* 2945–2955.

Tettamanti, M., Manenti, R., Della Rosa, P. A., Falini, A., Perani, D., Cappa, S. F., & Moro, A. (2008). Negation in the brain: Modulating action representations. *NeuroImage, 43,* 358–367.

Trope, Y., & Liberman, N. (2003). Temporal construal. *Psychological Review, 110,* 403–421.

Trope, Y., & Liberman, N. (2010). Construal-level theory of psychological distance. *Psychological Review, 117,* 440–463.

Trope, Y., Liberman, N., & Wakslak, C. (2007). Construal levels and psychological distance: Effects on representation, prediction, evaluation, and behavior. *Journal of Consumer Psychology, 17,* 83–95.

Van Dam, W. O., Rueschemeyer, S.-A., & Bekkering, H. (2010). How specifically are action verbs represented in the neural motor system: An fMRI study. *NeuroImage, 53,* 1318–1325.

Wakslak, C. J., Trope, Y., Liberman, N., & Alony, R. (2006). Seeing the forest when entry is unlikely: Probability and the mental representation of events. *Journal of Experimental Psychology: General, 135,* 641–653.

Wang, J., Conder, J. A., Blitzer, D. N., & Shinkareva, S. V. (2010). Neural representation of abstract and concrete concepts: A meta-analysis of neuroimaging studies. *Human Brain Mapping, 31,* 1459–1468.

Wimmer, H., & Perner, J. (1983). Beliefs about beliefs: Representation and constraining function of wrong beliefs in young children's understanding of deception. *Cognition, 13,* 103–128.

Yeo, B. T. T., Krienen, F. M., Sepulcre, J., Sabuncu, M. R., Lashkari, D., Hollinshead, M., . . . Buckner, R. L. (2011). The organization of the human cerebral cortex estimated by intrinsic functional connectivity. *Journal of Neurophysiology, 106,* 1125–1165.

CHAPTER 16

Perceiving Future Time across Adulthood

Frieder R. Lang
Franziska Damm

Temporal experience is part and parcel of human development across the lifespan. It reflects an individual's sense of change or stability over the course of his or her life. Any passing of time over the life course extends from a definable and remembered past to an unknown and undefined future of one's remaining life. Temporal characteristics of future time with regard to an individual's life course exist purely in the mind as a subjective construal or as a fantasy that may or may not turn out to be realistic, accurate, or adaptive with regard to functional outcomes (Lang, Weiss, Gerstorf, & Wagner, 2013; Oettingen, 2012; Oettingen & Mayer, 2002). This chapter focuses on the adaptive role of future-related temporal experience across adulthood. We review in what ways perceptions of future time contribute to adaptation processes across adulthood, as aging-related challenges often involve a change of perspectives toward one's personal future. For example, retirement is known to be associated with anticipating an increased wealth of time, more control over time use, or being freed from time pressure (Ekerdt & Koss, 2016; Münch, 2016). In this chapter, it is considered whether and to what extent the subjective construal of future time involves context-related adaptation to changing gain-loss dynamics across adulthood. Perceptions of future time (PFT) are defined as a multidimensional construct that involves a broad set of time-associated cognitions related to the finitude, pace, and valence of an individual's remaining time in life. Specifically, it is argued that the dimensional patterns of how individuals age differentially perceive future time reflects adaptive cognitive strategies that may protect against aging-related losses and threats associated with the finitude of life.

PFT comprise a diversity of phenomena in human cognition and behavior: They build on the human awareness of the finitude of life and on the human capacity to anticipate the future (Carstensen, 2006; Hoppmann, Infurna, Ram, & Gerstorf, 2015; Kastenbaum, 1961; Lang, 2000; Nuttin, 1985). Moreover, perceptions of future time have a strong impact on how individuals engage in goals, planning, thoughts, or activities in the near or in the more distant future (Carstensen, 2006; Lang & Carstensen, 2002; Oettingen, 2012; Oettingen & Mayer, 2002; Zimbardo & Boyd, 1999).

Over the course of more than five decades of psychological research, PFT were considered and discussed in relation to a broad range of time-cognitive constructs such as perceived causality (Faro, McGill, & Hastie, 2010), perceptions of time progression (Friedman & Janssen, 2010; John & Lang, 2016), perceived control (Cohen, 1954), setting of goals (Nuttin, 1985), concreteness of goals (Liberman & Trope, 2008), flexibility of goal adjustment (Brandtstädter & Rothermund, 2003), ambiguity (Brothers, Chui, & Diehl, 2014), decision making (Löckenhoff, 2011), temporal discounting (Hershfield, 2011; Klineberg, 1968), or self-continuity (Rutt & Löckenhoff, 2016).

According to the theory of socioemotional selectivity (Carstensen, 1995, 2006), perceptions of future time are pivotal for the understanding of the changes in motivation and emotion across adulthood. The theory suggests that observable aging-associated changes in motivation, cognition, and behavior reflect adaptation to a dwindling of the remaining time in life. When individuals perceive their remaining lifetime as coming to an end, they are likely to set new priorities that entail a shift from future-oriented goals, such as information acquisition, to more present-oriented goals, such as emotion regulation. Accordingly, perceiving a limited future time was consistently found to be associated with motivational shifts, social preferences, and positive emotion regulation across adulthood (Carstensen, Isaacowitz, & Charles, 1999). Moreover, such motivational and emotional changes were found to predict positive aging outcomes, such as health and subjective well-being (Carstensen, 1995; Fung & Carstensen, 2006, Lang & Carstensen, 2002).

Consistent with socioemotional selectivity theory, the model of selection, optimization, and compensation (SOC; Baltes, 1997) assumes a broad perspective on how human individuals adapt to aging-related challenges across the lifespan. According to the SOC model, there exist three interwoven adaptive strategies that are assumed to play a moderating role in protecting the self against the possible detrimental effects of perceiving one's time in life as vanishing. *Selection* involves a narrowed set of preferences and choices that in turn are typically directed toward minimizing negative while maximizing positive future experience. *Optimization* relates to the increased use of means and resources that serve to improve one's cognitive or behavioral resources. *Compensation* refers to actions or thoughts that serve to counterbalance actual or anticipated threats or losses of future time. Together, selection, optimization, and compensation reflect strategies by which individuals may positively adapt to increasing scarcity of lifetime across adulthood (Lang & Rohr, 2015; Lang, Rohr, & Williger, 2011). The model may also be applied to the question of how individuals age differentially and adaptively manage the challenges associated with perceptions of future time across adulthood. For example, an individual may decide to focus on making the best out of the available remaining time in life by focusing on a smaller number of interests (selection), thus increasing the time he or she is able to invest in these more specific meaningful activities of daily life (optimization; Lang, Rieckmann, & Baltes, 2002). Furthermore, when perceiving a threat to the self or loss of time in the future, he or she may increasingly savor the present time and simultaneously devalue a prospective negative future (compensation; Lang et al., 2013).

This chapter focuses on the structure of perceiving future time (PFT) and on how PFT contributes to cognitive adaptation in the process of aging. In this vein, the theoretical concepts of SOC are discussed with regard to how individuals perceive their future time. Specifically, this chapter addresses three main questions:

1. What are the dimensions of PFT across adulthood?
2. What are the age-associated changes in PFT?
3. How do the dimensions of PFT contribute to positive aging outcomes?

We discuss to what extent perceptions of future time reflect adaptive responses to aging-related challenges such as the awareness of finitude of life. The chapter begins with an overview of theoretical considerations and premises of existing concepts of future time perspective in the literature. Empirical illustrations will be given for how each of the three dimensions of PFT, that is, extension, valence, and pace, may contribute to adaptive functioning across adulthood. The chapter ends with a future outlook regarding possible open issues concerning the role of future-related time perceptions in the aging process.

WHAT ARE THE DIMENSIONS OF PERCEIVED FUTURE TIME ACROSS ADULTHOOD?

Over the past five decades, a plethora of concepts concerning how individuals perceive future time emerged in the psychological sciences (Brandtstädter & Rothermund, 2003; Carstensen, 2006; Husman & Shell, 2008; Kastenbaum, 1961; Rakowski, 1979; Zimbardo & Boyd, 1999). Of specific interest to this chapter are perceptions of future time as they refer to aging-associated individual differences in the time-related cognitions of extension, pace, and valence of one's remaining future time in life.

PFT develop across the entire life span from early childhood until very late in life. In the first two decades of life, emerging perceptions of present and future time are strongly connected with the development of cognition, motivation, and self-regulation (Fraisse, 1963; Klineberg, 1968; Lessing, 1972). Within the first decades of life, individuals develop a differentiated and multifaceted future time perspective (for an overview, see Nurmi, 1991). However, this chapter focuses on changes across adulthood. From early adulthood to late life, awareness of time has been shown to play a major role in the process of positive aging, motivation, and adaptation (Brandtstädter & Rothermund, 2003; Brandtstädter, Rothermund, Kranz, & Kühn, 2010; Carstensen, 1995, 2006; Kastenbaum, 1961; Lang & Carstensen, 2002; Neugarten, 1968). For example, perceptions of future time are associated with aging-related changes in cognition, affect, motivation, and behavior across adulthood (Brandtstädter et al., 2010; Carstensen, 2006; Hicks, Trent, Davis, & King, 2011).

Taken together, most well-known concepts of PFT share some commonalities but also entail a few distinctions in regard to the central features and functions of temporal perceptions of the future. The essence of such theoretical considerations can be summarized in three central propositions of PFT across adulthood.

Concepts of Perceived Future Time That Rely on Spatial Analogies Fall Short

Most theoretical considerations of PFT make use of a more or less explicit parallelism with concepts of physical space, in particular with regard to the construct of perceived extension of future time. Such analogies imply that the psychological experience of future time follows similar behavioral rules to orientation in physical space. For example, Kurt Lewin (1942/1997) introduced the concept of life space as a system of temporal cognition that integrates an individual's perceived future, present, and past.

Consequently, in the tradition of the concept of life space, PFT were often related to physical dimensions of space, such as the extension or the density of future time. However, spatial allegories of time fall short and may even lead to misconceptions of the psychological role of future time. Some of these issues were already discussed as early as in the work of Henri Bergson (1889/1910). For example, Bergson claimed that there is no valid analogy between time and space because time always reflects a duration that cannot be divided into parts: "As far as deep-seated psychic states are concerned, there is no perceptible difference between foreseeing, seeing, and acting" (1889/1910, p. 198). In other words, perceptions of the future cannot be seen separately from perceptions of the presence or from present action. Consequently, individuals often perceive their personal futures as part of their concurrent selves—and they are more likely to do so the older they are (Rutt & Löckenhoff, 2016).

Moreover, whereas a physical space may be empty, individuals cannot think of their personal futures as empty. Even in the extreme case of boredom, hopelessness, world-weariness, or pessimism, there is still a future that involves the self (Pyszczynski, Holt, & Greenberg, 1987). One may, however, believe that beyond one's personal lifetime there is no future that contains the self. Clearly, this possible ending of one's self on earth reflects a perception of finitude and nearness to death that one may also describe in terms of a restricted *time horizon*. However, even then, when imagining a future as void of oneself, there still remains a future of existence of other organisms. For example, even a culture-pessimistic person who anticipates a possible near ending of the world is likely to agree that nature or at least carbon molecules will continue to exist in such a future.

More importantly, even the most nihilistic perception of future time is part of an individual's current state of mind. Perceptions of future time occur in the present. It reflects a truism that subjective perceptions of future time can never be void. Rather, future time perceptions may also reflect an oxymoron as they refer to an invisible and introspective phenomenon. The implicit contradiction of perceiving future time may also be metaphorically pictured as *perceiving a black bear in a lightless dark cave*. It may really be there or not. Although perceptions of future time may be illusionary and invisible, they are always "real in their consequences" (Thomas & Thomas, 1928, p. 572), and they reflect a core feature of the human mind. In this vein, PFT may be seen as serving as an indicator function in the process of aging that is comparable to a fuel gauge. There are at least three psychological indicators of such a *future-time gauge:* (1) the belief of having less time left in life reflects that time is running out, (2) the sense that time passes by fast indicates that less time is available, and (3) the anticipation that one's future will not bring improvements for oneself reflects limitations in the future. Here, the perceived extension of future time can be seen as a fundamental dimension that may serve to initiate an individual's adaptation to the challenges of approaching his or her own finitude. However, there is some controversy in the literature with regard to the dimensions of PFT that are relevant in the process of aging beyond the idea that the future time horizon is more or less extended or distant (Löckenhoff, 2011; Münch, 2016).

Pace of Time Reflects a Dimension of Perceived Future Time That Is Not Well Understood

Most theoretical concepts of PFT typically involve more than one dimension, but they often tend to neglect the role of pace of PFT. For instance, Brandtstädter and Rothermund (2003) proposed the dimensions of concreteness, valence, desirability, and controllability of a PFT, as well as an individual's acceptance of finitude. Earlier and similarly, Kastenbaum (1961) and Nuttin (1985) described PFT as involving the dimensions of coherence, density, and vividness of future time, in addition to its perceived extension. One may think about future time as filled with events or possibilities, or one may perceive one's future time as unstructured. Coherence, density, and vividness each may reflect aspects of the pace of future time. Pace of perceived time is also sometimes synonymously referred to as *perceived progression of time* or as *subjective acceleration of time.* Perceived pace of future time reflects how fast one experiences future time approaching or happening in one's everyday life. When experiencing the passing of time, this necessarily implies that one is more or less explicitly aware of future time.

In contrast to the multidimensional views on the structure of perceived time, Zimbardo and Boyd (1999, 2009) proposed a unified theory of time perspective. According to this theory, PFT involve the experience of present time (e.g., subjective progression of time), as well as the experience of past time (e.g., past orientation). Consequently, temporal cognition at present, even a remembrance of the past, may entail future-related thought. Again, this involves that the pace of present time experience is part and parcel of PFT. Concurrent experience of time may depend on what a person anticipates for his or her future. For example, when a person believes him- or herself "to be in a hurry," this implies that there is little time left to accomplish a current task or errand. Also, when a person feels that "time stands still," a possible implication is that there is not much hope for a better future (i.e., "nothing changes").

In this vein, the concept of PFT also relates to issues of self-regulation and delay discounting (Hershfield, 2011; Steinberg et al., 2009; Vohs & Schmeichel, 2003). For example, in their thoughts about the future, individuals may feel that a better future has already come and thus may lack the energy to actually reach out for the better future in actuality (Oettingen & Mayer, 2002; Oettingen, Mayer, & Portnow, 2016). Consequently, subjective experience of time progression in everyday life can reflect a critical dimension of PFT. It shapes how much time individuals experience to have left in the immediate future time. However, it remains an open question in what ways pace of future time (e.g., subjective acceleration of time) is associated with perceived extension of future time or actually reflects a distinct and independent dimension of PFT.

Perceived Future Time Involves Affective Valence

Most theories agree that PFT may never be conceived as emotionally neutral or meaningless. The perceived valence of the future involves a positive or a negative expectation or attitude toward one's remaining time in life. For example, one may anticipate things getting better in the future. This implies that the present time is evaluated less positively than the future time. In contrast, when one expects things to get worse in the future, the present is savored or evaluated positively. Cognitively contrasting the future with obstacles in one's present reality was identified as a key in how individuals translate expectations of success into adaptive action consequences (cf. Oettingen, 2012).

Moreover, Cate and John (2007) distinguished between an approach-oriented focus on opportunity of future time and an avoidance-oriented focus on limitations of future time. In addition to the differentiation of positive versus negative valence of future time, Brothers et al. (2014) suggested that individuals may perceive the future time also as ambiguous or uncertain. It remains unclear, though, what the expected outcomes of such ambivalences in PFT are. For example, it can be argued that, depending on personality, some individuals tend to experience an ambiguous future as burdensome whereas others may experience the ambiguity of the future as neutral or indifferent (Aspinwall & Taylor, 1997).

Finally, valence of future time perspective has also been explored with respect to the *intertemporal* preferences that are associated with positive expectations about the future. In general terms, intertemporal choices might differ in regard to the type of benefits that individuals expect in the near or distant future. For example, they may expect immediate improvement or gains in the near future (e.g., of wealth or health), but they may also expect delayed improvement or payoffs after some time has passed (e.g., a year, a decade). Intertemporal choice or delay discounting reflects the extent to which individuals prefer receiving a larger benefit in the distant future over receiving an immediate but smaller benefit in the present (Hershfield, 2011). According to this, individuals might renounce an immediate gratification when expecting to receive greater rewards in the future (Hershfield, 2011; Löckenhoff, 2011; Rakowski, 1979). It was shown that there exist substantive individual differences in the length of PFT frames in which they are willing to discount possible immediate benefits for larger benefits (e.g., Löckenhoff, 2011). Consequently, delay discounting is strongly connected with perceptions of how much time one believes to have left when expecting to receive a future reward. When not much time is left in life, expecting a positive outcome in a distant future will appear to be less attractive in comparison to what can be achieved in the here and now. In this vein, it was suggested that the mode of how individuals think about the future is relevant with regard to possible adaptive outcomes. For example, Oettingen (2012; Oettingen, Pak, & Schnetter, 2001) observed that when individuals contrast positive future fantasies with thoughts about obstacles in the present reality, this activates functional expectations and the setting of goals that are more prone to success.

In sum, it is proposed that there are three major dimensions of PFT: (1) *Extension* reflects a perceived duration of remaining time before reaching an ending; (2) *pace* pertains to the subjective speed at which one is approaching one's future time; (3) *valence* involves an evaluation of one's future time, for example, with respect to hopes or fears. In the following section, we review how the extension, pace, and valence of perceptions of future time change across adulthood, and how such developmental patterns of temporal future experience hint at adaptive cognitive strategies in the aging process.

WHAT ARE CHANGES AND OUTCOMES OF PERCEIVED EXTENSION, PACE, AND VALENCE OF FUTURE TIME ACROSS ADULTHOOD?

Each of the three components of PFT show comparable but distinct patterns of change across adulthood. For example, older adults, as compared to young adults, generally report perceiving the future time as more limited, as more accelerated, and as bringing more negative consequences (Lang, Baltes, & Wagner, 2007; Lang & Carstensen, 2002; Lang et al., 2013). However, there are also contradictory and inconsistent findings about aging-related changes in PFT. For example, the experience of time in the aging process entails both a perceived limitation of future time and a sense of greater latitude in time (Ekerdt & Koss, 2016; Münch, 2016). One suggestion is that adults in the "third age" (e.g., 60–80 years) are more likely to experience latitude in the personal future time, whereas in the "fourth age" (e.g., above 80 years), individuals are likely to perceive their personal futures as constrained, limited, and undesirable.

Also, when anticipating a loss or an ending in one's future, one's current situation may or may not be viewed in more positive terms. For example, in early adulthood a negative future outlook may still imply that there is enough time in the future to counteract any adverse effects. In old age, though, it seems that perceiving remaining time in life as limited may have less detrimental consequences, but it was also observed to be associated with perceptions of accelerated pace of time (John & Lang, 2016) and with a more negative outlook on the future (Strough et al., 2016). Little is known about how the dimensions of perceived extension, valence, and pace of future time play together in the process of aging across adulthood.

In the following, we discuss empirical findings to date on age-related differences in the extension, pace, and valence of PFT. It is suggested that associations among perceived extension, pace, and valence of future time perceptions increase across adulthood: Perceiving one's time in life to be running out may involve an increased subjective pace of time experience, and also a more modest, humble, or realistic future outlook.

In a final section, it is argued that flexible experience of future time in old age involves cognitive strategies that protect against detrimental effects of PFT on subjective well-being in old age. Such adaptive strategies are associated with a narrowing of the future to an extended present, with a subjective accelerated time experience, and with a devaluation of anticipated future loss or limitation.

PERCEIVED EXTENSION OF FUTURE TIME: NARROWING CHOICES WHEN LIFE COMES TO AN END

There is long-standing and conclusive evidence that getting older is associated with a sense that one's time in life is running out (Carstensen, 2006; Cottle & Pleck, 1969; Lang & Carstensen, 2002; Lang, 2000; Hancock, 2010; Hoppmann et al., 2015). In midlife, individuals are beginning to think more often about how many years are left in life (Neugarten, 1968). Perceptions of limitations of remaining time in life thus reflect a "memento mori," a reminder that one has to die, as well as the awareness of "vanitas," a fundamental knowledge that one day all things in one's own life will vanish, including the self. Consequently, perceived extension of future time also refers to an individual's sense that time in life is finite and passing.

Perceived extension of future time was operationally defined and measured with constructs such as subjective time horizon (Löckenhoff, 2011), feelings of nearness to death (Lang, 2000), future time perspective (Lang & Carstensen, 2002), perceived residual life expectancy (Brandtstädter & Rothermund, 2003; Mirowsky & Ross, 2000), or desired longevity (Lang et al., 2007). To date it remains an open question whether such different operational measures of perceived extension of future time yield comparable findings, or whether they also reflect different facets of PFT extension.

Taken together, research on PFT extension suggests that the subjective experience of limited future time is a double-edged sword: On one side, limited future time perspective entails risks and challenges. When individuals realize that the end of their lives is approaching, this may entail alienation, a sense of "falling out of time" and of becoming disconnected with the world. Approaching death was found to be associated with social withdrawal or terminal decline and a personal indifference with regard to the future. Thus perceiving limited future time may also reflect a threat to an individual's purpose in life (Hicks et al., 2011) and may thus be associated with lower subjective well-being and even depression (Grühn, Sharifian, & Chu, 2016; Hoppmann et al., 2015).

On the other side, perceiving limitations in the time left in one's remaining life may activate adaptive processes, that—in consequence—contribute to improved subjective well-being (Carstensen, 2006). In this vein, it is argued that future-related temporal cognitions solicit adaptive emotional, motivational, and behavioral responses that protect against the detrimental effects of realizing a dwindling of one's future time. For example, when feeling near to death, older adults prioritized close social contacts and emotion-related social goals that were associated with positive aging outcomes (Lang, 2000; Lang & Carstensen, 2002). Thus perceiving future time may also be relevant in the process of adapting to aging-related challenges.

Little is known, though, about how PFT extension is reflective of how old one feels currently. For instance, it seems plausible that when individuals feel younger than their actual age, they may perceive that they have more time left in their lives. Self-perceptions of aging-related changes may activate thoughts about how much time one expects to have left in one's remaining life (Brothers, Gabrian, Wahl, & Diehl, 2016). Also, Weiss and Lang (2012) observed in an age-heterogeneous study on age-group identification that when older individuals identified with people of their own age group, they perceived having a more limited future time. In contrast, when older adults reported feeling different from *most people of the same age*, they experienced a more open-ended future time perspective.

A related issue pertains to how long individuals desire to live and what are the predictors of wanting to live long or not so long. In a series of studies with several representative age-heterogeneous national German samples, Lang et al.(2007) observed that desired life expectancy was only weakly associated with chronological age among adults between 20 and 90 years old. From early adulthood up to the age of 80 years, respondents typically expressed a wish to live until around the mid- to late eighth decade of their lives, on average, whereas, adults above age 85 on average desired to live a few more years. Notably, about 5% of the respondents did not want to report a desired life expectancy. Some people might refuse to consider their future time in terms of years of life expectancy and rather prefer to think of the future time as unpredictable and uncertain. This is reflected in another notable finding of this research on desired life expectancy.

In a second study, Lang and his colleagues (Lang et al., 2007) assessed how determined individuals in early, middle, and late adulthood were about their desire to reach a certain age. In this study, respondents, after reporting how long they want to live, rated on a 4-point scale how desirable it would be for them to reach this hypothetical age if they were "being confronted with a health problem resulting in frailty or the need for health care." About 75% of the respondents expressed that they would not find it desirable to reach their desired life expectancy when suffering severe health problems. Also, more than 75% agreed with the statement that they would like to decide on their own when and how to die (Lang et al., 2007; Study 2). Once more, such findings suggest that having a negative outlook on one's personal health in the future may also be associated with a devaluation of such negative future scenarios. These findings are also reflective of the risks for subjective quality of life that are associated with the anticipation of loss in old age or when nearing death. For example, when facing one's finitude and a nearness to death, individuals may respond to this with fear, worries, and even despair. Neglecting or ignoring such negative future outlooks while focusing on the present time may thus reflect one possible compensatory cognitive strategy that counteracts the threats of loss.

Such considerations are also consistent with findings of Brandtstädter and Rothermund (2003), who observed that the impact of perceived losses on subjective well-being was strongest when individuals felt close to the end of life (i.e., when they perceived that they had only a short residual life expectancy). However, such effects were found to be weaker when individuals expressed a strong level of flexible goal adjustment. In other words, when disengaging from goals and when lowering expectations, individuals maintained a stronger subjective well-being despite feeling near to death. Again, this points to temporal cognitions that protect against the negative or detrimental effects of experiencing a narrowing of one's remaining future time.

At times, older people are likely to subjectively extend their PFT beyond their personal lifetime on earth. This has been referred to as transcendent or spiritual future-thinking (Boyd & Zimbardo, 1997), reflecting a belief of some kind of continued existence after death. Transcendental future time perspective was found to be associated with religious beliefs but may also serve palliative functions when feeling that the time of one's death is approaching.

Another compensatory response to perceived limitation of future time relates to adopting a more generative attitude toward the future of others, for example, when investing more into the well-being of the next generations. Lang and Carstensen (2002) proved that when individuals perceive a narrowing in their future time perspective, they invest more in social goals of generativity toward others. Such a transformation of one's PFT reflects a flexible and functional response when dealing with risks of perceived finitude of life. This is also consistent with assumptions of the theory of symbolic self-completion (Gollwitzer & Kirchhof, 1998). When expecting life to come to an end, individuals may counteract such negative outlooks with a compensatory symbolic cognition that reflects a refusal to realize such a negative future prospect (see also Brandtstädter & Rothermund, 2003). For example, cherishing the moment or beginning a new leisure activity may reflect ways to maximize meaning of life in response to one's personal ending (Hicks et al., 2011).

A related issue of perceived time extension was addressed in research on temporal self-continuity across adulthood (Rutt & Löckenhoff, 2016): Participants rated perceived similarity of their current selves with past and future selves on a scale and with respect to self-descriptive adjectives. Participants rated similarity between their past and future selves for different temporal distances such as 1 month, 1 year, or 10 years. Findings suggested that older adults were more likely than younger adults to perceive continuity between their current selves and their past and future selves. These findings suggest that older adults appear to perceive an extended time frame of the present self. In other words, older adults were likely to embrace a broader time perspective in their current self-concepts. Although time horizons of the future time may be shrinking in old age, Rutt and Löckenhoff (2016) observed that older adults are experiencing an extended present (Carstensen, 2006).

Perceptions of future time comprise a class of future-directed temporal cognitions that occur in the present and that pertain to any time point or interval in the future, from seconds, days, months, or years to one´s entire lifetime (Fingerman & Perlmutter, 2001; John & Lang, 2016), and even to a possible eternity (Tornstam, 2005). Accordingly, Kurt Lewin (1942/1997) suggested that "the life space of an individual . . . includes the future, the present, and also the past. Actions, emotions, and certainly the morale of an individual at any instant depend upon his total time perspective" (1942/1997, p. 80). It is likely that the ability to perceive the future in terms of eternity is unique to the human species. Such mental extensions of one's PFT may serve to counterbalance possible detrimental effects of perceiving a nearness of death or a finitude of one's life.

Taken together, perceived extension of future time reflects critical challenges in the process of aging associated with acceptance of finitude, nearness of death, and mortality. However, there are also adaptive responses that may serve to protect against detrimental effects of such challenges and that contribute to positive aging outcomes. Such adaptive responses involve motivational change and intertemporal preferences toward maximizing short-term benefits, but they may also pertain to transcendental and transformational ways of cognitively extending the perceived future beyond one's lifetime.

Pace of Time Experience: Subjective Acceleration of Time as an Aging-Related Adaptation to Loss

Most people believe that time goes by faster when they get older. This phenomenon is reported in countless literature works from different historical epochs. Consistent with such lay conceptions, there exists a wealth of findings confirming a positive correlation between subjective acceleration of the experience of time and chronological age across adulthood (Friedman & Janssen, 2010; Wittmann & Lehnhoff, 2005). Subjective acceleration of time is often associated with challenges and risks of aging. For example, an accelerated pace of time may involve a risk of feeling unable to keep pace with the changes in one's surrounding environment. Connected feelings of subjective obsolescence were found to increase across adulthood (Brandtstädter & Rothermund, 2003) and to also be associated with depressive feelings.

Little is known about possible underlying psychological mechanisms that account for increases in subjective acceleration of time across adulthood. One explanation is related to possible declines of cognitive functioning across adulthood. For example, it appears plausible that cognitive slowing in old age is responsible for experiencing acceleration of time. However, such explanations may also reflect that there is some confusion about different constructs of psychological time. For example, most measures of *time perception* typically consist of cognitive performance tasks based on estimation or reproduction of an objective time interval in a controlled or laboratory setting (e.g., an estimated objective time interval of 30 seconds; Bschor et al., 2004). Thus time perception is often defined as a task-specific performance that may or may not prove correct. Indeed, measures of time perception (e.g., "press a button for 20 seconds") were found to be positively associated with cognitive performance. However, such measures of perception of time are distinct from the concept of *perceived pace of time* (e.g., a self-related rating of subjective acceleration of time). Self-reports on pace of future time reflect how individuals perceive the passing of time in everyday life contexts. Ratings of subjective acceleration of time (i.e., "How fast did time go by?") are typically not related with measures of cognitive performance (John & Lang, 2016). Moreover, ratings of perceived pace of time are found to be unrelated with performance in time perception tasks (Thoenes & Oberfeld, 2015). Thus it seems unlikely that cognitive decline may account for age-related increases of perceived pace of future time in old age.

Age differences in perceived pace of time are found to differ depending on length of time intervals (i.e., minutes, hours, days, months, years, decades): When considering relatively short time intervals of seconds or minutes, young and old adults do not differ much with respect to how fast they subjectively perceive the pace of time (Wittmann & Lehnhoff, 2005). However, when considering longer time intervals, age-related differences in perceived acceleration of time are typically observed to be larger. For example, when reflecting the previous 10 years, older adults compared with young adults were more likely to perceive that time has passed by faster (Friedman & Janssen, 2010). This suggests that in old age, individuals differentiate more strongly between short and long time intervals as compared with young adults.

Another possible explanation for aging-related differences in perceived pace of time relates to motivational changes across adulthood. According to such considerations, perceived pace of time in daily life depends on changes in the meaningfulness of everyday activities across adulthood. In old age, as compared with early adulthood, individuals will perceive subjective acceleration more strongly during meaningful, goal-relevant everyday activities. In contrast, age differences in subjective acceleration of time may be less pronounced during less meaningful everyday activities that are, for example, associated with regeneration or with consumption. John and Lang (2016) empirically investigated such an explanation for increases in subjective pace of time across adulthood in a series of studies.

In three studies including adults from 18 to 90 years of age, subjective acceleration of time was explored in relation to everyday activities during either the preceding day (i.e., the day-reconstruction method) or the following day (i.e., the tomorrow-construction method). In a first study, individuals reconstructed the day preceding the day of the interview. Respondents reported the activities they had undertaken during several episodes during the course of the preceding day and how fast they had experienced the time passing by. In general, two broad classes of activity patterns were distinguished: (1) productive activities involving social contact, household chores, work, or intellectual activities, and (2) regenerative–consumptive activities such as self-care, resting, eating, or physical exercise. There were no age differences in subjective acceleration of time during regenerative–consumptive activities. However, age differences of subjective time acceleration were observed during productive activities. Older adults, as compared with young adults, experienced time passing by faster during such productive activities. These associations were also related to perceiving one's remaining lifetime to be limited. Cognitive functioning did not account for the observed age differences (John & Lang, 2016, Study 2).

In an additional study with the newly developed *tomorrow-construction method,* a similar pattern of findings was observed when people had the task of anticipating subjective acceleration of time during the activities that they planned for the following day (John & Lang, 2016, Study 3). In this study, participants were randomly assigned to two experimental conditions and one control condition. In the first experimental condition, participants were instructed to plan for a productive day (i.e., *a day that provides opportunities to accomplish tasks*). In the second experimental condition, participants were instructed to plan for a regenerative day (i.e., *a day that provides opportunities to relax*). In the control condition, participants were just asked to plan the next day (without further instructions). Consistent with the above findings from the day-reconstruction method, age differences in anticipated subjective acceleration of time were more pronounced when planning activities for a "task day" as compared with the control condition (with no specific plans for the next day). Thus anticipation of pace of time in the near future did not differ substantively from perceptions of time during the preceding day.

Generally, planning to invest time in meaningful, productive activities is associated with perceiving time to pass by faster. These findings suggest that when older individuals perceive time to pass by faster, this may be a consequence of investing their personal time in meaningful activities and from making an optimal use of available time in everyday life. Subjective acceleration of time in daily life may thus reflect an optimization strategy of personal time use. It is an open question, though, whether subjective acceleration of time also contributes to positive affect and thus protects against possible detrimental effects of a more limited PFT.

In summary, getting older is associated with general increases in the pace or velocity of perceived everyday time. Such experience of subjectively accelerated time appears to reflect a preference for and optimization of meaningful activities in old age. For example, subjective time appears to go by faster only while one engages in or plans for desirable, productive, or meaningful activities. Thus subjective acceleration of time in old age reflects a temporal cognition that indicates an optimizing of time use in later adulthood. In this vein, subjective acceleration may reflect the maximization of meaningful positive experience and optimal use of time available in everyday life. On the downside, however, a pursuit of less desirable regenerative or consumptive everyday activities is associated with a sense that time goes by slowly or may even appear to stand still. This may also indicate that the future might appear to be less structured or ambiguous. When less desirable activities prevail in everyday activities of older adults, a decelerated, constrained, or extended experience of time also points to potential risks of aging-related losses (Lang et al., 2002).

Valence of Time Perspectives: Focusing on an Extended Present Time While Devaluing the Future?

Thinking about the future often provides a reference frame for evaluating one's current self against a hoped-for or feared-for self in an anticipated future (Cross & Markus, 1991; Oettingen, 2012). For example, a person may expect to feel better or worse in the future as compared with how she or he feels today. There is robust evidence that young adults hold more positive views about the future in comparison with older adults (Brandtstädter & Rothermund, 2003; Staudinger, Bluck, & Herzberg, 2003). Moreover, older individuals who have a more positive or optimistic attitude toward aging tend to feel better, engage in healthier lifestyles, and live longer (Levy, Slade, Kunkel, & Kasl, 2002; Tasdemir-Ozdes, Strickland-Hughes, Bluck, & Ebner, 2016). On the other side, such findings imply that pessimism and negative future outlooks may entail increased risks of despair, hopelessness, and resignation.

However, there are a few notable exceptions to this rule that point to possible benefits of a negative future outlook in old age. For example, a more negative future outlook was found to be associated with positive outcomes (Cheng, Fung, & Chan, 2009; Lachman, Röcke, Rosnick, & Ryff, 2008). Expectations of one's future may also be evaluated with regard to how accurate or realistic these expectations turn out to be. For example, an optimistic or pessimistic expectation about one's future self may turn out to become true after some time or turn out to be illusionary. People may have unrealistically low expectations for their remaining time in life and thus protect themselves against possible detrimental effects of a possible future loss (Norem & Cantor, 1986). Such defensive pessimism provides a resource for the process of coping with adversity or uncertainty, and it entails a sense of control over one's future time. For example, there is solid evidence that young adults often hold unrealistic positive future outlooks, in contrast to older adults, who are found to often hold more realistic, humble, or negative future expectations (Cheng et al., 2009; Lachman et al., 2008; Lang et al., 2013; Staudinger et al., 2003). Holding accurate beliefs about one's future time may also have an impact on positive aging outcomes.

Cheng and his colleagues (2009) observed an improvement in well-being over the course of a year when older adults held realistic or unrealistic negative expectations about their future physical selves. No such effect was observed with regard to the anticipated future *social* self. A negative outlook on one's future *physical* self may reflect a devaluation of the future. For example, the future *physical* self may appear less controllable than one's future *social* self. Older adults may lower their expectations about the future physical self, and—by doing so—protect themselves against negative effects of physical decline on well-being.

Consistent with this, Lang and colleagues (2013) examined age-associated changes in the accuracy of anticipation of future life satisfaction in a nationally representative sample of German adults between 18 and 90 years old over an extended period with repeated measurement. In this longitudinal study, participants rated their life satisfaction in the present (starting year) and reported how satisfied they expected to be in 5 years (target year). Such assessments of present and anticipated future life satisfaction were repeated six times over the course of 11 years. This procedure allowed a test of whether individuals' anticipations of future life satisfaction proved accurate and whether subsequent anticipations of future satisfaction changed over time.

In accordance with the theoretical expectations, young adults were observed to overestimate their future satisfaction, on average. Moreover, middle-aged adults were found to display more accurate anticipations, whereas older adults underestimated their future life satisfaction repeatedly and consistently over a time period of 11 years. This means that, even when subjective health and life satisfaction declined over time, older adults anticipated stronger declines in life satisfaction in their futures. In sum, across an extended period of time, older adults reported feeling more satisfied with their lives at present than they had expected 5 years earlier. Such findings may point to an adaptive cognitive strategy that protects against negative effects of anticipating aging-related losses. Older adults appear to focus on their present life situations while devaluing anticipated loss in the future. Such an underestimating of one's future life satisfaction and humble expectations were even found to be associated with reduced risks of disability and mortality among older adults (Lang et al., 2013). Feeling prepared for a possible future loss may imply that one perceives having predictive control over an otherwise unknown future, and this may contribute to improved coping capacities when confronted with aging-related challenges.

Underestimating one's life satisfaction in the future implies that the present is evaluated more positively (in relation to one's future outlook). It also implies that the present is given a stronger weight in evaluating one's current life satisfaction (e.g., "things will be bad in 5 years, but it is as good now as it can be"). Finally, when anticipating a potential loss in the future, individuals may find more relief in savoring or focusing on present time and engaging in meaningful activities in everyday life.

Such considerations appear to stand in contradiction to findings on age differences in time discounting across adulthood (Hershfield, 2011; Löckenhoff, 2011), which suggest that older adults are more likely than younger adults to delay immediate benefits in order to receive greater ones in the future. However, studies on age differences in time discounting often examined relatively short time intervals of delay of gratification, and time discounting differs depending on whether immediate outcomes are compared with possible (greater) gains or (smaller) losses in the future. At this point there is no conclusive evidence on age differences in time discounting regarding longer future time intervals—for example, when discounting anticipated gains in 5 years for a more immediate benefit.

To sum up, for older adults the valence of future time is also associated with anticipations of a potential negative course of the remaining time in life that entails the potential risks of despair and resignation. In later adulthood, individuals may expect no improvements in the remaining time in life. This may activate a compensatory focus on present time that involves savoring of the present time and a devaluation of a potential future.

FUTURE OUTLOOK AND SYNOPSIS

PFT refers to a broad set of age-associated temporal cognitions that reflect perceptions of more or less extended time horizons, subjective pace of time experience, and perceptions of future valence. Age-related differences in PFT mirror the challenges and risks resulting from an emerging negative gain–loss ratio across adulthood and late life (Baltes, 1997).

Getting older often involves the knowledge that time is running out and that loss experiences become more likely. In this vein, thinking about one's future may activate adaptive responses to such dwindling temporal resources. In this chapter, it has been suggested that PFT change across adulthood and that such age-related changes in PFT may not only entail risks but also trigger adaptive responses that contribute to positive aging outcomes. Specifically, it was suggested that PFT involve at least three age-related interwoven dimensions of temporal cognitions across adulthood, that is, PFT extension, subjective pace (or acceleration) of future time, and affective valence in temporal preferences.

Some of the above-reviewed empirical findings also speak to a seeming *aging paradox of simultaneously experiencing scarcity and wealth of time in old age*. On the one hand, aging individuals are known to experience the limitedness of their remaining lifetimes. On the other hand, older individuals often report subjective gains with respect to a possible deliberate and meaningful use of their time (e.g., Münch, 2016). The two seemingly contradictory perceptions of a simultaneous scarcity and wealth of future time are reflective of an ambivalence toward the future in old age. For example, older adults may experience negatively that their time in life is running out, but there is also a positive feeling of having some latitude of time use in everyday life. Thinking about one's future across adulthood appears to involve an increased flexibility with regard to whether one focuses on an extended present time or on a more distant and devalued future. Thus cognitive flexibility in PFT appears to reflect an adaptive response to challenges of the aging process. What are possible accounts for such a possible aging paradox of future-related temporal experience? One explanation is that dwindling temporal resources in old age are associated with at least two dynamically interwoven challenges associated with PFT across adulthood.

A first challenge pertains to the obvious boundaries of one's remaining time in life. In the course of aging, individuals approach an unknown, uncontrollable, indefinite, and ambiguous ending of their personal lives. It is a truism that no one knows when his or her life will end. The psychological implications of such a truism are not trivial, though, because people respond differentially and idiosyncratically to perceived lack of predictability of the future. Moreover, it is likely that, with increasing chronological age, subjective perceptions of one's remaining time in life, perceptions of anticipated losses in the future, or perceptions that time in daily life is rushing by become more strongly dependent on each other. For example, older adults who experience that their death is approaching may also anticipate losses in the future and may experience subjective obsolescence.

A second challenge pertains to the desire of maintaining autonomy or control in old age, irrespective or even in spite of resource losses (Baltes, 1997). Such striving for autonomy in old age was also observed in patterns of everyday activity in response to loss of resources (Lang et al., 2002). For example, older adults increasingly engaged in those activities that they experienced as meaningful while disengaging from less relevant activities. Consequently, older adults often report experiencing a sovereignty of time and a sense of personal control over use of time and sometimes also a wealth of personal time in everyday life. This is also reflective of narrative reports that older adults often feel more busy after having retired, while seeking to maintain structure and routines in their everyday lives (Ekerdt & Koss, 2016; Münch, 2016). Together, the two interwoven challenges of PFT across adulthood may reflect differential cognitive strategies in dealing with such challenges.

Rather than a paradox, the simultaneous and ambivalent experiences of scarcity and wealth of time in old age, as described above, may also involve a cognitive adaptation to increasing negative gain–loss ratios across adulthood. Perceptions of limited, accelerated, or undesirable remaining time in life may not be seen independently from aging-related loss experiences and self-perceptions in the aging process. Instead, they may reflect an individual's adaptive response to the risks and challenges that he or she faces in the process of aging. However, there are also potential positive outcomes when individuals respond adaptively to such risks and challenges. For example, when lifetime is running out, one might make more meaningful use of time in the activity patterns of everyday life (e.g., John & Lang, 2016; Lang et al., 2002), and, in turn, one may respond with more modest and realistic expectations about what the future will bring them (Lachman et al., 2008; Lang et al., 2013).

Thus, in summary, the three dimensions of extension, pace, and valence in PFT entail specific challenges and risks in the aging process, as well as potentials for positive aging outcomes. Having a negative future outlook may be associated with a risk of feeling despair, pessimism, and resignation. The feeling that future time is approaching quickly involves a sense of rush, urgency, and perceived obsolescence, associated with feelings of not being able to keep pace. Thus perceiving one's remaining lifetime to be limited also involves the risk of undesirable disengagement from social life. This may involve a sort of indifference or resignation. However, to all such known challenges in the aging process, there also exist protective and functional cognitive strategies that serve to reduce or soften the detrimental effects of perceiving one's future in terms of negative valence, accelerated pace, and limited remaining time.

What are such possible adaptive strategies to counteract the risks of future time perspective? Figure 16.1 proposes a preliminary theoretical framework of protective strategies against aging-associated challenges of future time perspective. The framework builds on the model of SOC and advances considerations of the theory of socioemotional selectivity. According to this preliminary framework, risks and demands emerge when perceiving a limited future or when expecting loss in the future. However, there are also adaptive cognitive and behavioral strategies that counterbalance the detrimental effects of limited, accelerated, or negative views on one's future time and that may be associated with positive outcomes.

One adaptive strategy when perceiving one's remaining time in life to be running out builds on the strategy of *selection* (e.g., Carstensen, 2006). Here, *selection* refers to changed preferences, a motivational shift toward an increased salience of emotional preferences, and seeking to maximize positive experience in response to limited future time. Consistent with this, it was found that individuals respond to a dwindling of remaining time in life with a stronger preference for positive social contact and emotional goals. This is associated with positive or protective effects on subjective well-being and social connectedness (Lang & Carstensen, 2002; Lang, 2000).

A second strategy, *optimization* of temporal experience, involves a behavioral pattern of enhanced experiences of time sovereignty and autonomy of time use in everyday life. It reflects everyday activities that contribute to behavioral competence,

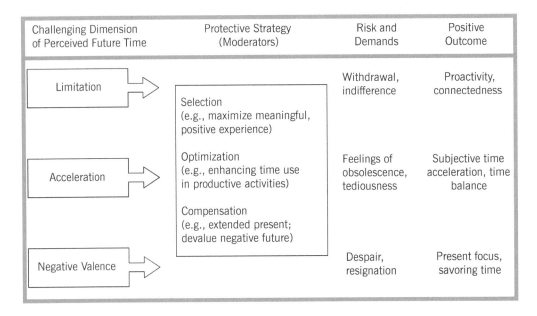

FIGURE 16.1. A preliminary framework of adaptation to perceived future time (PFT).

meaningful activities, and self-determination in daily life. In response to subjective threats to the ability to keep pace with time, individuals may invest time resources in productive, goal-related activities that contribute to enhanced meaning in life (John & Lang, 2016).

As a third strategy, *compensation* in PFT refers to palliative time-related cognitions in response to anticipated loss (e.g., Brandtstädter & Rothermund, 2003). For example, when expecting things to get worse in the future, individuals may shift their focus toward the present time, while devaluing a negative future loss. In other words, focusing on a positive present time may counterbalance possible threats of an anticipated future. This means that an older person may think that she or he wants to remain in the current moment as long as possible.

CONCLUSION

PFT reflect a major challenge in the process of aging. How individuals respond to PFT entails both risks and potentials for positive aging. PFT that are associated with experiencing limitations of one's personal future time, subjective acceleration of time, and a more negative, constrained outlook of remaining time in life entail many risks related to social withdrawal, despair, and feelings of obsolescence. However, such PFT were also observed to trigger functional adaptive thoughts, motivational changes, and behavior that protect against the threats associated with the finitude of life and anticipation of loss in the future. It is not well understood what the central intervening variables that secure positive consequences of challenging PFT across adulthood are. In this chapter, it was proposed that the model of SOC may serve as a framework that describes some of the functional and adaptive moderators that contribute to adaptive ways of dealing with undesirable and burdening aspects of PFT. According to this model, perceived challenges and risks of PFT may reflect a future-time gauge that can be refilled to generate adaptive strategies toward positive aging outcomes.

In addition, PFT also reflect domain-specific experiences of time that differ depending on the specific contexts of everyday life. For example, PFT with regard to one's personal functional health or autonomy may differ strongly from PFT regarding one's family and kinship. This possibly accounts for some of the ambivalence that older adults often experience with regard to their PFT. It is an open question to what extent there also exist domain-specific PFT across adulthood.

According to the proposed preliminary framework of PFT, adults may flexibly and differentially respond to perceived challenges and risks of future time. When perceiving scarcity in one domain (e.g., health), this may be responded to with domain-specific temporal perspectives such as narrowing the focus on the present and devaluing future loss. On the other hand, perceiving resource richness in other functional domains (e.g., family life) may entail open and positive future time perspectives. Another cognitive strategy in response to the finitude of life pertains to the experience of extending one's future time perspective beyond one's individual lifetime. Such transformational future time perspectives may mean that one takes responsibility or a legacy for future generations or shares concerns for one's offspring or may concern spiritual or transcendent thoughts about one's afterlife.

References

Aspinwall, L. G., & Taylor, S. E. (1997). A stitch in time: Self-regulation and proactive coping. *Psychological Bulletin, 121,* 417–436.

Baltes, P. (1997). On the incomplete architecture of human ontogeny: Selection, optimization, and compensation as foundation of developmental theory. *American Psychologist, 52,* 366–380.

Bergson, H. (1910). *Time and free will: An essay on the immediate data of consciousness* (F. L. Pogson, Trans.). London: Allen & Unwin. (Original work published 1889)

Boyd, J., & Zimbardo, P. G. (1997). Constructing time after death: A transcendental-future time perspective. *Time and Society, 6,* 35–54.

Brandtstädter, J., & Rothermund, K. (2003). Intentionality and time in human development and aging. In U. Staudinger & U. Lindenberger (Eds.), *Understanding human development* (pp. 105–124). New York: Springer.

Brandtstädter, J., Rothermund, K., Kranz, D., & Kühn, W. (2010). Final decentrations: Personal goals, rationality perspectives, and the awareness of life's finitude. *European Psychologist, 15,* 152–163.

Brothers, A., Chui, H., & Diehl, M. (2014). Measuring future time perspective across adulthood: Development and evaluation of a brief multidimensional questionnaire. *Gerontologist, 54,* 1075–1088.

Brothers, A., Gabrian, M., Wahl, H.-W., & Diehl, M. (2016). Future time perspective and awareness of age-related change: Examining their role in predicting psychological well-being. *Psychology and Aging, 31*(6), 605–617.

Bschor, T., Ising, M., Bauer, M., Lewitzka, U., Skerstupeit, M., Müller-Oerlinghausen, B., . . . Baethge, C. (2004). Time experience and time judgment in major depression, mania and healthy subjects: A controlled study of 93 subjects. *Acta Psychiatrica Scandinavica, 109,* 222–229.

Carstensen, L. L. (1995). Evidence for a life-span theory of socioemotional selectivity. *Current Directions in Psychological Science, 4,* 151–156.

Carstensen, L. L. (2006). The influence of a sense of time on human development. *Science, 312,* 1913–1915.

Carstensen, L. L., Isaacowitz, D. M., & Charles, S. T. (1999). Taking time seriously: A theory of socioemotional selectivity. *American Psychologist, 54,* 165–181.

Cate, R. A., & John, O. P. (2007). Testing models of the structure and development of future time perspective: Maintaining a focus on opportunities in middle age. *Psychology and Aging, 22,* 186–201.

Cheng, S.-T., Fung, H. H., & Chan, A. C. M. (2009). Self-perception and psychological well-being: The benefits of foreseeing a dark future. *Psychology and Aging, 24,* 623–633.

Cohen, J. (1954). The experience of time. *Acta Psychologica, 10,* 207–219.

Cottle, T. A., & Pleck, J. H. (1969). Linear estimations of temporal extensions: The effect of age, sex, and social class. *Journal of Projective Techniques and Personality Assessment, 33,* 81–93.

Cross, S., & Markus, H. (1991). Possible selves across the life span. *Human Development, 34,* 230–255.

Ekerdt, D. J., & Koss, C. (2016). The task of time in retirement. *Ageing and Society, 36,* 1295–1311.

Faro, D., McGill, A. L., & Hastie, R. (2010). Naive theories of causal force and compression of elapsed time judgments. *Journal of Personality and Social Psychology, 98,* 683–701.

Fingerman, K., & Perlmutter, M. (2001). Future time perspective and life events across adulthood. *Journal of General Psychology, 122,* 95–111.

Fraisse, P. (1963). *The psychology of time.* New York: Harper & Row.

Friedman, W. J., & Janssen, S. (2010). Aging and the speed of time. *Acta Psychologica, 134,* 130–141.

Fung, H. H., & Carstensen, L. L. (2006). Goals change when life's fragility is primed: Lessons learned from older adults, the September 11 attacks and SARS. *Social Cognition, 24,* 248–278.

Gollwitzer, P., & Kirchhof, O. (1998). The willful pursuit of identity. In J. Heckhausen & C. S. Dweck (Eds.), *Motivation and self-regulation across the life span* (pp. 339–423). New York: Cambridge University Press.

Grühn, D., Sharifian, N., & Chu, Q. (2016). The limits of a limited future time perspective in explaining age differences in emotional functioning. *Psychology and Aging, 31,* 583–593.

Hancock, P. A. (2010). The effect of age and sex on the perception of time in life. *American Journal of Psychology, 123,* 1–13.

Hershfield, H. E. (2011). Future self-continuity: How conceptions of the future self transform intertemporal choice. *Annals of the New York Academy of Sciences, 1235,* 30–43.

Hicks, J. A., Trent, J., Davis, W. E., & King, L. A. (2011). Positive affect, meaning in life, and future time perspective: An application of socioemotional selectivity theory. *Psychology and Aging, 27,* 181–189.

Hoppmann, C. A., Infurna, F. J., Ram, N., & Gerstorf, D. (2015). Associations among individuals' perceptions of future time, individual resources, and subjective wellbeing in old age. *Journals of Gerontology: Series B. Psychological Sciences and Social Sciences, 72*(3), 388–399.

Husman, J., & Shell, D. F. (2008). Beliefs and perceptions about the future: A measurement of future time perspective. *Learning and Individual Differences, 18,* 166–175.

John, D., & Lang, F. R. (2016). Subjective acceleration of time experience in everyday life across adulthood. *Developmental Psychology, 51,* 1824–1839.

Kastenbaum, R. (1961). The dimensions of future time perspective: An experimental analysis. *Journal of General Psychology, 65,* 203–218.

Klineberg, S. L. (1968). Future time perspective and the preference for delayed reward. *Journal of Personality and Social Psychology, 8,* 253–257.

Lachman, M. E., Röcke, C., Rosnick, C., & Ryff, C. D. (2008). Realism and illusion in Americans' temporal views of their life satisfaction. *Psychological Science, 19,* 889–897.

Lang, F. R. (2000). Endings and continuity of social relationships: Maximizing intrinsic benefits within personal networks when feeling near to death? *Journal of Social and Personal Relationships, 17,* 157–184.

Lang, F. R., Baltes, P. B., & Wagner, G. G. (2007). Desired lifetime and end-of-life desires across adulthood from 20 to 90: A dual-source information model. *Journals of Gerontology: Series B: Psychological Sciences and Social Sciences, 62,* P268–P276.

Lang, F. R., & Carstensen, L. L. (2002). Time counts: Future time perspective, goals, and social relationships. *Psychology and Aging, 17,* 125–139.

Lang, F. R., Rieckmann, N., & Baltes, M. M. (2002). Adapting to aging losses: Do resources facilitate strategies of selection, compensation, and optimization in everyday functioning? *Journals of Gerontology: Series B. Psychological Sciences and Social Sciences, 57*(6), 501–509.

Lang, F. R., & Rohr, M. (2015). Successful aging in societies of long living: The model of selection, optimization, and compensation. In J. Wright (Ed.), *International encyclopedia of the social and behavioral sciences* (2nd ed., pp. 667–672). Oxford, UK: Elsevier.

Lang, F. R., Rohr, M., & Williger, B. (2011). Modeling success in life-span psychology: The principles of selection, optimization, and compensation. In K. L. Fingerman, C. Berg, J. Smith, & T. Antonucci (Eds.), *Handbook of life-span development* (pp. 57–85). New York: Springer.

Lang, F. R., Weiss, D., Gerstorf, D., & Wagner, G. G. (2013). Forecasting life satisfaction across adulthood: Benefits of seeing a dark future? *Psychology and Aging, 28,* 249–261.

Lessing, E. E. (1972). Extension of personal future time perspective, age, and life satisfaction of children and adolescents. *Developmental Psychology, 6,* 457–468.

Levy, B. R., Slade, M. D., Kunkel, S. R., & Kasl, S. V. (2002). Longevity increased by positive self-perceptions of aging. *Journal of Personality and Social Psychology, 83,* 261–270.

Lewin, K. (1997). Time perspective and morale. In G. W. Lewin (Ed.), *Resolving social conflicts: Field theory in social science.* Washington DC: American Psychological Association. (Original work published 1942)

Liberman, N., & Trope, Y. (2008). The psychology of transcending the here and now. *Science, 322,* 1201–1205.

Löckenhoff, C. E. (2011). Age, time, and decision making: From processing speed to global time horizons. *Annals of the New York Academy of Sciences, 1235,* 44–56.

Mirowsky, J., & Ross, C. E. (2000). Socioeconomic status and subjective life expectancy. *Social Psychology Quarterly, 63,* 133–151.

Münch, A. (2016). Zeitliche Ambivalenz des Alter(n)s: Individuelles Handeln im Spannungsfeld von Zeitreichtum und Zeitarmut [Temporal ambivalences of aging: Individual patterns of time use in conflict between time wealth and time poverty]. *Zeitschrift für Gerontologie und Geriatrie, 49,* 10–14.

Neugarten, B. L. (1968). The awareness of middle age. In B. L. Neugarten (Ed.), *Middle age and aging* (pp. 93–98). Chicago: University of Chicago Press.

Norem, J. K., & Cantor, N. (1986). Defensive pessimism: Harnessing anxiety and motivation. *Journal of Personality and Social Psychology, 51,* 1208–1217.

Nurmi, J. (1991). How do adolescents see their future?: A review of the development of future orientation and planning. *Developmental Review, 11,* 1–59.

Nuttin, J. (1985). *Future time perspective and motivation.* Hillsdale, NJ: Erlbaum.

Oettingen, G. (2012). Future thought and behaviour change. *European Review of Social Psychology, 23,* 1–63.

Oettingen, G., & Mayer, D. (2002). The motivating function of thinking about the future: Expectations versus fantasies. *Journal of Personality and Social Psychology, 5,* 1198–1212.

Oettingen, G., Mayer, D., & Portnow, S. (2016). Pleasure now, pain later: Positive fantasies about the future predict symptoms of depression. *Psychological Science, 27,* 345–353.

Oettingen, G., Pak, H., & Schnetter, K. (2001). Self-regulation of goal setting: Turning free fantasies about the future into binding goals. *Journal of Personality and Social Psychology, 80,* 736–753.

Pyszczynski, T., Holt, K., & Greenberg, J. (1987). Depression, self-focused attention, and expectancies for positive and negative future life events for self and others. *Journal of Personality and Social Psychology, 52,* 994–1001.

Rakowski, W. (1979) Future time perspective in later adulthood: Review and research directions. *Experimental Aging Research, 5,* 43–88.

Rutt, J. L., & Löckenhoff, C. E. (2016). From past to future: Temporal self-continuity across the life span. *Psychology and Aging, 31,* 631–639.

Staudinger, U. M., Bluck, S., & Herzberg, P. Y. (2003). Looking back and looking ahead: Adult age differences in consistency of diachronous ratings of subjective wellbeing. *Psychology and Aging, 18,* 13–24.

Steinberg, L., Graham, S., O'Brien, L., Woolard, J., Cauffman, E., & Banich, M. (2009). Age differences in future orientation and delay discounting. *Child Development, 80,* 28–44.

Strough, J., Bruine de Bruin, W., Parker, A. M., Lemaster, P., Pichayayothin, N., & Delaney, R. (2016). Hour glass half-full or half-empty?: Future time perspective and preoccupation with negative events across the life span. *Psychology and Aging, 31,* 558–573.

Tasdemir-Ozdes, A., Strickland-Hughes, C. M., Bluck, S., & Ebner, N. C. (2016). Future perspective and healthy lifestyle choices in adulthood. *Psychology and Aging, 31,* 618–630.

Thoenes, S., & Oberfeld, D. (2015). Time perception in depression: A meta-analysis. *Journal of Affective Disorders, 175,* 359–372.

Thomas, W. I., & Thomas, D. S. (1928). *The child in America: Behavior problems and programs.* New York: Knopf.

Tornstam, L. (2005). *Gerotranscendence.* New York: Springer.

Vohs, K. D., & Schmeichel, B. J. (2003). Self-regulation and extended now: Controlling the self alters the subjective experience of time. *Journal of Personality and Social Psychology, 85,* 217–230.

Weiss, D., & Lang, F. R. (2012). "They" are old but "I" feel younger: Age-group dissociation as a self-protective strategy in old age. *Psychology and Aging, 27,* 153–163.

Wittmann, M., & Lehnhoff, S. (2005). Age effects in perception of time. *Psychological Reports, 97,* 921–935.

Zimbardo, P. G., & Boyd, J. N. (1999). Putting time into perspective: A valid, reliable individual-differences metric. *Journal of Personality and Social Psychology, 77,* 1271–1288.

Zimbardo, P. G., & Boyd, J. N. (2009). *The time paradox.* London: Rider.

PART III

GOALS AND PLANS

CHAPTER 17

Planning Out Future Action, Affect, and Cognition

Peter M. Gollwitzer
Christina Crosby

On Monday, there is an important meeting that you have to attend. Even though you are highly motivated to contribute to the meeting, you did not find the time to think about it during the week. So you reserve some time on the weekend to prepare for the meeting by setting and committing to goals that specify what you want to achieve in the meeting. In this chapter, we argue that doing so is just a first step toward a successful meeting. You need to take a further step. As successful goal striving commonly faces a host of challenges, we suggest that people better prepare themselves for prospective goal striving by making plans that specify how one wants to manage one's actions, feelings, and thoughts when certain challenges arise.

If–Then Planning

Successful goal striving is facilitated when the chosen goals are highly desirable and perceived as feasible (Gollwitzer, 1990). In other words, the goals that are striven for need to match the person's needs, higher order goals, and attitudes, as well as norms (e.g., regarding needs, see Hagger, Chatzisarantis, & Harris, 2006; Ryan & Deci, 2000; for higher order goals, see Gollwitzer & Kirchhof, 1998; and for attitudes and norms, see Ajzen & Fishbein, 1980), and they have to be in line with the person's control and self-efficacy beliefs (Ajzen, 1991; Bandura, 1977). It also matters how the chosen goals are framed; for instance, as promotion versus prevention goals (Higgins, 1997) or as performance versus learning goals (Dweck & Leggett, 1988). Finally, it is important that one feels committed to attaining the chosen goal (Oettingen, Pak, & Schnetter, 2001), as strong commitments help people to persist (i.e., "stay in the field"; Lewin, 1926).

However, successful goal striving also depends on how effectively people cope with the typical problems faced while they engage in goal striving: People need to get started with the initiation of goal-directed responses (i.e., they should not procrastinate), to shield their goal striving from distractions, and to quickly disengage from ineffective means, and they should not overextend themselves, because that would only handicap other important but currently nonfocal goal pursuits. In the present chapter, we argue that an incredibly powerful self-regulation strategy for effective goal striving is making "if–then" plans (i.e., forming implementation intentions) that spell out behavioral, affective, and cognitive goal-directed responses to potential critical situations ahead of time, prior to actually encountering them.

What Are If–Then Plans?

If–then plans (also referred to as implementation intentions; Gollwitzer, 1993, 1999) focus on the when, where, and how of striving toward one's goals. Ideally, they have the following format: "If the critical situation X is encountered, then I will perform the goal-directed response Y!" These implementation intentions are to be differentiated from goal intentions. The latter merely specify desired end states ("I want to achieve goal X!" or "I want to exert behavior X!"). In implementation intentions, on the other hand, the "if" component of an implementation intention specifies a future critical event or point in time, and the "then" component specifies how one will respond once these situational cues are actually encountered. Implementation intentions thus delegate control over the initiation of the intended response to a specified critical future situation (an opportunity that cannot be missed or an obstacle that needs to be overcome) by creating a link between this situation and a proper response that facilitates goal attainment.

Indeed, implementation intentions have been found to help people with their goal striving. Evidence that forming if–then plans enhances the rate of goal attainment has been obtained in many studies regarding a whole array of different domains, such as achievement, health, sports, and social relationships. A meta-analysis (Gollwitzer & Sheeran, 2006) involving more than 8,000 participants in 94 independent studies revealed a medium-to-large effect size ($d = 0.65$) of implementation intentions on the rate of goal attainment, and this on top of the effects of goal intentions (i.e., control participants who formed mere goal intentions). More recent meta-analyses focusing exclusively on goals of eating a healthy diet (Adriaanse, Vinkers, de Ridder, Hox, & de Wit, 2011) and engaging in physical activity (Belanger-Gravel, Godin, & Amireault, 2013) or on people's prospective memory performance (Chen et al., 2015) also demonstrate the beneficial effects of forming implementation intentions.

How Do Implementation Intentions Work?

The Mental Representation of the "If" Component

Because forming an implementation intention implies the selection of a prospective critical situation, the mental representation of this situation can be expected to become highly activated and hence more accessible. Such heightened accessibility of the situational cue specified in the "if" part of an implementation intention has been demonstrated in studies using different cognitive task paradigms. Webb and Sheeran (2004) used a cue-detection task and observed that the situational cues specified in implementation intentions were detected faster and more accurately than those that were not. Using a dichotic listening task paradigm, Achtziger, Bayer, and Gollwitzer (2012, Study 1) found that words describing the critical cue specified in the "if" part of an implementation intention were drawing attention toward them. When these critical words were presented to the nonattended ear, the shadowing performance in terms of enunciating the words presented in parallel on the attended ear did decrease. Moreover, using a cued-recall task in Study 2, participants more effectively recalled the available situational opportunities to attain a set goal given that these opportunities had been specified in if–then links, and this was true no matter whether the cued recall was requested 15 minutes or 24 hours later. Using a lexical decision task paradigm, Parks-Stamm, Gollwitzer, and Oettingen (2007) observed that implementation intentions not only increased the activation level of the specified critical cue but also diminished the activation level of nonspecified competing situational cues. Finally, a recent line of research looked at perceptual consequences of making if–then plans. In these studies, a well-established chronometric method was employed: the psychological refractory period (PRP) paradigm, combined with the locus-of-slack logic. The collected data (Janczyk, Dambacher, Bieleke, & Gollwitzer, 2015) support the idea that if–then plans even facilitate early perceptual processing and not just attentional responding to the specified critical cues.

In sum, various studies suggest that if–then plans enhance the activation of the mental representation of specified critical situational cues, making them more easily accessible. There are also some studies showing that the heightened accessibility of the mental representation of the critical cues specified in an implementation intention mediates the attainment of the respective goals (e.g., Aarts, Dijksterhuis, & Midden, 1999; Webb & Sheeran, 2007).

The Associative Link between the "If" Part and the "Then" Part

Gollwitzer (1999) postulated that forming implementation intentions creates a strong associative link between the critical situation specified in the "if" part and the goal-directed response specified in the "then" part. The consequence of such situation–response links he refers to as *strategic automaticity:* Even though if–then plans are formed intentionally, once the specified critical cue is encountered, it triggers the linked response in an automatic fashion. More specifically, the execution of the goal-directed response specified in the "then" component of the implementation intention is assumed to exhibit features of automaticity, including immediacy, efficiency, lack of need for a further conscious intent, and autonomous (i.e., stimulus-guided) responding.

Indeed, if–then planners were found to act more quickly (e.g., Gollwitzer & Brandstätter, 1997, Experiment 3), and this speed-up effect did still evince under high cognitive load and thus qualifies as efficient (e.g., Brandstätter, Lengfelder, & Gollwitzer, 2001). Also, a conscious intent to respond is not needed when the critical situation is encountered. Consistent with this last assumption, implementation intention effects were observed even when the critical cue was presented subliminally (e.g., Bayer, Achtziger, Gollwitzer, & Moskowitz, 2009). Finally, action control by implementation intentions is also associated with an enhanced autonomy of the specified critical response (i.e., a further feature of automaticity). Using a flanker task, Wieber and Sassenberg (2006) observed that the situational cue specified in the "if" part of an implementation intention still received attention when it was presented in a task that required ignoring it. In line with this finding, Schweiger Gallo, Pfau, and Gollwitzer (2012) observed that hypnotic instructions enriched with respective implementation intentions produced an increase in hypnotic responsiveness; importantly, this performance increase was accompanied by a felt involuntariness of responding.

In sum, various studies suggest that if–then planning strengthens the associative link between the specified critical cue and the specified response, thus promoting automatic responding to the critical situation. There are also some studies showing that the established associative links mediate the impact of forming implementation intentions on automatic responding (Webb & Sheeran, 2007, 2008).

Further Evidence for the Strategic Automaticity Hypothesis

There is a host of further research supporting the hypothesis that forming implementation intentions allows people to intentionally switch from effortful action control by goals to automatic action control by situational cues. This research can be grouped into three categories: assessing brain data, studying people who have particular difficulties with self-regulation, and demonstrating that implementation intentions still evince their beneficial effects when automatic habitual responses need to be outrun.

BRAIN DATA

In a functional magnetic resonance imaging (fMRI) study, Gilbert, Gollwitzer, Cohen, Oettingen, and Burgess (2009) had participants perform a prospective memory task. Prospective memory performance was assessed in terms of the frequency of acting on a presented prospective stimulus. Participants performed the task on the basis of goal intentions versus implementation intentions. Acting on goal intentions was associated with brain activity in the lateral rostral prefrontal cortex, whereas acting on implementation intentions was associated with brain activity in the medial rostral prefrontal cortex. Brain activity in the latter area is known to be associated with bottom-up (stimulus) control of action, whereas brain activity in the former area is known to be related to top-down (goal) control of action (Burgess, Dumontheil, & Gilbert, 2007). As automatic action control qualifies as highly stimulus driven, these brain data are in line with the data collected using cognitive task paradigms reported above, suggesting that action control by if–then plans is automatic. But do the brain processes triggered by implementation intentions actually mediate the observed facilitating effects on goal attainment? In the Gilbert et al. study (2009), the increased brain activity in the medial rostral prefrontal cortex closely matched the increase in prospective memory performance produced by forming implementation intentions.

CRITICAL SAMPLES

Further support for the strategic automaticity hypothesis (also referred to as the delegation of action control to situational cues hypothesis; Gollwitzer, 2014) comes from studies using critical samples—that is, individuals with poor self-regulatory abilities, such as people with schizophrenia and substance abuse disorders (Brandstätter et al., 2001, Studies 1 & 2), people with frontal lobe damage (Lengfelder & Gollwitzer, 2001), and children with attention-deficit/hyperactivity disorder (ADHD; Gawrilow & Gollwitzer, 2008).

Brandstätter et al. (2001, Study 1) assigned hospitalized opiate addicts under withdrawal the goal to write a short curriculum vitae (CV) before the end of the day; half of the participants formed a relevant implementation intention (they specified when and where they would start to write what), and the other half (control group) formed an irrelevant implementation intention (when and where they would eat what for lunch). Eighty percent of the participants with a relevant implementation intention had written a short CV at the end of the day, whereas none of the participants with an irrelevant implementation intention succeeded in doing so.

Implementation intentions also benefit children with ADHD. These children are known to have deficits in executive functions pertaining to (1) response inhibition, (2) task shifting, (3) working memory, and (4) dealing with delay aversion. Making respective if–then plans ameliorated all of these deficits (see Gawrilow & Gollwitzer, 2008; Gawrilow, Gollwitzer, & Oettingen, 2011a, 2011b). For example, with respect to response inhibition, performance in the presence of stop signals improved in children with ADHD who had formed implementation intentions (Gawrilow & Gollwitzer, 2008, Studies 1 & 2). This improved response inhibition was found to be reflected in electrocortical data. Typically, the P300 component evoked by NoGo stimuli has greater amplitude than the P300 evoked by Go stimuli; however, this difference is less pronounced in children with ADHD. Paul et al. (2007) found that if–then plans improved response inhibition and increased the P300 difference (NoGo minus Go) in children with ADHD.

IMPLEMENTATION INTENTIONS CONTROL HABITUAL RESPONSES

Assuming that the control of responses by implementation intentions is immediate and efficient, and adopting a simple horse race model (Adriaanse, Gollwitzer, de Ridder, de Wit, & Kroese, 2011), people should be in a good position to break reflexive responses by forming implementation intentions that spell out a response contrary to the reflexive response that is to be controlled. This hypothesis has been tested in numerous studies. Automatic biases, such as stereotyping, represent reflexive responses that can be in opposition to one's goals to be fair. Extending earlier work by Gollwitzer and Schaal (1998), Stewart and Payne (2008) found that implementation intentions designed to counter automatic stereotyping (e.g., "When I see a black face, then I will think 'safe'!") indeed reduced automatic stereotyping. Moreover, studies conducted by Schweiger Gallo, Keil, McCulloch, Rockstroh, and Gollwitzer (2009) with individuals suffering from arachnophobia (i.e., fear of spiders) showed that implementation intentions geared toward ignoring presented spider pictures or toward staying calm in the face of such pictures helped reduce the arousal in these participants, even though individuals with arachnophobia are known to reflexively experience arousal when confronted with spider pictures. Using dense-array electroencephalography (EEG), it was shown that implementation intentions specifying an ignore response significantly reduced the early activity in the visual cortex in response to spider pictures typically observed in individuals with arachnophobia, as reflected in a smaller P1 assessed at 120 milliseconds after a spider picture had been presented. Apparently, the strategically automated ignore response managed to outrun the reflexive fear response.

Finally, Cohen, Bayer, Jaudas, and Gollwitzer (2008, Study 2) found that if–then plans help decrease the advantage of habitual behavioral responses over nonhabitual ones as observed in a Simon classification task. In this type of task, classifying a stimulus (e.g., low vs. high tones) with the hand that corresponds to the location of the presented stimulus (i.e., to the left vs. right side of the person) is faster than classifying it with the noncorresponding hand. Specifying a noncorresponding response in an implementation intention that was geared toward fast responding alleviated this reduced speed of classifications made by the noncorresponding hand.

Still, forming implementation intentions may not always block reflexive habitual responses. Whether the reflexive response or the if–then guided response will "win the race" depends on the relative strength of the two behavioral orientations. For instance, if the reflexive response is based on strong habits and the if–then guided response is based on weak implementation intentions, the reflexive response will win over the if–then planned response (Webb, Sheeran, & Luszczynska, 2009); but the reverse should be true when weak habits are in conflict with strong implementation intentions. This implies that inhibiting strong reflexive responses requires the formation of strong implementation intentions (see later discussion).

Alternative Process Mechanisms?

Other potential process mechanisms than the ones described above have been explored. For instance, furnishing goals with implementation intentions might produce an increase in goal commitment or self-efficacy, which in turn may cause a heightened goal attainment. However, a meta-analysis of 66 implementation intention studies that assessed goal commitment or self-efficacy after the formation of if–then plans revealed negligible effects of making if–then plans on goal commitment and self-efficacy (Webb & Sheeran, 2008). Also, having to furnish goals with implementation intentions may be interpreted by the research participants as a hint that the experimenter wants them to do well on the goal at hand. However, no increase in experimenter demand is observed after the formation of implementation intentions (e.g., Schweiger Gallo et al., 2009). Finally, one might argue that implementation intentions have positive effects on goal attainment because they provide extra strategy knowledge. Several studies have critically tested this idea by using if–then plans that did not provide additional strategy information or by providing critical strategy information to participants who had formed mere goal intentions. However, the data did not support the alternative process hypothesis that enhanced strategy knowledge underlies implementation intention effects (e.g.,

Palayiwa, Sheeran, & Thompson, 2010; Webb, Ononaiye, Sheeran, Reidy, & Lavda, 2010).

Finally, the effects of implementation intentions may be understood as nothing more than specific goal effects, in line with Locke and Latham's (2013) goal-setting theory postulating that specific goals lead to better performance than "do your best" goals. The specificity that Locke and Latham are referring to in their extensive research, however, refers to the standards that people want to ultimately meet in their goals, and in their research they find that challenging, precisely defined standards promote goal attainment. In the case of implementation intentions, in contrast, the when, where, and how of goal striving is specified. Thus it is not the level or specificity of goal standards but rather the specificity of goal behavior that accounts for the goal attainment promoting effects of implementation intentions.

PLANNING FOR PROSPECTIVE GOAL STRIVING: THE SELF-REGULATION OF ACTION, AFFECT, AND COGNITION

We now report exemplary studies demonstrating that implementation intentions are very effective in helping people to use prospective situations (opportunities, obstacles) in the service of goal attainment. The studies are grouped in terms of which goal-directed responses were targeted by the if–then plans made by the research participants, that is, behavioral, affective, or cognitive goal-directed responses. For each of the three categories (action, affect, and cognition), we discuss at least two different types of self-regulatory problems and present the relevant research findings.

Future Planning and the Regulation of Action

When it comes to the self-regulation of goal-directed action, it is of primary importance that people initiate relevant behavioral responses (i.e., get started with goal striving) and stay on track until the goal is attained (i.e., shield goal striving from distraction). If–then planning has been found to facilitate meeting these demands of effective goal striving. Extensive research explored what types of if–then plans are best suited to facilitate getting started and staying on track. In this research, different kinds of negative influences on getting started and staying on track were analyzed, such as nonconscious influences from outside or inside the person, as well as performance handicaps people were painfully aware of. If–then planning stood its test, and it was discovered that it even managed to promote group performance in situations in which groups are known to fall behind individual performance.

Planning to Overcome Nonconscious Influences on Behavior

Implementation intentions have been shown to help individuals regain control over a variety of situational influences that affect our behavior outside of awareness, leading to negative consequences, such as driving too fast, overspending, and remaining attached to a failing course of action.

A plethora of studies have documented how human behavior can be primed outside of awareness (Bargh, 2013). Although these primes can at times be facilitative to goal striving, they can be deleterious at others. Gollwitzer, Sheeran, Trötschel, and Webb (2011) used implementation intentions to intervene when nonconscious primes were used to manipulate behavior. In one study, participants had to solve as many arithmetic problems as possible within a set time frame. In a 2 × 2 design, participants were first asked (or not) to form distraction-focused implementation intentions ("If I get distracted, then I will concentrate on the test even more!") and then were primed (or not) to behave prosocially. Later, while working on the arithmetic problems, participants were distracted by a presumed other participant (actually a confederate) asking for directions to the experimenter's office. When primed to behave prosocially, participants spent significantly more time attending to this distraction in comparison with those who had not received the prime. However, those who had formed the implementation intention described above were protected from this priming effect. In a further study, utilizing a driving simulator, Gollwitzer et al. (2011) looked at differences in driving speed and driving errors after some participants were randomly primed to be fast during an ostensibly unrelated prior task. Overall, participants who received the speed prime drove faster and made more driving errors than those who did not receive this prime. However, participants who had formed an implementation intention to control fast driving ("If I enter a curve, then I will slow down, and if I enter a straight road, then I will accelerate!") were shielded from the prime and did not increase their speed and error rate.

In addition to priming, other nonconscious processes, such as mimicry, can also affect our behavior. Behavioral mimicry (when at least two people are engaged in the same behavior) is quite ubiquitous in our social world (Chartrand & Lakin, 2013). Mimicry of others often occurs outside of awareness and is known to induce increased liking for the person who mimics us. This consequence may be to our advantage (e.g., when we want to make friends with people) and our disadvantage (e.g., when a salesperson mimics us to nudge us into buying things from her). Wieber, Gollwitzer, and Sheeran (2014, Study 2) used implementation intentions to buffer against mimicry effects when mimicry was being used for exploitative purposes. First, participants were given the intention to be thrifty, which was then furnished or not furnished with an implementation intention. At the end of the study, all participants were asked by the experimenter who mimicked them (or did not) whether they wanted to use some of the money they had received as compensation to purchase leftovers (e.g., chocolate) from other studies. As it turned out, mimicked participants supported with implementation intentions did not waste money on these leftovers.

The previous studies highlight the impact that nonconscious *external* influences can have on our behavior; however, our behavior can also be affected by *internal* biases that operate outside of our awareness. One such bias, often referred to as the *sunk-cost fallacy* (Arkes & Blumer, 1985), refers to our tendency to perseverate a failing course of action due to the amount of resources we have already invested (e.g., sitting through a terrible 2-hour movie just because you have already paid for the ticket and watched the first 30 minutes). Henderson, Gollwitzer, and Oettingen (2007) approached the sunk-cost fallacy by asking whether implementation intentions could help facilitate disengagement in sunk-cost situations. Participants were asked to form an implementation intention emphasizing abandonment of an unsuccessful means of goal pursuit: "If I receive disappointing feedback, then I'll switch my strategy!" All participants were first asked to solve trivia questions and to select one of three strategies that could, ostensibly, produce different performance outcomes. Participants were then asked to justify the choice of their strategy, a manipulation used by Bobocel and Meyer (1994) to enhance sunk-cost bias. Finally, they completed two sets of the trivia questions. By design, everyone experienced failure concerning the first set, and some participants experienced improvement in the second. After the second set, participants were given the choice to stick with the current strategy or to give up on it and make a change. Those in the control conditions fell prey to the sunk-cost fallacy and maintained their current strategies, regardless of whether or not their performance improved or continued to decline in the second set. Those with the implementation intention to switch when disappointing feedback was received were much more likely to change their strategies, regardless of whether or not performance was improving.

So far, we saw implementation intentions help individuals to act in their best interest despite the presence of a variety of situational contexts that, when left unchecked, threaten to derail their good intentions. In the next section, we look at how implementation intentions facilitate coping with more obvious threats to achievement.

Planning to Overcome Obstacles to Performance

We have just discussed ways in which implementation intentions can help us regain control over unconscious behavioral influences. Now we turn our attention to how implementation intentions can help us regain control when we are aware of our undesirable behavior that handicaps goal attainment. For example, oftentimes when we should be working to meet our goals, we might find ourselves sitting on the couch watching television instead. Perhaps this is because the television was on in the background and we glanced over for a second that turned into 2 hours. Perhaps this is because we are avoiding an important high-stakes task for fear of failing. Whatever the reason, we know that we should be working and are looking for help to get up off the couch. In a number of studies, implementation intentions have been shown to be an effective strategy to overcome such obstacles, whether they are external distractions, such as a television show (Wieber, von Suchodoletz, Heikamp, Trommsdorff, & Gollwitzer, 2011), or internal, such as doubts regarding one's future performance potential (Bayer & Gollwitzer, 2007; Thürmer, McCrea, & Gollwitzer, 2013).

Wieber et al. (2011) examined the effectiveness of using implementation intentions to remain focused on a primary task and avoid becoming consumed by appealing distractions. Children were asked to use a computer to categorize various images of animals and vehicles under two different distraction situations. In the first situation, distracting stimuli that varied in its attractiveness would appear directly in front of the children on the computer screen above the images they were tasked with classifying. In the second situation, a highly attractive animated movie played just to the left of the child, requiring that he or she turn away from the task at hand to view the movie. In the first scenario, an inverse relationship was found between the attractiveness of the distracting stimuli and the children's classification performance. However, for the children who had formed an implementation intention ("If there is a distraction, then I will ignore it!"), this inverse relationship disappeared as they were able to maintain high performance despite the attractiveness of the distraction. In the second scenario, in which an entertaining movie was constantly playing in the background, there was no difference between children with and without implementation intentions regarding how many times a child glanced at the movie screen. However, children who formed implementation intentions spent significantly less time looking overall, which resulted in better performance on the categorization task.

Thürmer et al. (2013) demonstrated that implementation intentions can also be used to curb self-handicapping. When the costs of failing at a given task are high, we can become distracted from the task itself and, instead, preoccupied with defending our sense of self-worth. This particular form of distraction often results in self-handicapping behaviors, by which we purposefully create obstacles to our future success (e.g., failing to study for an upcoming exam) as a way of protecting the self. Thürmer et al. (2013, Study 2) found that participants who formed implementation intentions ("And when I start with the test section of the task, then I will ignore my worries and tell myself: I can do it!") prior to a task ostensibly meant to assess intelligence and predict long-term career success chose to use their free time to better prepare for the upcoming task, in contrast to those who did not form such implementation intentions. Using a similar implementation intention also geared toward fostering self-efficacy, Bayer and Gollwitzer (2007) were able to even improve the performance on the Raven Intelligence Test in female high school students.

Planning to Overcome Obstacles to Group Performance

The previously discussed studies have all focused on individual action control and its shortcomings. We now point out that groups can fall victim to similar action control shortcomings and that these problems can be overcome by utilizing collective, group-based implementation intentions. An immediate question might be: Why should group implementation intentions be necessary if each group member could be given an individual implementation intention directed at the same aim?

The answer to this question is addressed in recent work by Thürmer, Wieber, and Gollwitzer (2017). They used triadic groups tasked with collectively holding up a heavy medicine ball for as long as possible. Groups were randomly assigned to form individual implementation intentions ("And if my muscles hurt, then I will ignore the pain and tell myself: I can do it!"), collective implementation intentions ("And if our muscles hurt, then we will ignore the pain and tell ourselves: We can do it!"), or an individual or collective control condition that received the same information without the if–then format ("We (I) will ignore our (my) muscle pain and tell ourselves (myself): We (I) can do it!"). Performance was measured as decrease in persistence compared with a baseline measure. Groups who formed implementation intentions performed significantly better than those who did not form implementation intentions, and groups who made collective plans performed better than those who made individual if–then plans. Moreover, collective implementation intentions appeared to foster more intensive group interaction and communication than individual implementation intentions. Thürmer et al. (2017) went on to show that when open communication is allowed within a group, collective implementation intentions are more effective than individual implementation intentions; however, when group communication is impeded, individual implementation intentions produce better performance outcomes. Therefore, whether collective or individual if–then plans are most beneficial will depend on the group context.

Just like individuals, groups have a tendency to fall prey to the sunk-cost fallacy and escalate commitment to failing courses of action. Wieber, Thürmer, and Gollwitzer (2015) were interested in whether implementation intentions, which had been shown to reduce escalating commitment in individuals, could prevent groups from making ill-advised investments. Participants were grouped into triads and asked to simulate a city council committee tasked with overseeing the funding of a local project. In three stages, the triad was asked to invest more of the city's budget into the project (despite the fact that the costs began to outweigh the benefits as time went on). Participants were told that the money that was not invested in the project would go toward other important city costs (such as hospital and school maintenance). Whereas control condition participants continued to invest large proportions of their city budget into the failing project, those in the collective implementation intentions condition ("If we are about to make an investment decision, then we will judge the project as neutral observers who are not responsible for earlier decisions!") invested significantly less money during the second and third stages. This implementation intention apparently empowered the groups to distance themselves from the initial investment, thus curtailing future investments.

A benefit to group decision making is that groups can make better informed decisions than any single individual by pooling the knowledge of all group members together—but group members often fail to capitalize on this advantage. Thürmer, Wieber, and Gollwitzer (2015) explored whether collective implementation intentions could overcome this common group oversight. Participants were again placed into triads tasked with making the optimal choice among multiple fictitious job applicants. Prior to any group discussion, individual participants were given limited information that would lead to a suboptimal candidate choice. The truly optimal candidate would only become apparent after considering all of the collective group knowledge. Groups that made a collective implementation intention to consider all of the available information prior to making their final choice detected the ideal applicant more frequently than groups that did not form this collective implementation intention (despite having access to all of the collective information).

Future Planning and Affect Regulation

Implementation intentions' self-regulatory benefits for action control extend into emotion regulation (summaries by Sheeran, Webb, Gollwitzer, & Oettingen, in press; Webb, Schweiger Gallo, Miles, Gollwitzer, & Sheeran, 2012). Implementation intentions allow people to take control of their affect in one of two ways: via either a direct or indirect path. In the direct path, implementation intentions focus on down- or up-regulating an anticipated critical emotion (e.g., reducing anticipated disgust or enhancing prospective happiness): "If I feel disgust (joy), then I will tell myself: Stay calm! (Enjoy your happiness!)." In the indirect path, implementation intentions are used to prevent the elicitation of the critical emotion: "If somebody utters a stinging (nice) comment then I tell myself: He didn't mean it that way!" For this purpose, one can also make an if–then plan to ignore the comment altogether. In the following, we discuss a number of studies that used different kinds of implementation intentions to control future emotions.

Planning to Regulate Disgust

In general, upsetting stimuli are associated with negative valence and high arousal, whereas pleasant stimuli are associated with moderate arousal but positive valence (e.g., Lang, Bradley, & Cuthbert, 1999). Thus it is the combination of the negative valence and high arousal that can make a stimulus unpleasant; if either of these components were to be reduced, the stimulus should not be as upsetting. Using disgusting objects as stimuli, Schweiger Gallo, McCulloch, and Gollwitzer (2012) targeted each of these components in isolation using either indirect implementation intentions ("And if I see blood, then I will take the perspective of a physician!") to reduce negative valence without altering arousal or direct implementation intentions ("And if I see blood, then I will stay calm and relaxed!") to reduce arousal without changing valence. Participants were exposed to a series of images consisting of equal proportions of positive, neutral, and disgusting pictures and asked to provide valence and arousal ratings for each image. As predicted, in comparison with control participants, the ratings of disgusting images made by participants who had formed indirect implementation intentions showed significantly reduced negative valence ratings with no difference regarding arousal. When the direct implementation intentions had been formed, participants showed decreased arousal to disgusting images in comparison with control participants but showed no difference in their valence ratings. These results emphasize the precision with which implementation intentions can be used to regulate anticipated affect. In line with this finding, Schweiger Gallo et al. (2009) observed that regulating disgust with implementation intentions did not come at an emotional cost to the experience of other emotions. The disgust-regulating implementation intentions did not create an overall flat affect in participants; rather, participants were still able to fully enjoy the positive affect associated with the pleasant images.

Further evidence for the precision with which implementation intentions can operate is presented in a recent study focusing on the emotion of *grima* (Schweiger Gallo, Fernández-Dols, Gollwitzer, & Keil, 2017). *Grima,* a Spanish word with no perfectly corresponding word in English, refers to the unpleasant feelings associated with distressingly high-pitched, squeaky sounds, such as hearing somebody's fingernails scratch a chalkboard. Schweiger Gallo et al. (2017) found that although *grima* is most similar to feelings of disgust (*asco* in Spanish), it does possess unique characteristics, such as being specifically elicited by auditory stimuli and varying in certain physiological responses (e.g., differential changes in heart rate). To test whether implementation intentions would allow discerning regulation of such similar negative emotions as *grima* and *asco,* Schweiger Gallo et al. (2017) had participants (native Spanish speakers) listen to pleasant and unpleasant stimuli (which included sounds uniquely associated with *grima* or *asco*) and asked them to rate associated valence and arousal. Prior to this listening task, some participants formed a *grima*-specific implementation intention ("And if I hear a *grima*-eliciting sound, then I will ignore it!"). Participants with this implementation intention geared toward down-regulating *grima* were able to successfully weaken the *grima*, but not the disgust, experience. In other words, the effect of the implementation intentions held true for the *grima*-eliciting sounds only, not for disgust-related sounds.

Planning to Regulate Anxiety

In a number of studies, implementation intentions have also been shown to successfully reduce anxiety (e.g., Parks-Stamm, Gollwitzer, & Oettingen, 2010; Schweiger Gallo et al., 2009; Stern, Cole, Gollwitzer, Oettingen, & Balcetis, 2013). As we have already discussed the studies by Schweiger Gallo et al. (2009) with participants with arachnophobia, we focus here on sports performance anxiety and text anxiety, utilizing different types of implementation intentions.

Stern et al. (2013) looked at regulating anxiety for a golf-putting task (Study 1) and a dart-throwing task (Study 2). In order to induce anxiety, participants' performances were filmed, ostensibly for experts to analyze and critique. However, before engaging in the respective tasks, participants were asked to generate their own personalized implementation intentions. Given that people respond differently under pressure, this guaranteed that participants were able to target personally relevant anxiety-related affective states (e.g., "If I feel irritated, then I will tell myself to relax"). In comparison to participants who did not form an implementation intention to regulate their anxiety (adjusting for individual differences in previous experience), those who did were significantly less anxious (as measured by objective coders blind to conditions) and perceived their targets to be closer (i.e., less difficult). As a result, participants in the implementation intentions condition performed significantly better than those whose anxiety went unregulated.

Although the varying types of implementation intentions discussed thus far appear to work equally well, it is important to point out that not all forms of implementation intentions can be expected to effectively control one's affective responses. Before having participants complete a math test designed to tax working memory while being distracted by entertaining commercials on the same screen, Parks-Stamm et al. (2010) had participants complete a scale of general test anxiety. Next, participants formed either the implementation intentions of "If I hear or see the commercials, then I will ignore them!" or "If I hear or see the commercials, then I will increase my efforts on the math task!" Although the type of implementation intention did not matter for those with low test anxiety, for those who were highly anxious about exams, the implementation intention focusing on increasing effort on the task diminished their performance. Apparently, forming implementation intentions that are geared toward increasing one's efforts is counterproductive for individuals who are already shaken by high test anxiety. Similarly, Gollwitzer and Schaal (1998) observed that highly motivated individuals experienced reduced performance when using an effort-focused implementation intention to overcome disruptive stimuli.

Planning to Regulate Counterproductive Positive Emotions

The previous sections focused on down-regulating unpleasant emotions such as anxiety and disgust; however, it can sometimes be necessary to down-regulate positive emotions to achieve one's goals. Although positive moods are generally thought to be desirable and beneficial, positive moods can also make us more susceptible to reliance on heuristics and stereotypes (e.g., Beukeboom & Semin, 2005). Thus a positive mood can be a barrier to one's good intentions to judge other people in an accurate, nonstereotypical way. Bayer, Gollwitzer, and Achtziger (2010), capitalizing on the known regulatory benefits of implementation intentions, investigated whether implementation intentions could be used to prevent enhanced stereotypical judgments during positive affective states. Participants watched either a film clip of stand-up comedy (to induce a positive mood) or a documentary (to induce a neutral mood) prior to judging two women in hand-painted sketches. Participants were asked to choose from different statements describing the women in the sketches and were provided with multiple-choice answers, with one gender-stereotypical choice for each image. Some participants also formed an implementation intention designed to prevent the consequential effects of a positive mood ("Whenever I analyze a given person, then I will ignore her gender!"). Participants with a positive mood induction chose less stereotypical descriptions when they had formed this implementation intention—actually as few as participants without a positive mood. In contrast, when no such implementation intention had been formed, participants with a positive mood induction showed the common effect that positive mood enhances stereotyping.

Anger can be looked at as a positive emotion when it comes to asserting oneself. For example, romantic relationships benefit when a partner does not hide but discloses his or her anger (Baumeister, Stillwell, & Wotman, 1990), and in the business domain it has been found that conveyed anger during negotiations often leads opponents to yield (van Kleef, Dreu, & Manstead, 2004). However, when engaged in ultimatum bargaining in which one party has the power to propose how a lump of money sitting on the table is to be shared, anger over unfair offers (i.e., the proposer taking an unequally large share of the money) commonly leads the receiver to reject the proposed offer, ending up with even less money (Güth, Schmittberger, & Schwarze, 1982). From an economic perspective, this is a foolish retort, given that getting something is always better than getting less (or even nothing at all). Kirk, Gollwitzer, and Carnevale (2011) used an ultimatum game task paradigm to study the regulation of anger by implementation intentions. Participants had to play the role of the receiver, and it was explained that if the proposed offer was rejected, then the proposer and the receiver would only receive a minor part of the offer the proposer had made. Before receiving a series of unfair offers, some participants formed the implementation intentions of either "If I feel any negative emotions, then I will tell myself: Stay calm!" or "If I receive an offer, then I will tell myself: This is an opportunity to make money!" There were no significant differences found between the two types of implementation intentions, but the acceptance rate of unfair offers was higher in receivers who had formed either of the two implementation intentions in comparison with those who did not.

Future Planning and the Regulation of Cognition

Dual-process models of thinking segment cognitive processing into two separate modes of thought: reflective and impulsive (e.g., Strack & Deutsch, 2004). Reflective processes are more effortful, requiring slow, deliberate, and conscious consideration, whereas impulsive processes require less cognitive effort and are quick, automatic, and often operate outside of awareness via previously formed cognitive associations. Implementation intentions are uniquely situated within dual-process models in that people can use them to strategically plan ahead of time whether they want to be guided by a reflective or reflexive thought process when they enter a critical prospective situation (Martiny-Huenger, Bieleke, Oettingen, & Gollwitzer, 2016). In the following, we present studies demonstrating this, and show that implementation intentions can be used to control not only the thinking process but also the content of thoughts.

Planning to Change One's Mode of Thought

In the research by Henderson et al. (2007), reported earlier, on people's readiness to switch between strategies (means) of performing a given task, a further implementation intention was used that read like this: "If I receive disappointing feedback, then I'll think about how things have been going with my strategy!" For participants who had formed this reflection implementation intention, it was found that the decision to switch one's strategy for performing the task at hand reflected not just the failure feedback that was received regarding the first set of items but also whether there was any improvement (positive feedback) or not in performing the second set of items.

Encouraged by this finding suggesting that if–then plans can help people to engage in reflection, Doerflinger, Martiny-Huenger, and Gollwitzer (2017; Study 1) explored the effectiveness of using implementation intentions to facilitate a reflective thinking process when making decisions about ongoing investments. In a first experiment, given the hypothetical role of a chief financial officer, participants had to decide which of two departments within the company should receive a large sum of money as an initial investment. Next, participants were told that 5 years later, their chosen department was either thriving and profitable or not. Participants were then provided a second sum of money to be divided up between the two departments as they wished. It turned out that only participants who received negative feedback and were equipped with an implementation intention to deliberate before making a reinvestment decision ("If the situation looks unfavorable, then I will deliberate thoroughly!") invested significantly less money to the department that was initially chosen. Those in the negative feedback condition who did not make the deliberation plan made reinvestment decisions similar to those in the positive feedback condition—behaving as if their initially chosen department were thriving instead of failing. In two follow-up experiments, using a poker game in which participants could earn actual cash, a reflective implementation intention was tested against an impulsive implementation intention ("If the situation looks unfavorable, then I will decide quickly and spontaneously!"). There was a significant main effect of perceived probability. The more likely it looked that one had a losing hand, the higher the odds were that participants would fold and end the round instead of increasing their investment; importantly, however, this relationship was stronger for those who formed a reflective rather than an impulsive implementation intention.

Like Kirk et al. (2011), Bieleke, Gollwitzer, Oettingen, and Fischbacher (2017) also sought to help individuals profit from any financial opportunity, even one below their ideal marker of fairness. Using an ultimatum task paradigm, participants received 10 ultimatum offers that varied in equitability. Participants were given either a reflection-focused implementation intention ("If I start acting in a hasty way, then I will tell myself: Use your brain!") or an impulsivity-focused one ("If I start pondering at length, then I will tell myself: Listen to your guts!"). Participants of the two implementation intention conditions significantly differed in their response times to unfair offers, with participants with the reflection-focused plan taking more time before making a decision. Moreover, those who formed reflection-focused implementation intentions were more likely to accept the unfair offers, that is, to opt for making more profitable decisions.

Planning to Change Future Thought Content

Although reasoning outcomes can be improved by implementing a more reflective thought process (as seen in the preceding section), this may not always be possible, as reasoning sometimes runs off too quickly for reflection to get in between. In these situations, however, people still have the option of "programming" the content of their thoughts ahead of time.

Although racial bias, such as believing that minorities are more violent and dangerous, can be overcome with deliberate thought, engaging in effortful reflection is not always possible, and there can be disastrous consequences when split-second decisions are called for. There are frequent examples of the cost of split-second decisions in the form of headlines regarding lethal force used by police officers in which the victim is significantly more likely to be black or Hispanic than white (Buehler, 2017). Provided that these split-second decisions happen in the realm of impulsive, automatic processing that is hard to moderate (Strack & Deutsch, 2004), there is the question of whether content-focused implementation intentions qualify as an alternative. Luckily, research by Mendoza, Gollwitzer, and Amodio (2010) provides a positive answer. They hypothesized that racial disparity in the use of deadly force is reduced if the shooter is able to remove racial content (which is irrelevant to the decision of whether or not force should be used) from his or her thoughts. To test this hypothesis, Mendoza et al. (2010) had participants engage in a shooter task in which they were shown images of black and white males holding either a weapon object (e.g., a gun) or a nonweapon object (e.g., a cell phone) with the instruction to quickly shoot any armed targets. To ensure that decisions were made so quickly that deliberate thinking could not take place, participants received an error message if they slowed down their responses. Results replicated previous findings indicating an overall racial bias in shooter tasks (Correll et al., 2007). There were, however, significantly fewer shooting errors made overall, and particularly in trials with unarmed and black targets, by participants who had made if–then plans ("If I see a person, then I will ignore his race!" and "If I see a person with a gun, then I will shoot! If I see a person with an object, then I will not shoot!") compared with control participants without such plans.

Another kind of automatic, cognitive bias that people often fall prey to is that of social projection, whereby we assume that other people hold similar beliefs and attitudes to our own (e.g., "I like sushi; so other people must like sushi, too"). Although such projection can have its benefits, such as increased feelings of closeness (Robbins & Krueger, 2005), it can also have costs (e.g., when projecting that the majority of people smoke cigarettes hinders behavior change). Given the fact that social projection can have positive as well as negative consequences, A. Gollwitzer, Schwörer, Stern, Gollwitzer, and Bargh (2017) explored whether implementation intentions could be used for both intensifying and reducing social projection. They found that implementation intentions could successfully up-regulate ("If I'm asked to estimate what percentage of people agree with me, then I will remember that other people are similar!") as well as down-regulate ("If I'm asked to estimate what percentage of other people agree with me, then I will remember that other people are different!") this cognitive bias.

OPEN QUESTIONS

Even though research on the effects of if–then plans on the rate of goal attainment and the underlying processes of these effects has been quite extensive since the time when the concept of implementation intentions was first introduced (Gollwitzer, 1993), there are still a host of research questions that need to be addressed.

Potential Moderators

Moderators of if–then plan effects on goal attainment have been targeted so far with respect to features of the implementation intentions formed, the superordinate goal, the person, and the context in which implementation intentions are formed and executed.

Features of If–Then Plans

Only if–then plans to which people feel highly committed can be expected to guide people's actions (Achtziger et al., 2012). The person with an if–then plan that carries high commitment no longer feels that there is a choice to be made when the critical situation is encountered. The action to be taken in the critical situation has been determined ahead of time and the person is now on autopilot—the planned action will be triggered directly by the specified situational cue.

Implementation intentions may, however, differ in their format. For instance, when it comes to shielding an ongoing goal pursuit from internal and external disruptions, a variety of different if–then plans can be used. Take the example of a person whose goal is to stay friendly to a neighbor who keeps making outrageous requests. She may form suppression-oriented implementation intentions, such as "If my neighbor approaches me with an outrageous request, then I will not get upset!" The "then" component of such suppression-oriented implementation intentions does not have to be worded in terms of not showing (i.e., negating) the critical behavior (in the present example, getting upset); it may alternatively specify a replacement behavior (" . . . then I will respond in a friendly manner!") or focus on ignoring the critical cue altogether (" . . ., then I'll ignore her request!"). Research by Adriaanse, van Oosten, de Ridder, de Wit, and Evers (2011) suggests that negation implementation intentions are less effective than the latter two types (i.e., replacement and ignoring if–then plans). One can also form implementation intentions geared toward stabilizing the ongoing focal goal pursuit at hand. For instance, "If the first part of my paper is finished, then I'll immediately turn to the second part!" Bayer et al. (2010) demonstrated the effectiveness of such if–then plans in a series of studies showing that if–then plans geared toward stabilizing an ongoing goal pursuit effectively blocked the disruptive effects of self-doubts, inappropriate moods, and ego depletion. Recent research shows that the ongoing goal pursuit can also be stabilized in a more general way (Kroese, Adriaanse, Evers, & De Ridder, 2011; van Koningsbruggen, Stroebe, Papies, & Aarts, 2011) by specifying the disruptive stimulus in the "if" part and a reminder of the goal at hand in the "then" part: " . . . then I will remind myself that my paper has a deadline that I want to meet!"

When forming implementation intentions, strong associative links between the critical situation and the goal-directed response have to be created. This is achieved most easily when implementation intentions use an if–then format. Simply specifying the when, where, and how of goal striving is a suboptimal way of creating strong associative links. Chapman, Armitage, and Norman (2009) observed that, for the goal to increase fruit and vegetable intake, inducing implementation intentions using an if–then format had a greater impact than stimulating implementation intentions by asking research participants to list the when, where, and how of acting toward the goal.

For if–then plans to be effective, it is also important that people specify the critical situational cue in a way so that it is readily detected when it is actually encountered. Even though concrete specifications may appear to be superior in this respect than abstract specifications, this may not always be true. Think, for example, of the specification of internal cues. Specifying as the critical cue the state of getting irritated may seem rather abstract, but the individual (e.g., a tennis player who wants to stay calm when he is falling behind in the game; Achtziger, Gollwitzer, & Sheeran, 2008) knows exactly what is implied and will thus easily identify this state when it occurs. When it comes to appropriate specifications of the "then" component of an if–then plan, it seems crucial to pick a response that is highly instrumental to goal attainment. Also, it needs to be a response the person feels capable of executing in the critical situation (i.e., for which self-efficacy is high; Wieber, Odenthal, & Gollwitzer, 2010).

Features of the Planning Person

Various relevant personality attributes have been discussed (Gollwitzer, 2014). The personality attribute of socially prescribed perfectionism seems to undermine implementation intention effects on goal progress, whereas for participants who score high on self-oriented perfectionism no such effects are observed. Possibly, social perfectionists fail to commit and stick to implementation intentions because they are very sensitive to the fact that the preferences of others often change unexpectedly and that their high readiness to respond to such changes in a flexible manner may be undermined by strong commitments to a fixed if–then plan. Moreover, the willingness to make if–then plans and reliably enact them seems to be reduced in highly impulsive individuals. For individuals high in urgency, it was found that implementation intentions fail to promote goal attainment when the situational context is emotionally charged. Making if–then plans and acting on them is heightened, however, in individuals high in conscientiousness and those with a propensity to manage their time and money effectively.

Features of the Targeted Goal

Many studies report that participants who form implementation intentions perform better than participants who only form goal intentions, in particular when the goals at hand are difficult rather than easy (Gollwitzer & Sheeran, 2006). In addition, having a strong goal commitment in place is a prerequisite for the positive effects of implementation intentions on goal attainment. Sheeran, Webb, and Gollwitzer (2005, Study 1) report that weak goal commitments undermine the effectiveness of if–then plans. This observation is in line with findings by Koestner, Lekes, Powers, and Chicoine (2002) showing that implementation intentions evince stronger effects when they are formed in the service of self-concordant goals. People also refrain from acting on their if–then plans when the respective goal is not activated in the situation at hand (Sheeran et al., 2005, Study 2).

Features of the Context

One important contextual feature is the emotional state of the person when forming if–then plans and when enacting them. Anger is an emotional state with positive effects on plan formation and enactment (Maglio, Gollwitzer, & Oettingen, 2014). It creates a strong sense of control that facilitates both the making of firm plans and the decisive acting on them. Another relevant contextual feature seems to be the person's mindset. When a person is deliberating on the pros and cons of pursuing a goal, he or she experiences a deliberative mindset (Gollwitzer, 2012) that is characterized by enhanced open-mindedness. As implementation intentions affect behavior by automatic bottom-up action control, deliberative mindsets undermine this type of action control—eliminating the common beneficial effects that implementation intentions have on goal attainment (Wieber, Sezer, & Gollwitzer, 2014).

Considering All of These Moderators at Once

In sum, many factors have been found to enhance or weaken action control by implementation intentions. Most studies so far have focused on one of these factors at a time. But future research might want to address the question of how these factors interact, as is exemplified by a recent set of studies reported by Hall, Zehr, Ng, and Zanna (2012). They examined the joint influence of goal strength, executive control resources (ECR), and differentially supportive environmental conditions on the effectiveness of implementation intentions geared toward enhancing physical exercise. The beneficial effects of implementation intentions turned out to be more potent under challenging environmental conditions, and implementation intentions were of special benefit for those with initially low ECRs. More recent research by Hall, Zehr, Paultzki, and Rhodes (2014), also examining the interaction of potentially undermining factors of implementation intention effects, found that in old to very old people, low ECRs undermine the positive effects of implementation intentions on physical activity.

Such a comprehensive approach is also called for when it comes to sticking two different types of self-regulation strategies together to create a powerful behavior-change intervention. For instance, having mental contrasting precede the formation of implementation intentions makes great sense, as it puts the prerequisites for if–then plan effects into place. Mental contrasting (Oettingen, 2000, 2012; Oettingen et al., 2001) implies juxtaposing fantasies about desired future outcomes with obstacles of present reality. This strategy not only creates strong goal commitments and vigorous goal striving in individuals with high expectations of success but also guarantees the identification of personally relevant obstacles that can then be specified as the critical cues in the "if" component of implementation intentions. Moreover, it helps to identify instrumental responses to be specified in the "then" component. Finally, mental contrasting has been found to create a readiness for making plans that link obstacles to instrumental goal-directed responses (Kappes, Singmann, & Oettingen, 2012). As implementation intentions are known to unfold their beneficial effects when the commitment to both the goal and the respective implementation intention is high, mental contrasting guarantees that these prerequisites are in place.

However, sticking two self-regulatory behavior change tools together may not always be beneficial. Various studies explored whether combining self-affirmation with the formation of implementations would intensify behavior-change effects. Whereas self-affirmation plus if–then plan formation worked well in some intervention studies (e.g., reducing alcohol consumption; Ferrer, Shmueli, Bergman, Harris, & Klein, 2012; eating more fruits and vegetables; Harris et al., 2014), it did not help in others (e.g., promoting exercise behavior; Jessop, Sparks, Buckland, Harris, & Churchill, 2014). Possibly, whenever the information provided with regard to the behavior change at issue turns out to threaten the person's self-integrity, a self-affirmation exercise prior to forming implementation intentions may be helpful, as it reduces self-defensiveness and thus encourages making binding if–then plans. If the information is nonthreatening, however, a self-affirmation exercise may not be helpful, as it may curb the perceived necessity to make goal-promoting if–then plans; one feels already pretty good about oneself and one's goal striving does not seem to need a boost.

Costs of If–Then Planning?

Given the many benefits of forming if–then plans, one wonders about potential costs. Such costs may be expected when recognizing and quickly seizing an alternative opportunity is essential for achieving the goal at hand. Indeed, Masicampo and Baumeister (2012) report that when participants were assigned a task goal in the lab, making an if–then plan hindered participants' ability to capitalize on a presented alternative opportunity for achieving the goal. But is the failure to use alternative opportunities actually a cost in terms of reaching the goal for which the implementation intention has been formed? Note that the goal is still attained even though an alternative opportunity to realize the goal has not been seized. Therefore, from a goal-attainment perspective, speaking of costs only makes sense when a better opportunity is not seized. So the question arises whether opportunities that promise easier or more beneficial goal attainment than the one specified in one's implementation intention will indeed stay unused. Interestingly, research on this question shows that implementation intention participants seem to have no problems with making effective use of unexpectedly arising better opportunities (Gollwitzer, Parks-Stamm, Jaudas, & Sheeran, 2008). Analogous research analyzing the use of alternative goal-directed responses shows that implementation intentions also seem to allow people to stay open to the use of responses that are of higher, or at least equivalent, instrumentality.

Moreover, as discussed above, implementation intentions respect the strength of the superordinate goal and its state of activation. This means that people can be expected to sensitively adjust their goal striving to the strength and activation of the goal at hand. They should stop striving for goals they have attained and halt striving in inappropriate contexts. So there is no need to fear that if–then-guided goal striving is rigidly repeated again and again only because the critical situation is encountered repeatedly or that people rigidly act on their if–then plans in inappropriate situations. Recent research also shows that if–then-guided goal striving is quite sensitive to failure feedback (Gollwitzer et al., 2008; Legrand, Bieleke, Gollwitzer, & Mignon, 2017). The feedback only needs to be articulate and severe so that the person acting on an if–then plan respects it. Still, future research might want to investigate how if–then plans can be worded in a way so that rigidity is kept at a minimum. One route we can imagine to be effective is using "if" and "then" specifications that are rather inclusive (e.g., "If I get anxious, then I will tell myself: Be confident!"), covering many different critical situations and many instrumental responses.

Conclusion

B. F. Skinner proposed in 1971 that in order to change behavior, the environment must be structured in such a way as to reward desirable behaviors. This implies that who we are and what we do is purely the result of the situations we find ourselves in. However, given the limited control we have on the world around us, Skinner's perspective paints quite a bleak outlook for anyone looking to change his or her behavior in the future. But as we have discussed in the present chapter, implementation intentions allow us to commandeer prospective situations to our personal benefit by linking them to desired, goal-directed responses.

References

Aarts, H., Dijksterhuis, A., & Midden, C. (1999). To plan or not to plan?: Goal achievement or interrupting the performance of mundane behaviors. *European Journal of Social Psychology, 29,* 971–979.

Achtziger, A., Bayer, U. C., & Gollwitzer, P. M. (2012). Committing to implementation intentions: Attention and memory effects for selected situational cues. *Motivation and Emotion, 36,* 287–303.

Achtziger, A., Gollwitzer, P. M., & Sheeran, P. (2008). Implementation intentions and shielding goal striving from unwanted thoughts and feelings. *Personality and Social Psychology Bulletin, 34,* 381–393.

Adriaanse, M. A., Gollwitzer, P. M., de Ridder, D. T. D., de Wit, J. B. F., & Kroese, F. M. (2011). Breaking habits with implementation intentions: A test of underlying processes. *Personality and Social Psychology Bulletin, 37,* 502–513.

Adriaanse, M. A., van Oosten, J. M., de Ridder, D. T., de Wit, J. B., & Evers, C. (2011). Planning what not to eat: Ironic effects of implementation intentions negating unhealthy habits. *Personality and Social Psychology Bulletin, 37,* 69–81.

Adriaanse, M. A., Vinkers. C. D. W., de Ridder, D. T. D., Hox, J. J., & de Wit, J. B. F. (2011). Do implementation intentions help to eat a healthy diet?: A systematic review and meta-analysis of the empirical evidence. *Appetite, 56,* 183–193.

Ajzen, I. (1991). The theory of planned behavior. *Organizational Behavior and Human Decision Processes, 50,* 179–211.

Ajzen, I., & Fishbein, M. (1980). *Understanding attitudes and predicting social behavior.* Englewood Cliffs, NJ: Prentice-Hall.

Arkes, H. R., & Blumer, C. (1985). The psychology of sunk cost. *Organizational Behavior and Human Decision Processes, 35,* 124–140.

Bandura, A. (1977). Self-efficacy: Toward a unifying theory of behavioral change. *Psychological Review, 84,* 191–215.

Bargh, J. A. (Ed.). (2013). *Social psychology and the unconscious: The automaticity of higher mental processes.* New York: Psychology Press.

Baumeister, R. F., Stillwell, A., & Wotman, S. R. (1990). Victim and perpetrator accounts of interpersonal conflict: Autobiographical narratives about anger. *Journal of Personality and Social Psychology, 59,* 994–1005.

Bayer, U. C., Achtziger, A., Gollwitzer, P. M., & Moskowitz, G. (2009). Responding to subliminal cues: Do if–then plans cause action preparation and initiation without conscious intent? *Social Cognition, 27,* 183–201.

Bayer, U. C., & Gollwitzer, P. M. (2007). Boosting scholastic test scores by willpower: The role of implementation intentions. *Self and Identity, 6,* 1–19.

Bayer, U. C., Gollwitzer, P. M., & Achtziger, A. (2010). Staying on track: Planned goal striving is protected from disruptive internal states. *Journal of Experimental Social Psychology, 146,* 505–514.

Belanger-Gravel, A., Godin, G., & Amireault, S. (2013). A meta-analytic review of the effect of implementation intentions on physical activity. *Health Psychology Review, 7,* 23–54.

Beukeboom, C. J., & Semin, G. R. (2005). Mood and representations of behaviour: The how and why. *Cognition and Emotion, 19,* 1242–1251.

Bieleke, M., Gollwitzer, P. M., Oettingen, G., & Fischbacher, U. (2017). Social value orientation moderates the effects of intuition versus reflection on responses to unfair ultimatum offers. *Journal of Behavioral Decision Making, 30,* 569–581.

Bobocel, D. R., & Meyer, J. P. (1994). Escalating commitment to a failing course of action: Separating the roles of choice and justification. *Journal of Applied Psychology, 79,* 360–363.

Brandstätter, V., Lengfelder, A., & Gollwitzer, P. M. (2001). Implementation intentions and efficient action initiation. *Journal of Personality and Social Psychology, 81,* 946–960.

Buehler, J. W. (2017). Racial/ethnic disparities in the use of lethal force by US police, 2010–2014. *American Journal of Public Health, 107,* 295–297.

Burgess, P. W., Dumontheil, I., & Gilbert, S. J. (2007). The gateway hypothesis of rostral PFC (Area 10) function. *Trends in Cognitive Sciences, 11,* 290–298.

Chapman, J., Armitage, C. J., & Norman, P. (2009). Comparing implementation intention interventions in relation to young adults' intake of fruit and vegetables. *Psychology and Health, 24*, 317–332.

Chartrand, T. L., & Lakin, J. L. (2013). The antecedents and consequences of human behavioral mimicry. *Annual Review of Psychology, 64*, 285–308.

Chen, X. J., Wang, Y., Liu, L. L., Cui, J. F., Gan, M. Y., Shum, D. H., & Chan, R. C. (2015). The effect of implementation intention on prospective memory: A systematic and meta-analytic review. *Psychiatry Research, 226*, 14–22.

Cohen, A.-L., Bayer, U. C., Jaudas, A., & Gollwitzer, P. M. (2008). Self-regulatory strategy and executive control: Implementation intentions modulate task switching and Simon task performance. *Psychological Research, 72*, 12–26.

Correll, J., Park, B., Judd, C. M., Wittenbrink, B., Sadler, M. S., & Keesee, T. (2007). Across the thin blue line: Police officers and racial bias in the decision to shoot. *Journal of Personality and Social Psychology, 92*, 1006–1023.

Doerflinger, J., Martiny-Huenger, T., & Gollwitzer, P. M. (2017). Planning to deliberate thoroughly: If–then planned deliberation increases the adjustment of decisions to newly available information. *Journal of Experimental Social Psychology, 69*, 1–12.

Dweck, C. S., & Leggett, E. L. (1988). A social-cognitive approach to motivation and personality. *Psychological Review, 95*, 256–273.

Ferrer, R. A., Shmueli, D., Bergman, H. E., Harris, P. R., & Klein, W. M. P. (2012). Effects of self-affirmation on implementation intentions and the moderating role of affect. *Social Psychological and Personality Science, 3*, 300–307.

Gawrilow, C., & Gollwitzer, P. M. (2008). Implementation intentions facilitate response inhibition in children with ADHD. *Cognitive Therapy and Research, 32*, 261–280.

Gawrilow, C., Gollwitzer, P. M., & Oettingen, G. (2011a). If–then plans benefit delay of gratification performance in children with and without ADHD. *Cognitive Therapy and Research, 35*, 442–455.

Gawrilow, C., Gollwitzer, P. M., & Oettingen, G. (2011b). If–then plans benefit executive functions in children with ADHD. *Journal of Social and Clinical Psychology, 30*, 616–646.

Gilbert, S. J., Gollwitzer, P. M., Cohen, A.-L., Oettingen, G., & Burgess, P. W. (2009). Separable brain systems supporting cued versus self-initiated realization of delayed intentions. *Journal of Experimental Psychology: Learning, Memory, and Cognition, 35*, 905–915.

Gollwitzer, A., Schwörer, B., Stern, C., Gollwitzer, P. M., & Bargh, J. A. (2017). Down and up regulation of a highly automatic process: Implementation intentions can both decrease and increase social projection. *Journal of Experimental Social Psychology, 70*, 19–26.

Gollwitzer, P. M. (1990). Action phases and mind-sets. In E. T. Higgins & R. M. Sorrentino (Eds.), *The handbook of motivation and cognition: Foundations of social behavior* (Vol. 2, pp. 53–92). New York: Guilford Press.

Gollwitzer, P. M. (1993). Goal achievement: The role of intentions. *European Review of Social Psychology, 4*, 141–185.

Gollwitzer, P. M. (1999). Implementation intentions: Strong effects of simple plans. *American Psychologist, 54*, 493–503.

Gollwitzer, P. M. (2012). Mindset theory of action phases. In P. Van Lange, A. W. Kruglanski, & E. T. Higgins (Eds.), *Handbook of theories of social psychology* (Vol. 1, pp. 526–545). London: SAGE.

Gollwitzer, P. M. (2014). Weakness of the will: Is a quick fix possible? *Motivation and Emotion, 38*, 305–322.

Gollwitzer, P. M., & Brandstätter, V. (1997). Implementation intentions and effective goal striving. *Journal of Personality and Social Psychology, 73*, 186–199.

Gollwitzer, P. M., & Kirchhof, O. (1998). The willful pursuit of identity. In J. Heckhausen &

C. S. Dweck (Eds.), *Motivation and self-regulation across the life span* (pp. 389–423). Cambridge, UK: Cambridge University Press.

Gollwitzer, P. M., Parks-Stamm, E. J., Jaudas, A., & Sheeran, P. (2008). Flexible tenacity in goal pursuit. In J. Shah & W. Gardner (Eds.), *Handbook of motivation science* (pp. 325–341). New York: Guilford Press.

Gollwitzer, P. M., & Schaal, B. (1998). Metacognition in action: The importance of implementation intentions. *Personality and Social Psychology Review, 2*, 124–136.

Gollwitzer, P. M., & Sheeran, P. (2006). Implementation intentions and goal achievement: A meta-analysis of effects and processes. *Advances in Experimental Social Psychology, 38*, 69–119.

Gollwitzer, P. M., Sheeran, P., Trötschel, R., & Webb, T. (2011). Self-regulation of behavioral priming effects. *Psychological Science, 22*, 901–907.

Güth, W., Schmittberger, R., & Schwarze, B. (1982). An experimental analysis of ultimatum bargaining. *Journal of Economic Behavior and Organization, 3*, 367–388.

Hagger, M. S., Chatzisarantis, N. L. D., & Harris, J. (2006). From psychological need satisfaction to intentional behavior: Testing a motivational sequence in two behavioral contexts. *Personality and Social Psychology Bulletin, 32*, 131–148.

Hall, P. A., Zehr, C. E., Ng, M., & Zanna, M. P. (2012). Implementation intentions for physical activity in supportive and unsupportive environmental conditions: An experimental examination of intention–behavior consistency. *Journal of Experimental Social Psychology, 48*, 432–436.

Hall, P. A., Zehr, C., Paultzki, J., & Rhodes, R. (2014). Implementation intentions for physical activity behavior in older adult women: An examination of executive function as a moderator of treatment effects. *Annals of Behavioral Medicine, 48*, 130–136.

Harris, P. A., Brearley, I., Sheeran, P., Barker, M., Klein, W. M. P., Creswell, J. D., . . . Bond, R. (2014). Combining self-affirmation with implementation intentions to promote fruit and vegetable consumption. *Health Psychology, 33*, 729–736.

Henderson, M. D., Gollwitzer, P. M., & Oettingen, G. (2007). Implementation intentions and disengagement from a failing course of action. *Journal of Behavioral Decision Making, 20*, 81–102.

Higgins, E. T. (1997). Beyond pleasure and pain. *American Psychologist, 52*, 1280–1300.

Janczyk, M., Dambacher, M., Bieleke, M., & Gollwitzer, P. M. (2015). The benefit of no choice: Goal-directed plans enhance perceptual processing. *Psychological Research, 79*, 206–220.

Jessop, D. C., Sparks, P., Buckland, N., Harris, P. R., & Churchill, S. (2014). Combining self-affirmation and implementation intentions: Evidence of detrimental effects on behavioral outcomes. *Annals of Behavioral Medicine, 47*, 137–147.

Kappes, A., Singmann, H., & Oettingen, G. (2012). Mental contrasting instigates goal pursuit by linking obstacles of reality with instrumental behavior. *Journal of Experimental Social Psychology, 48*, 811–818.

Kirk, D., Gollwitzer, P. M., & Carnevale, P. J. (2011). Self-regulation in ultimatum bargaining: Goals and plans help accepting unfair but profitable offers. *Social Cognition, 29*, 528–546.

Koestner, R., Lekes, N., Powers, T. A., & Chicoine, E. (2002). Attaining personal goals: Self-concordance plus implementation intentions equals success. *Journal of Personality and Social Psychology, 83*, 231–244.

Kroese, F. M., Adriaanse, M. A., Evers, C., & De Ridder, D. T. D. (2011). "Instant success": Turning temptations into cues for goal-directed behavior. *Personality and Social Psychology Bulletin, 37*, 1389–1397.

Lang, P. J., Bradley, M. M., & Cuthbert, B. N. (1999). *International Affective Picture System*

(IAPS): Technical manual and affective ratings (Tech. Rep. No. A-4). Gainesville: University of Florida, Center for Research in Psychophysiology.

Legrand, E., Bieleke, M., Gollwitzer, P. M., & Mignon, A. (2017). Nothing will stop me?: Flexibly tenacious goal striving with implementation intentions. *Motivation Science, 3,* 101–118.

Lengfelder, A., & Gollwitzer, P. M. (2001). Reflective and reflexive action control in frontal lobe patients. *Neuropsychology, 15,* 80–100.

Lewin, K. (1926). *Vorsatz, Wille und Bedürfnis* [Intention, will, and need]. Berlin, Germany: Springer.

Locke, A. E., & Latham, G. (Eds.). (2013). *New developments in goal setting and task performance.* New York: Routledge.

Maglio, S. J., Gollwitzer, P. M., & Oettingen. G. (2014). Emotion and control in the planning of goals. *Motivation and Emotion, 38,* 620–634.

Martiny-Huenger, T., Bieleke, M., Oettingen, G., & Gollwitzer, P. M. (2016). From thought to automatic action: Strategic and incidental action control by if–then planning. In R. Deutsch, B. Gawronski, & W. Hofmann (Eds.), *Reflective and impulsive determinants of behavior* (pp. 69–84). New York: Psychology Press.

Masicampo, E. J., & Baumeister, R. F. (2012). Committed but close-minded: When making a specific plan for a goal hinders success. *Social Cognition, 30,* 37–55.

Mendoza, S. A., Gollwitzer, P. M., & Amodio, D. M. (2010). Reducing the expression of implicit stereotypes: Reflexive control through implementation intentions. *Personality and Social Psychology Bulletin, 36,* 512–523.

Oettingen, G. (2000). Expectancy effects on behavior depend on self-regulatory thought. *Social Cognition, 18,* 101–129.

Oettingen, G. (2012). Future thought and behavior change. *European Review of Social Psychology, 23,* 1–63.

Oettingen, G., Pak, H., & Schnetter, K. (2001). Self-regulation of goal setting: Turning free fantasies about the future into binding goals. *Journal of Personality and Social Psychology, 80,* 736–753.

Palayiwa, A., Sheeran, P., & Thompson, A. (2010). "Words will never hurt me!": Implementation intentions regulate attention to stigmatizing comments about appearance. *Journal of Social and Clinical Psychology, 29,* 575–598.

Parks-Stamm, E. J., Gollwitzer, P. M., & Oettingen, G. (2007). Action control by implementation intentions: Effective cue detection and efficient response initiation. *Social Cognition, 25,* 248–266.

Parks-Stamm, E. J., Gollwitzer, P. M., & Oettingen, G. (2010). Implementation intentions and test anxiety: Shielding academic performance from distraction. *Learning and Individual Differences, 20,* 30–33.

Paul, I., Gawrilow, C., Zech, F., Gollwitzer, P. M., Rockstroh, B., Odenthal, G., . . . Wienbruch, C. (2007). If–then planning modulates the P300 in children with attention-deficit/hyperactivity disorder. *NeuroReport, 18,* 653–657.

Robbins, J. M., & Krueger, J. I. (2005). Social projection to ingroups and outgroups: A review and meta-analysis. *Personality and Social Psychology Review, 9,* 32–47.

Ryan, R. M., & Deci, E. L. (2000). Self-determination theory and the facilitation of intrinsic motivation, social development, and well-being. *American Psychologist, 55,* 68–78.

Schweiger Gallo, I., Fernández-Dols, J., Gollwitzer, P. M., & Keil, A. (2017). Grima: A distinct emotion concept? *Frontiers in Psychology, 8,* Article 131.

Schweiger Gallo, I., Keil, A., McCulloch, K. C., Rockstroh, B., & Gollwitzer, P. M. (2009). Strategic automation of emotion regulation. *Journal of Personality and Social Psychology, 96,* 11–31.

Schweiger Gallo, I., McCulloch, K. C., & Gollwitzer, P. M. (2012). Differential effects of various types of implementation intentions on the regulation of disgust. *Social Cognition, 30*, 1–17.

Schweiger Gallo, I., Pfau, F., & Gollwitzer, P. M. (2012). Furnishing hypnotic instructions with implementation intentions enhances hypnotic responsiveness. *Consciousness and Cognition, 21*, 1023–1030.

Sheeran, P., Webb, T. L., & Gollwitzer, P. M. (2005). The interplay between goal intentions and implementation intentions. *Personality and Social Psychology Bulletin, 31*, 87–98.

Sheeran, P., Webb, T. L., Gollwitzer, P. M., & Oettingen, G. (in press). Self-regulation of affect-health behavior relations. In D. M. Williams, R. E. Rhodes, & M. T. Conner (Eds.), *Affective determinants of health-related behaviors*. New York: Oxford University Press.

Skinner, B. F. (1971). *Beyond freedom and dignity*. New York: Penguin Books.

Stern, C., Cole, S., Gollwitzer, P. M., Oettingen, G., & Balcetis, E. (2013). Effects of implementation intentions on anxiety, perceived proximity, and motor performance. *Personality and Social Psychology Bulletin, 39*, 623–635.

Stewart, B. D., & Payne, B. K. (2008). Bringing automatic stereotyping under control: Implementation intentions as efficient means of thought control. *Personality and Social Psychology Bulletin, 34*, 1332–1345.

Strack, F., & Deutsch, R. (2004). Reflective and impulsive determinants of social behavior. *Personality and Social Psychology Review, 8*, 220–247.

Thürmer, J. L., McCrea, S. M., & Gollwitzer, P. M. (2013). Regulating self-defensiveness: If–then plans prevent claiming and creating performance handicaps. *Motivation and Emotion, 37*, 712–725.

Thürmer, J. L., Wieber, F., & Gollwitzer, P. M. (2015). A self-regulation perspective on hidden profile problems: If–then planning to review information improves group decisions. *Journal of Behavioral Decision Making, 28*, 101–113.

Thürmer, J. L., Wieber, F., & Gollwitzer, P. M. (2017). Planning and performance in small groups: Collective implementation intentions enhance group goal striving. *Frontiers in Psychology, 8*, Article 603.

van Kleef, G. A., De Dreu, K. D. W., & Manstead, A. S. R. (2004). The interpersonal effects of anger and happiness in negotiations. *Journal of Personality and Social Psychology, 86*, 57–76.

van Koningsbruggen, G. M., Stroebe, W., Papies, E. K., & Aarts, H. (2011). Implementation intentions as goal primes: Boosting self-control in tempting environments. *European Journal of Social Psychology, 41*, 551–557.

Webb, T. L., Ononaiye, M. S. P., Sheeran, P., Reidy, J. G., & Lavda, A. (2010). Using implementation intentions to overcome the effects of social anxiety on attention and appraisals of performance. *Personality and Social Psychology Bulletin, 36*, 612–627.

Webb, T. L., Schweiger Gallo, I., Miles, E., Gollwitzer, P. M., & Sheeran, P. (2012). Effective regulation of affect: An action control perspective on emotion regulation. *European Review of Social Psychology, 23*, 143–186.

Webb, T. L., & Sheeran, P. (2004). Identifying good opportunities to act: Implementation intentions and cue discrimination. *European Journal of Social Psychology, 34*, 407–419.

Webb, T. L., & Sheeran, P. (2007). How do implementation intentions promote goal attainment?: A test of component processes. *Journal of Experimental Social Psychology, 43*, 295–302.

Webb, T. L., & Sheeran, P. (2008). Mechanisms of implementation intention effects: The role of goal intentions, self-efficacy, and accessibility of plan components. *British Journal of Social Psychology, 47*, 373–395.

Webb, T. L., Sheeran, P., & Luszczynska, A. (2009). Planning to break unwanted habits: Habit strength moderates implementation intention effects on behaviour change. *British Journal of Social Psychology, 48,* 507–523.

Wieber, F., Gollwitzer, P. M., & Sheeran, P. (2014). Strategic regulation of mimicry effects by implementation intentions. *Journal of Experimental Social Psychology, 53,* 31–39.

Wieber, F., Odenthal, G., & Gollwitzer, P. M. (2010). Self-efficacy feelings moderate implementation intention effects. *Self and Identity, 9,* 177–194.

Wieber, F., & Sassenberg, K. (2006). I can't take my eyes off of it: Attention attraction of implementation intentions. *Social Cognition, 24,* 723–752.

Wieber, F., Sezer, L. A., & Gollwitzer, P. M. (2014). Asking "why" helps action control by goals but not plans. *Motivation and Emotion, 38,* 65–78.

Wieber, F., Thürmer, J. L., & Gollwitzer, P. M. (2015). Attenuating the escalation of commitment to a faltering project in decision-making groups: An implementation intention approach. *Social Psychology and Personality Science, 6,* 587–595.

Wieber, F., von Suchodoletz, A., Heikamp, T., Trommsdorff, G., & Gollwitzer, P. M. (2011). If–then planning helps school-aged children to ignore attractive distractions. *Social Psychology, 42,* 39–47.

CHAPTER 18

Mindsets Change the Imagined and Actual Future

Carol S. Dweck
David S. Yeager

People's beliefs are a fundamental part of their personality and motivation, although this is often unrecognized. People's foundational beliefs about themselves, others, and the world can powerfully shape their goals, the vigor and effectiveness of their goal pursuit, their recurrent patterns of behavior, and, in the end, their well-being. In this chapter, we spotlight beliefs about the self and others, particularly people's implicit theories or mindsets about human attributes (Burnette, O'Boyle, VanEpps, Pollack, & Finkel, 2013; Dweck & Leggett, 1988; Schleider, Abel, & Weisz, 2015; Yeager & Dweck, 2012). Focusing on the areas of intellectual achievement and social relations, we demonstrate the impact of conceiving of human attributes as fixed traits, as opposed to malleable qualities that can be developed. And we show how the impact of these beliefs stems, in large part, from the way they lead people to think about the future.

Our basic thesis is that believing in fixed traits (holding an *entity theory* or a *fixed mindset*) means that the judgments you make about yourself and others can potentially be lasting judgments. That is, the way people are now, in terms of their basic qualities, may well be the way they will always be. Needless to say, this can have strong repercussions for people's concerns in the present and their hopes and fears about the future.

In contrast, believing that basic qualities can be developed (holding an *incremental theory* or a *growth mindset*) means that any current judgments you make about yourself and others are subject to revision in the future. If people have the potential to learn and change, you have to be open to that possibility and even work toward it going forward—toward that more promising future.

The plan of the chapter is as follows. Using research on mindsets about intelligence and personality, we show that:

- The two mindsets orient people toward different goals: *performance goals* that are typically about validating the self right now versus *learning goals* that have a time dimension and are about mastering new challenges and improving the self.
- The two mindsets lend different meanings to difficulty, setbacks, and even effort: In one mindset they are measures of fixed qualities; in the other they are a natural part of learning and carry valuable information about how to move forward more successfully.
- Existing individual differences in mindsets can predict important intellectual and social outcomes over time.
- Interventions to promote a growth mindset about intelligence or personality, by focusing people away from permanent judgments and toward the potential for change in the future, can bring about changes in motivation, behavior, and outcomes, including increases in academic performance and reductions in aggression, stress, or the onset of depression.

We conclude by noting the implications of this research for the design of learning and working environments that are cultures of development rather than cultures of judgment—cultures in which people can focus on larger, longer term contributions instead of small, immediate, safe successes. We also pinpoint implications for psychological interventions in general, suggesting that successful psychological interventions are often ones that give people new beliefs, motivations, or self-regulatory skills that allow them to look beyond a problematic present and think constructively about (as well as work toward) a better future.

WHAT ARE THE FIXED AND GROWTH MINDSETS?

Do people believe that their intelligence (or their personality) is a fixed trait, or do they believe it is a quality that can be cultivated through learning and experience?

For intelligence, we find this out by asking people to agree or disagree with a series of statements, such as: "Your intelligence is something basic about you that you can't really change" or "No matter who you are, you can substantially change your level of intelligence" (Dweck, 1999; Dweck, Chiu, & Hong, 1995). If people tend to agree more with statements like the first one, they are endorsing a *fixed mindset*, that is, the idea that intelligence is a fixed entity. In contrast, if they tend to agree more with statements like the second, they are reflecting a *growth mindset*, that is, the idea that intellectual ability can be increased through learning. Analogously, to measure a fixed mindset of personality, people tell us how much they agree or disagree with statements such as: "The kind of person someone is is something very basic about them and it can't be changed very much" (Chiu, Hong, & Dweck, 1997; Dweck, 1999).

Can people hold different mindsets in different areas? Most definitely. Mindsets about intelligence reliably load on a different factor than mindsets about personality or moral character (Dweck et al., 1995). Intelligence mindsets correlate with personality mindsets at approximately $r = .30$—conceptually meaningful, but clearly not the same construct (Dweck et al., 1995). Recently, Schroder, Dawood,

Yalch, Donnellan, and Moser (2016) measured mindsets in many domains in a large sample of college students. They, too, found evidence for some shared variance across the different mindsets but also a great deal of domain-specificity, with the more domain-specific measures typically being the better predictors of outcomes of interest within that domain.

Furthermore, even within one domain, such as intellectual ability, people can believe that their language ability can be developed but that their math ability is fixed, or vice versa. (Note that holding a fixed mindset is quite different from having high or low confidence in your ability; you can believe that your ability is fixed at a high level or a low level; Dweck & Leggett, 1988).

There is something else we have come to appreciate over time. Even within an area, these mindsets can be quite dynamic, even when there is significant stability in the dominant mindset over time. Someone can hold a growth mindset much of the time, but certain events, such as highly challenging tasks, important setbacks, or harsh criticism, can push them into a fixed mindset—that is, can lead them, at least temporarily, to feel that their fundamental abilities are fixed and are now in question. If, on the other hand, they are able to remain in a growth mindset, they can still question their level of current ability but then ask what they need to do to develop it further.

Nonetheless, people's endorsement of the mindset statements, such as those presented above, usually give us a good idea of where they stand on the mindset continuum. The one exception is among people who have become familiar with the mindset concept, as has happened with many educators. In these cases, people may come to believe that agreement with the growth mindset item is the preferable answer, and so their survey responses become less predictive of their behaviors (Hooper, Yeager, Haimovitz, Wright, & Murphy, 2016). We are now working to address this by developing new, less direct measures.

However, mindsets are not simply an individual-difference variable. They are beliefs that can be primed or induced. They can be induced, for example, by telling people that the task they are about to perform either is a measure of a fixed ability or involves a skill that can be learned through practice (e.g., Martocchio, 1994). They can be induced by giving people persuasive articles to read that convey intelligence as either something inherent and unchangeable or something that can be increased through hard work, good strategies, and mentoring from others (e.g., Hong, Chiu, Dweck, Lin, & Wan, 1999; Nussbaum & Dweck, 2008). They can also be taught in more long-term ways by means of mindset interventions, that is, workshops that teach a growth mindset, its different ramifications, and how to apply it to the relevant situations, be they academic (e.g., Aronson, Fried, & Good, 2002; Blackwell, Trzesniewski, & Dweck, 2007; Good, Aronson, & Inzlicht, 2003; Paunesku et al., 2015; Yeager, Romero, et al., 2016), social (Yeager et al., 2014; Yeager, Miu, Powers, & Dweck, 2013; Yeager, Trzesniewski, & Dweck, 2013), work-related (Heslin, Latham, & VandeWalle, 2005), or health-related (Burnette & Finkel, 2012; Burnette et al., 2013).

MINDSETS CREATE DIFFERENT PSYCHOLOGIES

A view of the future is inherent in the definition of the mindsets. People in a fixed mindset may expect that current traits, performance, or behaviors will simply persist into the future, whereas people in a growth mindset believe that people have the potential to develop their attributes over time and become different in the future (Chiu et al., 1997; Yeager, Trzesniewski, Tirri, Nokelainen, & Dweck, 2011).

In this section, we convey how the mindsets, each with their different views of the present and future, set up different "meaning systems"—psychological frameworks in which the same things have different values and different meanings (Hong et al., 1999; Molden & Dweck, 2006). It is through these meaning systems that people with similar skills end up exposing themselves to different experiences, reacting to similar experiences in different ways, and achieving different levels of academic and social success, as well as different levels of well-being.

Goals: What Do People Want?

Freud famously asked, "What do women want?" (Jones, 1955). Here we ask, "What do people want?," and we show that what people want for themselves—their goals—can be meaningfully affected by their mindsets. This makes sense. If you believe that your intelligence is simply fixed, then you want to show it in a favorable light. You want to embark on tasks that ensure success, and you want to avoid tasks that pose a risk of struggle, mistakes, or failure. This means that when you think about the future, you have to carefully think of all the little and big land mines you have to avoid.

However, if you believe that your intelligence is something you can develop, you can worry less about how you fare on any given task in the short run and instead orient more toward developing your abilities over time. In other words, you can be more oriented toward growing into the person you would like to become in the future.

Intelligence Mindsets and Intellectual Goals

Blackwell and colleagues (2007) conducted a longitudinal study of adolescents making the difficult transition to seventh grade, a perfect time to examine the impact of mindsets. At the beginning of this transitional year, they measured students' intelligence mindsets and their achievement goals (among other things) and then monitored their grades in math over the next 2 years. Students with more of a growth mindset, compared with those with more of a fixed mindset, were significantly more oriented toward learning goals—goals that favor longer-term learning over shorter-term performance. Specifically, they more strongly endorsed statements such as "I like schoolwork that I'll learn from even if I make a lot of mistakes." We return to this study below.

In a related vein, Robins and Pals (2002) conducted a longitudinal study of college students, measuring their intelligence mindsets (among other things) and tracking their self-esteem across the last 3 years of college. Consistent with the findings from Blackwell et al. (2007), students with growth mindsets were more focused on learning goals ("The knowledge I gain in school is more important than the grades I receive"), whereas those with fixed mindsets were more focused on performance goals, worrying more about their grades and how they reflected on their ability. It is not that students in a growth mindset don't care about grades; they may simply care more about the learning (cf. Grant & Dweck, 2003).

Research by Cury, Elliot, Da Fonseca, and Moller (2006) lends further support and then goes on to demonstrate the direct, causal effect of mindsets. In a first study, Cury et al. (2006) found that students' growth versus fixed mindsets of intelligence predicted adolescents' learning versus performance goals, which accounted for their higher versus lower math grades. In a second study, they showed that orienting adolescents toward a growth (vs. fixed) mindset of intelligence before taking an intelligence test led to higher scores on the test by influencing their achievement goals.

Finally, Hong et al. (1999) caught entering college students at a pivotal moment in their academic careers. These students were enrolling at the University of Hong Kong, an elite school in which all of the classes were conducted in English. Unfortunately, not all of the entering students were proficient in English. On registration day, Hong and colleagues (1999) asked these freshman how likely they would be to take a remedial English course if the faculty offered it. Among the students who were not proficient in English, those who held a growth mindset of intelligence replied with a resounding yes—they wanted to learn—but the nonproficient students with a fixed mindset of intelligence were not as enthusiastic. It was as though they preferred to hide their deficiency rather than expose it, even if the deficiency put their future college career in jeopardy.

Importantly, these goals do not just operate when we are faced with a choice of tasks. They can affect our moment-to-moment decisions as we perform a task. Ehrlinger, Mitchum, and Dweck (2016) found that, as people worked on a task, those with more of a fixed mindset deployed their attention toward the easier problems rather than the harder ones. As a result, they ended up with distorted, overly high, views of their abilities on the task—views that suited their immediate need to feel intelligent. Those with a growth mindset deployed their attention to hard problems as well as easy ones, thus gaining a more realistic view of their abilities—a view that suited their longer-term learning goals. That is, an accurate view of their current knowledge and skills could direct their future learning more effectively.

Nussbaum and Dweck (2008) provide another example of people shoring up their current sense of their intelligence at the expense of learning. They oriented college students toward either a fixed or a growth mindset by having them read an article that espoused one view of intelligence or the other. Then, after a very difficult task on which students did poorly, they were given a choice. They could look at the strategies of students who had done better than they had (and learn from them) the strategies of students who had done even worse than they had (and feel better about their abilities). Compared with those in a growth mindset, those in a fixed mindset indeed looked more at the strategies of students who had done even worse than they had—and in fact felt better about themselves as a result.

An important question arises: If those with a fixed mindset believe that ability is unchangeable, why do they have to keep validating it over and over? For example, if they have already proven that they are smart, why can't they ride off into the sunset and take on new challenges? The answer seems to be that every new task or new course represents a new measure of their intelligence. Maybe they were smart enough for algebra but not for calculus; maybe they were smart enough for high school chemistry but not college chemistry; maybe they were smart in their former school but not in this new, more selective school. In other words, maybe their fixed intelligence was ample for past, easier tasks but not for harder ones. This is what keeps people with a fixed mindset focused on tasks that will yield positive judgments in the here and now and not necessarily on the tasks that will best equip them with the skills they need in the future.

Personality Mindsets and Social Goals

In a similar fashion, people's mindsets about their socially relevant personality traits can shape the goals they have for their social lives. When people hold more of a fixed mindset of personality, they tend to focus on validating their positive social traits and on avoiding situations in which they might be "outed" as socially deficient in some way. Although, of course, people don't want to humiliate themselves, an overly strong focus on these goals can keep them from situations in which they could grow and develop their social skills.

For instance, Erdley, Loomis, Cain, and Dumas-Hines (1997, Study 2) measured fourth- fifth-, and sixth-grade children's personality mindsets. Then they assessed the goals that the children would pursue in difficult social situations, such as deciding who to invite to a birthday party. Children with more of a fixed mindset of personality endorsed more performance-oriented goals—goals that ensured success (such as inviting people you were sure would say yes) but that provided little opportunity to expand their social network or practice new social skills. Using similar measures to the Erdley et al. (1997) research, Rudolph (2010) found that children with a fixed mindset were more likely to report performance versus learning goals in a social setting. They focused more on judgments from peers and less on growing or developing their relationships with peers.

Beer (2002) extended these ideas to a specific personality trait: shyness. In a series of studies she showed that shy people vary in the extent to which they endorse fixed mindset statements such as "My shyness is something about me that I can't change very much." She then assessed shy people's goals in a novel social situation that involved getting to know a stranger during a 5-minute social interaction. First, shy people with a fixed mindset were less likely to adopt learning goals for the upcoming interaction. That is, they were less likely to opt for an interaction in which they would "learn some social skills applicable beyond the laboratory setting" but risked appearing awkward on the videotape of the interaction. Next, shy individuals with more of a fixed mindset of shyness reported using more avoidant strategies (avoiding eye contact, or asking questions to turn attention away from themselves), and coding of their interactions showed that they in fact used these avoidant strategies more frequently. In the end, their interactions with a new person were rated as less successful.

More recent studies extended these findings to the goals people adopt when they are pursuing clinical treatments. One study (Schroder, Dawood, Yalch, Donnellan, & Moser, 2015) found that those with more of a fixed mindset of anxiety said that, if they struggled with mental health problems, they would choose medication as a treatment, rather than therapy or therapy plus medication. Therapy might seek to teach people skills for managing their problems, but, from the perspective of a fixed mindset, when anxiety is not changeable, that learning goal may seem less appealing and less fruitful. Another study examined actual responses to a clinical treatment (Valentiner, Jencius, Jarek, Gier-Lonsway, & McGrath, 2013). Exposure therapy is among the most effective means for reducing social anxiety, but it is aversive because it requires people to confront their fears in vivo. For people to benefit, they need to have a goal of learning from the exposure. Unsurprisingly, then, clinically socially anxious individuals with a fixed mindset about shyness ended up with only about half the benefit of the exposure therapy reaped by those with a growth mindset.

Summary

People in a fixed versus growth mindset contemplate the future in different ways as they formulate their goals (see Sevincer, Kluge, & Oettingen, 2014). In one meaning system, people have to worry about all the ways they can fail intellectually or socially and then guard against them. They do not want to earn a negative label in their own eyes or in the eyes of others. In the other meaning system, people are freer to consider what they want to learn, how they would like to grow, and who they want to become in the future. Of course, they need to plan how to do this effectively, but this involves strategizing about growth, not constantly guarding against the self-invalidating power of mistakes and setbacks.

What Does Failure Mean?

What does failure mean and what does it make people do? Why are people who endorse a fixed mindset so afraid to venture out of their comfort zone to learn new and challenging things? We have glimpsed the answer, but let us take a full look at it.

Intelligence Mindsets and the Meaning of Failure

In the study by Blackwell et al. (2007), we saw that adolescents with different mindsets favored different goals. Here we note that their mindsets were also significant predictors of how they understood difficulty and reacted to it. Reacting to a vignette depicting academic failure, students with a fixed mindset were more likely to attribute the academic setback to deficient ability: "I wasn't smart enough" or "I'm just not good at this subject." For them, this sums it up: My ability has been measured and found wanting—perhaps forever.

So what did they do with this bad news? Compared with those with more of a growth mindset, they endorsed strategies that limited their future learning but allowed them to save face, such as: "I would spend less time on this subject from now on," "I would try not to take this subject ever again," and "I would try to cheat on the next test." Feeling devoid of ability, students in a fixed mindset were left with fewer recipes for success.

However, those with a growth mindset, in line with their belief in malleable ability, more often faced the academic setback with a constructive plan: "I would work harder in this class from now on" and "I would spend more time studying for the tests." This is perfectly sensible given their meaning system. It is not surprising, then, that their more learning-oriented goals, their more positive interpretations of failure, and their more productive reactions to failure predicted increasing math grades over time compared with their peers with a fixed mindset (see also Hong et al., 1999).

The Robins and Pals (2002) research confirms these disparate reactions to difficulty. In their study of college students, those with fixed mindsets were more likely to attribute an academic setback to a lack of ability, whereas those with growth mindsets attributed disappointing grades to their effort and study skills. In line with these different meanings, a fixed mindset was predictive of more "helpless" responses ("When I fail to understand something, I become discouraged to the point of wanting to give up"), whereas a growth mindset was predictive of more positive, constructive responses ("When something I am studying is difficult, I try harder"). In this longitudinal study, the primary outcome was students' self-esteem trajectory over the college years. Independent of their grades and independent of their prior level of self-esteem, those with fixed mindsets were on a downward self-esteem spiral relative to those with growth mindsets. Again, this means that in the face of similar outcomes, a fixed mindset creates a meaning system in which a negative judgment is forever and people act accordingly. A growth mindset, regardless of current difficulties, leaves open the possibility of a brighter future and motivates people to work for it.

Can we observe these processes in the brain? Moser, Schroder, Heeter, Moran, and Lee (2011; see also Mangels, Butterfield, Lamb, Good, & Dweck, 2006) monitored college students' online processing of errors via their event-related potentials (ERPs) during an ongoing task. As students made and detected their errors on this task, the ERP activity of those with growth mindsets revealed heightened attention to and processing of their errors, which then predicted increased performance on the next trials. That is, those with growth mindsets processed the errors more deeply and exerted greater control to correct them compared with those with fixed mindsets. The brains of those with a fixed mindset showed little activity in the relevant brain area, perhaps suggesting a flight from rather than an embracing of the errors. Thus the meaning people take from failure can have an important impact on how (or whether) they use errors or failures to help prepare for the future.

Personality Mindsets and the Meaning of Rejection

Just as academic failure can signal to people in a fixed mindset of intelligence that they are "dumb," so social failure can signal to people in a fixed mindset of personality that they are deficient, "losers," or "not likable." Whether you are trying to make friends or are in a close relationship, setbacks or rejections, and the permanent labels they imply within a fixed mindset, can be especially wounding and can lead to less constructive actions.

Specifically, Howe and Dweck (2016), studying adults' attributions for rejection in close relationships, showed that those in a fixed mindset believed that rejection revealed their true, enduring self. As a result, they tended to carry this burden with them and let it affect their future relationships. Those in a growth mindset, in contrast, were more likely to view rejection as something they could learn from. In a study with children, Erdley et al. (1997, Study 1) found that in response to a (hypothetical) social rejection—not being selected as a pen pal—children in a fixed mindset entertained more fixed-trait attributions, such as "It made me wonder: Am I a likable person?"

Being in a fixed mindset can also lead people to attribute fixed traits to those who reject or offend them. That is, an entity theory predicts a tendency to make dispositional rather than situational attributions for behavior (Chiu et al., 1997; cf. research on lay dispositionism, Ross & Nisbett, 1991) Yeager et al. (2011) found that peer rejection led to the attribution that the peers were "bad people" when peers had made fun of them and started rumors about them in school. Assigning meaning to rejection in terms of fixed traits can then elicit more extreme social emotions. Adolescents with a fixed mindset expressed both greater *shame* toward themselves and greater *hatred* toward peer rejecters (Yeager et al., 2011; cf. Halperin, Russell, Trzesniewski, Gross, & Dweck, 2011). These attributions and negative emotions can lead to helpless or aggressive responses that do not solve the problem. It is not surprising, then, that a fixed mindset predicts greater stress and depression (Miu & Yeager, 2015; Yeager et al., 2011, 2014).

Summary

By giving undue weight and significance to negative events, people in a fixed mindset can remain mired in the present or past. In addition, these negative events give them information about what they are not capable of doing or being in the future, rather than information about how to reach their future goals more effectively.

INTERVENTIONS: MINDSETS CAN CHANGE THE FUTURE

By allowing people to transcend the here and now and plan for a better future (and a better self in the future), a growth mindset can potentially lead to better intellectual and social-emotional outcomes. We have already seen in the longitudinal studies, such as the Blackwell et al. (2007) and the Robins and Pals (2002) studies, that those with a growth mindset earned higher grades and experienced higher self-esteem over time than did those with a fixed mindset. Such findings pose the question of whether teaching a growth mindset would allow more people to reap these benefits.

Changing Intelligence Mindsets

The first research to examine this question was a study by Aronson et al. (2002). In this research, college students were taught different ideas about intelligence. One group was taught a growth mindset—the idea that intelligence is expandable and that every time they learned new things, their brains formed new connections. They saw a film that illustrated this idea, they discussed it, and, in order to help them internalize the message, they mentored a younger student using growth mindset principles. Another group was taught the theory of multiple intelligences, with the message being not to worry if you lack intelligence in one area, because you may still have it in other areas. They, too, mentored younger children in terms of this theory. Finally, there was a third, no-treatment control group. Students who learned a growth mindset earned significantly higher grades that semester than students in the other two groups. Importantly, for African American students, the growth mindset also led to a significant increase in how important academics were in their lives and in how much they enjoyed their academic work.

In a later study, Blackwell et al. (2007, Study 2) gave seventh graders an eight-session workshop. All of the students in the workshop received lessons on study skills, but half of them also received several sessions on the growth mindset and how to apply it to their schoolwork. The growth mindset workshop, but not the control workshop, halted the decline in math grades shown prior to the intervention. In addition, teachers, blind to condition singled out significantly more of the children in the growth mindset group as showing enhanced motivation to learn and improve.

Finally, a recent study by Paunesku et al. (2015) showed that teaching a growth mindset could be implemented on a large scale to improve student performance. Students from 13 high schools, diverse in their sizes and student populations, completed an online module that was condensed from the Blackwell et al. (2007) materials. Compared with a control condition, struggling students who learned a growth mindset and how to apply it earned significantly higher grades by the end of the semester. Recent replication studies (e.g., Yeager, Romero, et al., 2016; Yeager, Walton, et al., 2016) also show the feasibility of these large-scale interventions and highlight their role in promoting educational equity for underserved minorities and students at risk for school dropout.

Changing Social-Personality Mindsets

To date, most personality-mindset interventions have addressed mindsets in adolescents dealing with social stress (Yeager et al., 2014; Yeager, Lee, & Jamieson, 2016; Yeager, Miu, et al., 2013; Yeager, Trzesniewski, et al., 2013). These studies show that learning about people's potential for change can provide a basis for people to imagine a better future.

Growth mindset of personality interventions, such as those cited above, teach adolescents that people do not do things just because of traits that they have; they do things because of thoughts and feelings that they have—thoughts and feelings that live in the brain. Next, adolescents learn that the brain can change and grow new or stronger connections when people have life experiences that cause them to reconsider their behavior or change their values. Finally, adolescents learn that many former students like them have read and used this message to deal with their social difficulties and that they might find it helpful to do so, as well. The intervention seeks to go beyond the platitude of "people can change" and instead provide a mechanism, based in the neuroscience of adolescence, for the potential for change.

A first evaluation of this growth mindset of personality intervention tested for immediate effects (Yeager et al., 2011). Following a scenario of potential humiliation at the hands of peers—one in which the participant had done something embarrassing and now peers were starting rumors about him or her online—adolescents in the growth-mindset group showed a lower desire for revenge and a reduced belief that fantasizing about vengeance would make them feel better.

Subsequent evaluations of growth mindset interventions have put adolescents in socially difficult situations—such as an experience of ostracism via Cyberball (Williams & Jarvis, 2006) or the Trier Social Stress Test (Kirschbaum, Pirke, & Hellhammer, 1993)—and found that the growth mindset of personality reduced aggressive retaliation (Yeager, Trzesniewski, & Dweck, 2013), self-reports of stress, and physiological stress responses (Schleider & Weisz, 2016; Yeager et al., 2014; Yeager, Lee, & Jamieson, 2016). For example, Yeager, Lee, and Jamieson (2016) showed that adolescents who were taught a growth mindset of personality appraised themselves as having the resources to meet the demands of a strong socially evaluative stressor (on the Trier Social Stress Test, Kirschbaum et al., 1993; see Blascovich & Mendes, 2010; Jamieson, Mendes, & Nock, 2013; Seery, 2013, for more on stress-inducing appraisals). Growth mindset participants furthermore showed improved cardiovascular responses to a stressor—by showing less constriction in the blood vessels and a more efficient heart—as well as lower levels of cortisol, a stress hormone that indicates feeling strongly negatively evaluated by others.

Can such effects endure over time? There is some encouraging evidence that they can, although these interventions are undergoing even more extensive testing. Yeager, Trzesniewski, et al. (2013) delivered an in-person workshop to mostly ninth- and tenth-grade adolescents attending a high school with high levels of peer aggression. Over the course of six classroom sessions, students received lessons on the brain and, in particular, on how personality can change during high school or after. One month after the sessions ended, Yeager, Trzesniewski, et al. (2013) found that adolescents responded less aggressively to Cyberball ostracism—that is, they allocated less punishment (less disliked spicy hot sauce) to the peer who had excluded them. Three months after the treatment, teachers who were blind to condition also nominated more students in the growth mindset treatment for improvements in their conduct toward peers and teachers in school.

Later experiments have attempted shorter and more scalable versions of the growth mindset of personality treatment: one-session guided reading and writing exercises completed via the computer. These have reduced levels of cortisol on high-stress days up to a week later (Yeager, Lee, & Jamieson, 2016), reduced stress and self-reported depressive symptoms at 8- to 9-month follow-up (Miu & Yeager, 2015; Yeager et al., 2014) and even improved grade point average in core classes over the first year of high school (Yeager et al., 2014; Yeager, Lee, & Jamieson, 2016). If replications in larger samples continue to find promising results for the online growth mindset of personality intervention, it could eventually represent a promising way to help young people create a more hopeful future, despite their current social difficulties.

Summary

Online or in-person workshops that teach students a growth mindset and how they can use it in their lives have the potential to change how students think about the future and to change what actually happens to them in the future in terms of their academic motivation and achievement, their social relations, and their mental health.

THINKING ABOUT THE FUTURE

We have seen how orienting people toward a growth mindset—the idea that even our most basic attributes are capable of growth—can prevent them from becoming mired in the inevitable setbacks and failures that occur. Instead, this mindset encourages them to keep their eye on a more positive future and to think about how to bring it about.

We suggest that this is true not just at the level of the individual, but also at the level of organizations and even nations. New work by Canning, Murphy, Emerson, Chatman, et al. (2017) demonstrates that whole organizations, in this case large corporations, can embody a fixed or a growth mindset. In this research, companies that embodied a growth mindset (those that, according to employees, believed in and valued the development of everyone's abilities) were seen as supporting far more risk taking in the service of future innovation than companies that believed in and valued fixed talent. The growth mindset companies, by supporting and rewarding creativity, were able to create environments—"cultures of development"—in which people said they could focus on longer-term learning. Employees in the fixed mindset companies were, instead, more likely to report widespread cheating and hoarding of information, presumably in the service of proving oneself to be one of the talented few. An important task for the future is to understand how to create growth mindset cultures, be they in schools or business organizations, that work to spur the development of abilities in the many, rather than seeking to simply find the few who are identified early on as "talented" (see Dweck & Hogan, 2016, for how Microsoft has taken up this challenge).

More generally, as people enter a new place or role—a new college, a new job, a new relationship, and so on—they reasonably wonder what it will be like for them. That is, they try to discern what their future will look like. The mindsets provide a set of starting assumptions for individuals engaging in that future-oriented thinking. A fixed versus growth mindset can determine people's projections about whether their new environment is one that will allow growth and learning from mistakes, or one that will rush to put them in a box that defines their potential. It will be exciting in new research to identify transition points in people's lives and to try to help people carry their productive mindsets with them, or rapidly acquire new, more constructive mindsets upon arrival (e.g., Yeager, Walton, et al., 2016).

Research by Halperin et al. (2011) takes this idea to another level. Halperin et al. (2011) proposed that people could see whole groups or nations as embodying inherent, fixed characteristics or as capable of growth and change. They then tested whether instilling mindsets about groups could change Israelis' and Palestinians' attitudes toward each other. Importantly, they found that learning a growth mindset about groups led to less animosity and greater willingness to entertain serious compromises for the sake of peace on the part of both groups. These longstanding adversaries were now, at least for the moment, willing to glimpse a future that was different from the past.

Thinking about psychological interventions in general (see Walton, 2014; Yeager & Walton, 2011), we propose that successful psychological interventions are often ones that, by teaching new beliefs, motivations, or self-regulatory skills, allow people to see beyond a problematic present and begin to work toward a more promising future. By doing so, these interventions underscore the tremendous power of people's psychology to shape their futures. But they also underscore the malleability of our psychology and the promise this malleability holds for helping people envision and attain productive and fulfilling futures.

REFERENCES

Aronson, J. M., Fried, C. B., & Good, C. (2002). Reducing the effects of stereotype threat on African American college students by shaping theories of intelligence. *Journal of Experimental Social Psychology, 38,* 113–125.

Beer, J. S. (2002). Implicit self-theories of shyness. *Journal of Personality and Social Psychology, 83,* 1009–1024.

Blackwell, L. S., Trzesniewski, K. H., & Dweck, C. S. (2007). Implicit theories of intelligence predict achievement across an adolescent transition: A longitudinal study and an intervention. *Child Development, 78,* 246–263.

Blascovich, J., & Mendes, W. B. (2010). Social psychophysiology and embodiment. In S. T. Fiske, D. T. Gilbert, & G. Lindzey (Eds.), *Handbook of social psychology* (5th ed., Vol. 1, pp. 194–227). New York: Wiley.

Burnette, J. L., & Finkel, E. J. (2012). Buffering against weight gain following dieting setbacks: An implicit theory intervention. *Journal of Experimental Social Psychology, 48,* 721–725.

Burnette, J. L., O'Boyle, E. H., VanEpps, E. M., Pollack, J. M., & Finkel, E. J. (2013). Mindsets matter: A meta-analytic review of implicit theories and self-regulation. *Psychological Bulletin, 139,* 655–701.

Canning, E. A., Murphy, M. C., Emerson, K., Chatman, J. A., Dweck, C. S., & Kray, L. J. (2017). *Organizational mindsets shape corporate culture, trust, and commitment.* Unpublished manuscript, Indiana University.

Chiu, C., Hong, Y., & Dweck, C. S. (1997). Lay dispositionism and implicit theories of personality. *Journal of Personality and Social Psychology, 73,* 19–30.

Cury, F., Elliot, A. J., Da Fonseca, D., & Moller, A. C. (2006). The social-cognitive model of achievement motivation and the 2 × 2 achievement goal framework. *Journal of Personality and Social Psychology, 90,* 666–679.

Dweck, C. S. (1999). *Self-theories: Their role in motivation, personality, and development.* Philadelphia: Taylor & Francis/Psychology Press.

Dweck, C. S., Chiu, C., & Hong, Y. (1995). Implicit theories and their role in judgments and reactions: A world from two perspectives. *Psychological Inquiry, 6,* 267–285.

Dweck, C. S., & Hogan, K. (2016). How Microsoft uses a growth mindset to develop leaders. *Harvard Business Review.* Available at *https://hbr.org/2016/10/how-microsoft-uses-a-growth-mindset-to-develop-leaders.*

Dweck, C. S., & Leggett, E. L. (1988). A social-cognitive approach to motivation and personality. *Psychological Review, 95,* 256–273.

Ehrlinger, J., Mitchum, A. L., & Dweck, C. S. (2016). Understanding overconfidence: Theories of intelligence, preferential attention, and distorted self-assessment. *Journal of Experimental Social Psychology, 63,* 94–100.

Erdley, C. A., Loomis, C. C., Cain, K. M., & Dumas-Hines, F. (1997). Relations among children's social goals, implicit personality theories, and responses to social failure. *Developmental Psychology, 33,* 263–272.

Good, C., Aronson, J., & Inzlicht, M. (2003). Improving adolescents' standardized test performance: An intervention to reduce the effects of stereotype threat. *Journal of Applied Developmental Psychology, 24,* 645–662.

Grant, H., & Dweck, C. S. (2003). Clarifying achievement goals and their impact. *Journal of Personality and Social Psychology, 85,* 541–553.

Halperin, E., Russell, A. G., Trzesniewski, K. H., Gross, J. J., & Dweck, C. S. (2011). Promoting the Middle East peace process by changing beliefs about group malleability. *Science, 333,* 1767–1769.

Heslin, P. A., Latham, G. P., & VandeWalle, D. (2005). The effect of implicit person theory on performance appraisals. *Journal of Applied Psychology, 90,* 842–856.

Hong, Y., Chiu, C., Dweck, C. S., Lin, D. M.-S., & Wan, W. (1999). Implicit theories, attributions, and coping: A meaning system approach. *Journal of Personality and Social Psychology, 77,* 588–599.

Hooper, S. Y., Yeager, D. S., Haimovitz, K., Wright, C., & Murphy, M. C. (2016, March–April). *Creating a classroom incremental theory matters. But it's not as straightforward as you might think.* Paper presented at the meeting of the Society for Research on Adolescence, Baltimore, MD.

Howe, L. C., & Dweck, C. S. (2016). Changes in self-definition impede recovery from rejection. *Personality and Social Psychology Bulletin, 42,* 54–71.

Jamieson, J. P., Mendes, W. B., & Nock, M. K. (2013). Improving acute stress responses: The power of reappraisal. *Current Directions in Psychological Science, 22,* 51–56.

Jones, E. (1955). *Sigmund Freud: The life and work: Vol. 2. The years of maturity 1901–1919.* London: Hogarth Press.

Kirschbaum, C., Pirke, K.-M., & Hellhammer, D. H. (1993). The "Trier Social Stress Test": A tool for investigating psychobiological stress responses in a laboratory setting. *Neuropsychobiology, 28,* 76–81.

Mangels, J. A., Butterfield, B., Lamb, J., Good, C., & Dweck, C. S. (2006). Why do beliefs about intelligence influence learning success?: A social cognitive neuroscience model. *Social Cognitive and Affective Neuroscience, 1,* 75–86.

Martocchio, J. J. (1994). Effects of conceptions of ability on anxiety, self-efficacy, and learning in training. *Journal of Applied Psychology, 79,* 819–825.

Miu, A. S., & Yeager, D. S. (2015). Preventing symptoms of depression by teaching adolescents that people can change: Effects of a brief incremental theory of personality intervention at 9-month follow-up. *Clinical Psychological Science, 3,* 726–743.

Molden, D. C., & Dweck, C. S. (2006). Finding "meaning" in psychology: A lay theories approach to self-regulation, social perception, and social development. *American Psychologist, 61,* 192–203.

Moser, J. S., Schroder, H. S., Heeter, C., Moran, T. P., & Lee, Y.-H. (2011). Mind your errors: Evidence for a neural mechanism linking growth mind-set to adaptive posterror adjustments. *Psychological Science, 22,* 1484–1489.

Nussbaum, A. D., & Dweck, C. S. (2008). Defensiveness versus remediation: Self-theories and modes of self-esteem maintenance. *Personality and Social Psychology Bulletin, 34,* 599–612.

Paunesku, D., Walton, G. M., Romero, C., Smith, E. N., Yeager, D. S., & Dweck, C. S. (2015). Mindset interventions are a scalable treatment for academic underachievement. *Psychological Science, 26,* 284–293.

Robins, R. W., & Pals, J. L. (2002). Implicit self-theories in the academic domain: Implications for goal orientation, attributions, affect, and self-esteem change. *Self and Identity, 1,* 313–336.

Ross, L., & Nisbett, R. E. (1991). *The person and the situation: Perspectives of social psychology* (2nd ed.). London: Pinter & Martin.

Rudolph, K. D. (2010). Implicit theories of peer relationships. *Social Development, 19,* 113–129.

Schleider, J. L., Abel, M. R., & Weisz, J. R. (2015). Implicit theories and youth mental health problems: A random-effects meta-analysis. *Clinical Psychology Review, 35,* 1–9.

Schleider, J. L., & Weisz, J. R. (2016). Reducing risk for anxiety and depression in adolescents: Effects of a single-session intervention teaching that personality can change. *Behaviour Research and Therapy, 87,* 170–181.

Schroder, H. S., Dawood, S., Yalch, M. M., Donnellan, M. B., & Moser, J. S. (2015). The role of implicit theories in mental health symptoms, emotion regulation, and hypothetical treatment choices in college students. *Cognitive Therapy and Research, 39,* 120–139.

Schroder, H. S., Dawood, S., Yalch, M. M., Donnellan, M. B., & Moser, J. S. (2016). Evaluating the domain specificity of mental health-related mind-sets. *Social Psychological and Personality Science, 7,* 508–520.

Seery, M. D. (2013). The biopsychosocial model of challenge and threat: Using the heart to measure the mind. *Social and Personality Psychology Compass, 7,* 637–653.

Sevincer, A. T., Kluge, L., & Oettingen, G. (2014). Implicit theories and motivational focus: Desired future versus present reality. *Motivation and Emotion, 38,* 36–46.

Valentiner, D. P., Jencius, S., Jarek, E., Gier-Lonsway, S. L., & McGrath, P. B. (2013). Pretreatment shyness mindset predicts less reduction of social anxiety during exposure therapy. *Journal of Anxiety Disorders, 27,* 267–271.

Walton, G. M. (2014). The new science of wise psychological interventions. *Current Directions in Psychological Science, 23,* 73–82.

Williams, K. D., & Jarvis, B. (2006). Cyberball: A program for use in research on interpersonal ostracism and acceptance. *Behavior Research Methods, Instruments, and Computers, 38,* 174–180.

Yeager, D. S., & Dweck, C. S. (2012). Mindsets that promote resilience: When students believe that personal characteristics can be developed. *Educational Psychologist, 47,* 302–314.

Yeager, D. S., Johnson, R., Spitzer, B. J., Trzesniewski, K. H., Powers, J., & Dweck, C. S. (2014). The far-reaching effects of believing people can change: Implicit theories of personality shape stress, health, and achievement during adolescence. *Journal of Personality and Social Psychology, 106,* 867–884.

Yeager, D. S., Lee, H. Y., & Jamieson, J. P. (2016). How to improve adolescent stress responses: Insights from integrating implicit theories of personality and biopsychosocial models. *Psychological Science, 27,* 1078–1091.

Yeager, D. S., Miu, A. S., Powers, J., & Dweck, C. S. (2013). Implicit theories of personality and attributions of hostile intent: A meta-analysis, an experiment, and a longitudinal intervention. *Child Development, 84,* 1651–1667.

Yeager, D. S., Romero, C., Paunesku, D., Hulleman, C. S., Schneider, B., Hinojosa, C., . . . Dweck, C. S. (2016). Using design thinking to improve psychological interventions: The case of the growth mindset during the transition to high school. *Journal of Educational Psychology, 108,* 374–391.

Yeager, D. S., Trzesniewski, K. H., & Dweck, C. S. (2013). An implicit theories of personality intervention reduces adolescent aggression in response to victimization and exclusion. *Child Development, 84,* 970–988.

Yeager, D. S., Trzesniewski, K. H., Tirri, K., Nokelainen, P., & Dweck, C. S. (2011). Adolescents' implicit theories predict desire for vengeance after peer conflicts: Correlational and experimental evidence. *Developmental Psychology, 47,* 1090–1107.

Yeager, D. S., & Walton, G. M. (2011). Social-psychological interventions in education: They're not magic. *Review of Educational Research, 81,* 267–301.

Yeager, D. S., Walton, G. M., Brady, S. T., Akcinar, E. N., Paunesku, D., Keane, L., . . . Dweck, C. S. (2016). Teaching a lay theory before college narrows achievement gaps at scale. *Proceedings of the National Academy of Sciences of the USA, 113,* E3341–E3348.

CHAPTER 19

Long-Range Thinking and Goal-Directed Action

Edwin A. Locke

This chapter discusses long-range thinking, including long-range goal setting. Because thinking long range involves an awareness of and the regulation of action across time, I start with a brief explanation of what time is.

WHAT IS TIME?

Time is a relationship; time is motion, or, more precisely, a change in relationship between entities (Rand, 1990, p. 259). One observes one entity moving in relation to another. A plausible definition of time would be "the measurement of relative motion." To actually measure time requires a unit of measurement (e.g., the motions of a certain atom).

How does this apply to human life? Life is limited in duration, which means that you can only take a finite number of actions before you die. Thus you have to choose what values to pursue and how to prioritize them.

If you are free to act, your choices affect not only how long you will live but the meaning of your life. Meaning is created by human beings making value choices. *The meaning of your life is the totality of the goals and values that you choose and pursue.*

WHY DO HUMANS NEED TO THINK AND ACT LONG RANGE?

Animals function, and normally function successfully, at the sensory-perceptual level. Their sense organs are usually much more acute that those of humans. They are often stronger and faster. They can digest (survive off of) many foods that humans cannot digest, for example, grass. Each day follows the same basic pattern: sleep, wake up, look for food and water, avoid enemies, look for mates (depending on the season), play with others like themselves, rest, and so forth. Although they cannot project the future or think long range, they can survive unless the environment to which they have adapted changes radically in some way. They live off of nature, including each other in the case of carnivores. Functioning short range works long range for them because repeating the same thing each day has been successful from an evolutionary perspective.

Human beings cannot long survive in this manner. Early hominids were hunter–gatherers, but even this required primitive tools, planning, and coordination. But gifts of nature of the kind humans can utilize (e.g., fruits, berries, wild animals) are limited. Hunter–gatherers did not live very long, and population growth was very gradual.

Over millennia, humans learned to shape the earth to their needs. A major breakthrough was the invention of agriculture, along with the breeding of livestock. These required enormous conceptual work and a future time perspective, for example, finding and planting seeds, studying the soil, irrigation, storage, food processing, division of labor, trade, facts about animal care and breeding, and so forth. Future planning was required. It takes seeds time to grow and animals to breed. The seasons have to be taken into account. Seeds have to be saved for the next year's crops. Methods of irrigation have to be invented. Animal reproduction and mortality have to be tracked and managed. Advanced civilizations were made possible by the discovery of reason in philosophy and its applications, such as modern science and technology.

It is obvious that long-range planning in an industrial civilization is radically more complicated and much more critical and requires an even longer time perspective than in the case of primitive societies. For example, effectively managing wealth creation, education, and health require decades of planning; those who fail to do so will find themselves disadvantaged or worse.

Long-range planning is volitional; it is done by choice. (For a detailed discussion and validation of the nature of volition, see Peikoff, 1991). Unfortunately, a substantial number of people, though they "get by" for a time, do not choose to or do not know how to do the long-range thinking needed to make them thrive.

What is the problem? A major factor is sacrificing or ignoring, in varying degrees, the future for the present. Many people do what feels good now. Of course, everyone has to live in the present; thinking long range while ignoring the present would be irrational, actually suicidal. If you do not survive in the short range, then there is no long range. Imagine eating 300 calories a day to prevent gaining weight, to save money on food, and to leave more time for studying. One would not live very long.

But the same is true of the opposite. Focusing too much on immediate gratification is harmful. Years ago some now-famous studies called the Marshmallow Studies were conducted with children (Mischel, 2014). Children were invited to a laboratory session and given the choice of helping themselves to one marshmallow now or waiting 15 minutes and getting two marshmallows. (Cookies and pretzels were also used). There have been many variations on this original study, and long-term follow-ups have shown, in short, that those who postponed gratification in the marshmallow setting did better in life years later. Questionnaire studies by

Zimbardo and Boyd (2009) with adults found that people who were more future oriented routinely did better in life than those who lived mainly in the present, whether the outcome was education, income, job level, health, self-esteem, (lower) risk taking, and (less) addiction to alcohol and drugs. But none of the above authors discussed how long-range thinking was to be accomplished.

It must be noted that *postponing gratification by itself is not sufficient to create a successful life*, despite popular claims to the contrary. Not doing something now is a negative; it is refraining from certain actions. But to live you have to do something. *To achieve a successful life you have to choose, pursue, and attain goals.* Postponing gratification is only relevant in this context; you need to postpone or give up some values in the present in order to attain longer-range goals. You need to save some money today to have money tomorrow. You need to give up some leisure time in order to become educated. You need to give up some foods or some amounts of food in order to be healthy later.

GOAL-SETTING THEORY

Locke and Latham (1990, 2002), the developers of goal-setting theory, obviously view life as a goal-directed process. Goal theory was based on close to 400 studies using close to 90 tasks, 40,000 participants in seven countries besides the United States, and numerous outcome measures. Several hundred additional studies have been conducted since 1990 (see Locke & Latham, 2013, for a review of studies done since 1990). Goal setting works at the individual, team, and unit levels and even in small, entrepreneurial companies (Locke & Latham, 2013). Goal theory has been applied to work domains (e.g., human resource management), as well as non-work domains such as sports, negotiation, health promotion, psychotherapy, education, and self-development (Locke & Latham, 2013).

Goals, to be most effective, should be specific and difficult (challenging.) Specificity prevents vagueness. Maximum specificity is usually a matter of using numbers: for example, try for a score of X rather than trying to "do your best." Challenge arouses effort. The degree of challenge one undertakes should depend on context. No one has the energy to make every single goal in life difficult. One has to choose how to expend one's energy. The degree of challenge needs to be integrated with one's chosen priorities and the number of goals one has. Goals can be set for learning as well as for performance outcomes (Seijts, Latham, & Woodwark, 2013). Goals affect emotion; goals are at the same time something to shoot for and the standard for satisfaction.

There are four main causal mediators of goal effects. Goals direct attention and action toward goal-relevant outcomes. They arouse both effort and persistence commensurate with what the goal requires. They motivate the use of known task strategies, the attempt to discover new strategies (which may or may not be effective), or the development of needed skills. Learning goals are most helpful when useful new strategies have to be discovered. (Task knowledge and skill is also a goal moderator; see later discussion).

Critical goal moderators include feedback and commitment (Klein, Cooper, & Monahan, 2013). Goals do not work well unless one can track progress (Locke & Latham, 1990; Ashford & De Stobbeleir, 2013). Commitment starts with values, including one's value hierarchy. Goals that are considered more important (higher priority) are more likely to be attained than goals that are less important (Edmister & Locke, 1987). In the realm of practical values, there are many options: what type of career one wants, how far one wants to rise, what standard of living one desires, one's desire for a partner and children, and so forth. Values are hierarchical; this sets one's priorities. If one does not formulate them consciously, the subconscious does it automatically, although in the latter case there will be fuzziness, confusions, lack of constancy, and contradictions. This will undermine commitment to purposeful action.

The second causal factor fostering commitment is task- or domain-specific confidence or self-efficacy (Bandura, 1997). Confidence is acquired by learning (practice, experience), effort, and knowledge. Self-efficacy is the obverse of anxiety and self-doubt (Bandura, 1986). In addition to facilitating commitment, self-efficacy affects the difficulty of the goals one chooses, the quality of the task strategies one employs, and one's response to feedback (Locke & Latham, 1990). Negative feedback does not lead to lowered performance if self-efficacy is sustained (Bandura, 1997). It is likely that self-efficacy is even more important with respect to long-term goals than to short-term goals. Long-term goals are dependent on a long sequence of plans and actions, compared with short-term goals. For those with low efficacy for short-term goals, longer-term goals would be experienced as especially daunting. If one cannot manage day to day or week to week, one will not feel confident of managing year to year or decade to decade. On the other hand, building efficacy for short-term challenges should yield greater confidence about managing the future.

A third goal moderator is task knowledge or skill (which, as noted, is also a mediator). Goals are ends that require a means. Plans, strategies, or skills are the means of attaining goals. Sometimes the plan can be simply to pay attention to the goal and put forth effort and attention (Locke & Latham, 1990). However, as noted earlier, sometimes these do not suffice. One needs to formulate task-specific and possibly new strategies or to acquire new skills (Locke & Latham, 1990; Seijts et al., 2013; Wood, Whelan, Sojo, & Wong, 2013). For example, weight loss requires specific dietary policies and exercise. Saving money requires settling on an amount, a specific source of funds, and an investment strategy. Education requires finding the right institution, getting admitted, and learning how to study (Locke, 1998).

People can successfully pursue multiple goals as long as they are prioritized and/or orchestrated (Sun & Frese, 2013). In theory, goals can be set for moral self-development (for a discussion of ethics, see Peikoff, 1991) education, income, money management, health, romance, career progress, friendship, and children. As to age, the time span for future planning and its content obviously changes over time. The time perspectives and goal priorities of a 15-year-old, a 45-year-old, and a 75-year-old will obviously differ. Carstensen and her colleagues have found that older people who see their remaining "time" as limited are more likely to choose emotionally meaningful goals and the company of familiar social partners, whereas younger people are more focused on discovering new knowledge (e.g., Carstensen, Isaacowitz, & Charles, 1999).

What is hard for many people is integrating their choices and actions so as to benefit themselves in both the present and the future. Why is that so hard? Let's begin by seeing why long-range thinking can be difficult.

Why Is Long-Range Planning So Difficult for Many People?

The Present Is Real and Concrete

It is directly perceived and experienced automatically. *The future is not yet real and thus is not directly perceived.* It is not here now. The concept of the future is an abstraction formed by projecting what will or could happen. The future is a potential that is not yet actualized but will become so. It will become the present only as the present becomes the past.

Dealing with the Present Requires Attention and Energy

If you do not deal successfully with the present, there is no future. Many problems and worries are properly about issues in the present. Further, emotions include action tendencies (Locke, 2009a), wanting to approach desired objects and avoid objects appraised as undesirable. No one wants to give up present pleasures unless there is a compelling reason. No one wants to endure pain or frustration. Long-range thinking requires consciously setting aside time during the present for future planning. One has to engage in foresight (Bandura, 1986, 1997).

Many People Have Not Acquired the Skills Needed to Think Long Range

For example, long-range thinking requires focusing on a range of time spans: tomorrow, next week, next month, next year, and years down the road. This requires not just projection but cognitive integration, which includes an understanding of causal connections between present and future actions and between different future actions. It also requires mentally concretizing (imagining) the future. Lack of skill in contemplating the future may arouse fear and self-doubt, which may lead to avoidance. People may not know how to cope with conflicts between the present and the future.

Long-Range Thinking, Because It Is Not Automatic, Requires Volitional Mental Effort

Of course, dealing with the present requires thought, but grasping the present starts with sense perception, which is automatic. Projecting into the future is conceptually demanding; not everyone wants to do it.

Long-Range Thinking, Because It Has to Be Integrated with the Present, Requires Prioritization

Every action is a choice among possibilities. If you spend all your money now, you will not have that same money later. If you want to get educated, you cannot spend all your spare time each day on Internet games. If you want to lose or control weight, you cannot chronically ignore eating habits and exercise. Because life offers so many options and life circumstances are always changing in some respect, prioritization can be difficult.

Children learn to develop foresight by learning about causality, that is, that actions have consequences, starting with how their own actions affect people or objects—for example, crying, asking, rolling a ball. Gradually they learn to extend the time span, though this requires increasing effort. As the child grows into adult-hood, life gets more complicated. Adults are responsible for their own futures. The time scale needed to be in control expands to encompass, ideally at least, the whole rest of their lives.

Many education and career choices may need to be made to keep up with an ever-changing economy. Income has to meet expenses and take into account future needs, for example, the cost of rearing children and retirement needs. People need to choose a career, or at least a preliminary career. They need to think about their diets. The effect of eating habits may begin to have negative effects and put them at increasing risk for illness. These and many other values are relevant to life happiness.

Techniques to Facilitate Long-Range Thinking

Visualizing the Future

Using imagination, people can mentally visualize what they want their future to be like. For example, one might visualize a good income, an interesting career, a romantic partner (Locke & Kenner, 2011). One can visualize, by observing the world around him or her, what it is like to live in poverty versus living well (without being a millionaire). One can visualize negatives to avoid, for example, lying, heavy drinking, wild spending, or breaking the law.

Visualizing in this way is, in effect, fantasizing. However, an important research program by Oettingen (e.g., see Oettingen, 2014; Oettingen, Wittchen, & Gollwit-zer, 2013) and her colleagues has shown that fantasizing alone does not bring about the wanted future. Engaging in fantasy alone can lead to a subconscious belief that the future state has already been achieved and that therefore no action is necessary.

To be effective, the fantasy or wish has to be followed by additional cognitive processes. First, the individual has to be specific about the outcome desired; a vague wish is like a vague goal (Locke & Latham, 1990); it is not very effective. It does not specify just what the outcome is supposed to be. Second, the individual needs to consider possible obstacles (internal or external) to attaining the goal. This process, which involves mentally contrasting the desired state with the present reality, makes it explicit that some action must be taken—that wishing as such is not going to be sufficient. Third, once obstacles are identified, the individual needs to develop a specific plan or plans to attain the goals. Ideally, the plan will be accompanied by or be part of an "if–then" intention to implement the plan. Such an implementation intention involves making a conscious decision about when and where to take goal-relevant action; for example, "if situation X arises, then I will do Y." The needed action may often be taken later, without further conscious thought (Gollwitzer & Sheeran, 2006). As in the case of goal-setting theory (Locke & Latham, 1990, 2013), a number of factors may moderate the effectiveness of the implementation, for example, the strength of the intention, commitment, personality, the number of intentions, external (environmental) support, feedback (Gollwitzer, 2014). Clearly more research is required here.

Case Example.

Darlene realized that her weight was getting a bit out of control. She wanted to lose some pounds. She realized that the main obstacle was the actual presence of ice cream in the home; whenever she opened an ice cream container, she could not stop until she finished it. So she resolved to never have ice cream in the house. If she saw ice cream in the store, then she would pass it by. When she went to the store thenceforth, she was able to ignore the ice cream section without further thought. That solved the problem.

An additional factor that is critical to success in goal-directed action and intentional implementation is self-efficacy (basically what Oettingen, 2014, calls "expectancy"), which refers to task- or domain-specific confidence (Bandura, 1997). Thousands of studies testify to the beneficial effects of self-efficacy on effective task performance. The most powerful and direct means of gaining self-efficacy is through learning (enactive mastery), including directed practice to build skill level; social persuasion may also foster efficacy. To the degree that any of the foregoing cognitive processes or conditions are absent (or are considered in the wrong order, such as listing obstacles before wishes), the attainment of future goals or intentions (wishes, fantasies) is undermined. An interesting finding with respect to fantasy research is that high self-efficacy is beneficial only if mental contrasting is engaged in (Oettingen, 2012, 2014).

Oettingen's program involves both conscious and subconscious elements, as does almost all human activity (Locke, 2015). Both goal theorists and implementation theorists have done studies in which action is subconsciously primed, but that research is outside the scope of this chapter. (Latham, Brcic, & Steinhauer, 2017, have found that priming is partially mediated and moderated by conscious goals and conscientiousness, respectively).

Tying Proximal to Distal Goals

Locke and Latham (1990) reviewed the literature through that date comparing the effects of proximal (short-term) vs distal (long-term) goals. The results were inconsistent. In these studies, proximal and distal goals were not always used together. Latham and his colleagues, in more recent years, looked at whether proximal goals would facilitate the attainment of logically related distal goals when people had both. Latham and Seijts (1999) found that the two together were more effective than "do your best" goals. Seijts and Latham (2001), however, did not find this with learning goals. There appear to be various mediators at work, such as self-efficacy and task strategies, especially with learning goals. It is possible that proximal goals could slow people down if they are ahead of schedule to reach their distal goals.

Much more research needs to be done regarding the ideal time periods for proximal goals and distal goals, including the ideal intervals between them. Further, there are very few, if any, studies testing the benefits of proximal goals for long-term life goals, although there would seem to be obvious applications. For example, weekly or monthly savings deposit goals could be the means of attaining the needed retirement assets or backup funds in case of job loss or other emergencies. (It has been estimated that about two-thirds of the U. S. population do not plan sufficiently for retirement.) Weekly weight loss or eating goals could be set to help attain yearly or life goals for weight loss, which could benefit health or fitness. Taking a series of courses and studying conscientiously each day could lead to a degree that could lead to future job and career attainments. Opting out in sixth grade and not building skills for the future may have poor results down the road.

Through repetition, working toward proximal goals can become habit. Habits are at least partly subconscious, so exercising them on a regular basis does not require a great deal of conscious thought; but, contrary to popular belief, it often takes a conscious decision to set the habit in motion—for example: "I need to exercise every day but maybe I do not need to do it right now—oops—better do it." Conscious choice is the prime mover in everyday life (Locke, 2015).

Case Example.

Wes was an ambitious young employee of a technology company, He wanted to move to the top. He was intelligent, rational, and of good character. He set himself the everyday goal of doing each job he was assigned to do better than anyone in that organization had ever done it before. He wanted to move ahead in the company. After doing this for many years, he became CEO and succeeded in that role too.

Self-set work goals have been found to affect performance (in this case, promotions) over a 25-year time span (Howard, 2013). These goals involved managers' career aspirations. Presumably, these managers had shorter-term goals that involved performing well on a daily, weekly, or monthly basis, as implied in the preceding case example.

Proximal–distal goal setting also applies to organizations. At Google, the company's distal goal early on was to "organize the world's information" (Bock, 2015, p. 5), and they certainly are achieving that. ("Googling" today means finding almost anything you want on the Internet). But CEO Larry Page wants the company to keep growing and innovating and thus sets quarterly goals for the company. Employees are expected to make sure their own work goals are in sync with the company goals. The company also encourages "crazy, ambitious" goals (p. 155) to motivate creative thinking, even though they might not be reached. General Electric used the same idea and called them "stretch goals" (Kerr & Lepelley, 2013). These were used to stimulate creative thinking, but managers were not penalized for failing to reach them.

We can assume that the ideal time span for proximal and distal goals depends on the context. Personal or work goals can be daily, weekly, monthly, quarterly, or annual, with links between the shorter and longer spans made as needed. The links can extend as far into the future as wanted or needed based on the outcome desired—for example, healthy teeth in old age can be facilitated by daily brushing (and seeing the dentist annually).

Gaining Support

In pursuing goals, people can obtain useful guidance from others and then choose to utilize it. For example, managers can help new employees in a number of ways: through mentorship, through training to build confidence (self-efficacy; Bandura, 1997), by helping them cope with setbacks, or by showing them the long-range consequences of what they are doing on a given job, for example, building skills. A word of caution: There can be a fine line between support or mentorship and dependency. A good mentor will help the protégé to develop independence in order to make him or her ready for higher-level posts in the future. Some companies delegate more authority to new hires than they seem ready for—akin to sink or swim (Locke, 2008). The purpose here is to support self-development through extreme delegation.

Company support can also enhance the duration of goal-setting programs. Pritchard, Young, Koenig, Schmerling, and Dixon (2013) found that feedback/goal-setting programs set up by a consulting group had very positive effects. Even so, the duration of the programs varied a great deal as a result of the duration of management support. Some programs lasted up to 3 years. Managerial support was sometime withdrawn as a result of the misuse of stretch goals (penalizing failure) and personnel changes. (New managers often like to change everything to prove they are in charge). Latham and Baldes (1975) set up a goal-setting program for logging truck drivers that required them to load their trucks each day to a certain percentage of the maximum allowable level. The program had both management and union support. Follow-up inquiries revealed that it was successful for at least 7 years following the initial experiment.

Case Example.

Julio was from a Hispanic family who immigrated to the United States and at first knew nothing about such a thing as a college education. But Julio wanted to better himself and enrolled at a community college, at the same time as he held two jobs. At a loss as to what to do once admitted, Julio consulted a program director who managed a grant to help Hispanic students. The director became a mentor for Julio and guided him through several years of classes, despite delays and interruptions and various family emergencies. The director helped him get scholarship money and pointed out possible career paths. Unlike many of his peers, Julio took full advantage of the opportunities and advice offered to him. Julio did well in class, applied and was admitted to a prestigious 4-year university, and got a part-time job at a science institute. He is well on his way to a career in science.

Writing about Goals

Some people can function well by keeping their goals in their heads. But ideas in the mind can come and go, and goals held only as thoughts can become mushy or vague or be forgotten. It is often more effective to "objectify" goals by putting them in writing. For research on the benefits of writing about goals, see Travers (2013) and Morisano, Hirsh, Peterson, Pihl, and Shore (2010). These studies asked students to write at length about their personal life goals, which usually included but did not have to involve schoolwork. The reports encompassed many non-school aspects of their lives and characters, for example, self-esteem, stress relief, health, listening, conflict management, emotional regulation, and empathy. Objective outcome measures were taken in the Morisano et al. (2010) study and revealed that the writing process itself led to better academic performance. Writing about what one wants in the future (which has to involve thinking) brings goals into the directly perceivable present but also draws out value issues from the subconscious.

Case Example.

One student's personal goal statement from Travers (2013). "To improve my assertiveness by reducing the number of times I say yes to unreasonable requests by 75% so that I get what I want without denying the rights of others."

Seeking Feedback and Tracking

Effective goal setting requires tracking performance. This indicates whether progress is being made and may indicate that plans and strategies need revision. Keeping a table or graph or other visual records is helpful because progress is unambiguous and directly perceivable in quantitative form. Time is built into the process through making a time scale on the graph. Sometimes it is useful to seek feedback, such as on the job (Ashford & Tsui, 1991).

Using Role Models

Bandura (1986) has summarized the extensive search on role modeling as a means of learning. Role modeling is not simply imitation; it involves a variety of processes. These include: being able to observe (perceive, hear) what the role models do; retaining what was observed and rehearsing it; cognitive processing of what was observed, including integrating the observations into principles; observing the consequences of what actions the role model took; and being able to put what was learned into action. Role models who are most similar to the actor usually have the greatest effect.

Obvious role models are one's parents. One can look for qualities that benefited his or her childhood success and happiness—for example, affection, fairness, emphasis on cognitive development and education, clear behavioral guidelines, exercise, healthy eating habits, or effective listening. One can decide to reject the characteristics he or she did not like, such as meanness, smoking, dishonesty, neglect, irrational money management, failure to work for a living or develop job skills, and so forth.

Case Example.

Bob's father took no role in raising his kids. He cheated on his wife, then divorced her and married a model who was a gold digger and who ended up as a bitter alcoholic. He failed on many jobs because he never acquired the needed skills, though he was honest in his business dealings. Although he earned high salaries for a time, he did not save money and eventually filed for bankruptcy. At the time of his death, none of his children cared about him, and he was living on social security. His son Bob chose to be different in every respect. He helped raise his kids, never cheated on his wife, was very careful about money, and had a very successful career based on hard work and skill development. He rejected both parents' religious views and chose his own, secular philosophy.

Friends, teachers, and coworkers can also serve as positive and negative role models. Even fictional characters can be inspiring. Many Ayn Rand (1993) fans are inspired by the figure of Howard Roark in her novel *The Fountainhead* because he is honest, hardworking, and an intransigent, rational individualist who refuses to conform to mindless conventions.

Evaluating your Pleasures

Most people think of their pleasures as a given: "That's what I like." However, pleasures can be evaluated by asking this question: "Is this pleasure good for me or not, not just for today but for the long run?" Many people drift into pleasures rather than deliberately choosing them. Consider the couch potato who watches TV 5 hours or more every day. They may fail to ask themselves: "What do I like about these programs?" The motivation for their TV addiction may be negative, for example, reducing anxiety or avoiding having to make choices about their lives. They have the power to ask: "Am I getting something valuable out of every show?" They could ask themselves: "Are there others types of pleasures that would make my life better in the long run?" Hobbies are one example, but there are endless possibilities (e.g., other forms of art, reading, walking, sports). People who mentally stagnate become bored and also very boring to be with.

Learning to Introspect

Introspection is an important, and unfortunately a virtually forbidden, method of psychology (Locke, 2009b). Emotions as such are automatic, but they are not psychological primaries. Brain disorders aside, emotions stem from automatic subconscious appraisals based on stored knowledge and values (Locke, 2009a). For example, anger is based on the appraisal of some action or event that is perceived as unjust or morally wrong (assuming that one values justice). Guilt is based on the appraisal that one has violated one's moral code. Happiness is based on attaining values. Admiration is based on seeing a significant achievement by others. Because emotions are automatic, one can't change emotions by direct willpower; one has to deautomatize the sequence by correcting errors of judgment or knowledge or modifying one's values (e.g., with cognitive therapy). Viewing emotions as primaries can make one more likely to act short range, based on impulse; there is no tie to one's conscious values or self-concept or longer-range aspirations. Understanding that emotions have causes makes one less tempted to simply act on feelings of the moment and more likely to think about what is causing them and to decide what actions, if any, are in their best interests. Introspection can help one prioritize or reprioritize goals and values: "How should I expend my time today, this week, this year, for future years?"

Back to the issue of time: people frequently say, "I do not have time to do X." But it is important to identify exactly what this means, as time is not an actual entity that boxes you into a corner and thereby makes you feel helpless. *To say "I do not have time to do X" actually means that "I have higher priorities than X. There are more important actions that I want to take."* This opens up a whole new perspective: Time is not an intractable enemy. Time pressure can be a signal to check one's priorities;

this can lead to revising them, including giving up or postponing certain goals. Clinging to them could be undermining one's health and happiness.

Case Example.

Deborah wanted to do everything: go to school, work at a full-time job, do volunteer work, exercise, spend time with her boyfriend, take care of the apartment, do all the cooking and grocery shopping, and enjoy her hobbies. She was feeling anxious and exhausted. In effect, she was trying to be superwoman. She felt much better when she was convinced simply to give up some things (which eventually included her ne'er-do-well boyfriend). Having more time translated to taking fewer actions by eliminating the less important ones. Of course, some actions can be delegated.

Obviously, there is the other side to this coin. People can see their lives as slipping away, because they do too little or do things that mean nothing to them or fail to pursue what they really want. They are in motion, but what they do is not in line with their deepest goals and values and thus not a priority. They may get no pleasure from their careers or significant others or from leisure. Their short-range goals and actions are badly disconnected from what they want long range, and they may not allow themselves to be aware of the conflict. Introspection can put them on the path to reprioritization.

Dealing with "Temptations"

The term *temptation* is usually tied to religion (being tempted to disobey God and risk going to hell). But a temptation is simply a conflict, usually between the shorter term and the longer term. A student may be tempted to play a video game rather than do homework. An obese person may be tempted to eat a third pizza rather than control calorie intake. A spendthrift may be tempted, on the spur of the moment, to buy things he or she does not really need rather than saving for something more important. Of course, when thinking of temptation, most people associate it with infidelity. Consider two contrasting cases.

Peter was married to Andrea for 35 years. The couple turned out to be not really suited to each other and were in important respects unhappy a good part of the time. But neither cheated; furthermore, they were never seriously tempted to cheat, though they knew other attractive people. This was due to the fact that, independent of religious beliefs, both were people of the highest character and took pride in being honest. They could not seriously conceive of being unfaithful. There was no desire by either partner to even consider adultery. Finally, they split up, but the settlement was cordial. Both finally set a goal of finding a partner with whom they would be happier and both succeeded after considerable effort and stress.

Compare Peter and Andrea with David and Beth. Neither had any real philosophy, though they would sometimes attend church out of habit and conformity. Both drank a lot and liked to party. David "hooked up" one night because he felt like it. He did not confess, but Beth found out about it.

David said it was only one time and he would not do it again, but he did. So Beth decided to get her revenge by doing the same. The marriage ended in acrimony. Both acted on impulse rather than on principle. Their subsequent partners did not work out any better.

Temptation is not the human condition but the consequence of what kind of person one is, that is, what one makes of oneself or lets oneself become for better or for worse. (For a discussion of moral values, see Locke & Kenner, 2011, and Peikoff, 1991). Conflicts need to be resolved by fully understanding their causes through introspection (as discussed above). Further, there has to be commitment to the relationship (Locke & Kenner, 2011) and to moral principles.

CONCLUSION

Long-range thinking is essential for long-term survival and happiness. The conceptual (rational) faculty is one's main means of doing this. But because the future is not yet real, various means have to be used to bring about future goals, and these involve bringing the future into the present in various ways that can be logically connected to the future. This does not mean that one should or can give up the present; this would be fatal. Rather, it means the integration of the two. Work for happiness today and plan for how you will ensure that you continue to get it (and even more of it) as the years pass.

Of course, there are factors that block attempts to be happy both short and long term. The most obvious man-made danger is dictatorship. One's life is at the whim of rulers. One has no rights, and an individual and his or her loved ones can be disposed of as the dictator sees fit. The best bet is to escape if one can. Poverty also limits one's options, so a useful goal to set is to form a plan to earn more money. There are personal tragedies (illnesses, accidents, natural disasters) that cannot be controlled, although rational thinking and planning can sometimes help one to avoid or cope with them. Wartime injuries can ravage veterans, physically and psychologically. Some wonderful aids for injured people are service dogs and modern technology. Setbacks often require resetting one's priorities in line with new circumstances.

ACKNOWLEDGMENT

I am indebted to Dr. Ellen Kenner for her many helpful suggestions for this chapter.

REFERENCES

Ashford, S. J., & De Stobbeleir, K. E. M. (2013). Feedback, goal setting, and task performance. In E. A. Locke & G. P. Latham (Eds.), *New developments in goal setting and task performance* (pp. 51–64). New York: Routledge.

Ashford, S. J., & Tsui, A. S. (1991). Self-regulation for managerial effectiveness: The role of active feedback-seeking. *Academy of Management Journal, 34,* 251–280.

Bandura, A. (1986). *Social foundations of thought and action*. Englewood Cliffs, NJ: Prentice Hall.

Bandura, A. (1997). *Self-efficacy: The exercise of control*. New York: Freeman.

Bock, L. (2015). *Work rules!* New York: Twelve, Hachette Book Group.

Carstensen, L. L., Isaacowitz, D. M., & Charles, S. T. (1999). Taking time seriously: A theory of socioemotional selectivity. *American Psychologist, 54*, 165–181.

Edmister, R. O., & Locke, E. A, (1987). The effects of differential goal weights on the performance of a complex financial task. *Personnel Psychology, 40*, 505–517.

Gollwitzer, P. M. (2014). Weakness of the will: Is a quick fix possible? *Motivation and Emotion, 38*, 305–322.

Gollwitzer, P. M., & Sheeran, P. (2006). Implementation intentions and goal achievement: A meta-analysis of effects and processes. *Advances in Experimental Social Psychology, 38*, 69–119.

Howard, A. (2013). The predictive validity of conscious and subconscious motives on career advancement. In E. A. Locke & G. P. Latham (Eds.), *New developments in goal setting and task performance* (pp. 246–261). New York: Routledge.

Kerr, S., & Lepelley, D. (2013). Stretch goals: Risks, possibilities, and best practices. In E. A. Locke & G. P. Latham (Eds.), *New developments in goal setting and task performance* (pp. 21–31). New York: Routledge.

Klein, H. J., Cooper, J. T., & Monahan, C. A. (2013). Goal commitment. In E. A. Locke & G. P. Latham (Eds.), *New directions in goal setting and task performance* (pp. 65–89). New York: Routledge.

Latham, G. P., & Baldes, J. J. (1975). The "practical significance" of Locke's theory of goal setting. *Journal of Applied Psychology, 60*, 122–124.

Latham, G. P., Brcic, J., & Steinhauer, A. (2017). Toward an integration of goal setting theory and the automaticity model. *Applied Psychology: An International Review, 66*, 25–48.

Latham, G. P., & Seijts, G. H. (1999). The effects of proximal and distal goals on performance on a moderately complex task. *Journal of Organizational Behavior, 20*, 421–429.

Locke, E. A. (1998). *Study methods and study motivation*. New Milford, CT: Second Renaissance Books.

Locke, E. A. (2008). *The prime movers: Traits of the great wealth creators*. Irvine, CA: Ayn Rand Bookstore.

Locke, E. A. (2009a). Attain emotional control by understanding what emotions are. In E. A. Locke (Ed.), *Handbook of principles of organizational behavior* (pp. 145–160). New York: Wiley.

Locke, E. A. (2009b). It's time we brought introspection out of the closet. *Perspectives in Psychological Science, 4*, 24–25.

Locke, E. A. (2015). Theory building, replication, and behavioral priming: Where do we need to go from here? *Perspectives on Psychological Science, 10*, 408–414.

Locke, E. A., & Kenner, E. (2011). *The selfish path to romance*. Doylestown, PA: Platform Press.

Locke, E. A., & Latham, G. P. (1990). *A theory of goal setting and task performance*. Englewood Cliffs, NJ: Prentice Hall.

Locke, E. A., & Latham, G. P. (2002). Building a practically useful theory of goal setting and task performance. *American Psychologist, 57*, 705–717.

Locke, E. A., & Latham, G. P. (2013). *New developments in goal setting and task performance*. New York: Routledge.

Mischel, W. (2014). *The marshmallow test*. New York: Little, Brown.

Morisano, D. Hirsh, J. B., Peterson, J. B., Pihl, R. O., & Shore, B. M. (2010). Setting, elaborating, and reflecting on personal goals improves academic performance. *Journal of Applied Psychology, 95*, 255–264.

Oettingen, G. (2012). Future thought and behavior change. *European Review of Social Psychology, 23*, 1–63.

Oettingen, G. (2014). *Rethinking positive thinking: Inside the new science of motivation.* New York: Penguin Random House.

Oettingen, G., Wittchen, M., & Gollwitzer, P. (2013). Regulating goal pursuit through mental contrasting with implementation intentions. In E. A. Locke & G. P. Latham (Eds.), *New developments in goal setting and task performance* (pp. 523–548). New York: Routledge.

Peikoff, L. (1991). *Objectivism: The philosophy of Ayn Rand.* New York: Dutton.

Pritchard, R. D., Young, B. L., Koenig, N., Schmerling, D., & Dixon, N. W. (2013). Long-term effects of goal setting on performance with the productivity measurement and enhancement system (ProMES). In E. A. Locke & G. P. Latham (Eds.), *New developments in goal setting and task performance* (pp. 233–245). New York: Routledge.

Rand, A. (1990). *Introduction to objectivist epistemology.* New York: NAL.

Rand, A. (1993). *The fountainhead.* New York: Signet.

Seijts, G. H., & Latham, G. P. (2001). The effects if distal learning, outcome, and proximal goals on a moderately complex task. *Journal of Organizational Psychology, 22*, 291–307.

Seijts, G. H., Latham, G. P., & Woodwark, M. (2013). Learning goals: A qualitative and quantitative review. In E. A. Locke & G. P. Latham (Eds.), *New developments in goal setting and task performance* (pp. 195–212). New York: Routledge.

Sun, S. H., & Frese, M. (2015). Multiple goal pursuit. In E. A. Locke & G. P. Latham (Eds.), *New developments in goal setting and task performance* (pp. 177–194). New York: Routledge.

Travers, C. J. (2013). Using goal setting theory to promote personal development. In E. A. Locke & G. P. Latham (Eds.), *New developments in goal setting and task performance* (pp. 603–619). New York: Routledge.

Wood, R. E., Whelan, J., Sojo, V., & Wong, M. (2013). Goals, goal orientations, strategies, and performance. In E. A. Locke & G. P. Latham (Eds.), *New developments in goal setting and task performance* (pp. 90–114). New York: Routledge.

Zimbardo, P., & Boyd, J. (2009). *The time paradox.* New York: Free Press.

>>>>>>>>>>>>>>>>

CHAPTER 20

The Effect of Priming Goals on Organizational-Related Behavior
My Transition from Skeptic to Believer

Gary P. Latham

The purpose of this chapter is to review the literature on the effect of priming goals on organizational-related behavior. A prime is an environmental cue that activates a mental representation, stored in memory, in the absence of awareness. The mental representation, however, must be motivationally relevant or valued by the individual for goal pursuit to take place (Bargh, 1994). In reviewing this literature, the basis for my initial skepticism of the findings from research in social psychology on priming goals is explained, as well as my transition to that of a believer.

GOAL-SETTING THEORY

Together with Locke, I developed goal-setting theory (Locke & Latham, 1990, 2002, 2013; Latham & Locke, 2007, 2018). This inductively developed theory of motivation is based on approximately 400 experiments conducted in both laboratory and field settings (e.g., Latham & Locke, 1975). As of the early 2000s, there were more than 1,000 (Mitchell & Daniels, 2003). The essence of the theory is that the immediate determinant of behavior is an individual's *consciously* set goals. A core tenet of the theory is that a specific, high consciously set goal leads to higher performance than one that is easy, vague (such as to do one's best), or no goal at all. This assertion is conditional on four moderators: commitment, ability, feedback, and situational constraints/resources. That is, an individual must consciously *commit* to a difficult goal within his or her *ability* to attain. *Feedback* must be provided on what to continue, start, or stop doing to attain the goal. Finally, there must be no, or minimal, *situational constraints*; the person must have the *resources* necessary for goal attainment.

The mediators that explain the goal–performance relationship include the conscious *choice* of a goal, a *strategy* or *plan* to attain it, and the exertion of *effort*, as well as *persistence*, until the goal is attained. That is, the individual must choose a specific, high goal, develop a strategy or plan for attaining it, and then exert the requisite effort and persist in doing so until the goal is attained.

Of all the field experiments I have conducted on goal setting, my favorite involved engineers/scientists in the forest products industry (Latham, Mitchell, & Dossett, 1978). The field experiment, shown in Figure 20.1, involved a 3 × 3 + 1 factorial design. Consistent with goal-setting theory, the employees in the three do-your-best conditions performed no better than those in cell 10, even though they received praise (cell 7), public recognition (cell 8), or a monetary bonus (cell 9). The individuals in cell 10 did not know they were participating in an experiment. Those in the participative goal-setting conditions (cells, 4, 5, 6) had higher performance than the employees in the other conditions. Yet goal commitment was no higher when the employees were involved in setting their goals than when the goals were assigned by an employee's supervisor (cells 1, 2, 3). Goal difficulty level, however, was higher in the participatively set goal conditions than it was in the assigned goal conditions. Consistent with goal-setting theory, the higher a specific goal, the higher a person's job performance.

Scholars who reviewed the goal-setting literature have concluded that this cognitive theory, goal setting, is the most valid and practical theory of motivation in organizational psychology (Lee & Earley, 1992; Miner, 2003; Pinder, 1998). Thus it came as no surprise to me when I learned that there was a "replication crisis" in social psychology with regard to the findings from primed goal experiments (e.g., Pashler, Coburn, & Harris, 2012; Kahneman, 2012).

Social Psychology Experiments on Primed Goals

Arguably, the dominant framework for conducting experiments on priming goals is Bargh's (1994) automaticity model. As noted earlier, the model states that an external cue in the environment can activate a goal in the absence of awareness of

	Assigned Goal	Participative Goal	Do Your Best
Praise	1	4	7
Public Recognition	2	5	8
$	3	6	9

10

FIGURE 20.1. The effect of goals and rewards on behavior.

the goal's guiding role, and this goal will automatically influence choice, effort, and behavior if the situation allows its pursuit and the goal is valued by the individual. The critical difference between conscious and subconscious goal pursuit is that "unlike unconscious goal strivers, conscious goal strivers know why they do what they do" (Bargh, Gollwitzer, & Oettingen, 2010, p. 299). The model further states that conscious and subconscious goal pursuits follow the same processing stages, predict the same phenomena, and produce the same outcomes.[1]

Having spent my academic career inductively developing a theory of consciously set goals based on empirical experiments and correlational studies, I was highly skeptical that the automaticity model would be applicable in organizational settings. I was particularly skeptical of social psychology experiments in this domain. For example, Bargh, Chen, and Burrows (1996) primed the concept of *elderly* by having students who were randomly assigned to the experimental condition read a passage containing words such as *elderly* and *Florida*. Those in the control condition read a passage containing neutral words. When each participant left the laboratory, a research assistant, standing unobtrusively in the hallway, recorded the length of time it took for each participant to walk from the laboratory to the elevator. As hypothesized, the people primed with the stereotype of *elderly* walked significantly more slowly than those individuals in the control condition.

Dijksterhuis and van Knippenberg (1998) asked students to either write what they believed were the characteristics of either a professor or a soccer hooligan. Those randomly assigned to the primed professor condition answered more questions correctly from the game Trivial Pursuit than those who were thinking about a hooligan. Asking people to focus on the characteristics of a professor primed them with the determination to think before answering the questions.

Most incredible to me was the experiment by Fishbach, Friedman, and Kruglanski (2003). Female students in the experimental condition sat in a laboratory in which there were exercise and dieting magazines lying unobtrusively on a table.[2] On the table in another room were magazines about politics and economics. Some time later, a research assistant offered each participant the choice between a chocolate bar or an apple. Those in the experimental condition chose the apple with greater frequency than the chocolate. The magazines on exercise and dieting primed those students to eat healthy food. I personally have never chosen an apple over a chocolate bar. As I told an interviewer for the *Chronicle of Higher Education* (Bartlett, 2013), I viewed the results of priming experiments as "crap." Adding to my skepticism of findings from experiments in this domain is that there was often a failure to do a manipulation check for awareness. Also, I was suspicious of experimenter bias and demand effects. The short time frame (i.e., seconds, minutes) between the manipulation of a prime and the measurement of the dependent variable suggested

---

[1]Locke (2015) and I (Latham, Stajkovic & Locke, 2010) prefer the term *subconscious* to *unconscious*. The term *unconscious* was originally used by Freud to refer to information that could never become conscious; it could only be inferred through the analysis of dreams. *Subconscious* means information that is potentially conscious. It is material stored in memory that can be brought into awareness.

[2]A pilot study revealed that gender is a moderator. Females were found to be more concerned with their weight than males.

that the effect, if there indeed was one, was so fragile, so short-lived that it was irrelevant for goal setting in the workplace (Latham & Locke, 2012; Latham, Stajkovic, & Locke, 2010). Moreover, the dependent variables used in social psychology experiments regarding primed goals were typically of little or no relevance for work settings (e.g., time taken to walk from a laboratory to an elevator, choosing the correct answer to questions from a game, or choosing an apple to eat rather than a chocolate).

Priming Goals for Organizationally Relevant Tasks

Edwin Locke was as skeptical as I of the findings in social psychology on primed goals. Consequently, he agreed to do a laboratory experiment with Alex Stajkovic and Stajkovic's doctoral student, Eden Blair (Stajkovic, Locke, & Blair, 2006) to see whether they could replicate findings on priming using an organizationally relevant task, brainstorming.

College students were randomly assigned to conditions in a 2 (prime/no prime) × 3 (consciously set difficult goal, easy goal, or do your best) factorial design. Using priming methodology frequently utilized by Bargh (1989), the students were asked to make sentences out of scrambled words. Unbeknownst to them, many of the words in the experimental condition were achievement related (e.g., *wins, compete, success*), whereas the words in the control condition for making sentences were neutral in nature (e.g., *melts water when butter heated*). Much to Locke's surprise, there was a main effect for the primed goal for achievement, as well as for the consciously set difficult goal. Interrogation of each student at the end of the experiment revealed that none was aware of the hypothesized relationship between forming achievement-related sentences and subsequent task performance. There was also an interaction effect between the primed and the consciously set goal because the participants in the consciously set specific, easy goal condition stopped working when they attained their goal. When this condition is removed, the interaction effect is no longer significant.

To keep goal priming from coming further into the organizational psychology literature, I approached my doctoral student, Amanda Shantz, to do a field rather than a laboratory experiment. To minimize individual differences and to increase the probability of us obtaining null findings between conditions, we chose a "strong situation" (Mischel, 1968), namely a call center. A strong situation is one in which everyone behaves essentially in the same way. The effects of individual differences (e.g., personality) on the dependent variable are thus minimized. At a call center, all the employees are given the same instructions, prepared by management, to read when they are soliciting money from potential donors. The donated money is tracked by the center's computer. Thus there was no possibility for experimenter bias or contamination of this dependent variable, dollars pledged, by the subjectivity inherent in supervisory ratings of job performance. Therefore, no one could accuse us of "playing" with the data in order to obtain the null findings that we were sure that we would get.

We deemed it unlikely that management would allow us to request employees to make achievement-type sentences from scrambled words. Pavio (1986, 1991) found that behavior is affected by a cognitive system that is more responsive to pictures than to words. Choosing pictures can be readily applied to priming a goal in organizational settings. Consequently, we did a pilot study involving two different photographs plus a control condition to see whether one or both photographs resulted in employees brainstorming more ideas for a coat hanger than another. One did, namely a photograph of a person winning a race.[3]

The employees in the call center were then randomly assigned to a 2 (primed/control) × 2 (consciously set difficult goal/do-your-best) factorial design. The racer was portrayed in a backdrop, that is, the instructions for soliciting money were written across the photograph. The conscious difficult goal, set by management, for each employee was to raise $1,200 within the 3-hour work shift.

To our surprise, there was a main effect not only for the consciously set goal but also for the primed goal. Like Stajkovic et al. (2006), we used Bargh et al.'s (1996) funnel debriefing questionnaire to assess employee awareness of the primed goal–job performance relationship. Not only was every employee unaware of the hypothesis, but every employee reported not even noticing the photograph. They said they were too busy raising money to pay attention to the picture of the racer (Shantz & Latham, 2009).

My overall reaction to the results of this experiment was that I was too old and Shantz was too young to ruin our respective reputations by publishing these results. Thus we agreed that we would conduct two exact replications in two additional call centers.

As Molden (2014) noted, the advantage of an exact or direct replication is that it provides unambiguous information about the overall reliability of the phenomenon itself, whereas a conceptual replication that fails raises questions as to whether the failure means that the phenomenon is not robust or that it does not extend to the new conditions that were examined. Moreover, direct replications make it possible to correct Type 1 errors in the published literature.

At the end of a 4-hour work shift, employees in the second call center in the primed goal condition raised, on average, $455 versus $223 in the control condition. Employees in the primed goal condition in the third call center raised $584 versus $287 in the control condition (Shantz & Latham, 2011). These results clearly have practical as well as statistical significance.

To remove all doubt that these results might be due to experimenter bias or demand effects, a fourth field experiment was conducted in a fourth call center (Latham & Piccolo, 2012). Whereas Shantz was present in the first three call centers to ensure that the managers randomly assigned employees to conditions and to be alert for any evidence of employee awareness of the hypothesis while the employees were soliciting donations, neither Piccolo nor I were present when this fourth experiment took place. To remove any doubt regarding the fragile, short-term effect of a primed goal on behavior, the field experiment was conducted for an entire 4-day work week.

---

[3]The Stajkovic et al. (2006) brainstorming task with college students was for uses for a coat hanger. This task did little toward removing my skepticism of findings in this domain. Nevertheless, we used this task in our pilot study to see whether we could replicate their findings with adults before conducting an experiment in the workplace.

A projective test was used to determine whether the goals were primed in the subconscious. Three hypotheses were tested:

1. A primed context-specific goal, namely a photograph of employees performing the job, leads to a significantly higher number of work-related and achievement-related words in subsequent stories that people write than does a primed goal for general achievement, namely a photograph of a racer winning a race, or a no-prime control condition, as measured by the Thematic Apperception Test (TAT).
2. A primed goal for achievement (i.e., the photograph of a woman winning a race) leads to a significantly higher number of achievement-related words in subsequent TAT stories than a no-prime control condition.
3. A primed context-specific goal leads to significantly higher job performance than a primed goal for general achievement or a no-prime control condition.

In conducting this experiment, we did both an exact and a conceptual replication. The advantage of a conceptual replication is that it allows for the possibility of extending the original findings, as opposed to direct replications that simply reproduce them (Molden, 2014). Replication with variation also facilitates the search for mediators and moderators (Locke, 2015). Finally, with every difference that is introduced (e.g., independent and dependent variables, operationalization of a construct), the confirmatory power of the replication increases. This is because the phenomenon has been shown not to hinge on a particular set of operations but to generalize to a larger area of application (Chen & Latham, 2014; Stroebe & Strack, 2014).

The exact replication in this fourth experiment in a different call center consisted of the photograph of the racer as a prime, employing the same procedure, and using the same dependent variable, dollars, that was used by Shantz and Latham (2009, 2011). The conceptual replication consisted of a photograph of employees making calls to potential donors. This condition was included in order to test a core tenet of goal-setting theory, namely, that a specific goal is superior to a general goal for increasing subsequent performance. In this instance, we compared a context-specific prime, a photograph of three employees in a call center making telephone calls, with a general prime, the photograph of the racer. Consistent with goal-setting theory, employees in the context-specific prime condition raised 16% more money than those with the general prime and 85% more money than the employees in the control condition. The employees in the general prime condition raised 60% more money than those in the control condition. Again, these results revealed practical as well as statistical significance.

To determine whether the primed goals were in the subconscious, we used a projective test, the TAT, to see whether the two primes were increasing an employee's implicit need for achievement. McClelland (1987; McClelland & Winter, 1971) has argued that, unlike explicit motives that are in conscious awareness, implicit motives operate outside of awareness, in the subconscious.

To measure responses to the TAT, the Linguistic Inquiry and Word Count (Pennebaker, Francis, & Booth, 2001), a computerized dictionary, was used to count achievement and work-related words in the stories each employee had written about one or the other photograph. The photo of the call center employees elicited significantly more work-related and achievement-related words than were written in the stories by those employees who saw the racer or were in the control condition. Similarly, the employees who were primed with the photograph of the racer wrote stories with significantly more achievement words, but not work-related words, than those in the control condition. In summary, this experiment showed that the primed goal–performance relationship is not due to experimenter bias or demand effects, is not fragile but enduring, and primes the implicit need for achievement in the subconscious as measured by a projective test.

In addition to their field experiment, Shantz and Latham (2009) had also conducted a laboratory experiment involving students taking the TAT. They too found that the prime, the photograph of the racer, elicited the implicit need for achievement.

Learning versus Performance Goals

Goal-setting theory distinguishes between learning and performance goals. The former focuses on processes, procedures, or strategies (e.g., find X ways to increase the student evaluations of your teaching skills); the latter focuses on the desired outcome (e.g., get a mean of 6.0 or above on a 7-point scale from the students who are evaluating your teaching skills). These two types of goals are states. Hence they are not to be confused with Dweck's (Dweck & Leggett, 1988; Elliott & Dweck, 1988) theory of performance and learning goal orientations. They are traits. Whereas the primary focus of goal-setting theory is on motivation, the primary focus of goal orientation is on ability (Seijts, Latham, Tasa, & Latham, 2004). On tasks that require learning, Dweck and her colleagues found that children who have a performance goal orientation focus on the end result, have apprehensions of failure, and focus on the possible consequences of poor performance. When possible, they choose tasks on which they can show their competence at the expense of learning something new. Children with a learning-goal orientation prefer challenging tasks that will enable them to develop their competencies. Mistakes are viewed by them as part of the learning process.

Studies based on goal-setting theory show that regardless of an individual's goal orientation, a consciously set performance goal, a state, should be set when the person has the requisite ability to perform the task; a learning goal should be set when the individual lacks the knowledge and skill to perform the task (Winters & Latham, 1996; Seijts & Latham, 2011; Seijts et al., 2004). What had yet to be addressed is whether the same conclusion is true when these two goals are primed.

Chen and Latham (2014) sought the answer to this issue using a 2 (primed learning goal, control) × 2 (primed performance goal, control) × 3 (trials) factorial design. The participants were given a cover story regarding a complex scheduling task on which sheer effort and persistence would prove useless for performing effectively (i.e., " . . . the Office of the Registrar has requested you to complete class schedules. . . . This assignment is a good indicator of a person's problem-solving abilities."). The prime for the performance goal was the photograph of the racer. Based on the results from a pilot study, the prime for the learning goal was a photograph of Rodin's *The Thinker*. Consistent with the results obtained in experiments involving consciously set learning and performance goals, those with a learning goal that was primed performed significantly better than those with a performance goal that was primed. Neither priming the performance goal alone nor priming the two goals together had a beneficial effect on task performance.

This experiment provides strong support for the findings obtained by Dijksterhuis and van Knippenberg (1998) described earlier. In the Chen and Latham (2014) experiment, the primes were two photographs rather than a listing of the characteristics of a professor or a hooligan. The dependent variable was the acquisition of knowledge in order to perform the scheduling task rather than ascertaining the correct answer to questions on a multiple choice *test*. The results were the same in both experiments. People who were primed with the mental representation of intelligence/thinking, that is, *The Thinker*, performed better than those in the other two conditions.

Ganegoda, Latham, and Folger (2016) primed a goal for fairness in negotiations using a 10 × 10 matrix of words within which 8 of the 13 words in the experimental condition were fairness-related (e.g., *fair, ethical, integrity*). All 13 words in the no-prime matrix condition were fairness-neutral. The participants in both conditions were instructed to find as many words in the matrix as possible. Previous research had shown that negotiators hold egocentric fairness perceptions, equating "fair" with what benefits them (e.g., Babcock & Lowenstein, 1997; Thompson & Lowenstein, 1992). Hence they are reluctant to agree on an objectively fair settlement. Thus Ganegoda and colleagues (2016) used profit inequality as an indicator of the degree of fairness a negotiator demonstrates. The extent to which fairness/justice was salient in a negotiator's mind was measured by a 10-word fragment completion task developed by Van Prooijen, Van den Bos, and Wilke (2002). Five of the words were fairness-related (e.g., *just, honest*). For each word fragment, multiple correct words were possible (e.g., *un __ __ __ al* could be *unequal* or *unusual*). The results of this experiment showed that both a consciously set goal and a primed goal for fairness had additive effects on counteracting self-serving tendencies that typically arise during negotiations. The mediator for both types of goals was a heightened level of justice saliency.

Discussion

Six experiments, four conducted in field settings (Shantz & Latham, 2009, 2011; Latham & Piccolo, 2012), two in laboratory settings (Chen & Latham, 2014; Ganegoda et al., 2016), plus two enumerative reviews of the literature (Latham et al., 2010; Latham & Locke, 2012) have made it impossible for me to remain a skeptic of the primed goal–job-task-performance relationship. These six experiments include both exact and conceptual replications. The participants were unaware of the prime-performance hypothesis. This was not only evident in the funnel-debrief, but it was also particularly evident in the employees' great surprise when they were made aware of the hypothesis at the end of the debrief. The Latham and Piccolo (2012) experiment is especially noteworthy because it eliminated the rival hypotheses that the results can be explained by either experimenter bias or demand effects, as neither of us had any contact with the employees. The supervisor, who was instructed to randomly assign to the employees the instructions for soliciting money from potential donors, was given no explanation as to why some instructions contained no photograph, some contained a photograph of a racer, and some contained a photograph of employees making phone calls. Neither he nor any employee asked a question about the photographs. As noted earlier, the employees during the debrief stated that they were too busy making phone calls to pay attention to a photograph. Because the employees work in cubicles, no one noticed that some employees had a different photograph or that others had none. In short, the evidence is clear. Goals can be primed, and primed goals can increase job/task/fair performance. These findings are not restricted to an individual's performance.

Brcic and Latham (2016) conducted a quasi-experiment followed by two actual experiments to determine whether satisfaction with customer service can be primed in the absence of customer awareness of the effect of a prime on their affect. In all three instances, merely putting a yellow sticker of a smiling face on a sales receipt increased customer satisfaction with the service they received relative to that of customers in the control conditions, as measured by a subsequent survey of customer service satisfaction.

My colleagues and I are not the only ones in organizational psychology to show the positive effects that can occur as a result of priming the subconscious. Welsh and Ordóñez (2014) used Bargh's (1989) scrambled-word-sentence technique to prime ethical behavior. They found that doing so reduced the subsequent propensity of adults to behave unethically. The activation of an individual's moral standards, as measured by a questionnaire, mediated the subconscious prime–ethical behavior relationship. A subsequent experiment revealed that a primed goal for ethical behavior increased appropriate behavior only when the participants were not monitored. The moderator was monitoring in that priming was not necessary for inducing ethical behavior when people knew they were being observed. The two-way interaction between priming and monitoring suggest that both reduce unethical behavior, but there is little or no incremental effect on unethical behavior if both methods are used.

All of the priming experiments reviewed in this chapter thus far involved a supraliminal prime. That is, the participants could see the prime, but they were not aware of the effect of the prime on their behavior. Zdaniuk and Bobocel (2013) presented a prime subliminally, that is, below focal awareness. In their experiment, the participants completed three ostensibly unrelated tasks. First, they recorded their impressions of a fair and an unfair leader. Next, they completed a computer task in which they were subliminally exposed to the face of either a fair leader, an unfair leader, or a neutral person. Finally, the participants completed an in-basket task that required them to write a dismissal letter to an employee. The letters were content analyzed by judges who were blind to the condition to which a participant had been randomly assigned. Those who were subliminally presented the face of the unfair leader were less interactionally fair, as defined by expressions of remorse, than those who were presented the face of the fair leader or the neutral face. In short, fair–unfair behavior was elicited in the absence of an individual's awareness of the prime.

Practical Significance

A primary interest of organizational psychologists is to find ways of increasing an employee's job performance in fair and ethical ways. The studies reviewed in this chapter show that priming goals will increase job performance on tasks that are straightforward for employees (e.g., Latham & Piccolo, 2012), as well as those that are complex for them (Chen & Latham, 2014). Moreover, priming goals can ensure that an increase in an individual's performance does not occur at the expense of appropriate, fair, ethical behavior (Ganegoda et al., 2016; Welsh & Ordóñez, 2014).

An employee's cognitive resources are limited (Anderson, 1982; Miller, 1956). Thus of further practical significance for these findings for organizations is that a goal that is primed consumes fewer cognitive resources than a consciously set goal. Moreover, priming a goal is a straightforward way of increasing desirable job performance and, arguably most important, the effect of a primed goal and that of a specific, high goal that is consciously set have an additive effect on an individual's performance.

Theoretical Significance

Priming goals in general, and Bargh's automaticity model in particular, have provoked debate and skepticism (e.g., Bartlett, 2013; Doyen, Klein, Pichon, & Cleeremans, 2012; Shanks et al., 2013). The criticism has been so severe that priming advocates Dijksterhuis, van Knippenberg, and Holland (2014) have described this research area as "under siege."

The theoretical significance of the experiments in organizational psychology on priming, however, provide strong support for Bargh's (1994) automaticity model, which states, as previously noted, that conscious and subconscious goal pursuits follow the same processing stages, predict the same phenomena, and produce the same outcomes.

Contributing to the "siege" of the automaticity model and the empirical research supporting it is the lack of a theoretical framework. A theory specifies not only causal relationships but also the moderators regarding the boundaries or conditional variables for the causal relationships, as well as the mediators that explain those relationships. Goal-setting theory (Locke & Latham, 1990, 2013; Latham & Locke, in press) seems to be a likely candidate for providing this framework for conducting priming studies on organizational behavior. The evidence for this assertion includes the finding that a primed goal increased performance on the same tasks as a consciously set specific, high goal (e.g., Shantz & Latham, 2009). Consistent with goal-setting theory, a context-specific primed goal led to higher performance than either a general prime or a control condition (Latham & Piccolo, 2012). Consistent with empirical research on goal-setting theory, a primed learning goal led to higher performance on a task that was complex for people than did a primed performance goal (Chen & Latham, 2014). Both the automaticity model and goal-setting theory state that the goal must be motivationally relevant to and valued by the individual if it is to lead to goal pursuit (Higgins & Eitam, 2014; Locke & Latham, 2002). In addition, both the model and the theory state that only when the situation is favorable will goal pursuit occur (Locke & Latham, 1990).

As is the case with social psychology experiments on priming, to date the focus in organizational psychology on priming goals has been for the most part limited to identifying the different types of dependent variables that can be influenced by a prime. Only two experiments have identified a mediator (Ganegoda, et al., 2016; Welsh & Ordóñez, 2014) and only one has identified a moderator (Welsh & Ordóñez, 2014). Future research should systematically examine the mediators (e.g., conscious choice of goal difficulty level) and moderators (e.g., goal commitment) of goal-setting theory to determine their applicability to the automaticity model for priming organizationally related goals.

REFERENCES

Anderson, J. R. (1982). Acquisition of cognitive skill. *Psychological Review, 89,* 369–406.

Babcock, L., & Lowenstein, G. (1997). Explaining bargaining impasse: The role of self-serving biases. *Journal of Economic Perspectives, 11,* 109–125.

Bargh, J. A. (1989). Conditional automaticity: Varieties of automatic influence in social perception and cognition. In J. S. Uleman & J. A. Bargh (Eds.), *Unintended thought* (pp. 3–51) New York: Guilford Press.

Bargh, J. A. (1994). The four horsemen of automaticity: Awareness, efficiency, intention, and control in social cognition. In J. W. Wyer & T. K. Srull (Eds.), *Handbook of social cognition* (2nd ed., pp. 1–40). Hillsdale, NJ: Erlbaum.

Bargh, J. A., Chen, M., & Burrows, L. (1996). Automaticity of social behavior: Direct effects of traits construct and stereotype activation on action. *Journal of Personality and Social Psychology, 71,* 230–244.

Bargh, J. A., Gollwitzer, P. M., & Oettingen, G. (2010). Motivation. In S. T. Fiske, D. T. Gilbert, & G. Lindzey (Eds.), *Handbook of social psychology* (5th ed., pp. 268–316). New York: Wiley.

Bartlett, T. (2013, January 30). Power of suggestion. *Chronicle of Higher Education.* Available at *http://chronicle.com/article/Power-of-Suggestion/136907.*

Brcic, J., & Latham, G. P. (2016). The effect of priming affect on customer service satisfaction. *Academy of Management Discoveries, 2*(4), 392–403.

Chen, X. E., & Latham, G. P. (2014). The effect of priming learning vs performance goals on a complex task. *Organizational Behavior and Human Decision Processes, 125,* 88–97.

Dijksterhuis, A., & van Knippenberg, A. (1998). The relation between perception and behavior or how to win a game of Trivial Pursuit. *Journal of Personality and Social Psychology, 74,* 865–877.

Dijksterhuis, A., van Knippenberg, A., & Holland, R. W. (2014). Evaluating behavior priming research: Three observations and a recommendation. In D. C. Molden (Ed.), *Understanding priming effects in social psychology* (pp. 196–208). New York: Guilford Press.

Doyen, S., Klein, O., Pichon, C. L., & Cleeremans, A. (2012). Behavioral priming: It's all in the mind, but whose mind? *PLOS ONE, 7*(1), e29081.

Dweck, C. S., & Leggett, E. L. (1988). A social-cognitive approach to motivation and personality. *Psychological Review, 95,* 256–273.

Elliott, E. S., & Dweck, C. S. (1988). Goals: An approach to motivation and achievement. *Journal of Personality and Social Psychology, 54,* 5–12.

Fishbach, A., Friedman, R. S., & Kruglanski, A. W. (2003). Leading us not unto temptation: Momentary allurements elicit overriding goal activation. *Journal of Personality and Social Psychology, 84,* 296–309.

Ganegoda, D. B., Latham, G. P., & Folger, R. (2016). The effect of a consciously set and a primed goal on fair behavior. *Human Resource Management, 55,* 787–807.

Higgins, E. T., & Eitam, B. (2014). Priming . . . shmiming: It's about knowing when and why stimulated memory representations become active. In D. C. Molden (Ed.), *Understanding priming effects in social psychology* (pp. 234–251). New York: Guilford Press.

Kahneman, D. (2012). A proposal to deal with questions about priming effects. *Nature.* Available at *www.nature.com/polopoly_fs/7.6716.1349271308!/suppinfoFile/Kahneman%20Letter.pdf.*

Latham, G. P., & Locke, E. A. (1975). Increasing productivity with decreasing time limits: A field replication of Parkinson's law. *Journal of Applied Psychology, 60,* 524–526.

Latham, G. P., & Locke, E. A. (2007). New developments in and directions for goal setting. *European Psychologist, 12,* 290–300.

Latham, G. P., & Locke, E. A. (2012). The effect of subconscious goals on organizational behavior. In G. P. Hodgkinson & J. K. Ford (Eds.), *International review of industrial and organizational psychology* (Vol. 27, pp 39–63). Chichester, UK: Wiley.

Latham, G. P., & Locke, E. A. (2018). Goal setting theory: Controversies and resolutions. In D. Ones, N. Anderson, C. Viswesvaran, & H. Sinangil (Eds.), *Handbook of industrial, work & organizational psychology* (Vol. 2, pp. 103–124). London: SAGE.

Latham, G. P., Mitchell, T. R., & Dossett, D. L. (1978). The importance of participative goal setting and anticipated rewards on goal difficulty and job performance. *Journal of Applied Psychology, 63,* 163–171.

Latham, G. P., & Piccolo, R. F. (2012). The effect of context specific versus non-specific subconscious goals on employee performance. *Human Resource Management, 51,* 535–538.

Latham, G. P., Stajkovic, A., & Locke, E. A. (2010). The relevance and viability of subconscious goals in the workplace. *Journal of Management, 36,* 234–255.

Lee, C., & Earley, P. C. (1992). Comparative peer evaluations of organizational behavior theories. *Organization Developments Journal, 10,* 37–42.

Locke, E. A. (2015) Theory building, replication, and behavioral priming: Where do we go from here? *Perspectives in Psychological Science, 10,* 408–414.

Locke, E. A., & Latham, G. P. (1990). *A theory of goal setting and task performance.* Englewood Cliffs, NJ: Prentice Hall.

Locke, E. A., & Latham, G. P. (2002). Building a practically useful theory of goal setting and task motivation: A 35-year odyssey. *American Psychologist, 57,* 705–717.

Locke, E. A., & Latham, G. P. (2013). *New developments in goal setting and task performance.* New York: Routledge.

McClelland, D. C. (1987). *Human motivation.* New York: Cambridge University Press.

McClelland, D. C., & Winter, D. G. (1971). *Motivating economic achievement.* New York: Free Press.

Miller, G. A. (1956). Information theory. *Scientific American, 195,* 42–46.

Miner, J. (2003). The rated importance, scientific validity, and practical usefulness of organizational behavior theories: A quantitative review. *Academy of Management Learning and Education, 2,* 250–268.

Mischel, W. (1968). *Personality and assessment.* New York: Wiley.

Mitchell, T. R., & Daniels, D. (2003) Motivation. In W. Borman, D. Ilgen, & R. Klimoski (Eds.), *Handbook of psychology: Vol. 12. Industrial/organizational psychology* (pp. 225–254). New York: Wiley.

Molden, D. C. (2014). Understanding priming effects in social psychology: An overview and integration. In D. C. Molden (Ed.), *Understanding priming effects in social psychology* (pp. 252–258). New York: Guilford Press.

Pashler, H., Coburn, N., & Harris, C. R. (2012). Priming or social distance?: Failure to replicate effects on social and food judgment. *PLOS ONE, 7,* e42510.

Pavio, A. (1986). *Mental representations: A dual-coding approach.* New York: Oxford University Press.

Pavio, A. (1991). Dual coding theory: Retrospect and current status. *Canadian Journal of Psychology, 45,* 255–287.

Pennebaker, J. W., Francis, M. E., & Booth, R. J. (2001). *Linguistic inquiry word count.* Mahwah, NJ: Erlbaum.

Pinder, C. C. (1998). *Work motivation: Theory, issues and applications.* Upper Saddle River, NJ: Prentice Hall.

Seijts, G. H., & Latham, G. P. (2011). The effect of commitment to a learning goal, self-efficacy, and the interaction between learning goal difficulty and commitment on performance in a business simulation. *Human Performance, 24,* 189–204.

Seijts, G. H., Latham, G. P., Tasa, K., & Latham, B. W. (2004), Goal setting and goal orientation; An integration of two difficult yet related literatures. *Academy of Management Journal, 47,* 227–239.

Shanks, D. R., Newell, B. R., Lee, E. H., Balakrishnan, D., Ekelund, L., Cenac, Z., . . . Moore, C. (2013). Priming intelligence behavior: An elusive phenomenon. *PLOS ONE, 8,* e56515.

Shantz, A., & Latham, G. P. (2009). An exploratory field experiment of the effect of subconscious and conscious goals on employee performance. *Organizational Behavior and Human Decision Processes, 109,* 9–17.

Shantz, A., & Latham, G. P. (2011). Effect of primed goals on employee performance: Implications for human resource management. *Human Resource Management, 50,* 289–299.

Stajkovic, A. D., Locke, E. A., & Blair, E. S. (2006). A first examination of the relationships between primed subconscious goals, assigned conscious goals, and task performance. *Journal of Applied Psychology, 91,* 1172–1180.

Stroebe, W., & Strack, F. (2014). The alleged crisis and illusion of exact replications. *Perspectives on Psychological Science, 9,* 59–71.

Thompson, L., & Lowenstein, G. (1992). Egocentric interpretations of fairness and interpersonal conflict. *Organizational Behaviour and Human Decision Processes, 51,* 176–197.

Van Prooijen, J. W., Van den Bos, K., & Wilke, H. A. (2002). Procedural justice and status: Status salience as antecedent of procedural fairness effects. *Journal of Personality and Social Psychology, 83,* 1353–1361.

Welsh, D., & Ordóñez, L. D. (2014). Conscience without cognition: The effects of subconscious priming on automatic ethical behavior. *Academy of Management Journal, 57,* 723–742.

Winters, D., & Latham, G. P. (1996). The effect of learning versus outcome goals on a simple versus a complex task. *Group and Organization Management, 21,* 236–250.

Zdaniuk, A., & Bobocel, D. R. (2013). The automatic activation of (un)fairness behavior in organizations. *Human Resource and Management Review, 23,* 254–265.

CHAPTER 21

The Forward Rush

On Locomotors' Future Focus

Arie W. Kruglanski
Marina Chernikova
Katarzyna Jasko

Beethoven took more than 6 years to finish his Ninth Symphony; clearly, he was in no rush to accomplish his goal. In stark contrast, Mozart composed his last three symphonies in less than a month. Unlike Beethoven, Mozart appears to have been preoccupied with moving quickly toward his desired future states (i.e., completing symphonies). These anecdotes vividly exemplify how individuals can differ in their propensity to "rush forward" toward future goals and accomplishments. But what can explain these kinds of differences?

Regulatory mode theory posits two essential regulatory modes: locomotion and assessment (Higgins, 2012; Higgins, Kruglanski, & Pierro, 2003; Kruglanski et al., 2000). The locomotion mode represents the aspect of self-regulation concerned with motion and progress from state to state, whereas the assessment mode is the aspect of self-regulation concerned with critically evaluating goals and means. High locomotors are eager to initiate and maintain goal-driven behavior and dislike any interruptions that stand in their way. High assessors, on the other hand, are focused on carefully selecting both the right goal and the best means to that goal's attainment (Kruglanski et al., 2000). Locomotion is positively related to measures of Type A personality (Bortner, 1969), action (vs. state) orientation (Kuhl, 1985), and achievement orientation (Jackson, 1974); nonetheless, a variety of empirical tests have shown that locomotion is distinct from these constructs (Kruglanski et al., 2000). Similarly, assessment is positively correlated with social anxiety (Leary, 1983), fear of invalidity (Webster & Kruglanski, 1994), and public self-consciousness (Fenigstein, Scheier, & Buss, 1975); however, empirical tests have confirmed its divergent validity from these scales (Kruglanski et al., 2000). Locomotion and assessment are independent: Individuals can be high on one, high on both, or low on both. Prior studies on the two regulatory modes have shown that they can be measured as personality constructs (via the assessment and locomotion scales; see Table 21.1) or manipulated situationally (e.g., by asking participants to think back to times they acted like a locomotor or an assessor; Avnet & Higgins, 2003; Pierro, Pica, Klein, Kruglanski, & Higgins, 2013; Pierro, Presaghi, Higgins, & Kruglanski, 2009).

Of the two regulatory modes, locomotion in particular[1] is related to a greater attentiveness to and concern for the future (Kruglanski, Pierro, & Higgins, 2015). High locomotors are preoccupied with motion, and motion is typically oriented *forward* (i.e., toward the future). In other words, goal-directed motion generally entails moving from one's current (less desirable) state to a future state that is more desirable (Kruglanski, Jasko, et al., 2015). Locomotors' goal to maximize movement thus implies a focus on the future, where their movement is headed.

TABLE 21.1. Locomotion and Assessment Regulatory Mode Scales

Locomotion

1. I don't mind doing things even if they involve extra effort.
2. When I finish one project, I often wait a while before getting started on a new one. (*Reverse-coded*)
3. I am a "workaholic."
4. I feel excited just before I am about to reach a goal.
5. I enjoy actively doing things, more than just watching and observing.
6. I am a "doer."
7. When I decide to do something, I can't wait to get started.
8. By the time I accomplish a task, I already have the next one in mind.
9. I am a "low energy" person. (*Reverse-coded*)
10. Most of the time my thoughts are occupied with the task I wish to accomplish.
11. When I get started on something, I usually persevere until I finish it.
12. I am a "go-getter."

Assessment

1. I never evaluate my social interactions with others after they occur. (*Reverse-coded*)
2. I spend a great deal of time taking inventory of my positive and negative characteristics.
3. I like evaluating other people's plans.
4. I often critique work done by myself or others.
5. I often compare myself with other people.
6. I often feel that I am being evaluated by others.
7. I am very self-critical and self-conscious about what I am saying.
8. I rarely analyze the conversations I have had with others after they occur. (*Reverse-coded*)
9. I am a critical person.
10. I don't spend much time thinking about ways others could improve themselves. (*Reverse-coded*)
11. I often think that other people's choices and decisions are wrong.
12. When I meet a new person I usually evaluate how well he or she is doing on various dimensions (e.g., looks, achievements, social status, clothes).

---

[1]Assessment is largely irrelevant to an emphasis on the future, because assessors do not care about time *as such* any more than low assessors do; see Kruglanski, Pierro, and Higgins (2015) for a more detailed discussion of this.

A tendency to focus on the future can be manifested in multiple ways. Perhaps most obviously, it can lead individuals to plan more for the future and think less about the past (in that a past focus does not allow movement). Less obviously but of equal importance, a preoccupation with the future can lead individuals to *initiate* more future goal commitments, because such initiation allows them to maximize their motion toward various desired end states. Similarly, a focus on the future can cause individuals to *maintain* their future goal commitments, because such maintenance enables them to move toward their desired future states quickly and without interruption. In line with this reasoning, the following sections describe the impact of locomotion regulatory mode on individuals' tendencies to plan for the future, focus on the past, initiate future goal commitments, and maintain those commitments (see also Table 21.2).

LOCOMOTION AND FUTURE PLANNING

Individuals who are focused on the future should both contemplate it and try to make decisions that will benefit their future selves. Thus high locomotors should be more likely to plan for the future, work harder to ensure that their future selves will be provided for, and sacrifice their current desires for better outcomes in the future. Recent research supports these notions.

TABLE 21.2. Summary of Locomotion Effects

Future aspect	Effects of locomotion
Planning for the future	1. High locomotors are better at time management. 2. High locomotors are more likely to accumulate savings for retirement. 3. High locomotors get better grades and have higher achievement motivation. 4. High locomotors are less impulsive and have more self-control.
Forgetting the past	1. High locomotors experience less regret and less counterfactual thinking. 2. High locomotors experience less nostalgia. 3. High locomotors are less likely to commit the sunk-cost fallacy. 4. High locomotors prefer an individual who is assisting them with current goal attainment over an individual who assisted with past goal attainment.v 5. High locomotors are more willing to forgive themselves and others. 6. High locomotors are more committed to the goal of changing and better able to cope with organizational change.
Initiation of goal commitment	1. High locomotors are more morning-oriented. 2. High locomotors procrastinate less. 3. High locomotors are more likely to engage in delay discounting.
Maintenance of goal commitment	1. High locomotors prefer goals with high (vs. low) expectancy. 2. High locomotors prefer means that serve only one goal (vs. means that serve multiple goals). 3. High locomotors invest more time and effort into goal attainment. 4. High locomotors finish tasks more quickly and prefer organizational structures that facilitate faster goal completion. 5. High locomotors prefer to multitask.

Locomotion is significantly associated with measures of time management and the amount of control individuals perceive they have over their time. In two samples of students and employees, locomotion was positively related to overall perceived control of time, as measured by a subset of five items taken from the Time Management Behavior Scale (TMBS; Amato, Pierro, Chirumbolo, & Pica, 2014). The TMBS has three other subscales: Setting Goals and Priorities (which measures the tendency to set short- and long-term goals for the future), Mechanics of Time Management (which measures individuals' proclivity to make lists, arrange their schedules in advance, and plan ahead), and Preference for Organization (which measures the overall tendency to organize life and work environments; Macan, Shahani, Dipboye, & Phillips, 1990). In both the university student and employee samples, locomotion was positively and significantly related to each of the three TMBS subscales. Furthermore, the relationship between locomotion and perceived control of time was mediated by the subscale Setting Goals and Priorities, as well as the subscale Preference for Organization (Amato et al., 2014). These studies suggest that locomotors engage more in thinking about and planning for the future and that they experience greater control over their time as a result.

Individuals who are high on locomotion (and moderately high on assessment) are also more likely to accumulate greater savings for retirement. Researchers correlated individuals' locomotion scores with finance information from two national datasets: the HRS, which provides in-depth information on the finances of middle-age and older adults, and the MIDUS2, which provides similar information about wealth for individuals of all ages. Measured locomotion was associated with greater wealth accumulation for retirement when it was paired with a minimum level of assessment (Kim, Franks, & Higgins, 2013). These findings indicate that high (vs. low) locomotors not only spend time thinking about the far future but are also careful to ensure that their future selves will be provided for.

Doing well in school can considerably improve individuals' future prospects in life; consequently, those who are future-oriented should emphasize academic achievement. In this vein, there is a positive relationship between locomotion regulatory mode and academic engagement and achievement in college students. In one study, students' locomotion scores were significantly associated with their academic engagement, as assessed by the student version of the Utrecht Work Engagement Scale (UWES; Zhang & Gheibi, 2015). The UWES measure contains three subscales: Vigor, Dedication, and Absorption (Schaufeli, Salanova, González-Romá, & Bakker, 2002). Locomotion was significantly and positively associated with each of the subscales (Zhang & Gheibi, 2015). In another experiment, higher locomotion predicted higher grade-point averages in college students (for individuals who were also relatively high on assessment; Kruglanski et al., 2000). Locomotion is also significantly positively correlated with achievement motivation, as measured by the Achievement Motivation subscale of Jackson's (1974) Personality Research Form (Kruglanski et al., 2000). Thus, when making decisions in the academic realm, locomotors are likely to select options that will benefit their future selves in the long run.

Lastly, locomotion is negatively associated with impulsivity. In a sample of university students, locomotion exhibited a significant negative correlation with the Barratt Impulsiveness Scale, a common self-report scale of impulsive thoughts and behaviors (Shalev & Sulkowski, 2009; Spinella, 2007). Similarly, locomotion is positively associated with a measure of self-control (Struk, Scholer, & Danckert, 2015). These findings again attest to high locomotors' tendency to think about future consequences before giving in to momentary temptations.

In summary, activities such as making plans for the future and working to secure a comfortable future are means of ensuring that one is moving effectively toward his or her future goals. Given locomotors' preoccupation with forward motion and their desire to make progress on their goals, it is unsurprising that they are drawn to such future-oriented pursuits.

LOCOMOTION AND FORGETTING THE PAST

The flip side of an emphasis on the future is the propensity to think less about the past. In other words, those who concentrate on the future have less time and energy left over to pay attention to prior events. In accordance with this, individuals who are high on locomotion should be less likely to dwell on the past, make decisions biased by prior occurrences, feel regret at past choices, or hold grudges because of past occurrences. Locomotors should even be less susceptible to positive feelings regarding the past, such as the propensity to think wistfully about past events or to value friends who helped them in the past. Lastly, they should be eager to move on from the past by embracing change and innovation. Extant research offers consistent support for these notions.

Specifically, locomotors experience less regret and engage in less counterfactual thinking or in rumination about "what might have been." In one study, high locomotors who read a vignette with a negative outcome (an unfortunate purchasing decision) generated fewer counterfactuals regarding the scenario and felt that they would experience less regret if they were in the protagonist's place. In another study, participants described their own unfortunate purchasing decisions. Those who were high on locomotion generated fewer counterfactuals about the event; they also reported that they experienced less regret about the decision (Pierro et al., 2008). These studies indicate that those who are high on locomotion are less interested in analyzing the past, given that they spend less time dwelling on the past and thinking about what might have been.

Locomotors are less likely to experience nostalgia, defined as a sentimental longing or wistful affection for the past. In one experiment, participants completed three measures of proneness to nostalgia (Pierro, Pica, et al., 2013). The first was a nostalgia-relevant 3-item subscale of the Time Perspective Inventory, containing items such as "It gives me pleasure to think about my past" (Zimbardo & Boyd, 1999). The second measure was the 5-item Southampton Nostalgia Scale, containing questions such as "Generally speaking, how often do you bring to mind nostalgic experiences?" (Routledge, Arndt, Sedikides, & Wildschut, 2008). The third measure was the Batcho Nostalgia Inventory, in which participants rated the extent to which they missed 18 aspects of their past (e.g., "holidays I went on," "the way society was," and "my childhood toys"; Batcho, 1995). An individual-difference measure of locomotion was negatively associated with each of the nostalgia scales described above (Pierro, Pica, et al., 2013). In a separate study, situationally induced locomotion produced lower scores on a 3-item measure of state nostalgia, which asked participants to rate their agreement with statements such as "Right now, I am having nostalgic feelings" (Pierro, Pica, et al., 2013; Wildschut, Sedikides, Arndt, & Routledge, 2006). It appears, then, that locomotors are less inclined to think either negatively (i.e., with regret) or positively (i.e., with nostalgia) about the past.

An intriguing consequence of locomotors' lesser attachment to the past is their lower susceptibility to the sunk-cost fallacy. This fallacy is a decision-making bias that leads individuals to be unduly influenced by an unrecoverable past investment of money, even when ignoring the prior investment would lead to an objectively better outcome. In three studies, participants read a sunk-cost scenario such as the following:

> "As the president of an airline company, you have invested 10 million dollars of the company's money into a research project. The purpose was to build a plane that would not be detected by conventional radar, in other words, a radar-blank plane. When the project is 90% completed, another firm begins marketing a plane that cannot be detected by radar. Also, it is apparent that their plane is much faster and far more economical than the plane your company is building. The question is: Should you invest the last 10% of the research funds to finish your radar-blank plane?"

In all three studies, both measured and manipulated high locomotion led individuals to invest less money after reading a sunk-cost scenario (Amato, Chernikova, Pierro, Kruglanski, & Higgins, 2016). The fact that locomotors are less bound by previous decisions suggests that they put greater emphasis on their current and future choices.

Because they are more interested in the pursuit of future goals than in goals that have already been completed, high locomotors exhibit greater preference for individuals who serve as means to current (vs. past) goal attainments. In one study, college students were asked to list a friend who had helped them attain a goal in the past semester, as well as a friend who was helpful to attaining a future goal. High locomotors exhibited more positive affect toward a friend who was currently helping them as compared with the friend who was helpful in the past (Orehek, Fitzsimons, & Kruglanski, 2014). When high locomotors were experimentally induced to believe that they needed to make further progress on a goal, they felt more positively toward a friend helpful to that goal's attainment as compared with when they believed that they had already made enough progress on that goal (Orehek et al., 2014). These results offer evidence that individuals who are high on locomotion quickly forget those who helped them with past goal attainment and focus their attention only on those who are likely to be helpful to current or future goal attainment.

Due to their lesser propensity to dwell on the past, individuals who are high on locomotion are more willing to forgive themselves for past misdeeds. When participants were asked to recall a past experience when they had wronged someone else, those who were high on locomotion reported greater self-forgiveness regarding the situation (measured by the extent to which they felt accepting of themselves, forgiving of themselves, disliking of themselves [reverse-scored], and rejecting of themselves [reverse-scored]; Pierro, Pica, Kruglanski, & Higgins, 2014). High locomotion was also related to fast response times to self-forgiveness-related words in an adapted version of the Brief Implicit Association Test (Sriram & Greenwald, 2009), which indicates that self-forgiveness-related words are more accessible for locomotors (Pierro et al., 2014). In another study, a focus on the future was shown to play a mediating role in the relationship between locomotion and self-forgiveness: Locomotion was positively related to future focus (as measured by the Temporal Focus Scale; Shipp, Edwards, & Lambert, 2009), and future focus in turn predicted greater self-forgiveness (Pierro et al., 2014). These studies suggest that high locomotors are more willing to let go of the past by forgetting and forgiving any wrongs they have committed against others. In addition, they demonstrate that the mechanism underlying locomotors' tendency to forgive past wrongs is their greater focus on the future.

Importantly, individuals who are high on locomotion are also more forgiving of *others* who have wronged them. After reading a scenario involving a conflict with a friend, high locomotors reported a greater desire to reconcile with that friend (measured with items such as "I am motivated to reconcile with my partner") and felt less lingering unpleasantness regarding the conflict (measured with items such as "I have negative feelings as a result of this conflict"; Webb, 2012). This finding indicates that in their quest to move on from the past as quickly as possible, locomotors are quick not only to forgive their own wrongs but others' wrongs against them as well.

Lastly, high locomotors are more willing to accept and embrace change, which involves moving from a past state to a new (and potentially better) future state. Locomotion was positively correlated with a 5-item scale of commitment to change (Scholer & Higgins, 2012). The scale captures several elements of commitment to the goal of change: the determination to persist in changing, the intention to devote effort to change, and an unwillingness to abandon the pursuit of change (Klein, Wesson, Hollenbeck, Wright, & DeShon, 2001). It contains items such as "I am strongly committed to pursuing this goal [of change]." Locomotion scores also significantly predicted the likelihood of participants' wanting to switch from an old to a new experimental task. Participants spent 12 minutes alternating between two tasks: a fun task (playing a puzzle game that involves moving gems around on a screen) and a tedious task (counting X's and O's in a 40 × 40 grid). They were then given the option of either continuing to work on this combination of tasks or trying a new combination of tasks. High locomotors were more likely to try the new combination of tasks (Scholer & Higgins, 2012). In addition, individuals' locomotion orientation predicted the degree to which they experienced change as a positive event (measured by items such as: "Indicate the extent to which change in general is unpleasant/pleasant"; Scholer & Higgins, 2012). These studies show that a high locomotion orientation leads individuals to prefer change and progress over remaining stuck in the past.

Along the same lines, nurses who were high (vs. low) in locomotion were better able to cope with drastic changes in their professional roles on the job, as measured by a 12-item scale of coping with organizational change (Judge, Higgins, Thoresen, & Barrick, 1999; Kruglanski, Pierro, Higgins, & Capozza, 2007). Workers for the Italian Postal Service who were high in locomotion were more successful at adapting to far-reaching changes in the organization, which included downsizing, personnel reduction, and newly available incentives for transferring to alternative roles (Kruglanski, Pierro, Higgins, & Capozza, 2007). Similarly, workers for the Municipal City of Rome who were high in locomotion were better able to tolerate sweeping organizational reforms, which included a reorganization of incentive systems and the integration of various sectors (Kruglanski, Pierro, Higgins, & Capozza, 2007). Again, these results demonstrate that locomotors are willing and able to embrace change as a way of moving away from the past.

In short, the findings above suggest that locomotion-oriented individuals are generally uninterested in thinking about or lingering over the past. As the past is unchangeable, brooding over it forces one to stay in the same state, dwelling on the same things over and over again. Given their desire for swift forward motion, high locomotors are unsatisfied with such stasis; rather, they choose to move on from the past with impatient celerity, eagerly embracing novelty, change, and the future.

LOCOMOTION AND INITIATION OF GOAL COMMITMENT

Because locomotors enjoy moving toward desired future states, they should be more likely to initiate goal commitments, as these allow them to maximize such motion. Therefore, locomotors should prefer to begin their daily tasks as early as possible, avoid procrastination, and select goals that can be initiated immediately. Evidence in support of these claims can be found in multiple domains.

Rather than taking their time and sleeping in in the mornings, locomotors prefer to start their days early. In one study, participants were asked to respond to a morningness–eveningness scale, which included items such as "One hears about morning and evening types of people; which one of these types do you consider yourself to be?" (Smith, Reilly, & Midkiff, 1989). Individuals with a strong locomotion orientation were more likely to report being morning-oriented than evening-oriented (Pica, Amato, Pierro, & Kruglanski, 2015). These results suggest that one consequence of locomotors' preference for swift progress toward their future state is their desire to wake up as early as they can.

Individuals who are high on locomotion also avoid procrastinating on goals and tasks, preferring instead to start moving as soon as possible. Locomotion was negatively correlated with scores on the Tuckman Procrastination Scale (Tuckman, 1991), which measures the tendency to delay task initiation or completion using items such as "When I have a deadline, I wait until the last minute" (Pierro, Giacomantonio, Pica, Kruglanski, & Higgins, 2011). When insurance workers were asked to set three job-related goals for themselves for the following 3 months, locomotion was negatively associated with their actual procrastination on those goals, as measured 3 months later with the question "To what extent has the fulfillment of the goals [you listed] been postponed?" (Pierro et al., 2011). High locomotors also reported that they generally did not procrastinate when taking exams. In addition, locomotors were also less likely to actually postpone an upcoming exam they planned to take; this was mediated by their greater propensity to avoid distractions and focus on the task at hand (Pierro et al., 2011). Again, these results confirm the notion that locomotors do not like to sit still and do nothing; rather, they are constantly initiating motion toward their desired future states.

Finally, locomotion is positively correlated with delay discounting, or the tendency to prefer small but immediate rewards to larger but delayed rewards. When individuals had to make a series of hypothetical choices between smaller rewards they could obtain right away and larger rewards they would have to wait between 7 and 120 days for, locomotion was positively associated with the tendency to select the smaller but immediate rewards (Guo & Feng, 2015). This suggests that locomotors prefer to set goals (i.e., getting a candy bar) that can be initiated immediately, rather than goals that may require a delay.

To summarize, initiating goals and tasks offers individuals the opportunity to engage in immediate movement, because the beginning of a new project will generally require prompt activity and effort. This perfectly suits locomotion-oriented individuals' desire for brisk, future-oriented action. As a result, as can be seen above, locomotors are more likely to initiate new projects and goals.

LOCOMOTION AND MAINTENANCE OF GOAL COMMITMENT

High locomotors are concerned with maintenance of their goal commitments, as this allows them to move toward their desired future states without interruption. Given their preference for commitment maintenance, high locomotors should prefer goals with a higher attainment expectancy, because high expectancy signifies that they will most likely reach the desired state without problems. Locomotors should also invest more time and effort into their goals, as this increases their expectancy of goal attainment. Finally, high locomotors should complete tasks quickly and enjoy working on many goals at the same time, as this increases the speed with which they move toward their desired future states. These conjectures were explored in the studies considered in the following.

There is consistent evidence that locomotors prefer goals with high (vs. low) attainment expectancy. In one study, participants listed five attributes they wanted to attain (e.g., "being fit") and rated their expectancy of attaining each of those goals. High locomotors tended to select goals with higher attainment expectancy (i.e., goals that would be easier to achieve; Kruglanski et al., 2000). Locomotion is also positively correlated with optimism, or the increased expectancy of being able to attain one's goals (Kruglanski et al., 2000). These results are consistent with the idea that, because locomotors enjoy making progress toward their desired future states, they are most likely to select goals that allow them to make such progress without undue difficulties or delays.

In a similar vein, locomotors prefer means that serve a single goal (*unifinal* means) rather than means that serve multiple goals (*multifinal* means), because unifinal means offer a higher expectancy of goal attainment due to their perceived higher instrumentality (Zhang, Fishbach, & Kruglanski, 2007). In one experiment, participants read a paragraph that described either one advantage of consuming tomatoes (unifinal means condition) or two advantages of consuming tomatoes (multifinal means condition). When tomatoes were attached to one goal, locomotion was positively associated with the evaluation of tomatoes. When tomatoes were attached to two goals, however, locomotion was negatively associated with evaluations of tomatoes (Orehek, Mauro, Kruglanski, & van der Bles, 2012). In a second study, participants were asked to list either one goal or three goals that computers can serve. A modified affect misattribution procedure (Payne, Cheng, Govorun, & Stewart, 2005) was subsequently used to assess participants' evaluations of computers. Locomotors' implicit evaluations of computers were higher when computers were associated with one goal (vs. three goals). Another study showed that high locomotors reported greater thirst when the linkage between drinking water and a single goal was disproportionately strengthened through priming (in the unifinal means condition), rather than when the linkage between drinking water and two goals was made equal (the multifinal means condition). In the last experiment in this series, participants were offered the use of a pen that served either one goal (writing) or two goals (writing and serving as a laser pointer). High locomotors were significantly more likely to select the unifinal (vs. the multifinal) pen (Orehek et al., 2012). Thus locomotors are willing to select options that serve a single goal if it means that their expectancy of attaining it will be greater as a result.

Locomotion is related to greater investment of time and effort in goal attainment, as investing more effort increases the expectancy that the goal will be accomplished successfully. Studies using employee samples have shown that workers high in locomotion invested more effort into task accomplishment (Pierro, Kruglanski, & Higgins, 2006). In another series of studies conducted in organizational settings, Bélanger and colleagues (2015) demonstrated that employees who were high in locomotion were more highly committed to their work and exhibited fewer withdrawal (from work) behaviors. For example, locomotion was negatively related to absenteeism and lateness, whether those were self-reported or measured via organizational records. Locomotors were also more involved in the tasks they pursued: Even though locomotors were more prone to exhibiting workaholic tendencies, their greater job involvement served as a protective factor from work-related stress. Specifically, due to greater involvement in their work, high locomotors experienced less work-related burnout and psychological strain (De Carlo et al., 2014). Taken together, these findings illustrate locomotors' greater commitment to maintaining motion toward their desired future states.

High locomotors tend to move quickly toward goal attainment. When engaged in a proofreading task that involved checking writing samples to make sure they were congruent with a master copy, high locomotors finished the task significantly faster than low locomotors (Kruglanski et al., 2000). Locomotion was also positively associated with measures of Type A personality, which is characterized by impatience and the desire to get things done quickly (Friedman & Rosenman, 1959; Kruglanski et al., 2000). High locomotors even prefer organizational structures that facilitate faster goal completion. For example, Kruglanski, Pierro, and Higgins (2007) showed that individuals with a stronger locomotion orientation prefer a more directive and forceful leader, presumably because a leader of this kind stimulates faster initiation of goal commitment and completion of goal pursuit (whereas a more considerate and deliberative leader may unnecessarily prolong the decision-making process). Thus high locomotors clearly do not wait to get things done but prefer to progress steadily toward their desired end states.

Locomotors enjoy making progress on several goals in quick succession; they therefore view multitasking as an attractive strategy, as multitasking involves rapidly switching back and forth between tasks (Han & Marois, 2013). In line with this finding, one experiment showed that high locomotors reported a greater preference for multitasking (Pierro, Giacomantonio, Pica, Kruglanski, & Higgins, 2013).

In another experiment, locomotors were more satisfied when they were given the opportunity to complete several tasks at the same time (as compared with being asked to work on each task separately; Pierro, Giacomantonio, et al., 2013). These studies suggest that locomotors are devoted to accomplishing as many goals as they can in any given time period.

In review, maintaining goal commitments allows an individual to move rapidly toward his or her desired future states. High locomotors are especially eager to experience such feelings of goal progress and goal-oriented motion. As a result, locomotors will make every effort to maintain their goals, including using strategies such as multitasking, choosing high-expectancy goals, and investing more time and energy into goal pursuit.

GENERAL DISCUSSION

The studies described above demonstrate that locomotion regulatory mode can influence how individuals think about the future and pursue their goals. In fact, the locomotion orientation affects nearly every aspect of a person's thoughts and actions, from the types of attentional processes they evince to the extent to which they value different activities and outcomes. More specifically, locomotion has been shown to make individuals plan more for the future, focus less on the past, and be more likely to initiate and maintain future goal commitments. These findings can have both positive and negative implications for high locomotors and their interaction partners. They also offer myriad new directions for future research.

Practical Implications

As can be seen from the wide variety of findings reviewed above, locomotion can often be highly beneficial. Nonetheless, the extant research on locomotion also suggests that there are many circumstances in which locomotion could actually lead to detrimental outcomes. As such, the fact that it is possible to situationally induce locomotion becomes critically important, as there are numerous tasks and environments in which it might be advantageous to either raise or lower individuals' locomotion levels. Previous situational manipulations of regulatory mode have attempted to put individuals into a locomotion mindset by having them think about times in the past when they acted like locomotors (e.g., when they finished one project and immediately got started on another; Avnet & Higgins, 2003). Other methods that have proven successful at inducing active goal pursuit are mental contrasting and implementation intentions (which, combined, are known as the MCII approach; Gollwitzer, 2014; Kappes, Wendt, Reinelt, & Oettingen, 2013; Kappes & Oettingen, 2014; Oettingen, 2012; Sevincer, Busatta, & Oettingen, 2014). These latter methods, too, have the potential to effectively induce a locomotion orientation because they simultaneously augment goal commitment and increase one's tendency to act toward a goal. Some situations in which such manipulations could be useful are discussed below.

Locomotors possess many characteristics that managers are likely to find appealing, such as the propensity for planning and organization, as well as intense engagement in tasks and reduced procrastination. Thus using locomotion as a criterion in the recruitment process, as well as strategically inducing a high-locomotion mindset in employees when specific tasks require it, could be a wise strategy for organizational leaders. However, given that locomotors strongly emphasize the pace of their work, less measurable aspects of performance quality (e.g., creativity) may be traded in for more readily quantifiable aspects of their work (e.g., speed of task completion). More specifically, there can be a downside to locomotors' focus on expectancy and single-minded goal pursuit. For instance, generating creative ideas often requires the risky strategy of considering incidental information which—on the surface—may appear unrelated to the problem at hand. Indeed, broader attentional focus is known to be related to a more creative idea generation (Ward, Patterson, & Sifonis, 2004). Thus, if locomotors focus only on the most goal-relevant and easily accessible options and avoid exploring potentially risky paths, they may miss out on objectively superior routes to their goals. Therefore, it seems that the ideal employee should be high in locomotion *and* have other complementary qualities that will balance his or her level of locomotion (e.g., assessment; Chernikova et al., 2016; Lo Destro, Chernikova, Pierro, Kruglanski, & Higgins, 2015; Kruglanski et al., 2000). Regulatory mode manipulations have the potential to help employers attain this goal (cf. Avnet & Higgins, 2003).

Locomotors are less positive in their evaluations of past events and individuals who helped them to attain past goals. This tendency to downplay the past could have both positive and negative social consequences for locomotors. For example, lack of gratitude toward former helpers may be negatively perceived by others. Moreover, if locomotors' interaction partners recognize that they are valued as means to these individuals' goals, they may balk and withdraw from the relationship. Ultimately, this could undermine the quality of locomotors' social interactions; people who are struggling with such social issues may actually benefit from a *low*-locomotion induction. On the other hand, due to locomotors' greater inclination to forgive, they may have better relations with people who have wronged them in the past; as a result, individuals who are struggling to forgive others may profit from a *high*-locomotion induction. Interestingly, it is also possible that the combination of these two tendencies could lead to locomotors having less polarized attitudes toward other people on the basis of the past history of their relations. They may be more positive toward people who hurt them but also less positive toward people who helped them.

Another consequence of locomotors' reduced focus on the past could be a propensity to learn less from past experience. Research on deliberate practice has shown that acquisition of expertise in a given domain requires a thorough analysis of one's past experience (Ericsson, Krampe, & Tesch-Römer, 1993). The latter involves paying attention to feedback, which is needed to understand what one must do differently. If high locomotors are unlikely to focus on the past, they may consequently learn less from their past experience and perhaps be prone to repeating the same mistakes. Again, in such a situation, a *low*-locomotion induction would appear to be valuable.

There are many other domains, such as those of health, education, sports achievement, and others, in which high levels of locomotion can be either more or less advantageous, depending upon the situation and the structure of the task in question. Delineating the best way to manipulate locomotion, as well as the specific circumstances under which low (vs. high) locomotion might be the most useful, is a task for future research to undertake.

FUTURE RESEARCH DIRECTIONS

Future research could examine additional consequences of locomotors' tendency to privilege the future over the past. For instance, given their inclination to avoid dwelling on the past, locomotors should be less susceptible to the endowment effect (Kahneman, Knetsch, & Thaler, 1991). That is, locomotors may counterintuitively value things they already own *less* than things they could potentially own in the future. Likewise, given their greater openness to change, locomotors may be less prone to biases that reflect greater attachment to the status quo, such as the mere existence bias (Eidelman, Crandall, & Pattershall, 2009) or the proneness toward loss aversion (Kahneman et al., 1991). In the political domain, locomotion should be negatively correlated with measures of conservatism, as conservatives are more attached to traditional social conditions and more averse to social change (Jost, Glaser, Kruglanski, & Sulloway, 2003). In the domain of health, high locomotors might actually prove to be in better physical health than their low-locomotor counterparts, due in part to their desire to move frequently and keep moving continuously (which should translate into increased physical activity) and in part to their tendency to forgive and forget past wrongs (which has been linked to better overall health; McCullough, 2000).

Given that locomotors plan more and feel greater control over their time, future research could investigate whether they are less prone to some planning biases and more accurate in time estimation concerning their completion of future tasks. Moreover, their time estimation errors, if any, should lie in the underestimation of the amount of time that they will need to complete a task. This assumes that the locomotors' motivation to move quickly through tasks would lead to the expectancy that they will be able to do so.

High (vs. low) locomotors are faster in goal pursuit, less prone to procrastination, more hard working, and more persistent in their goal striving; in short, they appear to be better at self-regulation. However, the mediating mechanisms driving those effects are not yet clear, and future research should attempt to illuminate them. For instance, future studies can examine the construal level (Trope & Liberman, 2011) at which locomotors naturally represent their goals. Given that locomotors enjoy goal attainment more, they may be more inclined to represent their long-term goals in terms of many small, concrete, and easily attainable subgoals. Such a strategy would multiply the experience of goal accomplishment, which is something that locomotors enjoy; at the same time, it would translate into better overall performance. In addition, the concept of goal attainment may have strong motivational value for locomotors. As a result, high locomotors may exhibit a steeper goal-gradient effect; that is, they may increase their effort expenditure as they get closer to their goals (Hull, 1932; Liberman & Förster, 2008).

It could also be of interest to investigate moderators of locomotors' apparent tendency toward determined goal persistence. For instance, a counterintuitive consequence of locomotors' emphasis on swift goal achievement could be quicker withdrawal from a goal if its attainment expectancy decreases. When obstacles interfere with locomotors' smooth progress toward goal attainment, they may be faster to abandon that objective and move on to a new goal that promises fewer impediments and delays.

SOME APPARENT CONTRADICTIONS

The careful reader may have noticed two seeming contradictions in the research reviewed in this chapter. First, some studies have shown that locomotors enjoy multitasking because it involves rapidly switching back and forth between tasks (Pierro, Giacomantonio et al., 2013). But—in apparent contradiction to this—other research has come to the conclusion that locomotors prefer means that serve a single goal at one time to means that serve multiple goals at one time, because the former are perceived as more instrumental (Orehek et al., 2012). However, this inconsistency can be explained by paying close attention to the features of each task environment. When a multitasking situation involves switching back and forth between means in order to achieve multiple tasks (as in the Pierro, Giacomantonio, et al., 2013 study), it allows and encourages movement; as a result, locomotors should prefer to multitask in this environment. However, when a situation involves choosing between one means that either serves one or multiple goals (as in the Orehek et al., 2012, study), there is only a single means in both cases, and no task switching or movement between means is possible. In that situation, locomotors' focus is switched to the instrumentality of the means in question—which affords the smoothest, most certain movement.

A second potential contradiction lies in the existence of studies showing that locomotion is negatively associated with impulsivity and positively associated with self-control (Shalev & Sulkowski, 2009; Spinella, 2007; Struk et al., 2015), whereas other studies show that locomotion is also positively correlated with the tendency to prefer small, immediate rewards to large, delayed rewards (Guo & Feng, 2015). Nonetheless, much like the first one, this contradiction is only apparent. Although the inability to resist momentary rewards in order to attain long-term goals has been treated as a symptom of impulsive behavior (Tangney, Baumeister, & Boone, 2004), we argue that it is not the failure to adhere to long-term goals that drives this effect among locomotors. Rather, locomotors may choose smaller rewards because they care less about the overall value of their strivings and more about movement as such. As a result, when locomotors have the option to engage in action *right now* by choosing to receive something in the present as opposed to in the future, locomotors will jump on that chance and select the immediate option. Locomotors' greater self-control presumably resides in their resistance to distractions and temptations once they are moving toward a salient objective. So the apparent contradiction between the findings is accounted for by the fact that locomotors are wont to initiate movement as soon as possible and to maintain it without interruptions until the end is reached. Nevertheless, these conjectures are merely speculative; future experiments should be conducted in order to investigate the moderating variables that influence when locomotors will tend to exhibit self-control versus impulsivity.

CONCLUSION

In summary, locomotion regulatory mode is an important determinant of individuals' orientation toward the future. A wide variety of research findings has demonstrated the impact of locomotion on future-oriented thinking, planning, goal pursuit, and behavior. Nonetheless, many aspects of locomotors' preoccupation with the future remain unexplored and could be profitably investigated in future research.

ACKNOWLEDGMENT

Katarzyna Jasko's work on this project was supported by the Polish Ministry of Science and Higher Education (the Mobility Plus project 1115/MOB/13/2014/0).

REFERENCES

Amato, C., Chernikova, M., Pierro, A., Kruglanski, A. W., & Higgins, E. T. (2016). *Getting stuck on sunk costs or letting them go: Regulatory mode and the sunk cost fallacy.* Unpublished manuscript, University of Rome—La Sapienza.

Amato, C., Pierro, A., Chirumbolo, A., & Pica, G. (2014). Regulatory modes and time management: How locomotors and assessors plan and perceive time. *International Journal of Psychology, 49,* 192–199.

Avnet, T., & Higgins, E. T. (2003). Locomotion, assessment, and regulatory fit: Value transfer from "how" to "what." *Journal of Personality and Social Psychology, 39,* 525–530.

Batcho, K. I. (1995). Nostalgia: A psychological perspective. *Perceptual and Motor Skills, 80,* 131–143.

Bélanger, J. J., Pierro, A., Mauro, R., Falco, A., De Carlo, N., & Kruglanski, A. W. (2015). It's about time: The role of locomotion in withdrawal behavior. *Journal of Business and Psychology, 31,* 265–278.

Bortner, R. W. (1969). A short rating scale as a potential measure of pattern A behavior. *Journal of Chronic Diseases, 22,* 87–91.

Chernikova, M., Lo Destro, C., Mauro, R., Pierro, A., Kruglanski, A. W., & Higgins, E. T. (2016). Different strokes for different folks: Effects of regulatory mode complementarity and task complexity on performance. *Personality and Individual Differences, 89,* 134–142.

De Carlo, N. A., Falco, A., Pierro, A., Dugas, M., Kruglanski, A. W., & Higgins, E. T. (2014). Regulatory mode orientations and well-being in an organizational setting: The differential mediating roles of workaholism and work engagement. *Journal of Applied Social Psychology, 44,* 725–738.

Eidelman, S., Crandall, C. S., & Pattershall, J. (2009). The existence bias. *Journal of Personality and Social Psychology, 97,* 765–775.

Ericsson, K. A., Krampe, R. T., & Tesch-Römer, C. (1993). The role of deliberate practice in the acquisition of expert performance. *Psychological Review, 100,* 363–406.

Fenigstein, A., Scheier, M. F., & Buss, A. H. (1975). Public and private self-consciousness: Assessment and theory. *Journal of Consulting and Clinical Psychology, 43,* 522–527.

Friedman, M., & Rosenman, R. H. (1959). Association of specific overt behavior pattern with blood and cardiovascular findings: Blood cholesterol level, blood clotting time, incidence of arcus senilis, and clinical coronary artery disease. *Journal of the American Medical Association, 169,* 1286–1296.

Gollwitzer, P. M. (2014). Weakness of the will: Is a quick fix possible? *Motivation and Emotion, 38,* 305–322.

Guo, Y., & Feng, T. (2015). The mediating role of LPFC–vmPFC functional connectivity in the relation between regulatory mode and delay discounting. *Behavioural Brain Research, 292,* 252–258.

Han, S. W., & Marois, R. (2013). The source of dual-task limitations: Serial or parallel processing of multiple response selections? *Attention, Perception, and Psychophysics, 75,* 1395–1405.

Higgins, E. T. (2012). *Beyond pleasure and pain: How motivation works.* New York: Oxford University Press.

Higgins, E. T., Kruglanski, A. W., & Pierro, A. (2003). Regulatory mode: Locomotion and assessment as distinct orientations. *Advances in Experimental Social Psychology, 35,* 293–344.

Hull, C. L. (1932). The goal-gradient hypothesis and maze learning. *Psychological Review, 39,* 25–43.

Jackson, D. N. (1974). *Personality research form manual.* Goshen, NY: Research Psychologists Press.

Jost, J. T., Glaser, J., Kruglanski, A. W., & Sulloway, F. J. (2003). Political conservatism as motivated social cognition. *Psychological Bulletin, 129,* 339–375.

Judge, T. A., Higgins, C. A., Thoresen, C. J., & Barrick, M. R. (1999). The Big Five personality traits, general mental ability, and career success across the life span. *Personnel Psychology, 52,* 621–652.

Kahneman, D., Knetsch, J. L., & Thaler, R. H. (1991). Anomalies: The endowment effect, loss aversion, and status quo bias. *Journal of Economic Perspectives, 5,* 193–206.

Kappes, A., & Oettingen, G. (2014). The emergence of goal pursuit: Mental contrasting connects future and reality. *Journal of Experimental Social Psychology, 54,* 25–39.

Kappes, A., Wendt, M., Reinelt, T., & Oettingen, G. (2013). Mental contrasting changes the meaning of reality. *Journal of Experimental Social Psychology, 49,* 797–810.

Kim, H., Franks, B., & Higgins, E. T. (2013). Evidence that self-regulatory mode affects retirement savings. *Journal of Aging and Social Policy, 25,* 248–263.

Klein, H. J., Wesson, M. J., Hollenbeck, J. R., Wright, P. M., & DeShon, R. P. (2001). The assessment of goal commitment: A measurement model meta-analysis. *Organizational Behavior and Human Decision Processes, 85,* 32–55.

Kruglanski, A. W., Jasko, K., Chernikova, M., Milyavsky, M., Babush, M., Baldner, C., . . . Pierro, A. (2015). The rocky road from attitudes to behaviors: Charting the goal systemic course of actions. *Psychological Review, 122,* 598–620.

Kruglanski, A. W., Pierro, A., & Higgins, E. T. (2007). Regulatory mode and preferred leadership styles: How fit increases job satisfaction. *Basic and Applied Social Psychology, 29,* 137–149.

Kruglanski, A. W., Pierro, A., & Higgins, E. T. (2015). Experience of time by people on the go: A theory of the locomotion–temporality interface. *Personality and Social Psychology Review, 20,* 100–117.

Kruglanski, A. W., Pierro, A., Higgins, E. T., & Capozza, D. (2007). "On the move" or "staying put": Locomotion, need for closure, and reactions to organizational change. *Journal of Applied Social Psychology, 37,* 1305–1340.

Kruglanski, A. W., Thompson, E. P., Higgins, E. T., Atash, M., Pierro, A., Shah, J. Y., . . . Spiegel, S. (2000). To "do the right thing" or to "just do it": Locomotion and assessment as distinct self-regulatory imperatives. *Journal of Personality and Social Psychology, 79,* 793–815.

Kuhl, J. (1985). Volitional mediation of cognition-behaviour consistency: Self-regulatory processes and action versus state orientation. In J. Kuhl & J. Beckman (Eds.), *Action control: From cognition to behaviour* (pp. 101–128). Berlin, Germany: Springer-Verlag.

Leary, M. R. (1983). Social anxiousness: The construct and its measurement. *Journal of Personality Assessment, 47,* 66–75.

Liberman, N., & Förster, J. (2008). Expectancy, value and psychological distance: A new look at goal gradients. *Social Cognition, 26,* 515–533.

Lo Destro, C., Chernikova, M., Pierro, A., Kruglanski, A. W., & Higgins, E. T. (2015). Practice benefits locomotors: Regulatory mode complementarity and task performance. *Social Psychological and Personality Science, 7,* 358–365.

Macan, T. H., Shahani, C., Dipboye, R. L., & Phillips, A. P. (1990). College students' time management: Correlations with academic performance and stress. *Journal of Educational Psychology, 82,* 760–768.

McCullough, M. E. (2000). Forgiveness as human strength: Theory, measurement, and links to well-being. *Journal of Social and Clinical Psychology, 19,* 43–55.

Oettingen, G. (2012). Future thought and behaviour change. *European Review of Social Psychology, 23,* 1–63.

Orehek, E., Fitzsimons, G. M., & Kruglanski, A. W. (2014). *Moving on means leaving behind: How locomotors devalue support providers.* Unpublished manuscript. University of Pittsburgh, Pittsburgh, PA.

Orehek, E., Mauro, R., Kruglanski, A. W., & van der Bles, A. M. (2012). Prioritizing association strength versus value: The influence of self-regulatory modes on means evaluation in single goal and multigoal contexts. *Journal of Personality and Social Psychology, 102,* 22–31.

Payne, B. K., Cheng, C. M., Govorun, O., & Stewart, B. D. (2005). An inkblot for attitudes: Affect misattribution as implicit measurement. *Journal of Personality and Social Psychology, 89,* 277–293.

Pica, G., Amato, C., Pierro, A., & Kruglanski, A. W. (2015). The early bird gets the worm: On locomotors' preference for morningness. *Personality and Individual Differences, 76,* 158–160.

Pierro, A., Giacomantonio, M., Pica, G., Kruglanski, A. W., & Higgins, E. T. (2011). On the psychology of time in action: Regulatory mode orientations and procrastination. *Journal of Personality and Social Psychology, 101,* 1317–1331.

Pierro, A., Giacomantonio, M., Pica, G., Kruglanski, A. W., & Higgins, E. T. (2013). Locomotion and the preference for multitasking: Implications for well-being. *Motivation and Emotion, 37,* 213–223.

Pierro, A., Kruglanski, A. W., & Higgins, E. T. (2006). Regulatory mode and the joys of doing: Effects of "locomotion" and "assessment" on intrinsic and extrinsic task-motivation. *European Journal of Personality, 20,* 355–375.

Pierro, A., Leder, S., Mannetti, L., Higgins, E. T., Kruglanski, A. W., & Aiello, A. (2008). Regulatory mode effects on counterfactual thinking and regret. *Journal of Experimental Social Psychology, 44,* 321–329.

Pierro, A., Pica, G., Klein, K., Kruglanski, A. W., & Higgins, E. T. (2013). Looking back or moving on: How regulatory modes affect nostalgia. *Motivation and Emotion, 37,* 653–660.

Pierro, A., Pica, G., Kruglanski, A. W., & Higgins, T. E. (2014). *Regulatory mode orientations and self-forgiveness.* Unpublished manuscript, University of Rome "La Sapienza."

Pierro, A., Presaghi, F., Higgins, T. E., & Kruglanski, A. W. (2009). Regulatory mode preferences for autonomy supporting versus controlling instructional styles. *British Journal of Educational Psychology, 79,* 599–615.

Routledge, C., Arndt, J., Sedikides, C., & Wildschut, T. (2008). A blast from the past: The terror management function of nostalgia. *Journal of Experimental Social Psychology, 44,* 132–140.

Schaufeli, W. B., Salanova, M., González-Romá, V., & Bakker, A. B. (2002). The measurement of engagement and burnout: A two-sample confirmatory factor analytic approach. *Journal of Happiness Studies, 3,* 71–92.

Scholer, A. A., & Higgins, E. T. (2012). Commitment to change from locomotion motivation during deliberation. *Motivation and Emotion, 36,* 114–129.

Sevincer, A. T., Busatta, P. D., & Oettingen, G. (2014). Mental contrasting and transfer of energization. *Personality and Social Psychology Bulletin, 40,* 139–152.

Shalev, I., & Sulkowski, M. L. (2009). Relations between distinct aspects of self-regulation to symptoms of impulsivity and compulsivity. *Personality and Individual Differences, 47,* 84–88.

Shipp, A. J., Edwards, J. R., & Lambert, L. S. (2009). Conceptualization and measurement of temporal focus: The subjective experience of the past, present, and future. *Organizational Behavior and Human Decision Processes, 110,* 1–22.

Smith, C. S., Reilly, C., & Midkiff, K. (1989). Evaluation of three circadian rhythm questionnaires with suggestions for an improved measure of morningness. *Journal of Applied Psychology, 74,* 728–738.

Spinella, M. (2007). Normative data and a short form of the Barratt Impulsiveness Scale. *International Journal of Neuroscience, 117,* 359–368.

Sriram, N., & Greenwald, A. G. (2009). The brief Implicit Association Test. *Experimental Psychology, 56,* 283–294.

Struk, A. A., Scholer, A. A., & Danckert, J. (2015). A self-regulatory approach to understanding boredom proneness. *Cognition and Emotion, 30,* 1388–1401.

Tangney, J. P., Baumeister, R. F., & Boone, A. L. (2004). High self-control predicts good adjustment, less pathology, better grades, and interpersonal success. *Journal of Personality, 72,* 271–324.

Trope, Y., & Liberman, N. (2011). Construal level theory. In P. A. M. van Lange, A. W. Kruglanski, & E. T. Higgins (Eds.), *Handbook of theories of social psychology* (Vol. 1, pp. 118–134). London: SAGE.

Tuckman, B. W. (1991). The development and concurrent validity of the procrastination scale. *Educational and Psychological Measurement, 51,* 473–480.

Ward, T. B., Patterson, M. J., & Sifonis, C. M. (2004). The role of specificity and abstraction in creative idea generation. *Creativity Research Journal, 16,* 1–9.

Webb, C. (2012, June). *Motivations for reconciliation: Regulatory mode, individual differences, and evolutionary considerations.* Paper presented at the 25th annual conference of the International Association for Conflict Management, Stellenbosch, South Africa. Available at *https://papers.ssrn.com/sol3/papers.cfm?abstract_id=2086538.*

Webster, D. M., & Kruglanski, A. W. (1994). Individual differences in need for cognitive closure. *Journal of Personality and Social Psychology, 67,* 1049–1062.

Wildschut, T., Sedikides, C., Arndt, J., & Routledge, C. (2006). Nostalgia: Content, triggers, functions. *Journal of Personality and Social Psychology, 91,* 975–993.

Zimbardo, P. G., & Boyd, J. N. (1999). Putting time in perspective: A valid, reliable individual-differences metric. *Journal of Personality and Social Psychology, 77,* 1271–1288.

Zhang, P., & Gheibi, S. (2015). The gloomy picturesque empowering leadership through the lens of work engagement. *European Scientific Journal, 11,* 385–401.

Zhang, Y., Fishbach, A., & Kruglanski, A. W. (2007). The dilution model: How additional goals undermine the perceived instrumentality of a shared path. *Journal of Personality and Social Psychology, 92,* 389–401.

>>>>>>>>>>>>>>>>>>>>

CHAPTER 22

Where I Ideally Want to Be versus Where I Ought to Be

Regulatory Focus and the Future

James F. M. Cornwell
E. Tory Higgins

One of the most important aspects of being human is our capacity to make choices concerning in which direction to take our lives into the future—the sense of "becoming" that we all possess (Higgins, 2005). People have a sense of where they are and of where they are motivated to be, now and in the future. The inherent indeterminacy of the future has given rise to a number of theories of human decision making that try to predict the kinds of options that people prefer, which in turn predict the choices they will make for moving into the future. It is critical, then, to understand what motivates people's choice preferences. We propose that a combination of regulatory focus and relating one's perceived status quo to a potential future state is a major contributor to individuals' preference for one option over alternatives.

In this chapter, we discuss how individuals' regulatory focus influences their preferences about which goals to pursue and how to pursue them and how their choices are also influenced by the relation between their current state and the status quo. In the following section, we provide some historical background for the development of regulatory focus theory, including information about how regulatory focus is operationalized and assessed. We also discuss how having a promotion focus versus a prevention focus differs in the psychological significance of the relation between one's current state and the status quo. We then review research on how individuals' choice preferences vary as a function of their regulatory focus and whether they perceive themselves to be at, below, or above the status quo. We finish the chapter by applying this understanding to two case examples: risk taking in the marketplace and the United States 2016 presidential primaries.

REGULATORY FOCUS: ITS DEVELOPMENT, ASSESSMENT, AND RELATION TO FUTURE END STATES

From Self-Discrepancy Theory to Regulatory Focus Theory

Regulatory focus theory originally grew out of self-discrepancy theory. According to self-discrepancy theory, individuals' self-concepts are composed of three distinct "selves." The *actual-self* is the sense of who the individual is at the current moment. Two distinct alternatives also exist: the *ideal-self* and the *ought-self*. The ideal-self comprises people's hopes, wishes, and aspirations for themselves, whereas the ought-self comprises people's beliefs about their duties, obligations, and responsibilities. According to self-discrepancy theory, all individuals are motivated to close the gap between their actual selves and both their ideal and ought selves, although the emphasis on ideals versus oughts can vary (Higgins, 1987).

This theory necessarily incorporates the future. When reflecting on the degrees to which their actual selves are discrepant from their ideal and ought selves, individuals are implicitly declaring their beliefs concerning not only where they are but where they *ideally want* to be and where they *ought* to be. Failure to attain these ideals and oughts creates two distinct forms of negative affect. Actual–ideal discrepancies create dejection-related forms of negative affect, such as feeling sad, discouraged, or blue, whereas actual–ought discrepancies create agitation-related forms of negative affect, such as feeling anxious, worried, or nervous (Higgins, 1987). Thus, in order to reduce these discrepancies, individuals are motivated to approach their ideal and ought selves and to avoid any further discrepancy from those particular end-states.

Assessing and Operationalizing Regulatory Focus

Research on self-discrepancy was eventually expanded into a general theory of goal pursuit called *regulatory focus theory*. According to regulatory focus theory, approach and avoidance motives are subdivided into promotion and prevention motives (Higgins, 1997, 1998). Individuals are motivated to approach both gains (end-states exceeding the status quo) and non-losses (end-states that maintain or restore the status quo). Similarly, individuals are motivated to avoid non-gains (end-states failing to move beyond the status quo) and losses (end-states failing to maintain the status quo). The distinction between gains and non-gains corresponds to the promotion focus, which takes aspirations, mastery, and growth (i.e., +1 gain end-states) as its primary referent for success and a failure to achieve such end-states (i.e., 0 non-gain end-states) as its referent for failure. The distinction between non-losses and losses corresponds to the prevention focus, which takes responsibilities, safety, and security (i.e., 0 non-loss end-states) as its primary referent for success and a failure to secure such end-states (i.e., –1 loss end-states) as its referent for failure (see Higgins, 2014; Higgins & Cornwell, 2016).

Compared with self-discrepancy theory, regulatory focus theory has a broader range of applicability. Self-discrepancy was typically assessed chronically through self-report (see Higgins, 1987; Higgins, Klein, & Strauman, 1985). In contrast, not only are there means to assess the degree to which individuals identify as being more effective in the domains of promotion or prevention (Higgins et al., 2001) or which goals are more chronically accessible (Higgins, Shah, & Friedman, 1997), but regulatory focus can also be experimentally induced situationally. Merely focusing upon one's hopes and aspirations can induce an individual into a promotion state, and focusing upon one's duties and obligations can induce an individual into a prevention state (Freitas & Higgins, 2002). Thus regulatory focus is frequently operationalized as the form of self-regulatory goal (either ideals or oughts) that is currently more accessible either through a general chronic predominance of one set of goals over the other or through situational priming. This accessibility (or motivational relevance; see Eitam & Higgins, 2010), in turn, determines the motivational significance of one's current state vis-à-vis potential future end-states and thereby has important effects on which options individuals prefer for their path forward.

Regulatory Focus and the Future

Individuals in both a promotion focus and a prevention focus have specific choice preferences as a function of their current states relative to the status quo. Those with a strong promotion focus are primarily concerned with ensuring a better future relative to their current state (a gain) and will thus be more attuned to options involving advancement and growth. Moreover, those with a strong promotion focus will also be concerned with avoiding getting stuck at the status quo (a non-gain) and will thus be more likely to adopt approaches that will effect some sort of positive change, even if those approaches are themselves risky. Thus the promotion focus, motivationally speaking, acts as a kind of "push" from behind, aiming at any possible improvement and avoiding sticking to the status quo except in extreme circumstances. This tendency can even be seen in the etymology of its name; the word *promote* is itself derived from the Latin *promovere*, which means "to move forward." Consideration of the future is therefore of supreme importance for this self-regulatory system: The future is a better place to which an individual with a strong promotion focus would ideally like to move.

Notably, the future is also very important to those with a strong prevention focus, although in a different way. In colloquial parlance, the word *prevention* is sometimes conflated with the word *avoidance*. Indeed, some researchers have developed scales that incorrectly measure avoidance orientation and identify it as the prevention focus (see Summerville & Roese, 2008). However, the prevention focus is not merely concerned with avoiding negative outcomes or dealing with such negative outcomes as they arise. Instead, the word *prevention*, with respect to the prevention focus, is better understood according to its older meaning. *Prevent* means to act ahead of or to precede something—literally, the word *prevent* comes from the Latin *praevenire*, which means "to anticipate." Anticipating potential mistakes or potential losses in order to make sure they do not come to pass is precisely what prevention vigilance is all about. For those with a strong prevention focus, a future of non-losses is something to be secured and guarded.

Thus the "focus" of the prevention focus is a satisfactory status quo that is to be maintained now and in the future at all costs (a non-loss). The concern is a positive state of safety and security that is maintained and engaging in actions to make this happen (approach). It is *not* about avoiding an undesired end-state or inhibiting action (avoidance). Indeed, at times the maintenance of the status quo requires the approaching of negative or potentially threatening stimuli. Research on monkeys has found that those typically categorized as inhibited or "shy" (i.e., avoidance-oriented) were more likely to *approach* an unknown object placed in their environment than those categorized as risky or "bold" (i.e., approach-oriented; Franks et al., 2013) because they need to be vigilant to check on potential danger. Furthermore, research on rats has found that those preferring safety and security rather than gains (i.e., preferring an option that turned off the lights vs. an option that provided food) were actually the first to approach a noxious object placed into their environment in order to deal with it (Franks, Higgins, & Champagne, 2012). The behavior of both the monkeys and the rats is best understood as acting ahead of a potential problem in order to preserve a desirable status quo. Thus it is evident that, for different reasons, the future is of critical importance to both those with a strong promotion focus and those with a strong prevention focus.

PROMOTION AND PREVENTION PREFERENCES AT, BELOW, AND ABOVE THE STATUS QUO

A critical element of regulatory focus theory concerns the status quo. The status quo plays a crucial role in understanding the differences in how individuals with a strong promotion focus versus a strong prevention focus value potential future end-states (see Higgins, 2014). For those with a strong promotion focus, an end-state corresponding to a satisfactory status quo is perceived as a motivational failure (a non-gain), whereas for those with a strong prevention focus, an end-state corresponding to a satisfactory status quo is perceived as a motivational success (a non-loss). These different relations between the status quo and promotion versus prevention has been found to produce a number of significant effects.

Future End-States When at the Status Quo

Those with a strong prevention focus have a stronger attachment to the status quo than those with a strong promotion focus. Some decision theorists have suggested that individuals generally are reluctant to part with an object in their possession in exchange for an object of approximately equal value (e.g., Kahneman, Knetsch, & Thaler, 1991). This "endowment effect" is understood to be a regular deviation from purely rational decision making. Subsequent research has shown that, in fact, the endowment effect is primarily driven by those with a strong prevention focus. Liberman, Idson, Camacho, and Higgins (1999) found that those primed with a prevention focus were significantly less likely than 50% to be willing to exchange an endowed object (in this case, a pen or a mug) for an object of equal value. However, those primed with a promotion focus were *not* significantly different from 50%; that is, they were as likely to exchange the endowed object for the alternative as to keep the endowed object. Interestingly, Liberman et al. (1999) also found that in spite of the fact that those with a strong prevention focus were less willing to substitute their endowed object for an alternative compared with those with a strong promotion focus, there were no differences between the two foci with respect to the degree to which they liked the endowed object. Thus the differences that were found between promotion and prevention were entirely due to their different motivational relations to the status quo.

This general attachment or nonattachment to the status quo has major implications for the different strategies individuals use as they make decisions concerning their future actions. For example, research has shown that those with a strong promotion focus are more likely to generate a number of potential creative avenues of action (e.g., potential uses for a brick) compared with those with a strong prevention focus (Crowe & Higgins, 1997; Friedman & Förster, 2001). This has been confirmed in organizational contexts as well, with researchers finding that organizational leaders who are more promotion-focused tend to have subordinates who provided reports that were judged to be more creative (Wu, McMullen, Neubert, & Yi, 2008). This is consistent with the research noted above because those with a strong promotion focus would be more motivated to generate potential futures beyond the status quo, that is, to be open to new possibilities, whereas those with a strong prevention focus would be satisfied with maintaining the status quo (Friedman & Förster, 2001).

It is also worth noting that those with a strong prevention focus are more adept at analytical reasoning (Friedman & Förster, 2000), which involves careful movement from premises toward conclusions. In such cases, those with a strong promotion focus may be eager to jump to potential conclusions that may contain mistakes. This difference is consistent with evidence that individuals with a strong promotion focus have a preference for using their general feelings or intuitions when making decisions, whereas those with a strong prevention focus have a preference for using concrete reasons when making a decision (Pham & Avnet, 2004; Avnet & Higgins, 2006).

There are additional implications for those with a strong prevention focus. They should be more likely to treat their own past behaviors and those of others as establishing a status quo that needs to be maintained in the future. Indeed, research has shown that those with a strong prevention focus are more likely than those with a strong promotion focus to manage their own subordinates in the manner in which they themselves were managed, even when they did not approve of this management style (Zhang, Higgins, & Chen, 2011). Perhaps even more striking, having a prevention focus has been linked to the motivation to repeat past behaviors, regardless of whether these behaviors were ethical or unethical. That is, those who engaged in ethical behavior at one point in time (e.g., refusing to misreport a score on a test in order to improve the chances of winning a cash prize) were more likely to engage in ethical behavior again when given the opportunity if they had a strong prevention focus. But that is not all, because those prevention-focused individuals who engaged in *unethical* behavior at one point in time were also more likely to engage in unethical behavior at a subsequent time. This effect did not hold for promotion-focused individuals (Zhang, Cornwell, & Higgins, 2014).

This preference for maintaining versus moving beyond the status quo has important implications for whether individuals with a strong promotion or prevention focus will engage in risky or conservative tactics when making choices about future desired end-states. Generally speaking, research has found a strong association between risk-seeking tactics among those with a strong promotion focus and risk-aversive tactics among those with a strong prevention focus. For example, when engaging in a signal-detection task, those with a strong promotion focus showed a "risky" or lenient response bias (a higher proportion of hits and false alarms), whereas those with a strong prevention focus showed a "conservative" response bias (a higher proportion of misses and correct rejections; Crowe & Higgins, 1997). Research has extended this individual difference to group-level differences by showing that groups with a promotion focus showed less risk aversion on a subsequent task compared with groups with a prevention focus (Levine, Higgins, & Choi, 2000; Florack & Hartmann, 2007).

Other research has found that these effects extend beyond the lab to field-study contexts, showing behavioral correlates of these underlying tactics. For example, those with a strong prevention focus are more likely to limit their speeding violations compared with those with a strong promotion focus, and, in their actual behavior, they required greater gaps between oncoming cars before proceeding through a busy intersection than their promotion-focused counterparts (Hamstra, Bolderdijk, & Veldstra, 2011). Another study examining willingness to engage in unethical behavior found that those induced into a promotion focus were more likely to cheat than those induced into a prevention focus, with the effect driven primarily by differences in attitudes toward risk where cheating is risky (Gino & Margolis, 2011). All of this research confirms a general association between the promotion focus and risky tactics on the one hand and the prevention focus and conservative tactics on the other.

But this is not the whole story. Given the importance of the psychological status quo in understanding how individuals with a strong promotion focus or prevention focus view the future, it is important to also understand the motivational significance of risky and conservative choices for individuals' current states relative to the status quo. In all of the previous studies participants were engaging in this prospective decision making from the vantage point of the psychological status quo "0." Therefore, risks were evaluated in terms of their likelihood of either moving beyond the current status quo "0" (for the promotion focus) or falling below the current status quo "0" (for the prevention focus). What if the current state was not the status quo "0"? What tactical choices would individuals with promotion and prevention foci make if, instead of currently being at "0," they found themselves to be currently beneath the status quo ("−1") or to have currently advanced well beyond the status quo ("+1")? Would their psychological experience of potential future end-states, and therefore their tactical approaches to decision making, change? This important question was addressed in two recent lines of research.

Future End-States When below the Status Quo

As noted above, the major difference between promotion and prevention foci is their orientation toward the status quo. Possible futures are understood as being increasingly or decreasingly motivationally engaging insofar as they serve the purposes of each motivational system as it relates to the status quo: for the prevention focus, maintaining the status quo; for the promotion focus, exceeding the status quo. The intriguing research question that arises from this is whether this distinction flows from a general preference those with a strong prevention focus have toward conservative tactics and a general preference those with a strong promotion focus have toward risky tactics, or whether the difference between the two groups with respect to tactics flows from the difference between the two systems' relation to the status quo.

Each theoretical approach would make its own distinct empirical prediction. The first theoretical approach would assume that regardless of the current status relative to the status quo, those with a strong prevention focus would continually adopt more conservative tactics, and those with a strong promotion focus would continually adopt more risky tactics. Alternatively, Scholer, Zou, Fujita, Stroessner, and Higgins (2010) predicted that the key to the prevention focus was its attachment to a satisfactory status quo. Therefore, if someone with a strong prevention focus were to fall *below* the status quo, then he or she would adopt whatever tactics were deemed necessary to restore that original status quo, *even if those tactics involved risk*. Thus the motivational power of the possible futures represented by risky and conservative tactics would reverse for those with a strong prevention focus when they were psychologically below the status quo. The future in which the status quo is restored becomes so motivationally engaging that those with a strong prevention focus would do whatever was necessary in order to obtain it.

Scholer and colleagues (2010) tested this possibility by setting up an experiment in which participants would have the opportunity to decide between a conservative and a risky choice after finding themselves in a state of loss. At the beginning of the experiment, participants had their regulatory focus measured using the Regulatory Focus Strength Measure (Higgins et al., 2001). Following this task, participants were compensated $5 and then were told that they could continue with a second task in which they would invest that $5, potentially increasing or decreasing their overall payoff—or even end up owing the experimenter money if they lost more than $5.

Those who elected to invest their money were given a choice of stocks to choose from, and then they watched what happened to their selected stock. At the end of the period, participants were told their stock was down $9, placing them *beneath* their original status quo. The primary question was whether, under this loss ("–1") condition, those with a strong prevention focus would maintain their typical preference for a conservative tactic or, instead, would switch to a risky tactic if that tactic was necessary to restore their lost status quo. Specifically, participants were given the opportunity to choose between a conservative option (75% chance of winning $7; 25% chance of losing $10) and a risky option (25% chance of winning $20; 75% chance of losing $4). Importantly, in this case, only the risky option had the possibility of returning individuals to their status quo. Scholer et al. (2010) found that those with a strong prevention focus preferred the risky option over the conservative option under these circumstances. Also of interest, those with a strong promotion focus showed no preference for either option, suggesting that neither was particularly motivating, as neither option provided the possibility of substantially exceeding the status quo to achieve a better state (get to "+1"; see the next section for an example of what is perceived as exceeding the status quo from a promotion-focused perspective).

Other studies by Scholer and colleagues (2010) further clarified the motives of the prevention-focused individuals in these circumstances. They found, for example, that this particular reversal of tactics was only true of those with a strong prevention focus when they experienced a loss, not when they experienced a gain. Furthermore, when below the status quo, they did not favor the risky option over the conservative option if neither option had a chance of restoring their lost status quo or if both options could restore the status quo. Indeed, in the latter case, in which both options could restore the status quo, they preferred the conservative option because it made restoring the status quo more likely. That is, they were not interested in a risky option that could exceed the status quo when a conservative option had a higher likelihood of restoring the status quo.

These additional findings are important because they make clear what determines the risk choices of prevention-focused individuals. They are *not* risk seeking in the domain of losses. They will choose a risky option over a conservative option when that is the only way to restore a satisfactory status quo. Indeed, in another study in which they were in the domain of losses and the risky option was the only way to return to the status quo, when explicitly asked whether they liked or disliked the conservative option and liked or disliked the risky option, the prevention-focused participants said that they *disliked* the risky option *less*. They did *not* seek out risk because they liked it, but chose it despite its being disliked, when it was necessary to restore status quo.

In sum, for those with a strong prevention focus, the motivating power of possible future end-states (as represented by the different choice options) are not entirely the result of simply being at a current psychological state (i.e., being at a "–1" loss). Instead, what is critical is the degree to which the possible states represented by the choice options entail a high likelihood of restoring the desired status quo. Those futures that restore a status quo that has been lost will be far more motivating to a prevention-focused individual than alternative futures, including the possibility of exceeding the status quo at the risk of not simply restoring the status quo.

There is also recent evidence that other self-regulatory effects may be moderated by signals of being beneath the status quo rather than simply a general preference for particular tactics. For example, extending the research noted above that has generally found that individuals with a strong promotion focus tend to engage in more creative problem solving than those in a prevention focus, research has found that those with a strong prevention focus will also engage in more creative problem solving when they receive signals that they are currently in a state beneath the status quo (Baas, De Dreu, & Nijstad, 2011). This was achieved both by signaling the noncompletion of prevention goals (i.e., that a gap exists between participants' current state and the status quo) or an affective state signaling the same (i.e., fear—the emotional correlate of not being safe; see Higgins, 2001).

There may be a potential connection here as well for how people make judgments. For example, as noted above, research has shown that those with a strong promotion focus have a preference for using their intuitive feelings for making judgments, whereas those with a strong prevention focus prefer to use careful reasoning (Avnet & Higgins, 2006). "Going with your gut" can be considered a riskier method at arriving at a decision compared with careful analysis based on reasons, but perhaps being in a state of loss could cause those with a strong prevention focus to use more intuitive judgment tactics. Recent research has shown that those experimentally induced into a promotion focus are more likely to incorporate their feelings into their moral judgments than those induced into a prevention focus (i.e., they give harsher judgments in "moral dumbfounded" scenarios that people tend to perceive as wrong but cannot give an explanation as to why; Cornwell & Higgins, 2016). Could placing participants in a state of loss or signaling loss with affects such as fear (i.e., falling below a safe status quo) or disgust (i.e., falling below a clean status quo) reverse this effect for the prevention focus? Other research has indeed shown that when individuals are primed into a state of emotional disgust, their moral judgments can in certain cases become more intense (Schnall, Haidt, Clore, & Jordan, 2008). Additional research needs to be conducted to examine these hypothesized relations more directly.

Future End-States When above the Status Quo

From the above findings, it is clear that individuals with a strong prevention focus shift their tactics when they are beneath the status quo (i.e., in the domain of losses). What about individuals with a strong promotion focus? Will they shift their tactics when they are above the status quo (i.e., in the domain of gains)? Again, one possibility is that they will consistently prefer a risky tactic over a conservative tactic. However, as we just saw with prevention, it is also possible that there is a condition relating the current state to the status quo that will result in those with a strong promotion focus switching from preference for a risky tactic to preference for a conservative tactic. This condition might be one in which individuals with a strong promotion focus experience their current state as clear progress, a clear "+1," in relation to the status quo, where they began. Now there would be no need to be risky because a clear gain has already been made.

To determine which of these possibilities was correct, Zou, Scholer, and Higgins (2014) adopted a similar procedure to the one used to test preferences in the domain of losses that we described above. In this research, however, participants made subsequent bets after their stocks had achieved a gain. In this research, the stocks either achieved no gain, a small gain (£4), or a large gain (£20). After learning of their stock's performance, participants were given the option of taking a conservative position on their stock (100% chance of staying in the same place) or a risky position on their stock (50% chance of gaining £5; 50% chance of losing £5). Consistent with the tactical approach being driven by their preference for exceeding the status quo, those with a strong promotion focus preferred the conservative, rather than the risky, option when their stock had achieved a large enough gain to signal that clear progress had been made. Also, as expected in the domain of gains, there were no effects of any of these positions on the decision making of those with a strong prevention focus.

It is interesting to consider the above research in light of research on regulatory fit effects—the motivational engagement one achieves when the manner of one's goal pursuit is a fit with one's goal pursuit motivational orientation. Previous research has shown that the experience of success is a fit with the promotion focus because it sustains eagerness (and the experience of failure is a fit with the prevention focus because it sustains vigilance). Studies have found that this experience of success actually leads to greater engagement among those with a strong promotion focus, causing their eager strategic inclinations to be sustained rather than decline from being satisfied (Idson & Higgins, 2000). Additional findings from Zou et al. (2014) suggest that the choice preferences of promotion-focused individuals are more than just strengthened engagement from regulatory fit.

Zou et al. (2014) found that those who made a small gain in the first round of stocks were still motivationally engaged enough to prefer the risky tactic. In fact, it was only after a gain was so large that it clearly signaled progress, clearly signaled a move to "+1," that those with a strong promotion focus changed to choosing a conservative tactic. It may be that the experience of success as signaling that one is moving in the right direction without yet attaining "+1" (not enough gain yet) is motivationally engaging, causing one to maintain a risky disposition in the hopes of attaining "+1." In contrast, the experience of success as signaling *attainment* (success at reaching "+1;" a real gain) shifts the motivational focus to that of shoring up one's gains. In Zou et al. (2014), the preference for a conservative rather than a risky option following a large gain among those induced into a promotion focus was mediated by perceptions of progress, such that it was precisely those who believed that they had made substantial progress in the gains they achieved who switched from a risky to a conservative tactic. Therefore, it is this perception of progress that may be critical for individuals in a promotion focus. This issue of progress toward goals is further elucidated in the concluding section.

It is possible that the perception of progress could influence some of the other findings associated with the promotion focus. To take two of the examples cited above, perhaps those with a strong promotion focus would be less willing to engage in risky cheating following a substantial gain, as the possibility of negative consequences of being caught could take away that progress. It is also possible that those with a strong promotion focus will also engage in less creative processing of a situation after they feel they have arrived at an ideal solution to a problem. More research will need to be conducted to better understand the conditions and consequences of this important factor.

APPLYING THE FINDINGS: RISKY INVESTMENTS AND THE 2016 PRESIDENTIAL PRIMARIES

The preceding research shows the importance of understanding how those with a strong promotion or prevention focus evaluate choices that relate to possible future end-states and how the different ways they view these options are dependent both on their regulatory focus and on their perception of their current states relative to a psychological status quo "0." How might these findings be used to explain everyday phenomena? One example would be cases in the financial world, in which most investment advice tends to follow a "promotion-focused" set of investment tactics. Many managed portfolios associated with retirement or education funds are set up to purchase risky investments early and to switch to conservative investments as the final goal approaches (presumably, after years of gains have been achieved). This follows the findings with respect to the promotion focus in the domain of gains, noted earlier.

What about the domain of losses? In the lead-up to most major recessions, we find investors whom everyone tends to see as careful and cautious stewards of their investments suddenly risking, and losing, millions of dollars of their banks' money. Why would these careful investors behave in such a risky manner? One possibility was that the investors initially found that they had lost some money, and, in trying to restore this initial loss, they chose more risky investments. When they lost more money from these risky investments, they chose even more risky investments to recoup their losses . . . and so on and so on. This pattern is a fine example of a prevention-focused investor—careful and cautious—who finds himself down and wanting to recover his losses by taking whatever risks are necessary to do so.

Let us now consider more fully another example from recent political events. What happened in the 2016 Democratic and Republican primaries selecting who would compete in the election for President of the United States? It surprised and puzzled many pundits, and, of course, there are many plausible explanations that help us to understand what happened to some extent. We suggest that regulatory focus may also have played a role in what happened. In the 2016 primaries, each party, the Democrats and the Republicans, was split into two roughly evenly sized groups supporting two different kinds of candidates. Just as the value of different potential choices leading to different end-states is a product of participants' regulatory focus and their current positions relative to the psychological status quo, we believe that the cleavages within the Democrats and within the Republicans could be understood in terms of the regulatory focus of conservatives and liberals and their perceptions of their current states (at the time of voting) relative to the nation's status quo.

On the Republican side, the GOP electorate was relatively evenly divided between two more traditional Republican presidential candidates, Ted Cruz and John Kasich, on the one hand, and a very nontraditional candidate, Donald Trump, on the other. Everyone with an eye on politics seemed to be trying to understand what drove support for these different kinds of candidates. In particular, Donald Trump seemed like a risky candidate to put forward for President, especially when compared to the safer, more traditional candidates put forward in past elections, such as Mitt Romney and John McCain. What was going on? It is possible that our previous description of how the prevention focus works may provide some of the answer.

Those who are on the more conservative end of the political spectrum tend to have a stronger prevention focus than political liberals (Cornwell & Higgins, 2013). This prevention focus should typically be associated with the motivation to preserve and sustain the status quo with the adoption of conservative rather than risky tactics. This can be seen in the past selection of relatively safe and non-risky Presidential candidates with experience and clear track records of support for policies that preserve the American status quo against major internal and external threats. In past elections, this has led to the nomination of relatively safe and conservative (in the tactical sense) candidates for President in the GOP. Mitt Romney, John McCain, George W. Bush, Bob Dole, and others fit this persona. John Kasich in the 2016 election embodied this traditional approach. Ted Cruz may have been a more conservative version of this consensus and often used more strident rhetoric than Kasich, but he still generally comported himself in public in the traditions of a tactically conservative, safe candidate by sticking to the main ideological positions of the Republican Party platform without a major deviation.

Donald Trump represented a clear break from this historical Republican approach. His temperament and behavior were all very unlike anyone the Republican Party has put forward for President in the past, and yet he received the support of almost half of the GOP primary electorate, and eventually won the nomination. The difference between Trump supporters and supporters of more traditional candidates may actually have been partially motivational in nature and related to their perceptions of their positions relative to the status quo. Specifically, because the Republican electorate are generally prevention-focused conservatives, it is possible that those who preferred the more conservative tactic of choosing a more traditional candidate (i.e., Cruz, Kasich) perceived themselves and the nation as being at or close to the status quo, whereas those who preferred the more risky tactic of choosing a nontraditional candidate (i.e., Trump) perceived themselves and the nation as having fallen far below the status quo.

There are no data directly available to test this hypothesis, but it is notable that factors that significantly predicted which counties voted for Trump on Super Tuesday were higher unemployment, lower prevalence of college degrees, greater declines in manufacturing since 1999, and, most distressingly, a greater increase in the white mortality rate since 1999 (Guo, 2016). Each of these factors could signal to the voters that they were falling below the status quo that in previous times they had been able to maintain. However unlikely it was for Trump to succeed at that time in the primary campaign, his candidacy could have represented for them a means by which they could restore the status quo. Indeed, Trump's campaign theme was, "Make America Great Again." By saying "again," this motto presupposed that it is *not* great *now* as it was in the past. America being great was the status quo for these Americans, and this status quo had been lost. It was time to take any risk, including supporting a risky nontraditional candidate, to restore America's greatness (and restore their lives). A more traditional, conservative candidate such as Cruz or Kasich did not go far enough to restore the lost status quo. Thus these Republican voters' prevention orientation, combined with their perceptions of the current state as a "–1," far below a satisfactory status quo, motivated them to make the risky Trump choice when considering their future and the nation's future.

What, then, happened on the Democratic side? Hillary Clinton, for her part, made the case for her candidacy on her years of experience and her knowledge of the internal workings of government. She was the more traditional candidate, and choosing her was the conservative tactical choice. Bernie Sanders, in contrast, presented himself as a more radical candidate, one more closely in tune with the aspirational ideals of the Democratic Party than his opponent—a major advance to the "+1" dream. Indeed, Sanders referred to his campaign and purpose as starting "a political revolution."

This divide between Democratic liberals can again be understood in terms of a difference among Democratic voters in how they perceived the current state of themselves and the nation in relation to the status quo. To understand this difference, it is important to consider how these voters viewed the achievements of the Obama Administration. The research on regulatory focus and political ideology noted earlier found an association between the promotion focus and political liberalism (Cornwell & Higgins, 2013). Thus, generally speaking, political liberals were highly motivated to move to a state that is perceived as exceeding the current status quo. Barack Obama ran his 2008 candidacy on a platform of "hope and change," which are two elements very closely tied to the promotion focus. Many voters were motivated, therefore, to support the President in his efforts to move the country beyond the status quo toward what they perceived as a better state. The status quo of comparison for these voters would be when Barack Obama took office in 2008. The critical question from the perspective of these voters was: Have we advanced substantially beyond that status quo? Have we made real progress? We know from the findings of Zou et al. (2014), discussed earlier, that when promotion-focused individuals perceive that real progress has been made, they prefer tactically conservative options. This option would be Hillary Clinton. On the other hand, when they do *not* perceive that real progress has been made, they prefer tactically risky options. This option would be Bernie Sanders.

Again, there are no data directly collected that could be used to evaluate this question. However, exit polls have clearly shown that among those who wanted the next President to continue the policies begun under the Obama Administration (signifying a belief that these policies had provided substantial gains or real progress), Hillary Clinton led by a substantial margin (ABC News Analysis Desk, 2016). In contrast, among those who wanted to break with these policies in favor of more liberal ones (signifying a belief that these policies had *not* provided substantial gains or real progress), Bernie Sanders led by a substantial margin (ABC News Analysis Desk, 2016). Thus, like Republican voters, Democratic voters' regulatory focus orientation (promotion, in their case) interacted with their perceptions of their current state in relation to the status quo to influence their choice as President to ensure the future they wanted for themselves and the nation.

It is important once again to note that there were likely a multiplicity of factors going into any given individual's choice of whom to vote for in the 2016 presidential primaries, with an equivalent number of plausible explanations for this intriguing sociopolitical phenomenon. However, we felt it was worth highlighting because it so clearly illustrates the primary concern of this chapter: the dynamics surrounding promotion and prevention regulatory foci, their relations to the current state and the status quo, and the evaluation of potential future end-states as represented in choice options.

CONCLUSIONS AND FUTURE DIRECTIONS

Bringing the story full circle to the origins of regulatory focus theory, it is worth noting that the effects surrounding the status quo highlighted in this chapter are unsurprising when considering the growth of regulatory focus theory out of self-discrepancy theory. Self-discrepancy theory determined not only that different discrepancies (i.e., actual–ideal vs. actual–ought) result in different kinds of affect experiences, but also that the degree of discrepancy from those ideal and ought selves was related to the intensity of that experienced affect (Higgins, Bond, Klein, & Strauman, 1986). Similarly, theoretical developments in motivation by Carver and Scheier (1990, 1998) note that motivational intensity is often inversely related to the amount of progress toward the attainment of its associated goal (recall that "progress" acted as a mediator in one of the studies conducted by Zou et al., 2014).

Thus it is possible that a preference for the "risky" versus the "conservative" behavioral tactic derives, in part, from the degree of motivational intensity produced by how much one's current state deviates from one's desired end-state—that is, higher motivation from a greater discrepancy (or lower motivation from a smaller discrepancy) leads to a stronger (weaker) preference for a risky tactic; that is, when is it worth taking a chance? This is certainly consistent with the results previously discussed, as being in a state of loss creates *more* distance from the desired end-state of a prevention focus (i.e., non-loss), and thus more risk preference, whereas making progress creates *less* distance from the desired end-state of a promotion focus (i.e., gain), and thus less risk preference. It is also worth noting that the focus for which the domain was irrelevant (losses and non-losses for promotion; gains and non-gains for prevention) saw no consistent switching effects dependent upon one's position vis-à-vis the status quo. It needs to be emphasized, however, that, for the prevention focus, the shift from a conservative to a risky tactic occurred only when the risky option was the only option with the chance of achieving the goal of a restored status quo. Thus the story is not just about motivational intensity as a function of the distance from the desired end-state. Further research will be needed to understand better the underlying mechanisms for the choice preferences of promotion-focused and prevention-focused individuals as a function of the relation between the current state and the status quo.

Additional future research is also needed to address what occurs after these decisions are made. Many goal pursuits involve both the selection of means and the mustering of the motivation to implement those means in order to achieve the desired future end-states. There are ways in which manipulating one's sense of the status quo could not only change one's sense of the *progress* toward achieving one's goals, but also the amount of *commitment* one is willing to make in order to achieve them (see Fishbach & Dhar, 2005). For example, research on mental contrasting has shown that mentally comparing a potential desired future with one's current state can influence behavior change (Oettingen, 2012). There could be an important moderating effect of regulatory focus depending on whether one views the potential future as existing at, below, or above the status quo. For example, a prevention-focused individual may not be willing to invest commitment into behavior change if she or he mentally contrasts a future state that exceeds the status quo, particularly if such a change would prove difficult or would carry risks. Similarly, a promotion-focused individual may not be willing to invest commitment if he or she mentally contrasts a future positive state that is at the status quo. These possibilities could be examined given that Oettingen, Mayer, and Thorpe (2010), have found that mental contrasting can be used to enhance commitment to reach desired futures that exist at, below, or above the status quo.

Another question is whether people with a chronic promotion focus would spontaneously mentally contrast about improving the status quo and those with a prevention focus would spontaneously mentally contrast about keeping the status quo (Sevincer & Oettingen, 2013). If not, the use of implementation intentions (see Gollwitzer, 2014) may be the most effective way to bring about behavior change. People would not need to rely on the kinds of commitment that could arise out of a fit between a person's chronic focus and the potential future that the person mentally contrasts (see, e.g., Tam & Spanjol, 2011).

The manner in which people consider several possible options leading to potential future end-states and select one in particular over alternatives is one of the most studied aspects of human psychology. As we have shown, the degree to which individuals will have a preference for one possible choice over alternatives is a product of both individuals' regulatory focus *and* their perceptions of their current state relative to the status quo. Research has shown how the combination of these two factors is a critical element in decision making and can be used to help explain otherwise puzzling real-world phenomena. We have noted areas in which researchers, armed with this knowledge, can continue to advance our understanding of human choice and commitment to those choices. Our choices of which future end-states to pursue and how to pursue them are crucial aspects of what makes us human, and motivation science is one avenue by which we can better understand these critical capacities.

REFERENCES

ABC News Analysis Desk. (2016, March 15). Mini Super Tuesday Democratic exit poll analysis. *ABC News*. Retrieved from *http://abcnews.go.com/Politics/live-mini-super-tuesday-democratic-exit-poll-analysis/story?id=37666687*.

Avnet, T., & Higgins, E. T. (2006). How regulatory fit affects value in consumer choices and opinions. *Journal of Marketing Research, 43,* 1–10.

Baas, M., De Dreu, C. K. W., & Nijstad, B. A. (2011). When prevention promotes creativity: The role of mood, regulatory focus, and regulatory closure. *Journal of Personality and Social Psychology, 100,* 794–809.

Carver, C. S., & Scheier, M. F. (1990). Origins and functions of positive and negative affect: A control-process view. *Psychological Review, 97,* 19–35.

Carver, C. S., & Scheier, M. F. (1998). *On the self-regulation of behavior.* New York: Cambridge University Press.

Cornwell, J. F. M., & Higgins, E. T. (2013). Morality and its relation to political ideology: The role of promotion and prevention concerns. *Personality and Social Psychology Bulletin, 39,* 1164–1172.

Cornwell, J. F. M., & Higgins, E. T. (2016). Eager feelings and vigilant reasons: Regulatory focus differences in judging moral wrongs. *Journal of Experimental Psychology: General, 145,* 338–355.

Crowe, E., & Higgins, E. T. (1997). Regulatory focus and strategic inclinations: Promotion and prevention in decision-making. *Organizational Behavior and Human Decision Processes, 69,* 117–132.

Eitam, B., & Higgins, E. T. (2010). Motivation in mental accessibility: Relevance of a Representation (ROAR) as a new framework. *Social and Personality Psychology Compass, 4,* 951–967.

Fishbach, A., & Dhar, R. (2005). Goals as excuses or guides: The liberating effect of perceived goal progress on choice. *Journal of Consumer Research, 32,* 370–377.

Florack, A., & Hartmann, J. (2007). Regulatory focus and investment decisions in small groups. *Journal of Experimental Social Psychology, 43,* 626–632.

Franks, B., Higgins, E. T., & Champagne, F. A. (2012). Evidence for individual differences in regulatory focus in rats, *Rattus norvegicus. Journal of Comparative Psychology, 126,* 347–354.

Franks, B., Reiss, D., Cole, P., Friedrich, V., Thompson, N., & Higgins, E. T. (2013). Predicting how individuals approach enrichment: Regulatory focus in cotton-top tamarins (*Sanguinus oedipus*). *Zoo Biology, 32,* 427–435.

Freitas, A. L., & Higgins, E. T. (2002). Enjoying goal-directed action: The role of regulatory fit. *Psychological Science, 13,* 1–6.

Friedman, R. S., & Förster, J. (2000). The effects of approach and avoidance motor actions on the elements of creative insight. *Journal of Personality and Social Psychology, 79,* 477–492.

Friedman, R. S., & Förster, J. (2001). The effects of promotion and prevention cues on creativity. *Journal of Personality and Social Psychology, 81,* 1001–1013.

Gino, F., & Margolis, J. D. (2011). Bringing ethics into focus: How regulatory focus and risk preferences influence (un)ethical behavior. *Organizational Behavior and Human Decision Processes, 115,* 145–156.

Gollwitzer, P. M. (2014). Weakness of the will: Is a quick fix possible? *Motivation and Emotion, 38,* 305–322.

Guo, J. (2016, March 4). Death predicts whether people vote for Donald Trump. *The Washington Post.* Retrieved from *www.washingtonpost.com/news/wonk/wp/2016/03/04/death-predicts-whether-people-vote-for-donald-trump.*

Hamstra, M. R., Bolderdijk, J. W., & Veldstra, J. L. (2011). Everyday risk taking as a function of regulatory focus. *Journal of Research in Personality, 45,* 134–137.

Higgins, E. T. (1987). Self-discrepancy: A theory relating self and affect. *Psychological Review, 94,* 319–340.

Higgins, E. T. (1997). Beyond pleasure and pain. *American Psychologist, 52,* 1280–1300.

Higgins, E. T. (1998). Promotion and prevention: Regulatory focus as a motivational principle. In M. P. Zanna (Ed.), *Advances in experimental social psychology* (Vol. 30, pp. 1–46). New York: Academic Press.

Higgins, E. T. (2001). Promotion and prevention experiences: Relating emotions to non-emotional motivational states. In J. P. Forgas (Ed.), *Handbook of affect and social cognition* (pp. 186–211). Mahwah, NJ: Erlbaum.

Higgins, E. T. (2005). Humans as applied motivation scientists: Self-consciousness from "shared reality" and "becoming." In H. S. Terrace & J. Metcalfe (Eds.), *The missing link in cognition: Origins of self-reflective consciousness* (pp. 157–173). New York: Oxford University Press.

Higgins, E. T. (2014). Promotion and prevention: How "0" can create dual motivational forces. In J. W. Sherman, B. Gawronski, & Y. Trope (Eds.), *Dual-process theories of the social mind* (pp. 423–438). New York: Guilford Press.

Higgins, E. T., Bond, R. N., Klein, R., & Strauman, T. (1986). Self-discrepancies and emotional vulnerability: How magnitude, accessibility, and type of discrepancy influence affect. *Journal of Personality and Social Psychology, 51,* 5–15.

Higgins, E. T., & Cornwell, J. F. M. (2016). Securing foundations and advancing frontiers: Prevention and promotion effects on judgment and decision making. *Organizational Behavior and Human Decision Processes, 136,* 56–67.

Higgins, E. T., Friedman, R. S., Harlow, R. E., Idson, L. C., Ayduk, O. N., & Taylor, A. (2001). Achievement orientations from subjective histories of success: Promotion pride versus prevention pride. *European Journal of Social Psychology, 31,* 3–23.

Higgins, E. T., Klein, R., & Strauman, T. (1985). Self-concept discrepancy theory: A psychological model for distinguishing among different aspects of depression and anxiety. *Social Cognition, 3,* 51–76.

Higgins, E. T., Shah, J., & Friedman, R. (1997). Emotional responses to goal attainment: Strength of regulatory focus as moderator. *Journal of Personality and Social Psychology, 72,* 515–525.

Idson, L. C., & Higgins, E. T. (2000). How current feedback and chronic effectiveness influence motivation: Everything to gain versus everything to lose. *European Journal of Social Psychology, 30,* 583–592.

Kahneman, D., Knetsch, J. L., & Thaler, R. H. (1991). Anomalies: The endowment effect, loss aversion, and status quo bias. *Journal of Economic Perspectives, 5,* 193–206.

Levine, J. M., Higgins, E. T., & Choi, H.-S. (2000). Development of strategic norms in groups. *Organizational Behavior and Human Decision Processes, 82,* 88–101.

Liberman, N., Idson, L. C., Camacho, C. J., & Higgins, E. T. (1999). Promotion and prevention choices between stability and change. *Journal of Personality and Social Psychology, 77,* 1135–1145.

Oettingen, G. (2012). Future thought and behaviour change. *European Review of Social Psychology, 23,* 1–63.

Oettingen, G., Mayer, D., & Thorpe, J. (2010). Self-regulation of commitment to reduce cigarette consumption: Mental contrasting of future with reality. *Psychology and Health, 25,* 961–977.

Pham, M. T., & Avnet, T. (2004). Ideals and oughts and the reliance on affect versus substance in persuasion. *Journal of Consumer Research, 30,* 503–518.

Schnall, S., Haidt, J., Clore, G. L., & Jordan, A. H. (2008). Disgust as embodied moral judgment. *Personality and Social Psychology Bulletin, 34,* 1096–1108.

Scholer, A. A., Zou, X., Fujita, K., Stroessner, S. J., & Higgins, E. T. (2010). When risk-seeking becomes a motivational necessity. *Journal of Personality and Social Psychology, 99,* 215–231.

Sevincer, A. T., & Oettingen, G. (2013). Spontaneous mental contrasting and selective goal pursuit. *Personality and Social Psychology Bulletin, 39,* 1240–1254.

Summerville, A., & Roese, N. J. (2008). Self-report measures of individual differences in regulatory focus: A cautionary note. *Journal of Research in Personality, 42,* 247–254.

Tam, L., & Spanjol, J. (2012). When impediments make you jump rather than stumble: Regulatory nonfit, implementation intentions, and goal attainment. *Marketing Letters, 23,* 93–107.

Wu, C., McMullen, J. S., Neubert, M. J., & Yi, X. (2008). The influence of leader regulatory focus on employee creativity. *Journal of Business Venturing, 23,* 587–602.

Zhang, S., Cornwell, J. F. M., & Higgins, E. T. (2013). Repeating the past: Prevention focus motivates repetition, even for unethical decisions. *Psychological Science, 25,* 179–187.

Zhang, S., Higgins, E. T., & Chen, G. (2011). Managing others like you were managed: How prevention focus motivates copying interpersonal norms. *Journal of Personality and Social Psychology, 100,* 647–663.

Zou, X., Scholer, A. A., & Higgins, E. T. (2014). In pursuit of progress: Promotion motivation and risk preference in the domain of gains. *Journal of Personality and Social Psychology, 106,* 183–201.

CHAPTER 23

To Approach or to Avoid

Integrating the Biopsychosocial Model of Challenge
and Threat with Theories from Affective Dynamics
and Motivation Science

Jeremy P. Jamieson
Andrew J. Elliot

A fundamental, evolved process is the ability to assess the adaptive significance of environmental stimuli and respond accordingly (e.g., Orians & Heerwagen, 1992). Even single-cell organisms approach hospitable and avoid harmful stimuli (Schneirla, 1959). In humans, multiple psychological processes, including (but not limited to) appraisals, beliefs, and goals, are involved in evaluating and assessing external and internal cues and directing downstream behaviors. In fact, a common theme across myriad models of attention, motivation, emotion, and health is explaining why, how, and when humans approach appetitive stimuli and avoid aversive stimuli.

To achieve a deep understanding of approach and avoidance motivation, we argue for an integrative approach to psychological science—advancing research by synthesizing and consolidating existing models. Toward this end, the current chapter uses the biopsychosocial (BPS) model of challenge and threat as a nexus for integrating research on the extended process model of emotion regulation, implicit theories, and achievement goals to elucidate how psychological factors feed-forward to produce approach and avoidance responses both immediately and in the future.

A focus on "future" processes is integral to the BPS model of challenge and threat and, indeed, is integral to any motivationally oriented model of human behavior. Anticipated positive and negative possibilities and their associated implications energize and orient individuals in an appetitive or aversive manner. Once energized, individuals commonly direct their behavior proactively by pursuing goals and strategies that help them attend to their desires and fears (Elliot &

Covington, 2001; Higgins, 2013; Lewin, 1935). The behavior of even basic organisms is influenced by anticipated future possibilities, but the hallmark of human behavior is the complexity and flexibility of future-based thinking, planning, and acting (Cacioppo, Gardner, & Berntson, 1997; Tolman, 1932).

The BPS Model of Challenge and Threat

Before outlining some avenues of integration, we first provide an overview of the BPS model of challenge and threat. BPS models, broadly construed, were initially formulated by George Engle at the University of Rochester in 1977 and are influential in medicine, health, and affective science. BPS models posit that psychological processes, situational factors, and biological systems interact to determine health and behavioral outcomes. In medicine and clinical science, BPS models afford a means for physicians and clinicians to understand how subjective experiences and psychological processes contribute to diagnosing and treating mental and physical health problems (see Borrell-Carrió, Suchman, & Epstein, 2004, for a review). In affective science, the *BPS model of challenge and threat* focuses on motivational processes of approach and avoidance to understand acute stress responses (see Blascovich, 2008; Jamieson, 2017; Seery, 2011, for reviews).

Challenge and threat theory has roots in Lazarus and colleagues' *appraisal theory of emotion* (see Lazarus & Folkman, 1991, for a review), which argued that multiple processes, such as sensory information from the body, past experiences and expectations regarding future events, and situational factors contribute to how individuals appraise environmental stimuli, which then direct subsequent emotional experience (e.g., Lazarus, DeLongis, Folkman, & Gruen, 1985). Two levels (or stages) of appraisal processes were delineated: *primary* and *secondary* (Folkman, Lazarus, Dunkel-Schetter, DeLongis, & Gruen, 1986). Primary appraisals indicate whether anything important is at stake (i.e., does the situation matter for well-being?), and secondary appraisals evaluate coping options to minimize harm and/or maximize gain (Lazarus & Folkman, 1991).

Primary appraisals are not "primary" because they always come first in the temporal sequence; rather, they are primary because they confer personal relevance and signal that the situation has the *potential* to elicit emotional responses (Lazarus & Smith, 1988). Moreover, primary and secondary appraisals can be interdependent (Lazarus & Folkman, 1984). For example, primary appraisals might suggest a threatening situation with the potential for harm, such as staring down a steep, icy ski slope. However, if secondary appraisals indicate that one can cope with the threat, such as through skiing expertise and experience, then threat is diminished. Alternatively, challenging situations can become threatening if coping resources are not sufficient to meet perceived demands. For instance, consider a high-achieving student about to take a final exam in a course. Because of her or his high level of prior performance throughout the semester, this situation may be initially appraised as challenging. However, she or he did not study at all for this particular exam. So, during the test, secondary appraisal processes indicate that the student does not have the knowledge to perform well, eliciting threat (Jamieson, Hangen, Lee, & Yeager, 2017).

Building on the appraisal model, researchers sought to ground *challenge* and *threat* cognitions and responses in physiological systems, which led to the development of the BPS model of challenge and threat (e.g., Blascovich, 1992). In Lazarus's appraisal model, "challenge" and "threat" referred to primary appraisals rooted in perceptions of gain (challenge) and loss (threat) potential, and secondary appraisals assessed coping and response options. The BPS model of challenge and threat integrated these levels of appraisals that produced challenge or threat responses: coping resources > situational demands = challenge; situational demands > coping resources = threat. Based on the ratio of demand to resource appraisals, responses can fall anywhere on the continuum from extreme challenge to extreme threat (and in between). The motivational distinction between challenge and threat responses is rooted in this resource–demand ratio. Challenge states are presented as approach motivated and threat states as avoidance motivated. That is, when one appraises coping resources to exceed the demands presented by the situation, these cognitive processes direct the body to enact approach-oriented responses and behaviors, whereas when demands exceed resources, the body enacts avoidance-oriented responses and behaviors (e.g., Beltzer, Nock, Peters, & Jamieson, 2014; Jamieson & Mendes, 2016; Jamieson, Valdesolo, & Peters, 2014).

However, the specific *content* of the resource and demand appraisals in the BPS model of challenge and threat varies substantially across situations and people (see Blascovich & Mendes, 2000, for a review). For example, resource appraisals could include perceptions of knowledge, ability, or skills that are independent of perceptions of demands such as danger, difficulty, or effort. Consider a student taking an important mathematics exam. This student has performed well in previous math courses and considers him- or herself as being knowledgeable in mathematics. However, when receiving the exam, the student perceives that these particular questions are at the limit of (or even exceed) his or her ability and will take a lot of effort to complete successfully. In such a situation, resource appraisals would be high (ability/knowledge), but demand appraisals would also be high (difficulty/effort).

Alternatively, appraisals can index bipolar factors. For instance, familiarity–uncertainty or safety–danger factors represent anchors along a single continuum, and one's placement on these bipolar continua impact both resources *and* demands: As familiarity increases and uncertainty decreases, resource appraisals increase and demand appraisals decrease (Blascovich, 2008). Referring back to the example of the student taking a difficult math exam, the student could be differentially familiar with multiple types of problems (e.g., Is the test composed of word problems or equations?) that could appear on the exam. If the student has little experience completing mathematics word problems, she or he may be more likely to appraise high demands and lower resources if, upon being handed the exam, she or he sees that the test is composed solely of unfamiliar word problems.

In the BPS model of challenge and threat appraisal, processes elicit differential physiological response patterns, which influence subsequent cognitive appraisals and/or feed-forward to affect behavioral outputs (see Blascovich & Mendes, 2010, for a review). To provide a brief summary, both challenge and threat responses are accompanied by activation of the sympathetic–adrenal–medullary (SAM) axis, but threat also strongly activates the hypothalamic–pituitary–adrenal (HPA) axis.

Thus, when individuals appraise challenge, the production of catecholamines resulting from SAM activation increases ventricular contractility (increasing heart rate), constricts veins (facilitating return of blood to the heart), and elicits vasodilation (decreasing resistance in the peripheral vasculature; Brownley, Hurwitz, & Schneiderman, 2000). More downstream, these changes are indicated by increased cardiac output (e.g., Blascovich, Mendes, Hunter, & Salomon, 1999). On the other hand, when individuals appraise threat, HPA axis activation tempers SAM effects, resulting in reduced (or little change in) cardiac output and increased resistance in the peripheral vasculature (for reviews, see Blascovich, 2008; Blascovich & Mendes, 2010; Seery, 2011).

The BPS model of challenge and threat maps the sequence of responses in *specific* motivated-performance situations. However, the world does not exist as a sequence of distinct, well-defined situations that are mutually exclusive of one another. Rather, processes (cognitive, affective, physiological, and behavioral) at one time can influence how the individual engages with and responds to subsequent situations she or he encounters both immediately and far into the future. Thus, appraisal processes—and challenge and threat responses—should not be conceptualized as static, only applicable to particular situations. Rather, these motivated responses are dynamic. Factors that modify or change responses in one situation can have far-reaching effects (e.g., Jamieson, Mendes, Blackstock, & Schmader, 2010; Jamieson, Peters, Greenwood, & Altose, 2016; Yeager, Lee, & Jamieson, 2016). Along these lines, we suggest that future avenues of research should seek to more fully synthesize BPS-derived challenge–threat appraisals and responses with dynamic models of emotion regulation, such as Gross's (2015) extended process model.

THE EXTENDED PROCESS MODEL OF EMOTION REGULATION

Recent updates to the classic process model of emotion regulation (e.g., Gross, 2002) emphasize the temporal dynamics of appraisal processes for determining affective or emotional responses (see Gross, 2015, for a review). Central to this extended process model is the notion that a valuation system—demand and resource appraisals are types of valuation appraisals—can be activated for extended periods of time to shape future outcomes (Ochsner & Gross, 2014). To illustrate, attributes of the external environment ("the World" in the extended process model) necessitate engagement of Perceptual processes (or selective attention to salient environmental cues). Perceptions then trigger Valuations (attributions, appraisals, etc.), which produce Action outputs (behaviors, decisions, physiological responses, etc.). Targets of Actions are attributes of "the World," and resulting changes in situational factors lead to a second cycle that is Perceived, Valued, and Acted upon (e.g., Sheppes, Suri, & Gross, 2015). This cyclical process then repeats itself over time. For instance, a Valuation process at Cycle 1 can "snowball" to influence processes in future cycles (see Figure 23.1). Such a regulatory system helps explain how appraisal-based cognitive-behavioral therapies can have long-lasting benefits (e.g., Barrett, Duffy, Dadds, & Rapee, 2001).

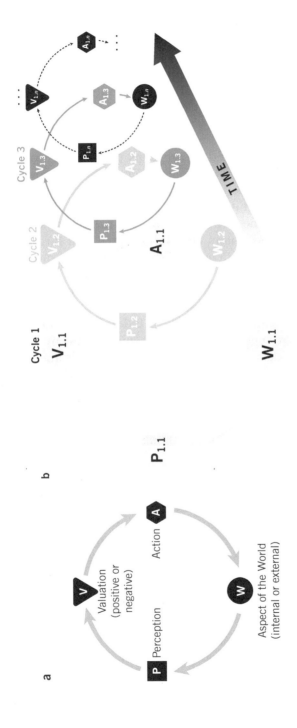

FIGURE 23.1. (a) The World (W) (notably, motivated-performance situations) gives rise to Perception (P) processes that include orienting responses. Valuations (V) based on perceptions give rise to Actions (A), which alter situational factors (i.e., "the World"). (b) Valuation processes, which include appraisals, unfold over time to shape behavioral and cognitive outputs/processes into the future (see Cycles 1, 2, 3, etc.), as shown in the spiral depiction. Adapted from Gross (2015); Oschner and Gross (2014); and Sheppes, Suri, and Gross (2015).

To synthesize the BPS model of challenge and threat with this extended process model, BPS-derived demand–resource appraisals integrate well with Valuation processes in the cyclical emotion regulation and experience chain. That is, people first assess whether situations constitute a motivated performance context that requires instrumental responding (similar to primary appraisals in Lazarus's model) and then weigh perceived demands against perceived coping resources to determine whether to respond with approach-motivated challenge or avoidance-motivated threat. Thus, the "value" of appraisals for the organism is to orient motivated behavior—either approach or avoidance in a basic sense.

However, we emphasize that the Valuation system is not *only* composed of appraisals of demands and resources. The complex human Valuation system includes myriad processes, and even appraisals are not singular operations. For instance, appraising whether one possesses sufficient coping resources to address demands in a given motivated-performance situation involves multiple cognitive operations, including (but not limited to) orienting attention toward demanding aspects of the situation, engaging "self" processes for assessing self-relevance, recalling episodic memories of past (if any) experiences of similar situations, and using prefrontal processes to sustain goals and "meaning" in the case of reappraisal (see Ochsner, Silvers, & Buhle, 2012; Schmitz & Johnson, 2007; Silvers, Buhle, & Ochsner, 2013, for reviews and similar arguments). Thus a myriad of cognitive factors interact to determine how individuals evaluate their place in a given situation and enact regulation strategies (see also Webb, Schweiger Gallo, Miles, Gollwitzer, & Sheeran, 2012).

The multiple cognitive operations inherent in the Valuation system allow multiple, flexible response options both across people and within people across time given the same environmental inputs. To illustrate, whereas one person might exhibit challenge in an acute stress situation, another could respond with threat based primarily on differences in appraisals of demands and resources (see Jamieson, Mendes, & Nock, 2013, for a review). Then previous challenge–threat responses (which are based on appraisals) could alter the content of future appraisals. For example, if a student appraises demands as exceeding resources in one math evaluation context, she or he will respond with avoidance-motivated threat and is likely to perform poorly. Then, when the student encounters a future math testing situation, her or his demand and resource appraisals will be shaped by this previous experience—the domain of math could be perceived as more demanding and knowledge/ability as insufficient. In fact, the aforementioned reciprocal process could help explain high levels of math anxiety and the dearth of women and minorities in science, technology, engineering, and mathematics (STEM) professions in American society (e.g., Jamieson et al., 2016; Putwain, Daly, Chamberlain, & Sadreddini, 2016; Putwain, Sander, & Larkin, 2013).

By placing BPS-derived appraisal processes in the context of the extended process model of emotion regulation, we can begin to understand how (brief) reappraisal interventions can exert long(er)-term effects on behavior and performance. For instance, recent studies have provided initial support for the notion that changing appraisals (valuations) at one time can improve future affective responses in subsequent social stress contexts (e.g., Jamieson et al., 2010; Jamieson et al., 2016). In this line of research, the arousal experienced during stressful situations is reappraised as a functional *coping resource* that aids performance. That is, signs of stress arousal are reinterpreted as coping tools, which facilitate challenge appraisals to affect subsequent physiological, affective, and motivational processes.

One of the first studies in this line of inquiry tested the effects of appraisals on Graduate Record Examination (GRE) performance in the lab and then 1–3 months later in the field (Jamieson et al., 2010). During an initial lab session, participants were randomly assigned to receive reappraisal instructions (vs. no instructions) and then performed a GRE practice test. Reappraisal participants outperformed controls on the quantitative section of the GRE. Then, 1–3 months later, participants provided their score reports from their actual GREs. Reappraisal participants again outperformed controls on the quantitative section without any boosters delivered after the lab session. Extending findings to the classroom, a double-blind experiment at a community college demonstrated that teaching students to appraise their stress arousal as a coping tool reduced test anxiety and improved exam performance by increasing perceptions of coping ability (Jamieson et al., 2016). Thus reappraisal instructions improved future academic outcomes through (presumably) reciprocal processes highlighted by the extended process model: Changing valuations at Cycle 1 altered responses at Cycle 1, which then fed forward to improve perceptions, valuations, and responses at Cycle 2, and so forth.

Existing research on stress reappraisal manipulations derived from the BPS model of challenge and threat, however, has most frequently focused on measuring physiological and cognitive effects in the short term within a given domain (e.g., Beltzer et al., 2014; Jamieson, Nock, & Mendes, 2013); the long-term, iterative effects of reappraisal remain speculative and need future research attention. In addition to affecting future psychological, physiological, and behavioral functioning via dynamic appraisal processes, it is possible that more "meta level" belief systems—which themselves could remain stable—may affect multiple situations both in the present and the future. In this regard, *implicit theories of personality* hold great promise for integration with the BPS model of challenge and threat.

IMPLICIT THEORIES OF PERSONALITY

Implicit theories are typically classified as representing *entity* or *incremental* beliefs (see Dweck & Leggett, 1988). An individual holding an entity theory endorses the belief that personality, intelligence, and other characteristics are fixed and immutable. This belief system asserts that the domain or attribute of interest can remain stable across situations and over time. For instance, an entity theorist believes that people are innately intelligent or not and that intellectual ability does not grow or improve with study and hard work in academics. Alternatively, an individual who holds an *incremental* theory believes in the potential for growth and change in traits, intelligence, and so forth. So, rather than endorsing the belief that people are either smart or not smart, the incremental theorist believes that intelligence grows (and/or diminishes) throughout the lifespan based on engagement, studying and learning, and approaching new knowledge and experiences.

Previous research highlights the negative consequences of holding an entity theory. For instance, in an entity theory of personality, social threats are viewed as diagnostic of long-term, lasting social realities. Thus, from a BPS perspective, the entity theorist should appraise negative evaluative social stress situations as highly demanding because status or reputation hangs in the balance, but he or she may also perceive such situations as exceeding coping resources because no amount of resources can overcome a fixed, deficient identity. Hence appraisals of demands exceed resources—producing the experience of threat. Moreover, this entity theory can "bleed over" into other social situations and domains, potentially negatively affecting close relationships, academic and career success, and/or civic engagement, to name a few possibilities. On the other hand, an incremental theory of personality—the belief that people can grow and change—prevents "fixed" trait attributions. Social evaluative stress (e.g., peer exclusion or victimization) is not seen as permanent because coping resources and situational demands (traits, ability, people) are malleable. Thus experiences of social adversity may be seen as opportunities for improvement (Yeager, Trzesniewski, & Dweck, 2013).

Developing methods to instill a more incremental theory of personality has the potential to improve responses across multiple social domains (and across time). Along these lines, two double-blind, randomized, placebo-controlled experiments (a laboratory study and a longitudinal field experiment) tested whether manipulating implicit theories of personality could improve stress appraisals and stress responses as defined by the BPS model of challenge and threat (Yeager et al., 2016). In Study 1, adolescents were randomly assigned to receive either incremental theory of personality (IToP)—the belief that people have the potential to change—or control instructions before completing a stressful speech task that included negative social feedback. Relative to controls, the IToP instructions decreased appraisals of task demands (the negative social situation was appraised as more manageable), increased resource appraisals (adolescents perceived that they could better cope with the stressor), and improved in vivo physiological and behavioral responses (i.e., better speech task performance). Thus the implicit theories intervention successfully operated on situation-specific stress appraisals as outlined by the BPS model to improve stress responses. Notably, the process through which an implicit theory of personality enacted positive change (i.e., stress appraisals) was similar to how the aforementioned arousal reappraisal approach improved acute stress responses.

Study 2 extended findings to a naturalistic setting and examined medium- and long-term future effects of altering implicit theories beliefs. Ninth-grade students were randomly assigned to complete either an IToP intervention or control materials the first week of the semester, along with a baseline saliva sample assayed for cortisol—a catabolic stress hormone that is the end product of HPA activation. A week after the intervention, students reported daily stressful events and stress appraisals using a diary method, and cortisol was again assayed with follow-up saliva samples. Final grades were tracked 7 months later. The IToP intervention attenuated HPA-axis activation a week later (lower cortisol levels) on high-stress days, and also improved academic performance (GPA) 7 months later. Taken together, the data from this set of studies provided the first direct test of a synthesis of BPS and implicit theories models. Supporting this integrative approach, manipulating global beliefs about the capacity for people to grow and change directly affects situation-specific appraisal processes relevant to challenge–threat response patterns.

As depicted in Figure 23.2, implicit theories may be conceptualized as a "lens" through which to understand situation-specific challenge–threat appraisal processes

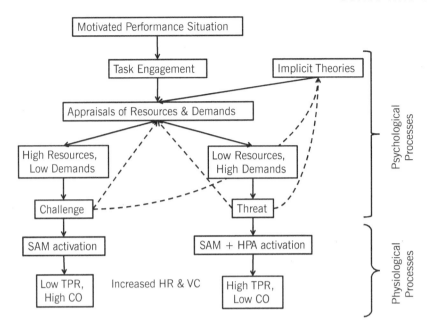

FIGURE 23.2. Integration of BPS and implicit theories models: Implicit theories are general belief systems depicted as operating on the appraisal processes delineated in the BPS model of challenge and threat. Dashed lines represent feedback (feed-forward) processes: Challenge–threat states are hypothesized to influence subsequent appraisals and beliefs. SAM, sympathetic–adrenal–medullary axis; HPA, hypothalamic–pituitary–adrenal axis; TPR, total peripheral resistance; CO, cardiac output; SV, stroke volume.

and subsequent motivated behavior. For instance, if one perceives resources (ability, intelligence, social coping, etc.) as fixed in a given domain (an entity theory in that domain—such as in an entity theory of personality), then challenge–threat appraisals will be particularly sensitive to perceptions of demands. That is, the "action" will be rooted in the demand side of the demand–resource ratio. Furthermore, appraisal-based interventions that target resource appraisals could also be moderated by implicit theories (i.e., less effective for those holding an entity theory).

However, in an incremental theory, the attributes of the lens may change, and this "shifting lens" could lead to (and subsequently be affected by) lower demand appraisals and increased resource appraisals. Thus the hypothesized integrative model (Figure 23.2) includes "feedback" paths (though feed-forward in a temporal sense), whereby *experiences* of motivated challenge–threat responses at one time point or in one situation can influence *future* beliefs and appraisals. However, as with hypothesized integrations of the BPS model and the extended process model of emotion regulation, no research has tested these cyclical paths.

In achievement or motivated-performance situations (the focus of the BPS model of challenge and threat), individuals not only have different theories or beliefs about intelligence or competence, but they also adopt and pursue different goals regarding competence. Thus a complete, integrated model of approach–avoidance motivation in any domain must account for this intentional, conative form of self-regulation. Specifically, consideration of the *achievement goal* construct vis-à-vis the BPS model may help shed new light on basic BPS processes.

ACHIEVEMENT GOALS

An achievement goal is a cognitive representation of a future competence-based possibility that one is committed to approach or avoid (Elliot & Fryer, 2008). Achievement goals vary according to two components: how competence is defined and how competence is valenced. Competence is defined in terms of the evaluative standard—the task/self or others—and competence is valenced in that it may be construed in terms of a positive possibility to approach (competence) or a negative possibility to avoid (incompetence). Crossing these two components produces four basic achievement goals in a 2 × 2 model (Elliot, 1999): mastery-approach goals (focused on doing well relative to task requirements or one's own performance trajectory), performance-approach goals (focused on doing well relative to others), mastery-avoidance goals (focused on not doing poorly relative to task requirements or one's own performance trajectory), and performance-avoidance goals (focused on not doing poorly relative to others). We suggest achievement goals and appraisals could interact to determine challenge (approach)–threat (avoidance) responses (see Figure 23.3). Below we review research supporting this possible integration.

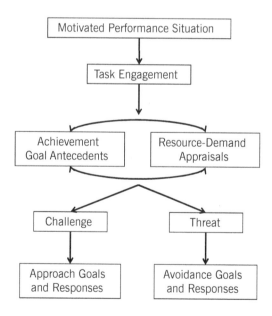

FIGURE 23.3. Hypothesized integration of BPS-derived appraisal processes and achievement goals. Note that the hypothetical model focuses only on psychological processes as delineated by the BPS model of challenge and threat. It does not include paths predicting physiological responses and feedback mechanisms, such as embodiment processes, from physiological–behavioral responses to psychological operations (for a review of those processes, see Blascovich & Mendes, 2010).

Achievement goals are situation-specific self-regulatory processes that emerge from dispositional and situational antecedents. Dispositional antecedents of achievement goals include variables such as need for achievement and fear of failure, whereas situational antecedents include variables such as task-based and normative evaluative structures (Elliot & Hulleman, 2017). These antecedent variables are presumed to influence (and may be influenced by) situational appraisals, which in turn lead to motivated responses such as challenge and threat, and accompanying achievement goals (Figure 23.3).

Once achievement goals are instantiated, they can then create a framework through which one interprets and experiences future achievement situations (Ames, 1992; Dweck, 1986; Nicholls, 1984; on the functionality of goals more generally, see Gollwitzer, 2014; Oettingen, 2012). Thus, regardless of the source of achievement goal adoption, the commitment to pursue a particular goal is thought to influence a multitude of affective, cognitive, and behavioral processes and outcomes. For example, in one set of studies, the positive focus stemming from mastery-approach and performance-approach goals of attaining academic competence was linked to appraising a specific course or exam as a challenge, and the negative focus stemming from performance-avoidance goals of not performing worse than others was linked to appraising the specific course or exam as a threat (McGregor & Elliot, 2002).

As with cyclical emotion-regulation processes (Gross, 2015), most achievement scenarios are not one-off experiences, but instead represent extended sequences. Thus, coping with these stressors is best viewed as a dynamic process (McGregor & Elliot, 2002). With regard to integrating goals and appraisals, achievement goals may operate as both antecedents of resource–demand appraisals and consequences of challenge–threat responses. Moreover, it is possible that goals serve both these roles sequentially and reciprocally. It is important to note, however, that the extant research on achievement goals and appraisals has focused almost exclusively on self-reported challenge and threat experiences, not BPS-derived resource and demand appraisals. Thus, additional research is needed to elucidate the interaction between goals and demand–resource appraisals in motivated-performance contexts.

Integration of achievement goals into the BPS model of challenge and threat also raises additional questions in need of empirical attention. For example, in the BPS model, approach-motivated challenge and avoidance-motivated threat are psychological states that act as anchors on a continuum of potential stress responses; one may be highly challenged (approach motivated), highly threatened (avoidance motivated), or anywhere in between. However, it is not possible to be highly challenged *and* highly threatened simultaneously at a single point in time. In contrast, in the achievement goal literature, multiple goal adoption is common. In fact, approach and avoidance goals may even be held at the *same time* (Law, Elliot, & Murayama, 2012). It would be interesting to explore how this apparent motivational ambivalence manifests at the physiological level within the BPS model and whether the physiological indicators of challenge and threat may be used to better understand the often high correlation observed between performance-approach and performance-avoidance achievement goals.

To illustrate, consider a student taking an exam. She or he could hold an approach goal stemming from the belief that she or he is highly knowledgeable in that particular domain but hold an avoidance goal rooted in the high difficulty of the particular exam items. As applied to the BPS model, such a scenario might elicit "indeterminate" downstream physiological responses defined by high levels of sympathetic arousal, but no clear challenge–threat autonomic response pattern (for an example, see Mendes, Reis, Seery, & Blascovich, 2003). In other words, the student might fall somewhere in the middle of the prototypical challenge–threat continuum because perceived resources and perceived demands are both high. Or challenge–threat responses to this scenario could be parsed temporally. That is, the student might begin the exam situation with a challenge response resulting from approach goals–high-resource appraisals, but then this response could transition in vivo to a more threat-oriented response because of avoidance goals–high-demand appraisals. Understanding the temporal sequence and dynamics of challenge and threat responses—and how these responses might be communicated between people (e.g., Waters, West, & Mendes, 2014)—is important for advancing research on the BPS model of challenge and threat and integrating and elucidating how goals and appraisals interact.

SUMMARY AND CONCLUSION

This chapter advocates for integrative science to advance psychological science. Toward this end, we started with the BPS model of challenge and threat and explored avenues through which this particular model may be integrated with influential theories in affective science, intervention research, and motivation. Not only was this exercise informative from the perspective of bridging models, but we believe this and similar efforts can be highly generative. Exploring how theories may be bridged has the potential to stimulate new research ideas and offer novel perspectives through which to understand existing data.

We emphasize, however, that the BPS model of challenge and threat is not some unique hub for *all* psychological integrations. Rather, this chapter represents an initial foray into how such integrations might be carried out. Once sufficient research has accumulated on the synthesis of particular models, it may then be possible to integrate the integrations to create more general models and facilitate the consolidation of major theories in psychology. Such an approach would be akin to meta-analytic researchers conducting a meta-analysis of meta-analyses (i.e. a mega-analysis). In the immediate future, the objective of the integrative exercise undertaken here (and future empirical studies resulting from this approach) is to advance psychological theory in novel and informative ways. Consolidating models that share common, or interactive, processes may also allow more accurate and process-focused predictions regarding future cognitions, emotions, and behaviors.

REFERENCES

Ames, C. (1992). Classrooms: Goals, structures, and student motivation. *Journal of Educational Psychology, 84,* 261–271.

Barrett, P. M., Duffy, A. L., Dadds, M. R., & Rapee, R. M. (2001). Cognitive-behavioral treatment of anxiety disorders in children: Long-term (6-year) follow-up. *Journal of Consulting and Clinical Psychology, 69,* 135–141.

Beltzer, M. L., Nock, M. K., Peters, B. J., & Jamieson, J. P. (2014). Rethinking butterflies: The affective, physiological, and performance effects of reappraising arousal during social evaluation. *Emotion, 14,* 761–768.

Blascovich, J. (1992). A biopsychosocial approach to arousal regulation. *Journal of Social and Clinical Psychology, 11,* 213–237.

Blascovich, J. (2008). Challenge and threat. In A. J. Elliot (Ed.), *Handbook of approach and avoidance motivation* (pp. 431–446). Mahwah, NJ: Erlbaum.

Blascovich, J., & Mendes, W. B. (2000). Challenge and threat appraisals: The role of affective cues. In J. Forgas (Ed.), *Feeling and thinking: The role of affect in social cognition* (pp. 59–82). New York: Cambridge University Press.

Blascovich, J., & Mendes, W. B. (2010). Social psychophysiology and embodiment. In S. T. Fiske, D. T. Gilbert, & G. Lindzey, *Handbook of social psychology* (Vol. 1, pp. 194–227). Hoboken, NJ: Wiley.

Blascovich, J., Mendes, W. B., Hunter, S. B., & Salomon, K. (1999). Social "facilitation" as challenge and threat. *Journal of Personality and Social Psychology, 77,* 68–77.

Borrell-Carrió, F., Suchman, A. L., & Epstein, R. M. (2004). The biopsychosocial model 25 years later: Principles, practice, and scientific inquiry. *Annals of Family Medicine, 2,* 576–582.

Brownley, K. A., Hurwitz, B. E., & Schneiderman, N. (2000). Cardiovascular psychophysiology. In J. T. Cacioppo, L. G. Tassinary, & G. G. Berntson (Eds.), *Handbook of psychophysiology* (2nd ed., pp. 224–264). New York: Cambridge University Press.

Cacioppo, J. T., Gardner, W. L., & Berntson, G. G. (1997). Beyond bipolar conceptualizations and measures: The case of attitudes and evaluative space. *Personality and Social Psychology Review, 1,* 3–25.

Dweck, C. S. (1986). Motivational processes affecting learning. *American Psychologist, 41,* 1040–1048.

Dweck, C. S., & Leggett, E. L. (1988). A social-cognitive approach to motivation and personality. *Psychological Review, 95,* 256–273.

Elliot, A. J., (1999). Approach and avoidance motivation and achievement goals. *Educational Psychologist, 34,* 149–169.

Elliot, A. J., & Covington, M. V. (2001). Approach and avoidance motivation. *Educational Psychology Review, 13,* 73–91.

Elliot, A. J., & Fryer, J. W. (2008). The goal concept in psychology. In J. Shah & W. Gardner (Eds.), *Handbook of motivational science* (pp. 235–250). New York: Guilford Press.

Elliot, A. J., & Hulleman, C. S. (2017). Achievement goals. In A. Elliot, C. Dweck, & D. Yeager (Eds.), *Handbook of competence and motivation: Theory and application* (2nd ed., pp. 43–60). New York: Guilford Press.

Folkman, S., Lazarus, R. S., Dunkel-Schetter, C., DeLongis, A., & Gruen, R. J. (1986). Dynamics of a stressful encounter: Cognitive appraisal, coping, and encounter outcomes. *Journal of Personality and Social Psychology, 50,* 992–1003.

Gollwitzer, P. M. (2014). Weakness of the will: Is a quick fix possible? *Motivation and Emotion, 38,* 305–322.

Gross, J. J. (2002). Emotion regulation: Affective, cognitive, and social consequences. *Psychophysiology, 39,* 281–291.

Gross, J. J. (2015). The extended process model of emotion regulation: Elaborations, applications, and future directions. *Psychological Inquiry, 26,* 130–137.

Higgins, E. T. (2013). *Beyond pleasure and pain: How motivation works.* Oxford, UK: Oxford University Press.

Jamieson, J. P. (2017). Challenge and threat appraisals. In A. Elliot, C. Dweck, & D. Yeager

(Eds.), *Handbook of competence and motivation: Theory and application* (2nd ed., pp. 175–191). New York: Guilford Press.

Jamieson, J. P., Hangen, E. J., Lee, H. Y., & Yeager, D. S. (2017). Capitalizing on appraisal processes to improve stress responses. *Emotion Review.*

Jamieson, J. P., & Mendes, W. B. (2016). Social stress facilitates risk in youths. *Journal of Experimental Psychology: General, 145,* 467–485.

Jamieson, J. P., Mendes, W. B., Blackstock, E., & Schmader, T. (2010). Turning the knots in your stomach into bows: Reappraising arousal improves performance on the GRE. *Journal of Experimental Social Psychology, 46,* 208–212.

Jamieson, J. P., Mendes, W. B., & Nock, M. K. (2013). Improving acute stress responses: The power of reappraisal. *Current Directions in Psychological Science, 22,* 51–56.

Jamieson, J. P., Nock, M. K., & Mendes, W. B. (2013). Changing the conceptualization of stress in social anxiety disorder: Affective and physiological consequences. *Clinical Psychological Science, 1*(4), 363–374.

Jamieson, J. P., Peters, B. P., Greenwood, E. J., & Altose, A. J. (2016). Reappraising stress arousal improves performance and reduces evaluation anxiety in classroom exam situations. *Social Psychological and Personality Science, 7,* 579–587.

Jamieson, J. P., Valdesolo, P., & Peters, B. J. (2014). Sympathy for the devil?: The physiological and psychological effects of being an agent (and target) of dissent during intragroup conflict. *Journal of Experimental Social Psychology, 55,* 221–227.

Law, W., Elliot, A. J., & Murayama, K. (2012). Perceived competence moderates the relation between performance-approach and performance-avoidance goals. *Journal of Educational Psychology, 104,* 806–819.

Lazarus, R. S., DeLongis, A., Folkman, S., & Gruen, R. (1985). Stress and adaptational outcomes: The problem of confounded measures. *American Psychologist, 40,* 770–779.

Lazarus, R. S., & Folkman, S. (1984). *Stress, appraisal, and coping.* New York: Springer.

Lazarus, R. S., & Folkman, S. (1991). The concept of coping. In A. Monat & R. S. Lazarus (Eds.), *Stress and coping: An anthology* (pp. 189–206). New York: Columbia University Press.

Lazarus, R. S., & Smith, C. A. (1988). Knowledge and appraisal in the cognition–emotion relationship. *Cognition and Emotion, 2,* 281–300.

Lewin, K. (1935). *A dynamic theory of personality.* New York: McGraw-Hill.

McGregor, H. A., & Elliot, A. J. (2002). Achievement goals as predictors of achievement-relevant processes prior to task engagement. *Journal of Educational Psychology, 94,* 381–395.

Mendes, W. B., Reis, H. T., Seery, M. D., & Blascovich, J. (2003). Cardiovascular correlates of emotional expression and suppression: Do content and gender context matter? *Journal of Personality and Social Psychology, 84,* 771–792.

Nicholls, J. G. (1984). Achievement motivation: Conceptions of ability, subjective experience, task choice, and performance. *Psychological Review, 91,* 328–346.

Ochsner, K. N., & Gross, J. J. (2014). The neural bases of emotion and emotion regulation: A valuation perspective. *Handbook of Emotion Regulation, 2,* 23–42.

Ochsner, K. N., Silvers, J. A., & Buhle, J. T. (2012). Functional imaging studies of emotion regulation: A synthetic review and evolving model of the cognitive control of emotion. *Annals of the New York Academy of Sciences, 1251,* E1–E24.

Oettingen, G. (2012). Future thought and behavior change. *European Review of Social Psychology, 23,* 1–63.

Orians, G. H., & Heerwagen, J. H. (1992). Evolved responses to landscapes. In J. H. Barkow, J. L. Cosmides, & J. Tooby (Eds.), *The adapted mind: Evolutionary psychology and the generation of culture* (pp. 555–579). New York: Oxford University Press.

Putwain, D. W., Daly, A. L., Chamberlain, S., & Sadreddini, S. (2016). "Sink or swim":

Buoyancy and coping in the cognitive test anxiety–academic performance relationship. *Educational Psychology, 36,* 1807–1825.

Putwain, D., Sander, P., & Larkin, D. (2013). Academic self-efficacy in study-related skills and behaviours: Relations with learning-related emotions and academic success. *British Journal of Educational Psychology, 83,* 633–650.

Schmitz, T. W., & Johnson, S. C. (2007). Relevance to self: A brief review and framework of neural systems underlying appraisal. *Neuroscience and Biobehavioral Reviews, 31,* 585–596.

Schneirla, T. (1959). An evolutionary and developmental theory of biphasic processes underlying approach and withdrawal. In M. Jones (Ed.), *Nebraska Symposium on Motivation* (pp. 1–42). Lincoln: University of Nebraska Press.

Seery, M. D. (2011). Challenge or threat?: Cardiovascular indexes of resilience and vulnerability to potential stress in humans. *Neuroscience and Biobehavioral Reviews, 35,* 1603–1610.

Sheppes, G., Suri, G., & Gross, J. J. (2015). Emotion regulation and psychopathology. *Annual Review of Clinical Psychology, 11,* 379–405.

Silvers, J. A., Buhle, J. T., & Ochsner, K. N. (2013). The neuroscience of emotion regulation: Basic mechanisms and their role in development, aging, and psychopathology. In K. N. Ochsner & S. Kosslyn (Eds.), *Oxford handbook of cognitive neuroscience: Vol. 2. The cutting edges* (pp. 52–78). New York: Oxford University Press.

Tolman, E. (1932). *Purposive behavior in animals and men.* New York: The Century.

Waters, S. F., West, T. V., & Mendes, W. B. (2014). Stress contagion: Physiological covariation between mothers and infants. *Psychological Science, 25,* 934–942.

Webb, T. L., Schweiger Gallo, I., Miles, E., Gollwitzer, P. M., & Sheeran, P. (2012). Effective regulation of affect: An action control perspective on emotion regulation. *European Review of Social Psychology, 23,* 143–186.

Yeager, D., Lee, H. Y., & Jamieson, J. P. (2016). Changing a simple belief alters adolescents' cardiovascular and neuroendocrine responses to social stress. *Psychological Science, 27,* 1078–1091.

Yeager, D. S., Trzesniewski, K. H., & Dweck, C. S. (2013). An implicit theories of personality intervention reduces adolescent aggression in response to victimization and exclusion. *Child Development, 84,* 970–988.

CHAPTER 24

Anticipating and Overcoming Unethical Temptation

Oliver J. Sheldon
Ayelet Fishbach

Although most people care deeply about maintaining a moral self-image, preserving a sense of integrity, and being perceived as ethical by others, people also commonly behave in ways that put these valued goals at risk. From education to sports to politics, bending ethical rules or behaving dishonestly for personal gain is commonplace. Although most unethical behavior is relatively minor in scale (Mazar, Amir, & Ariely, 2008), its prevalence is nevertheless concerning, for, in aggregate, even minor transgressions can cause significant social and economic damage. For instance, widespread academic dishonesty can raise doubts among employers about the value of a college degree (Happel & Jennings, 2008), and rampant tax evasion and corruption can deprive countries of billions of dollars in much-needed revenue (Cebula & Feige, 2012).

What explains why people sometimes succumb to ethical temptations (e.g., dishonesty, opportunities to cheat), and at other times resist them? Consistent with a growing body of literature documenting the central role of self-regulation in interpersonal and social functioning (Rawn & Vohs, 2006; Fitzsimons & Finkel, 2010), we argue that self-control, a future-looking response to anticipated temptation, plays a critical role in promoting ethical behavior. Indeed, ethical dilemmas pose a self-control conflict, presenting decision makers with a choice between two mutually exclusive courses of action, one of which offers immediate benefits and another of which offers more long-term benefits. In particular, they involve a choice between acting unethically to gain something that advances one's self-interest in the moment (e.g., money, power, status, a competitive advantage) versus acting ethically to obtain more long-term rewards, such as a moral self-image, ethical reputation, or social acceptance. Accordingly, it makes sense that factors shown to help people prepare in advance for and navigate self-control conflicts in other domains (e.g., health, finance) would likewise induce them to make more ethical decisions.

In this chapter, we review theory and recent research on counteractive self-control that supports this general argument, offering a self-control analysis of ethical decision making (Sheldon & Fishbach, 2011, 2015). Specifically, we discuss evidence from recent research, including our own, showing that ethical behavior is future oriented and requires anticipating a self-control conflict and planning its resolution. That is, we suggest that two general factors contribute to one's ability to overcome the temptation to behave unethically: identification of impending ethical dilemmas as posing a self-control conflict for one personally and selecting an appropriate self-control strategy to counteract ethical temptations. Broadly speaking, our analysis thus highlights the central importance of how people think about future ethical situations and how they plan for them in determining whether they successfully resist ethical temptations. Following this discussion, we conclude by noting implications for the existing literature on self-control and ethical decision making.

A SELF-CONTROL ANALYSIS OF ETHICAL DECISION MAKING

People experience a self-control conflict whenever they face a choice between two mutually exclusive courses of action, one offering them immediate benefits and another offering them long-term benefits (Baumeister & Heatherton, 1996; Hofmann, Friese, & Strack, 2009; Loewenstein, 1996; Mischel, Shoda, & Rodriguez, 1989). At present, much of the literature on self-control focuses on such intrapsychic problems as they arise within intrapersonal domains, such as health, fitness, finance, or academics. This might include a gym user's decision about whether to eat a slice of pizza versus a healthy salad after a vigorous workout or a student's decision about whether to stay home and prepare for class or join friends at the bar on a given evening. However, because people often internalize others' interests as their own long-term interests, they can also face such conflicts in more interpersonal domains, such as when deciding whether to behave selfishly or collaborate in bargaining encounters (Sheldon & Fishbach, 2011; Achtziger, Alós-Ferrer, & Wagner, 2015) or to retaliate against versus accommodate others in close relationships (Finkel & Campbell, 2001). In these contexts, people sometimes feel tempted to pursue short-term personal economic or emotional payoffs acquired by acting selfishly or vengefully, yet they also recognize that acting this way may compromise their ability to gain longer-term benefits for themselves and others associated with cooperation, such as maintaining ongoing relations marked by reciprocity and mutual support (Komorita & Parks, 1995; Schroeder, 1995).

Notably, many ethical dilemmas, particularly those involving a decision about whether to behave honestly, pose a similar type of problem (Monin, Pizzaro, & Beer, 2007). Specifically, such dilemmas typically present decision makers with a choice between behaving unethically so as to achieve some momentary benefit (i.e., dishonesty for immediate, selfish gain) or behaving ethically (i.e., honestly) so as to achieve a host of longer-term benefits. Such long-term benefits may include cultivating a moral self-image, a sense of integrity, and, to the extent that the decision is public, an ethical reputation and social acceptance. Consistent with this observation, research in the resource-depletion literature has shown that short-term impairments in self-control, brought about by the prior exertion of self-control in some unrelated domain (e.g., a cognitively taxing task, operating on little sleep) can lead to increased dishonesty (Barnes, Schaubroeck, Huth, & Ghumman, 2011; Christian & Ellis, 2011; Gino, Schweitzer, Mead, & Ariely, 2011; Mead, Baumeister, Gino, Schweitzer, & Ariely, 2009). Furthermore, work in the criminology literature has found that low self-control plays a key role in producing criminal, antisocial behavior (Gottfredson & Hirschi, 1990; Muraven, Podarsky, & Shmueli, 2006).

Given that ethical dilemmas can pose a self-control conflict, our self-control analysis suggests that two general factors contribute to people's ability to resist ethical temptations (e.g., the pull of dishonesty) and make ethical decisions in their everyday lives. First, it is critical that an individual identify the associated ethical dilemma in advance as posing a self-control conflict for him or her personally. After all, it is only to the extent that one identifies an ethical self-control conflict in the first place that one is likely to see any need to exercise self-control, that is, enact self-control strategies. Second, one must successfully implement self-control to overcome the temptation. This involves selecting and enacting an appropriate self-control strategy for the situation. In this sense, the ethical self-control process is a two-stage process geared toward future events. The person who anticipates future opportunities to engage in a certain tempting behavior must first identify the behavior as potentially problematic (e.g., unethical) and then tune his or her motivational system to counteract the influence of this temptation on behavior.

The resolution of conflict requires the implementation of ethical self-control strategies. These strategies, which may be conscious or unconscious, aim to bring about asymmetric shifts in motivational strength: an increase in one's motivation to behave ethically and a decrease in one's motivation to embrace unethical temptation. Overall, self-control is thus a future-oriented response. To overcome ethical temptations, having advance warning of and therefore anticipating the temptation is helpful, as this can facilitate choosing and enacting a self-control strategy best suited for the task at hand.

In the following, we elaborate on various factors that research shows can affect whether people identify future ethical dilemmas as posing self-control conflicts for them personally. We then move on to discuss in more detail how people can respond with self-control and hence behave more ethically once they identify a conflict. In Table 24.1, we summarize the principles governing each stage: identification of conflict and resolution of the conflict.

IDENTIFYING ETHICAL SELF-CONTROL DILEMMAS

Although one might assume that ethical self-control conflicts are self-evident, in fact, they are not always clear-cut. For example, if a person anticipates that a given behavior will only occur once, or that this behavior is socially acceptable, this behavior will not bear negatively on his or her self-concept, and, therefore, he or she may not identify it as posing a conflict in the first place. That is, this person may not recognize the future behavior as having the potential to jeopardize his or her moral self-image, sense of integrity, or ethical reputation. In this case, the individual may realize that the behavior could be considered unethical or even illegal in

TABLE 24.1. The Stages and Principles of Ethical Self-Control

Stage	Principles
Stage 1: Conflict Identification	1. Bracketing ethical decisions more broadly increases awareness of a conflict. 2. Higher psychological connectedness (i.e., perceived stability of one's personal identity over time) increases experienced conflict. 3. The more that a given unethical behavior seemingly reflects on the self (i.e., is perceived as self-diagnostic), the more likely one is to identify conflict.
Stage 2: Conflict Resolution	1. Advance warning of impending unethical temptation promotes ethical decisions. 2. Self-control strategies increase the motivational strength of behaving ethically and decrease that of behaving unethically.

certain circumstances (e.g., if no one else behaved in this manner) but, in the present context, simply view it as an isolated opportunity or as how things are done and hence as moral. For instance, if a job applicant assumes that bluffing in an upcoming negotiation with a potential employer about his or her current salary will be a one-time event, or if a student assumes that everyone else in a class is cheating, this person may fail to identify an ethical dilemma (and hence a conflict) in anticipating doing so him- or herself.

So what facilitates conflict identification in circumstances in which ethical dilemmas are less than clear-cut? In some cases, other actors, such as friends, family members, coworkers, or an organization to which one belongs will identify future conflicts directly for an individual. For example, many colleges now require students to sign an honor code before exams to promote the perception that cheating is unethical (Shu, Gino, & Bazerman, 2011), and many companies distribute written ethics standards to employees, with information on behaviors considered unethical, for this very same reason (Tenbrunsel, Smith-Crowe, & Umphress, 2003). At other times, however, such external prompts are absent in a situation, and several, more psychological, variables influence the likelihood that a given individual identifies a conflict. These include how people mentally bracket ethical choices, their level of psychological connectedness, and how self-diagnostic their behavior happens to be. We turn next to a discussion of this latter set of variables.

Viewing Ethical Decisions in Broad Brackets

Research on bracketing suggests that when decision makers confront a given temptation (ethical or otherwise), they can view it as either a single, isolated opportunity to act or as one of multiple similar temptations they will confront over time (e.g., as an opportunity to cheat on today's quiz or as one of eight such opportunities they will face over the semester). That is, they can bracket (or frame) the opportunity narrowly or broadly. Whenever the cost of acting on a single temptation is negligible (i.e., a one-time occurrence), framing the opportunity in relation to other, future opportunities to act can help people better identify a self-control conflict in the situation (Rachlin, 2000; Myrseth & Fishbach, 2009; Read, Loewenstein, &

Rabin, 1999). The reason is that viewing temptations in a wider frame (or bracket) can push people to consider the aggregate cost or consequences of acting on all such temptations for their long-term interests. For instance, in the ethical domain, one would expect that a committed, loyal spouse tempted to flirt with an attractive coworker would be more likely to resist this temptation when thinking about multiple subsequent opportunities she will likely have to flirt, compared with just the one faced presently. When viewed through a broad bracket, the potential long-term impact of flirting with this coworker for her sense of integrity is likely to seem more significant (i.e., costly).

Supporting this, prior research has shown that most people cheat "a little bit" when given the opportunity, in part because they view a single instance of cheating as having a negligible impact on their ethical self-concept (Mazar et al., 2008). Offering even more direct evidence of the impact of broad brackets, Sheldon and Fishbach (2015) recently had participants in one study read, evaluate the morality of, and report their intentions across six different everyday work situations, each describing an ethically questionable behavior (e.g., downloading copyrighted materials without paying on company time, intentionally pacing work slowly to avoid additional tasks, calling in sick when actually just tired, and taking office supplies home for personal use). Half were induced to view to these situations in a broad bracket (i.e., as interrelated decisions) by reading and responding to all dilemmas at once, on the same screen. The remainder were induced to view the situations in a narrow bracket (i.e., as isolated, unrelated events) by reading and responding to each of the dilemmas on a separate screen (e.g., answering questions on downloading copyrighted materials and then, on the next screen, on calling in sick, and then, on the next screen, on taking work supplies home for personal use). In this paradigm, a broad bracket causes people to consider multiple ethical decisions simultaneously, making it easier to identify that a person who engages in these various unethical actions would be unethical. In contrast, a narrow bracket leads them to consider these same ethical decisions in isolation from each other, making it difficult to recognize that a person who engages in each of these behaviors at different times would be, overall, unethical. Accordingly, the researchers found that participants who read, evaluated, and made decisions about the six situations in isolation from each other (narrow bracket) reported the situations as less morally relevant, and hence as posing less of an ethical dilemma (i.e., self-control conflict), than those who read and responded to them all at once (broad bracket). Importantly, participants assigned to the narrow-bracket condition also reported greater intentions to behave unethically in such situations. Together, these various findings thus point to the important role that choice bracketing can play in shaping whether or not people identify ethical temptations as posing a self-control conflict for them personally.

The Role of Psychological Connectedness

A second key factor that can influence whether people identify an impending ethical dilemma as posing a personal self-control conflict is their level of psychological connectedness. Similar to viewing ethical temptations in broad brackets, one's level of psychological connectedness shapes whether a person views an ethical decision (e.g., acting on the temptation to lie in a given situation) as related to other, future decisions he or she will make and, hence, as important. Psychological connectedness refers to the extent to which an individual views his or her personal identity (e.g., current personality, temperament, values, beliefs, preferences) as stable over time (Bartels & Rips, 2010). When it comes to acting on temptations (ethical or otherwise), the less stability people see in their own personal identity (i.e., the lower their psychological connectedness), the less likely they are to view actions or things they are currently tempted by as related or connected to things they will find tempting in the future. That is, the less likely they are to experience current temptations as posing a self-control conflict, and the more likely they are to view acting on them as simply isolated violations that do not reflect on the self. This perceived disconnect, in turn, is associated with a preference for immediate over delayed outcomes, presumably because acting on present temptations is not diagnostic of similar, future decisions one will make. For instance, van Gelder, Hershfield, and Nordgren (2013) found that when young adults (25–30 years old) confronted 40-year-old versions of themselves via a mental or virtual simulation task—a task designed to boost the vividness of (and hence connection to) their future selves—they were less likely to cheat than when they confronted a current version of themselves.

In other research, Sheldon and Fishbach (2015) found similar results, while also providing more direct evidence for the effect of psychological connectedness on conflict identification in an ethical domain. In one of their studies, they manipulated participants' psychological connectedness by directing half to read a (made-up) research report suggesting that one's personal identity is far more stable than most people realize (high connectedness) and directing the remainder to read a report suggesting one's personal identity is forever changing and unstable (low connectedness). Participants then completed a series of eight computerized proofreading tasks supposedly assessing their reading comprehension, verbal skills, and attention to detail. For each, they had to assign themselves to a short or long version of a written passage in need of proofreading by privately flipping a coin (labeled *short* on one side and *long* on the other), ostensibly to ensure random allocation. They learned that short versions of passages, to be assigned if the coin landed *short* side up, would always contain 2 spelling or grammatical errors. In contrast, long versions, to be assigned if the coin landed *long* side up, would always contain 10. After each coin flip, participants reported the results and completed the corresponding (short or long) task before moving on to proofread the actual paragraph. This paradigm poses an ethical dilemma: Give in to the temptation to assign oneself to short versions of passages (which entailed less work), even when one's coin flips might not warrant it (the unethical choice), or assign oneself to whatever versions of passages one's coin flips happened to indicate (the ethical choice). The total number of coin flips reported served as a measure of participants' ethicality (honesty) in this study. These researchers assumed that if the percentage of short-task assignments within a given condition was significantly higher than 50%, some participants in the condition were misreporting.

This study revealed that participants induced to feel high (vs. low) psychological connectedness behaved less dishonestly, on average: they were more likely to report being assigned, by coin flip, to 50% short tasks, which is the number of short tasks one would expect based on chance (see Figure 24.1). Interestingly, this effect of connectedness was only evident when participants anticipated the temptation to cheat

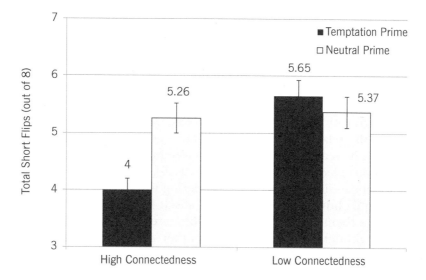

FIGURE 24.1. Effects of psychological connectedness and anticipating the temptation to cheat (temptation prime) of participants' reported number of "short" coin flips (out of eight). Only high-connectedness participants who were primed with temptation reported receiving the favorable outcome in the task 50% of the time (i.e., were honest). Reprinted with permission from Sheldon, O. J., & Fishbach, A. (2015). Anticipating and resisting the temptation to behave unethically. *Personality and Social Psychology Bulletin, 41*, 962–975.

in advance (a condition we discuss later, in the section on exercising self-control in response to ethical temptations). Notably, participants high in psychological connectedness also subsequently reported feeling more conflicted about choices they had made in the study, suggesting that they were more likely to identify an ethical self-control conflict.

The Self-Diagnosticity of Ethical Actions

Finally, a third key factor that can influence whether people identify a decision as an ethical dilemma that poses a personal self-control conflict is the self-diagnosticity of the action in question; that is, the degree to which the act reflects on one's self-concept. Given that one long-term benefit that people derive from behaving ethically is maintaining a moral self-image, people are more likely to identify an ethical self-control conflict when the act in question is seen as more diagnostic of who they really are (i.e., their "true" self). If one does not view a given act as particularly diagnostic, then one is unlikely to view it as reflecting all that badly on oneself.

A variety of recent research in behavioral ethics supports this notion. In one study, for instance, Touré-Tillery and Fishbach (2012) found that people follow ethical standards more carefully at the beginning and end of a sequence of actions compared with the middle of a sequence, in part because beginning and end positions are more salient and, therefore, appear more diagnostic. Specifically, using a similar coin-flip task as described above (Sheldon & Fishbach, 2015), these researchers found less cheating in the first and last trials of a 10-trial task compared with any position in the middle. This pattern emerged presumably because participants identified their decision to cheat at the beginning and end (vs. the middle) as posing a self-control dilemma (see Figure 24.2).

Similarly, other research has shown that directing people's attention to the self before exposing them to an ethical dilemma increases ethical behavior, presumably for the same general reason. For instance, signing one's name at the beginning of a form that one is tasked with completing decreases subsequent dishonest self-reports compared with doing so at the end (Shu, Mazar, Gino, Ariely, & Bazerman, 2012), while in the related domain of charitable giving, signing one's name when making a pledge increases commitment to subsequent giving compared with making an anonymous pledge (Koo & Fishbach, 2016). Additionally, one recent study found that when decision makers are considering whether to cheat, warning them against it by highlighting implications for the self (e.g., that they will be labeled a "cheater") makes them less likely to cheat compared with simply cautioning them against acting, without reference (direct or otherwise) to implications for the self (Bryan, Adams, & Monin, 2013). Taken together, such research suggests that the self-diagnosticity of an ethically questionable action can facilitate conflict identification.

EXERCISING SELF-CONTROL IN RESPONSE TO ETHICAL TEMPTATIONS

Assuming one has identified an upcoming situation as posing a self-control conflict, the next step required for overcoming this temptation and resisting the urge

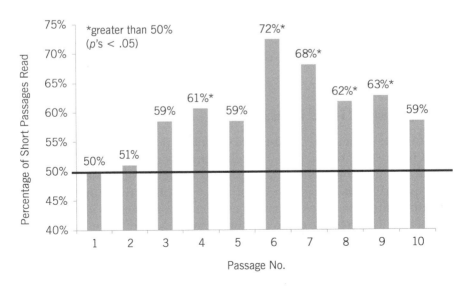

FIGURE 24.2. Percentages of participants who reported the favorable outcome of the coin flip and assigned themselves to the short proofreading passage, for each of the 10 passages in the sequence. Horizontal line at 50% value indicates chance level. * p < .05 (percentage greater than chance). Copyright © 2012 American Psychological Association. Reprinted by permission from Touré-Tillery, M., & Fishbach, A. (2012). The end justifies the means, but only in the middle. *Journal of Experimental Psychology: General, 141,* 570–583.

to behave unethically is to effectively exercise self-control. That is, one must select and enact a self-control strategy likely to sufficiently offset or counteract the influence of that temptation on goal pursuit, thereby helping to resolve the dilemma. Although several lines of research have identified preconditions for success at this stage and forms that such strategies can take, including the distinct literatures on mental contrasting (Oettingen, 2012) and implementation intentions (Gollwitzer, 2014), here we focus on recent work on counteractive control theory. According to counteractive control theory, one precondition for success at this stage is having advance warning of the impending temptation. Much the way a person preparing to lift a piece of furniture will put more force into doing so if he or she expects the furniture to be heavy, forewarning of impending temptations can prompt people (i.e., help them prepare) to put more force into overcoming these obstacles in goal pursuit (Fishbach & Trope, 2005; Fishbach, Friedman, & Kruglanski, 2003). Thus, when someone who values ethicality is told that the temptation to behave dishonestly in a future situation is likely to be strong, he or she is likely to react by exerting more effort to overcome this obstacle to his or her long-term goal of being an ethical person.

To demonstrate this point, Sheldon and Fishbach (2011) explored the process of self-control in social dilemmas (e.g., the Prisoner's Dilemma). Social dilemmas (or mixed-motive interactions, more generally) include two or more parties who face a conflict between the motives to compete and to cooperate with each other (Komorita & Parks, 1995; Schelling, 1960). Social dilemmas also pose a self-control conflict: compete in order to secure immediate, selfish benefits (e.g., short-term financial or social gain) versus cooperate so as to secure more long-term benefits both for the self and others (e.g., higher joint gains, a good reputation, ongoing relations marked by trust and reciprocity). Sheldon and Fishbach (2011) had participants choose between cooperation and competition. Before participants did so, half were warned that they would face significant obstacles to success in the impending task (i.e., that doing well would be difficult), and the other half were not. When participants were forewarned and thus anticipated barriers to achieving successful outcomes, they were more likely to cooperate, a pattern indicative of counteractive self-control. For example, one study used a six-round, increasing-sum Centipede game (Bornstein, Kugler, & Ziegelmeyer, 2004; Rosenthal, 1981), in which two players take turns choosing either to take a slightly larger share of an increasing pile of money (corresponding to a competitive move) or to pass the pile to a counterpart (corresponding to a cooperative move). The payoffs in this paradigm are arranged such that if Player 1 passes the pile and Player 2 passes it back, the size of the pile increases for both players. However, if Player 1 passes and Player 2 takes on the next round, Player 1 receives less than if he or she had taken the pile the round before (Figure 24.3 displays this payoff structure). In this game, there is a long-term incentive to trust that one's counterpart will not take immediately and to cooperate (pass), but on each round, a player feels tempted to compete (take) in order to secure current earnings. Participants played this game with an alleged "counterpart" who passed on all rounds, leaving the decision about whether to cooperate or defect to the participant. Supporting a counteractive control prediction, anticipating barriers to success (vs. no warning) increased the number of rounds participants passed before choosing to take the pile.

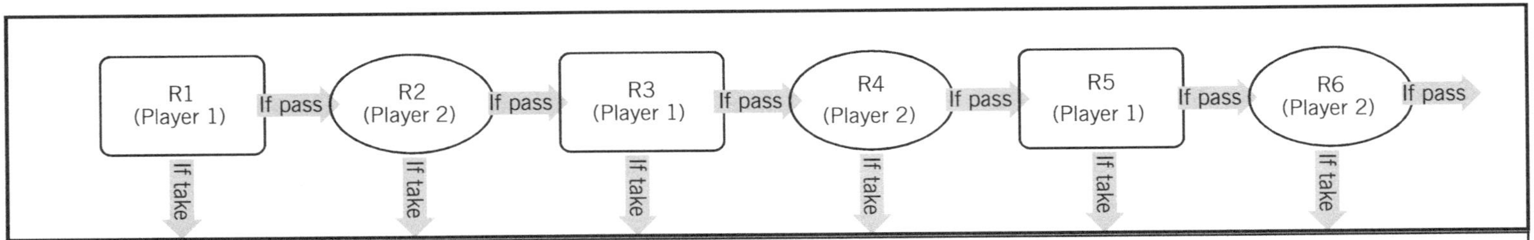

Player1's Payoff ($)	15	10	45	20	75	30	105
Player 2's Payoff ($)	5	30	15	60	25	90	35

FIGURE 24.3. The increasing-sum Centipede game: Graphical presentation of the choice and payoff structure for the six-round game. Copyright 2011 from Elsevier. Reprinted from Sheldon, O. J., & Fishbach, A. (2011). Resisting the temptation to compete: Self-control promotes cooperation in mixed-motive interactions *Journal of Experimental Social Psychology, 47,* 403–410.

With respect to actual strategies that people employ, when people fear that their long-term interests (e.g., their desire to be moral) are threatened by an impending temptation (e.g., an opportunity to satisfy some need through dishonesty), they proactively attempt to increase the motivational strength of behavior supporting their long-term interests and decrease that of the conflicting temptation. Although little prior work focuses directly on how people typically accomplish this within the ethical domain, prior research on counteractive control *does* speak to how they do so in other spheres (e.g., health, academics)—findings that presumably generalize to the domain of ethics. Specifically, the extant literature on counteractive control suggests that to induce such shifts, people rely on one or both of two broad types of strategies: behavioral strategies aimed at changing some feature of the choice situation or nonbehavioral (cognitive) strategies aimed at modifying the psychological meaning of the choice situation. The former can include strategies such as precommitting to one's long-term interests by restricting future choice sets, using penalties and rewards to change the relative value of acting on momentary temptations versus long-term interests, or proactively avoiding temptations and increasing one's proximity to objects or people that facilitate longer-term goals. Nonbehavioral strategies can include mentally activating constructs relevant to one's long-term interests while inhibiting temptation-related constructs, altering the perceived value of acting on temptations versus acting consistent with long-term interests, or changing the processing level at which temptations that conflict with long-term interests are construed. In the remainder of this section, we elaborate on these two general routes, and some of the strategies that exemplify them, in more detail.

Changing Features of the Ethical Choice Situation

Precommitting to Ethical Behavior

When faced with an impending conflict between one's long-term interests and some momentary temptation, one strategy that people motivated to exercise self-control sometimes adopt is to restrict the choices available to them in this future situation (Ainslie, 1992; Schelling, 1984, Thaler & Shefrin, 1981). For instance, in the domain of health, people often precommit to adhere to their long-term health interests and shield themselves from unhealthy temptation by stocking their pantries with more healthy and less unhealthy food than what they may later wish to consume. When confronting ethical dilemmas, it is likely that people sometimes turn to a similar strategy. For instance, the institution of marriage represents such a precommitment device. Those who wish to remain loyal to their romantic partners often make a binding, legal commitment through marriage. As it happens, dissolving a marriage is indeed significantly harder than ending a relationship without marriage.

Penalizing Unethical Choices and Rewarding Ethicality

Yet another strategy often employed by those who wish to counteract obstacles to goal pursuit is to alter the relative value of acting on momentary temptations versus long-term interests (Trope & Fishbach, 2000). This can be accomplished either by attaching contingent bonuses to acting in ways consistent with one's long-term interests or by imposing penalties on oneself for acting on conflicting temptations. For instance, when people wager with friends that they can finish a marathon, promise themselves a trip abroad should they successfully make it through college, or write contracts with others that preauthorize certain punishments should they deviate from a given goal, they are employing this strategy. When it comes to battling ethical temptations, people may occasionally adopt this same type of strategy. For instance, when writing up prenuptial agreements, couples engaged to be married might stipulate and agree to specific financial consequences (forfeiture of assets) that will result should they at some point divorce on grounds of adultery. They might do this in part as a means of motivating themselves to think twice before cheating in the context of their impending marriage.

Approaching Ethical Influences and Avoiding the Unethical

Finally, a third route by which people occasionally seek to modify features of impending conflicts to facilitate self-control is by distancing themselves from relevant temptations and establishing their proximity to objects likely to assist in achieving their long-term interests (Ainslie, 1992; Schelling, 1984; Thaler & Shefrin, 1981). Thus motivated students may choose to seclude themselves in the library rather than their rooms at home in order to facilitate studying and avoid being distracted by video games or television. Similarly, people commonly keep their distance from those who they believe might exert a "bad influence" (e.g., smokers), while maintaining proximity to those they consider helpful for pursuing long-term interests (e.g., health-conscious individuals; Fitzsimons & Shah, 2008). Given the prevalence of this strategy in other domains, it follows that people likely employ it to help them navigate certain ethical self-control conflicts as well. For instance, when choosing advisors, confidants, or role models, the ethical politician or leader might opt for only those individuals viewed as having the utmost integrity, in part to avoid any temptation to engage in morally questionable behavior him- or herself.

Modifying the Psychological Meaning of the Ethical Choice Situation

Whereas each of the strategies just discussed involves behaviorally modifying objective features of ethical self-control conflicts to facilitate ethical responding, other common self-control strategies involve purely cognitive operations aimed at modulating one's mental representations of self-control conflicts. Next, we describe three such strategies, although there are undoubtedly others.

Activating Constructs Related to Ethical Goals and Inhibiting Those Related to Unethical Temptations

One such strategy entails mentally activating thoughts related to long-term interests while inhibiting those related to conflicting temptations (Fishbach et al., 2003). Similar to a precommitment strategy, this strategy affects the relative availability of different options in the impending choice situation, only at the level of mental representations. Through mentally activating thoughts about long-term interests while inhibiting those about conflicting temptations, the proactive self-regulator increases the relative mental "availability" of behavior consistent with the former and decreases that of temptation-consistent behavior. For instance, one would expect that people with the goal of being ethical would activate concepts related to honesty (and suppress benefits associated with dishonesty) in situations in which they are tempted to act otherwise. Indeed, Fishbach and colleagues (2003) found that for religious individuals, subliminal presentation of concepts related to temptation (e.g., "drugs," "temptation") facilitated the recognition of concepts related to religious beliefs (e.g., "prayer," "Bible"), whereas subliminal presentation of concepts related to religious beliefs suppressed or inhibited recognition of concepts related to religious temptation. This pattern of asymmetric activation (temptations activate goals but goals inhibit temptations), in turn, ultimately increases the likelihood a person will successfully act in accordance with their long-term interests.

Altering the Perceived Value of Acting in Accordance with Ethical Goals versus Acting on Unethical Temptations

Another strategy that people employ to modulate how they represent self-control conflicts parallels that detailed earlier of using contingent bonuses and penalties to alter the actual value of the choice options, only this strategy seeks to alter the *perceived* (rather than objective) value of such options. Whereas imposing penalties and rewards makes temptation less tempting and goal-congruent actions more appealing, to spur increased personal resistance to impending temptations that conflict with long-term interests, this strategy acts to undermine the perceived value of the former and/or bolster the perceived value of the latter. In the academic domain, for instance, a motivated student might elaborate on what makes studying for an upcoming exam appealing (i.e., important, helpful, positive) and on what makes partying unappealing (i.e., unimportant, unhelpful, negative) as one strategy for decreasing the perceived value of partying and hence his or her motivation to do it (Myrseth, Fishbach, & Trope, 2009; Fishbach, Zhang & Trope, 2010). When confronting ethical dilemmas that pose a personal self-control conflict, people potentially do the same. That is, they may elaborate on what makes the ethical option worthier and the less ethical option unworthy in an effort to decrease the perceived value of behaving unethically. For example, to maintain their relationship commitment, individuals involved in dating relationships, relative to those who are not, tend to perceive opposite-sex persons as less physically and sexually attractive (Cole, Trope, & Balcetis, 2016; Simpson, Gangestad, & Lerma, 1990). In addition, they may perceive their relationship partners as more attractive after considering the attractiveness of single others.

Changing the Processing Level at Which Unethical Temptations and Ethical Goals Are Construed

Finally, yet another mental operation that people sometimes draw upon to strategically shift how motivated they are to act on long-term interests versus conflicting temptations is to change the processing level at which these two competing motivations are construed. A tempting glazed donut, for instance, can be viewed in a "cool," abstract, psychologically distanced way (e.g., as a sugary, round object), or it can be viewed in a "hot," concrete, psychologically proximal way (e.g., as a tasty, pleasure-inducing, doughy morsel; Fujita & Han, 2009; Fujita, Trope, Liberman, & Levin-Sagi, 2006; Metcalfe & Mischel, 1999). When people view impending temptations in the former manner, it can attenuate their motivational appeal, facilitating the ability to resist them. Conversely, when people view temptations in a hotter, concrete, and more proximal manner—the default manner in which they often view them—it can boost their appeal, making resistance to them more difficult (e.g., Fujita et al., 2006; Mischel & Baker, 1975). Thus one strategy that people sometimes employ to resist temptations (e.g., an upcoming opportunity to cheat), ethical or otherwise, is to proactively reconstrue them in a cooler, abstract, and more psychologically distanced manner. In addition, they reconstrue their goals (e.g., to be honest) in a psychologically close manner. Presumably, this helps people act in accordance with their long-term interests and, when applicable, behave ethically in such situations.

CONCLUSIONS

This chapter argues and presents evidence for the role of self-control in ethical decision making. As is the case in other spheres (e.g., health, finance), success at self-control in the ethical domain often depends on advance planning. The person who anticipates a future temptation has a better chance of resisting it than a person confronting a temptation in the present and without preparation. Specifically, the person who anticipates future temptation can identify the future situation as posing specific temptations and plan to enact various self-control strategies aimed at canceling out the threat posed by these upcoming temptations.

Broadly speaking, this chapter thus contributes to our understanding of ethical decision making by generating novel predictions about when people behave unethically. Namely, when conditions are such that people fail to identify impending ethical temptations, that is, when they are induced to think about such temptations in ways that mask how acting upon them will compromise long-term interests (e.g., bracket them narrowly), they become more likely to behave unethically. In addition, even if people identify the ethical problem, if they do not possess or if they fail to implement appropriate self-control strategies, unethical decisions become more likely.

The theory and findings reviewed here further contribute to the literature on future-oriented thinking, highlighting the importance of how people think about future ethical situations and how they plan for them in determining ethical behavior. In doing so, the theory and findings we discuss complement similar findings in the self-regulation literature. Specifically, they are consistent with research on mental contrasting and implementation intentions, which explores strategies for securing goal adherence. Mental contrasting involves mentally contrasting future desired states with the current obstacles that impede reaching the future states, and forming implementation intentions in the context of mental contrasting (MCII) involves making action plans that focus on surmounting the obstacles (Oettingen,

2012, 2014; Duckworth, Kirby, Gollwitzer, & Oettingen, 2013; Stadler, Oettingen, & Gollwitzer, 2010; see also Oettinger & Sevincer, Chapter 7, this volume). In MCII research, conflict identification can rise from mental contrasting, and implementation intentions help to overcome the obstacles once they arise. We note, however, that beyond such similarities, MCII research offers a prescriptive angle—a specific four-step structure that people can use to achieve success in any of their life domains. Our self-control model, in contrast, explores situational variables that facilitate anticipating a problem and planning a resolution (the two stages of self-control). Thus we do not offer a specific strategy of how to identify ethical dilemmas and solve them but, instead, are interested in when the situation encourages people to do so.

As with any endeavor, this chapter leaves certain questions unanswered. For instance, our analysis emphasizes the similarities between ethical and other self-control dilemmas, such as eating healthily versus unhealthily and saving versus spending. A remaining question, however, is whether ethical dilemmas also have unique characteristics that distinguish them from self-control problems in other domains. If they do, different or further interventions may at times be helpful for resolving them.

One possibility is that, for ethical dilemmas, identification is significantly harder because many, if not most, ethical violations are relatively easy to justify. Identification of ethical dilemmas can be especially difficult when the behavior in question appears to be normative, that is, within the social norm of a given society. For example, when students believe that everyone else cheats, then by cheating they merely maintain an even playing field, and when people believe domestic violence is common, abusing family members may appear "normal" and therefore less of a violation of some ethical principle. Indeed, at times, certain social norms even override the law in enabling unethical behavior. For example, drivers often violate the speed limit because they believe that the social norm (and thus the ethical decision) on a particular stretch of the road is to speed.

Lastly, we note that, unlike other dilemmas, in ethical self-control dilemmas, there are two types of long-term interests, both of which conflict with ethical temptation: the higher-order interests of the individual and the interests of society. For example, a person can cooperate (vs. compete) with others either because he or she recognizes it is in his or her best long-term interest to have a good reputation or high self-esteem, or because he or she recognizes that it is in the societal interest to have members of society cooperate with each other. In this way, ethical self-control dilemmas are unique because they are not limited to an intrapsychic conflict; rather, they also include internalized conflict between the interests of the self and societal interests.

Given these and perhaps other unique features of ethical self-control dilemmas, future work might accordingly focus more directly on the unique characteristics of such dilemmas to identify new interventions that contribute of the welfare of individuals and their society. Our hope is that the research discussed in this chapter, and its emphasis on the importance of how people think about future ethical situations and how they plan for them in determining ethical self-control, will help facilitate this endeavor.

References

Achtziger, A., Alós-Ferrer, C., & Wagner, A. (2015). Money, depletion, and prosociality in the dictator game. *Journal of Neuroscience, Psychology, and Economics, 8,* 1–14.

Ainslie, G. (1992). *Picoeconomics: The strategic interaction of successive motivational states within the person.* Cambridge, MA: Cambridge University Press.

Barnes, C. M., Schaubroeck, J., Huth, M., & Ghumman, S. (2011). Lack of sleep and unethical conduct. *Organizational Behavior and Human Decision Processes, 115,* 169–180.

Bartels, D. M., & Rips, L. J. (2010). Psychological connectedness and intertemporal choice. *Journal of Experimental Psychology: General, 139,* 49–69.

Baumeister, R. F., & Heatherton, T. F. (1996). Self-regulation failure: An overview. *Psychological Inquiry, 7,* 1–15.

Bornstein, G., Kugler, T., & Ziegelmeyer, A. (2004). Individual and group decisions in the Centipede game: Are groups more "rational" players? *Journal of Experimental Social Psychology, 40,* 599–605.

Bryan, C. J., Adams, G. S., & Monin, B. (2013). When cheating would make you a cheater: Implicating the self prevents unethical behavior. *Journal of Experimental Psychology: General, 142,* 1001–1005.

Cebula, R. J., & Feige, E. (2012). America's unreported economy: Measuring the size, growth, and determinants of tax evasion in the U.S. *Crime, Law and Social Change, 57,* 265–286.

Christian, M., & Ellis, A. (2011). Examining the effects of sleep deprivation on workplace deviance: A self-regulatory perspective. *Academy of Management Journal, 54,* 913–934.

Cole, S., Trope, Y., & Balcetis. E. (2016). In the eye of the betrothed: Perceptual downgrading in romantic self-control conflicts. *Personality and Social Psychology Bulletin, 42,* 879–892.

Duckworth, A. L., Kirby, T. A., Gollwitzer, A., & Oettingen, G. (2013). From fantasy to action: Mental contrasting with implementation intentions (MCII) improves academic performance in children. *Social Psychological and Personality Science, 4,* 745–753.

Finkel, E. J., & Campbell, W. K. (2001). Self-control and accommodation in close relationships: An interdependence analysis. *Journal of Personality and Social Psychology, 81,* 263–277.

Fishbach, A., Friedman, R. S., & Kruglanski, A. W. (2003). Leading us not unto temptation: Momentary allurements elicit overriding goal activation. *Journal of Personality and Social Psychology, 84,* 296–309.

Fishbach, A., & Trope, Y. (2005). The substitutability of external control and self-control in overcoming temptation. *Journal of Experimental Social Psychology, 41,* 256–270.

Fishbach, A., Zhang, Y., & Trope, Y. (2010). Counteractive evaluation: Asymmetric shifts in the implicit value of conflicting motivations. *Journal of Experimental Social Psychology, 46,* 29–38.

Fitzsimons, G. M., & Finkel, E. J. (2010). Interpersonal influences on self-regulation. *Current Directions in Psychological Science, 19,* 101–105.

Fitzsimons, G. M., & Shah, J. (2008). How goal instrumentality shapes relationship evaluations. *Journal of Personality and Social Psychology, 95,* 319–337.

Fujita, K., & Han, H. A. (2009). The effect of construal levels on evaluative associations in self-control conflicts. *Psychological Science, 20,* 799–804.

Fujita, K., Trope, Y., Liberman, N., & Levin-Sagi, M. (2006). Construal levels and self-control. *Journal of Personality and Social Psychology, 90,* 351–367.

Gino, F., Schweitzer, M., Mead, N., & Ariely, D. (2011). Unable to resist temptation: How self-control depletion promotes unethical behavior. *Organizational Behavior and Human Decision Processes, 115,* 191–203.

Gollwitzer, P. M. (2014). Weakness of the will: Is a quick fix possible? *Motivation and Emotion, 38,* 305–322.

Gottfredson, M. R., & Hirschi, T. (1990). *A general theory of crime.* Stanford, CA: Stanford University Press.

Happel, S. K., & Jennings, M. M. (2008). An economic analysis of academic dishonesty and its deterrence in higher education. *Journal of Legal Studies Education, 25,* 183–214.

Hofmann, W., Friese, M., & Strack, F. (2009). Impulse and self-control from a dual-systems perspective. *Perspectives on Psychological Science, 4,* 162–176.

Komorita, S. S., & Parks, C. D. (1995). Interpersonal relations: Mixed-motive interaction. *Annual Review of Psychology, 46,* 183–207.

Koo, M., & Fishbach, A. (2016). Giving the self: Increasing commitment and generosity through giving something that represents one's essence. *Social Psychological and Personality Science, 7,* 339–348.

Loewenstein, G. (1996). Out of control: Visceral influences on behavior. *Organizational Behavior and Human Decision Processes, 65,* 272–292.

Mazar, N., Amir, O., & Ariely, D. (2008). The dishonesty of honest people: A theory of self-concept maintenance. *Journal of Marketing Research, 45,* 633–644.

Mead, N., Baumeister, R. F., Gino, F., Schweitzer, M., & Ariely, D. (2009). Too tired to tell the truth: Self-control resource depletion and dishonesty. *Journal of Experimental Social Psychology, 45,* 594–597.

Metcalfe, J., & Mischel, W. (1999). A hot/cool-system analysis of delay of gratification: Dynamics of willpower. *Psychological Review, 106,* 3–19.

Mischel, W., & Baker, N. (1975). Cognitive appraisals and transformations in delay behavior. *Journal of Personality and Social Psychology, 31,* 254–261.

Mischel, W., Shoda, Y., & Rodriguez, M. I. (1989). Delay of gratification in children. *Science, 244,* 933–938.

Monin, B., Pizarro, D., & Beer, J. S. (2007). Deciding versus reacting: Conceptions of moral judgment and the reason–affect debate. *Review of General Psychology, 11,* 99–111.

Muraven, M., Podarsky, G., & Shmueli, D. (2006). Self-control depletion and the general theory of crime. *Journal of Quantitative Criminology, 22,* 263–277.

Myrseth, K. O. R., & Fishbach, A. (2009). Self-control: A function of knowing when and how to exercise restraint. *Current Directions in Psychological Science, 18,* 247–252.

Myrseth, K. O. R., Fishbach, A., & Trope, Y. (2009). Counteractive self-control: When making temptation available makes temptation less tempting. *Psychological Science, 20,* 159–163.

Oettingen, G. (2012). Future thought and behavior change. *European Review of Social Psychology, 23,* 1–63.

Oettingen, G. (2014). *Rethinking positive thinking: Inside the new science of motivation.* New York: Penguin Random House.

Rachlin, H. (2000). *The science of self-control.* Cambridge, MA: Harvard University Press.

Rawn, C. D., & Vohs, K. D. (2006). The importance of self-regulation for interpersonal functioning. In K. D. Vohs & E. J. Finkel (Eds.), *Self and relationships: Connecting intrapersonal and interpersonal processes* (pp. 15–31). New York: Guilford Press.

Read, D., Loewenstein, G., & Rabin, M. (1999). Choice bracketing. *Journal of Risk and Uncertainty, 19,* 171–197.

Rosenthal, R. W. (1981). Games of perfect information, predatory pricing, and the chain store paradox. *Journal of Economic Theory, 25,* 92–100.

Schelling, T. C. (1960). *The strategy of conflict.* Cambridge, MA: Harvard University Press.

Schelling, T. C. (1984). Self-command in practice, in policy, and in a theory of rational choice. *American Economic Review, 74,* 1–11.

Schroeder, D. A. (1995). *Social dilemmas: Perspectives on individuals and groups.* Westport, CT: Praeger.

Sheldon, O. J., & Fishbach, A. (2011). Resisting the temptation to compete: Self-control promotes cooperation in mixed-motive interactions *Journal of Experimental Social Psychology, 47,* 403–410.

Sheldon, O. J., & Fishbach, A. (2015). Anticipating and resisting the temptation to behave unethically. *Personality and Social Psychology Bulletin, 41,* 962–975.

Shu, L., Gino, F., & Bazerman, M. H. (2011). Ethical discrepancy: Changing our attitudes to resolve moral dissonance. In D. De Cremer & A. E. Tenbrunsel (Ed.), *Behavioral business ethics: Ideas on an emerging field* (pp. 221–240). London: Taylor & Francis.

Shu, L. L., Mazar, N., Gino, F., Ariely, D., & Bazerman, M. H. (2012). Signing at the beginning makes ethics salient and decreases dishonest self-reports in comparison to signing at the end. *Proceedings of the National Academy of Sciences of the USA, 109,* 15197–15200.

Simpson, J. A., Gangestad, S. W., & Lerma, M. (1990). Perception of physical attractiveness: Mechanisms involved in the maintenance of romantic relationships. *Journal of Personality and Social Psychology, 59,* 1192–1201.

Stadler, G., Oettingen, G., & Gollwitzer, P. M. (2010). Intervention effects of information and self-regulation on eating fruits and vegetables over two years. *Health Psychology, 29,* 274–283.

Tenbrunsel, A. E., Smith-Crowe, K., & Umphress, E. E. (2003). Building houses on rocks: The role of the ethical infrastructure in organizations. *Social Justice Research, 16,* 285–307.

Thaler, R. H., & Shefrin, H. M. (1981). An economic theory of self-control. *Journal of Political Economy, 89,* 392–406.

Touré-Tillery, M., & Fishbach, A. (2012). The end justifies the means, but only in the middle. *Journal of Experimental Psychology: General, 141,* 570–583.

Trope, Y., & Fishbach, A. (2000). Counteractive self-control in overcoming temptation. *Journal of Personality and Social Psychology, 79,* 493–506.

van Gelder J. L., Hershfield, H. E., & Nordgren, L. F. (2013). Vividness of the future self predicts delinquency. *Psychological Science, 24,* 974–980.

CHAPTER 25

The Road to Hell

An Overview of Research
on the Intention–Behavior Gap

Paschal Sheeran
Thomas L. Webb

Goals are mental representations of desired outcomes (Austin & Vancouver, 1996) such as "be healthy." Goal intentions are people's self-instructions to achieve these outcomes (e.g., "I will try to look after my health!"), whereas behavioral intentions are self-instructions to perform particular actions directed toward their attainment (e.g., "I intend to jog for 30 minutes each day!"; Triandis, 1980). Intentions capture both the level of the set goal or behavior (e.g., 30 minutes of jogging each day) and the person's commitment to attaining it (e.g., how determined one is to jog every day for 30 minutes). Although people's behavior may predominantly involve responses that are triggered automatically by situational cues (e.g., Bargh, 2006; Wood & Neal, 2007), intentional control can be crucial for securing long-term goals (Baumeister & Bargh, 2014; Kuhl & Quirin, 2011). The concept of intention has thus proved especially valuable for researchers concerned with *behavior change,* and interventions designed to promote public health, energy conservation, and educational and organizational outcomes generally rely on frameworks that construe intentions as a key determinant of behavior change (e.g., Ajzen, 1991; Bandura, 1996; Locke & Latham, 1992; Rogers, 1983).

Intentions offer very good prediction of behavior in prospective, correlational studies. Sheeran (2002) meta-analyzed 10 previous meta-analyses (422 studies in total) and observed a conventionally "large" sample-weighted average correlation between intentions measured at one time point and measures of behavior taken at a subsequent time point ($r_+ = 0.53$). Moreover, correlational tests indicate that intention offers superior prediction of behavior to other cognitions, including (explicit and implicit) attitudes, norms, self-efficacy, and perceptions of risk and severity (e.g., McEachan, Conner, Taylor, & Lawton, 2011; Sheeran, Harris, & Epton, 2014;

Sheeran, Gollwitzer, & Bargh, 2013), as well as personality factors (e.g., Chiaburu, Oh, Berry, Li, & Gardner, 2011; Poropat, 2009; Rhodes & Smith, 2006). These findings would seem to suggest that forming an intention helps if people are to initiate new behaviors or to alter courses of action that are no longer seen as desirable.

Is the Proverbial "Road to Hell" Paved with "Good" Intentions?

Correlations between measures of intentions taken at one time point and behavior that is measured at a subsequent time point do not indicate whether intentions predict *behavior change,* however—because past behavior is not taken into account (Sheeran, Klein, & Rothman, 2017). Past behavior could determine both intention and future behavior, and so bivariate associations between intention and behavior could be spurious (i.e., entirely due to the third variable, past behavior). In fact, four lines of evidence that go beyond bivariate correlational tests indicate that the impact of intention on behavior change is a great deal more modest than the average correlation between measures of intention and behavior of .53 would suggest.

First, to investigate how well intention predicts behavior after past behavior has been taken into account, Sheeran, Klein, and Rothman (2017) reanalyzed data from a meta-analysis of prospective, correlational studies of health behaviors (McEachan et al., 2011). The sample-weighted average correlations (r_+) between intention and behavior, past behavior and intention, and past behavior and behavior were .40, .44, and .48, respectively (minimum N = 21,786). Multiple regression analyses were conducted to determine the unique variance explained in behavior after past behavior was statistically controlled. Findings indicated that the average correlation between intention and *changes* in behavior was only r_+ = .21.

The second line of evidence used statistical simulations to assess the impact of an intervention that maximizes participants' intention scores on subsequent behavioral performance. Fife-Schaw, Sheeran, and Norman (2007) undertook such simulations using data from 211 participants in relation to 30 behaviors. Analyses of the raw data indicated that the median rate of translating intentions into action was 47% (i.e., less than one-half of intentions were enacted). The statistical simulation involved estimating the median rate of intention translation if all participants in the sample had the maximum possible score on the intention measure. Consistent with the idea that changing intention changes behavior, simulating maximum intention scores increased the rate of intention translation by 29% (from 47% to 76%). However, this simulation also reveals a substantial discrepancy between intention and behavior, as some 24% of maximized intentions are not translated into action. Even the "best" intentions may not be enacted, it seems.

The third line of evidence comes from experiments that change intentions (Rhodes & Dickau, 2012; Webb & Sheeran, 2006). Webb and Sheeran (2006) reviewed 47 interventions that (1) were successful in strengthening intentions among treatment participants as compared with control participants and (2) measured subsequent behavior for both groups. Findings showed that a medium-to-large-sized change in intentions (d_+ = 0.66) led to a small-to-medium-sized change in behavior (d_+ = 0.36). Taken together then, Sheeran, Klein, and Rothman's (2017) findings indicate that the average effect size for the impact of intention on behavior change is $r_+ = .21$ in correlational studies, while Webb and Sheeran's (2006) findings suggested that the effect size is $r_+ = .18$ in experimental studies. These effects are small to medium in magnitude, not large. It therefore seems fair to conclude that there is a substantial "gap" between intention and behavior.

These three lines of evidence demonstrate how large the intention–behavior gap is, but they do not indicate the source of the discrepancy between intentions and behavior. To investigate this issue, Sheeran (2002; Orbell & Sheeran, 1998) decomposed the intention–behavior relation into a 2 (intend to act vs. do not intend to act) ×2 (subsequently act vs. do not act) matrix. Using this matrix to analyze prospective studies of health behaviors showed that the median percentage of participants who intended to act and subsequently acted was only 53%, whereas the median percentage of participants who did not intend and did not act was 93%. Thus it is people who intend to act but fail to do so (termed *inclined abstainers*) who are mainly responsible for the intention–behavior gap (see Godin & Conner, 2008; Rhodes & de Bruijn, 2013, for equivalent findings). In sum, when past behavior is taken into account, statistical simulations are undertaken, experimental evidence is analyzed, or intention–behavior consistency is decomposed, findings in each case show just how well-paved with "good" intentions is the proverbial "road to hell."

CAN INTENTIONS AVOID THE ROAD TO HELL?: MODERATORS OF INTENTION–BEHAVIOR RELATIONS

Understanding why some people with strong intentions to act fail to do so whereas other people with equivalent intentions succeed (i.e., differences between *inclined abstainers* and *inclined actors*) has been the focus of considerable research during the past 15 years. Numerous factors have been observed to interact with goal or behavioral intentions in predicting outcomes, making it more or less likely that a focal intention will be translated into action. Four categories of moderating variables have been studied extensively: (1) actual and perceived control, (2) habits and experience with the behavior, (3) the basis of intention, and (4) properties of the respective intention. We consider each of these categories in turn.

Actual and Perceived Control

By definition, people can enact intentions only when they have actual control over performance of the behavior. Intentions to visit Mars next Tuesday or to speak fluent Mandarin by dinner time are not likely to be realized, because most people do not possess the requisite resources, ability, skills, cooperation, opportunity, or time (i.e., features of actual control) needed to realize these intentions. Empirical evidence, too, speaks to how features of actual control prevent intention realization. For example, Conner et al. (2013) observed that socioeconomic status, which may index people's access to resources or opportunities, moderated intention–behavior relations in three studies such that the intention–behavior relationship was attenuated among people with lower socioeconomic status (SES). DiBonaventura and Chapman (2008) and Martijn et al. (2008) found that blocked opportunities prevented the realization of intentions to obtain influenza vaccinations or complete an assignment, respectively. Sheeran, Trafimow, and Armitage (2003) offered a direct test by indexing actual control using assessments of control taken in the wake of performing the behavior. Findings showed that these assessments did not merely reflect self-serving bias for failures to enact intentions and reliably moderated the intention–behavior relation in two studies. Intentions were more consistent with behavior when participants had greater actual control over the focal behavior.

Of course, people generally do not intend to do impossible things, because beliefs about whether performing behaviors will be difficult or within their control are key determinants of intention formation (e.g., Ajzen, 1991; Bandura, 1998). Interestingly, however, evidence suggests that people's *perceptions* of the difficulty of performing the behavior or the extent to which they have control over behavioral performance (self-efficacy or perceived behavioral control) do not consistently moderate the intention–behavior relationship (Armitage & Conner, 2001; Sheeran, 2002). This may be because intentions measured when people are in a calm or satiated ("cold") state take insufficient account of how powerful are visceral states (e.g., arousal, hunger) at the moment of acting (Nordgren, van der Pligt, & van Harreveld, 2008) or because people generally underestimate the difficulty of performing behaviors (Buehler, Griffin, & Ross, 1994; DiBonaventura & Chapman, 2008; Sheeran et al., 2003). In short, perceptions of control may not accurately reflect actual control over behaviors, and interventions may be needed to bring perceptions in line with reality.

Mental contrasting is a powerful technique derived from fantasy realization theory (see Oettingen, 2012, for a review) that can serve to bring perceptions of control in line with actual behavior change. Mental contrasting involves, first, elaborating the most positive aspect of a desired future and, second, elaborating the most critical obstacle that, in reality, stands in the way of realizing that future. Compared with merely fantasizing (mentally indulging a desired future as if it has already been realized) or dwelling (ruminating about the negative aspects of reality that block one's path), mental contrasting activates expectations (i.e., judgments that the desired future is likely) that generate strong intentions to act (e.g., Oettingen, Pak, & Schnetter, 2001). Priming experiments have demonstrated that mental contrasting tethers thoughts about the desired future to the features of reality that stand in the way of that future (e.g., Kappes & Oettingen, 2014) in a manner that should promote more realistic intentions. Importantly, mental contrasting also links the obstacles in reality to the instrumental behaviors needed to overcome those obstacles (Kappes, Singmann, & Oettingen, 2012).

Habits and Experience

Ouellette and Wood (1998) proposed that behaviors that are performed repeatedly in stable contexts are liable to become habitual. Over time, features of the context (particular times, places, or people) become associated with the behavioral performance such that merely encountering these cues serves to trigger the behavior relatively automatically. The implication is that intention has less influence on behavior when the relevant sequence of actions has become a habit. Consistent with this idea, Ouellette and Wood's (1998) influential meta-analysis observed that intention better predicted nonhabitual behaviors (actions performed annually or biannually in unstable contexts) than habitual behaviors. Webb and Sheeran's (2006) meta-analysis of interventions that changed intentions obtained equivalent findings, and studies have found that interventions designed to change intentions to perform environmental behaviors (e.g., saving water, reusing shopping bags) are particularly effective when people have recently moved home (and habits have yet to develop) but are much less effective when participants have occupied the same residence for a long time and habits have formed (Thomas, Poortinga, & Sautkina, 2016; Verplanken & Roy, 2016).

Although numerous studies have found that habit or experience reduces the predictive validity of intentions, several other studies have observed precisely the opposite effect—that experience increases the consistency between intentions and behavior (e.g., Doll & Ajzen, 1992; Kashima, Gallois, & McCamish, 1993; Sheeran & Abraham, 2003). Experience may reduce the gap between intentions and behavior, because repeatedly performing a behavior serves to stabilize intention, which increases its likelihood of enactment. Experience with a behavior thus appears to have paradoxical effects on intention–behavior relations: Experience weakens intention–behavior consistency in some studies but strengthens intention–behavior consistency in other studies.

Sheeran, Godin, Conner, and Germain (2017) proposed a resolution of this paradox by hypothesizing that the impact of experience on the intention–behavior relationship is captured by an inverted U-shaped curve. That is, greater experience initially enhances the predictive validity of intention (because experience stabilizes intentions). After a certain point, however, greater experience reflects increased automatization of behavior, and so the predictive validity of intention declines. Support for the inverted-U hypothesis was observed in a longitudinal study of blood donation that used objective measures of both donation experience and behavior. Findings showed that, as experience with blood donation increased from low to moderate, the predictive validity of intention was enhanced, whereas intention's predictive validity declined as experience increased from moderate to high. Thus experience with a behavior can serve both to strengthen *and* weaken intention-behavior consistency.

The Basis of the Intention

Several factors that guide intention formation (i.e., form the basis of the intention) also influence how effectively those intentions are realized. Potentially important factors include attitudinal versus normative control, moral obligation, anticipated regret, want/should conflict, and identity relevance. Consistent with self-determination theory (SDT; e.g., Deci & Ryan, 2000), intentions based on personal beliefs about the outcomes of acting (i.e., attitudes) better predict behavior than intentions based on social pressure to act (i.e., norms; Sheeran & Orbell, 1999). Furthermore, intentions based more on feelings about performing the behavior (i.e., affective attitudes) than on thoughts about the behavior's instrumental consequences (i.e., cognitive attitudes) also better predict behavior (Keer, Conner, Van den Putte, & Neijens, 2014). Findings also indicate that greater feelings of moral obligation and greater anticipated regret about failing to act are associated with improved consistency between intentions and behavior. For example, in 5 studies of different health behaviors (e.g., smoking, physical activity, driving over the speed limit), Godin, Conner, and Sheeran (2005) observed better prediction of behavior when intentions were based more on moral norms than on attitudes. Abraham and Sheeran (2004) found that anticipated regret about not exercising moderated intention–behavior relations. The more regret that participants expected to experience if they did not exercise, the greater was the likelihood that their intentions were translated into behavior (for equivalent findings, see Conner, Sandberg, McMillan, & Higgins, 2006; Sheeran & Orbell, 1999). Moreover, making regret salient at the moment of intention formation (by measuring anticipated regret prior to measuring intentions) has been found to improve the translation of intentions to exercise into action (Abraham & Sheeran, 2004; see also Godin, Germain, Conner, Delage, & Sheeran, 2014).

Many intentions present a conflict between what people want to do and what they feel that they should do (termed *want/should conflicts*; Milkman, Rogers, & Bazerman, 2008). Taylor, Webb, and Sheeran (2014) proposed that such conflicts can lead people to justify indulgence to themselves and therefore undermine the realization of their "good" intentions. Focus groups and open-ended surveys were used to identify the different ways that people justify the consumption of desirable, but unhealthy, foods. Common justifications included thinking that one deserves a treat (e.g., "I've had a hard day, I need a treat!"), construing tempting food as irresistible ("It's too good to say 'no' to!"), interpreting indulgence as an exception to the norm ("Once in a while is OK!"), and believing that one will compensate for the indulgence later ("I'll do some exercise tomorrow to make up for it!"). Justifications for indulgence were found to moderate the intention–behavior relation in both the lab and the field, such that participants who often justified indulgence were less likely to act on their intentions to reduce consumption. In short, evidence suggests that people sometimes willingly undermine their own intentions by justifying so doing to themselves (see also de Witt Huberts, Evers, & de Ridder, 2012; Prinsen, Evers, & de Ridder, 2016).

The extent to which intentions are relevant to the persons' identity and current concerns (Klinger, 1971, 1975, 1977) can influence the likelihood that they are enacted. Two aspects of identity relevance have been studied in relation to the intention–behavior gap. The first concerns self-schemas—people's self-concepts in domains of enduring investment and concern. For instance, people are designated as possessing an exerciser self-schema if they rate "exercising regularly," "being physically active," and "keeping in shape" as both self-descriptive and important to their image of themselves (Kendzierski, 1990). Sheeran and Orbell (2000) found that, even after controlling for past behavior, people who possessed an exerciser self-schema better translated their intentions to exercise into action compared with participants who did not possess a relevant self-schema.

The second aspect of identity relevance concerns whether a focal behavioral intention serves people's overarching identity goals. For instance, the goal of being a "good" professor is served by many different intentions and behaviors (e.g., publishing papers, advising graduate students, managing a lab), and these intentions and behaviors are symbols of possessing that identity. According to self-completion theory (SCT; Wicklund & Gollwitzer, 1982), when identity symbols are noticed by other people, they give the person a sense of possessing the identity (i.e., a sense that their identity is complete). Ironically, however, if behavioral intentions qualify as identity symbols and those intentions are noticed by others, then evidence suggests that people are less likely to act because they feel that they already possess the relevant identity and so no longer need to actually perform the behavior relevant to attaining that identity. For example, Gollwitzer, Sheeran, Michalski, and Seifert (2009) found that participants whose intentions were acknowledged by other people felt a stronger sense of possessing the relevant identity and acted less intensively on their intentions than participants whose intentions were kept private. Consistent with SCT, these effects were observed when participants were strongly committed to the overarching identity goal and behavioral intentions indeed qualified as symbols of the aspired-to identity.

Properties of Intention

It is well established that the correlation between intention and behavior grows weaker as the time interval between the measurement of intention and behavior increases (e.g., Sheeran & Orbell, 1998). This is likely because intentions change as a result of new information or because alternative activities become more important. To understand properties of intention that make for durable intentions and enhance prediction of behavior, researchers have drawn from the literature on attitude strength. Studies of intention properties measure not only the direction and intensity of intentions (e.g., "I intend to jog for 30 minutes each day!"), but also other features of the intention, such as accessibility (indexed by how quickly people respond to questions about their intentions), certainty (e.g., "I am certain that my intention to jog will not change!"), and temporal stability (e.g., the within-participants correlation between measures of intention taken at two time points prior to the measurement of behavior). The distinctiveness of temporal stability, certainty, and accessibility as properties of intention is supported by principal-components analysis (Cooke & Sheeran, 2013).

Several lines of research indicate that intention stability is a superior indicator of intention strength compared with accessibility or certainty. First, intention stability is a more powerful moderator of the intention–behavior relation than the other indicators (Conner & Godin, 2007; Cooke & Sheeran, 2013; Sheeran & Abraham, 2003; see Cooke & Sheeran, 2004, for a meta-analysis). In one study, temporal stability of intention improved the consistency between measures of intention and behavior that were taken 6 years apart (Conner, Norman, & Bell, 2002). Second, temporal stability is associated with improved processing of goal-relevant information and increased resistance to attacks on intention. For instance, Cooke and Sheeran (2013) found that, compared with participants with unstable intentions, participants with stable intentions to exercise showed improved memory for exercise-related information in a surprise recall task. Participants with stable intentions were also less influenced by a manipulation designed to alter their intentions. Stable intentions have also been found to attenuate the relationship between people's past behavior and their future behavior, making it more likely that people act on their intentions and not merely on the basis of habit (Sheeran, Orbell, & Trafimow, 1999). Finally, evidence indicates that intention stability mediates the influence of other moderators of the intention–behavior relationship (Keer et al.,

2014; Sheeran & Abraham, 2003). In particular, attitudinal versus normative control, anticipated regret, self-schemas, experience with the behavior, and intention certainty were each associated with more stable intentions and no longer moderated the intention–behavior relation once the terms representing the interactions between these factors and intention stability were included in the equation (see also Turchik & Gidycz, 2012). Thus, although several categories of moderator variables have been tested, accumulated evidence suggests that temporal stability of intention best predicts how well intentions are translated into action.

WHAT HAPPENS ON THE ROAD TO HELL? POTENCIES AND PROBLEMS IN REALIZING INTENTIONS

Motivational Processes That Support Intention Realization

Forming intentions instigates motivational processes that support the realization of those intentions (for a review, see Johnson, Chang, & Lord, 2006). For instance, the processing of information relevant to the intention is accorded priority, as exemplified by Goschke and Kuhl's (1993) demonstration of *intention superiority* effects, whereby information that is relevant to the respective goal is activated to a greater degree than irrelevant information. Johnson et al. (2006) meta-analyzed evidence on the processing of goal-related information and found support for three hypotheses. First, goals were found to prime closely related information. In particular, goal activation reduced response latencies to information related to the goal ($d_+ = -0.34$) and increased the likelihood that this information would be accessed ($d_+ = 0.46$). Second, Johnson et al. (2006) found that activating a goal curbed the activation of competing goals ($d_+ = -0.22$), an effect that was more pronounced the stronger and more passionate were participants' intentions to pursue the goal (Shah, Friedman, & Kruglankski, 2002; Bélanger, Lafrenière, Vallerand, & Kruglanski, 2013). Fishbach, Friedman, and Kruglanski (2003) also observed the opposite relation—that priming competing goals heightened the activation of the focal goal (e.g., images of chocolate heightened the accessibility of the goal of controlling one's weight)—though the effect was observed only among people who are successful at self-regulating their behavior (see also Stroebe, van Koningsbruggen, Papies, & Aarts, 2013). Third, once goals have been attained or the window of opportunity for their attainment has passed, Johnson et al. (2006) observed that information related to the goal no longer receives greater activation ($d_+ = -0.20$ to -0.43 in various paradigms), thus freeing resources to pursue other goals.

Self-Regulatory Problems

Research on the intention–behavior gap makes it clear, however, that these motivational processes do not guarantee that intentions are realized. Gollwitzer and Sheeran (2006) specified various self-regulatory problems—challenges in aligning one's thoughts, feelings, and actions with the focal intention—that people face as they strive to achieve goals and perform intended behaviors. These challenges may be encountered during different phases of goal pursuit and may embrace failures to (1) get started, (2) keep ongoing goal pursuit on track, (3) call a halt to goal striving that has become futile, and (4) conserve capability for future goal striving. Key problems encountered in getting started with goal pursuit include forgetting to act, missing opportunities to act, and failing to engage in preparatory behaviors. For example, Einstein, McDaniel, Williford, Pagan, and Dismukes (2003) observed that after a delay of merely 5 seconds, 8% of their (young, healthy) participants forgot to enact an intended behavior, and this proportion increased to 24% when their attention was divided (leading the researchers to title their paper "Forgetting of intentions in demanding situations is rapid"). Forgetting to act is commonplace and has been implicated in not taking medication as planned (e.g., O'Carroll, Chambers, Dennis, Sudlow, & Johnston, 2014; Zogg, Woods, Sauceda, Wiebe, & Simoni, 2012) and in failing to perform intended energy-saving behaviors (Corradi, Priftis, Jacucci, & Gamberini, 2013).

Even if people do remember their intentions, they may still be thwarted because they miss good opportunities to act. Failing to capitalize on favorable conditions for acting seems especially likely when such opportunities are brief or infrequent (termed *short-fuse behaviors*; Dholakia & Bagozzi, 2006 or involve deadlines or when there are multiple ways to realize the intention and the person is undecided about the best means of attaining his or her goal. Experiencing "second thoughts" at the moment of acting (goal revision in situ) and procrastination can also cause people to miss opportunities to act. Goal revision in situ may occur when people have failed to anticipate the visceral drives present at the moment of acting (Nordgren et al., 2008), when they are ambivalent about acting, or when the presence of tempting alternative courses of action leads people to justify indulgence to themselves (Taylor et al., 2014). Procrastination appears to be both dispositionally and situationally determined (e.g., by low conscientiousness and task aversiveness) and is reliably associated with the intention–behavior gap (Steel, 2007).

Closely related to the problem of missing opportunities to act is the failure to engage in necessary preparatory behaviors. Many goals involve sequences of action, and completing actions earlier in the sequence may be a prerequisite for successful goal completion. For instance, condom use during sex demands preparatory behaviors to ensure that condoms are available (e.g., by buying, storing, or carrying condoms) and that one's partner agrees to using them (e.g., suggesting condom use, handling reluctance to use a condom; e.g., Sheeran, Abraham, & Orbell, 1999). Even strongly intending to use a condom does not ensure that the necessary preparatory behaviors are undertaken (Carvalho, Alvarez, Barz, & Schwarzer, 2015; van Empelen & Kok, 2008).

Having successfully started to strive for a goal, the next self-regulatory problem that people face is straying off track. Goal attainment often relies on frequent and consistent performance of goal-directed behaviors (e.g., repeatedly limiting calorie intake to lose weight). Goal pursuit can become derailed because people fail to monitor progress toward their goal or because unwanted influences become overwhelming. Evidence suggests that keeping track of progress toward goals (e.g., using a weight-loss diary) promotes intention realization (for reviews, see Harkin et al., 2016; Michie, Whittington, Abraham, McAteer, & Gupta, 2009), perhaps because progress monitoring serves to identify discrepancies between current and desired states (i.e., it signals the need to act; Myrseth & Fishbach, 2009) and maintains attention on the focal goal (Liberman & Dar, 2009). However, relatively few people monitor their household energy consumption, check their bank balances regularly, or keep track of what they are eating (Webb, Chang, & Benn, 2013). This motivated avoidance of progress monitoring is termed the *ostrich problem* and appears to be rooted in people's desire to maintain favorable views of themselves and their standing with respect to the goal (Webb et al., 2013).

Manifold unwanted influences can derail ongoing goal pursuit, including distractions, temptations, competing goals, disruptive thoughts and feelings, unwanted social influences, and low willpower. Distractions consume time or effort needed to realize the focal intention, whereas temptations are enticing stimuli that afford the opportunity to engage in behavior that is antithetical to the focal intention (e.g., the arrival of the dessert cart at a convention for chronic dieters; Hofmann, Baumeister, Förster, & Vohs, 2012). Competing goals not only arise when people realize that they have more things to do than they have time to do them but can also be automatically activated by situational features (i.e., without people being aware of the activation of the competing goal or its impact on behavior). For instance, priming the goal of moving fast in an ostensibly unrelated initial task was observed to undermine the enactment of intentions to drive safely (Gollwitzer, Sheeran, Trötschel, & Webb, 2011).

Unwanted thoughts and feelings can also disrupt efforts to enact intentions. Social anxiety (Webb, Ononaiye, Sheeran, Reidy, & Lavda, 2010) and test anxiety (Parks-Stamm, Gollwitzer, & Oettingen, 2010) both hamper performance. Worry about an upcoming psychotherapy appointment has been found to be associated with nonattendance, despite participants' having strong intentions to keep the appointment (Sheeran, Aubrey, & Kellett, 2007). In other studies, negative mood and high levels of arousal led to unintended risk behavior (Webb et al., 2010). Negative affect appears to undermine intention realization via multiple routes—by increasing the strength of temptations, by consuming working memory resources needed to monitor progress, and by prioritizing mood repair over acting on the focal intention (see Wagner & Heatherton, 2014, for a review). This is not to say that positive affect necessarily benefits intention realization, however. When people are in a positive mood, they are less successful in realizing their intentions to avoid stereotyping (Bayer, Gollwitzer, & Achtziger, 2010). It seems that positive affect and negative affect can both cause self-regulatory problems.

Unwelcome social influences can also disrupt the translation of intentions into action, often without people being aware of that influence. For instance, people may not realize how group settings and task instructions can lead to social loafing (i.e., lower effort and attainment by individuals when in a group than when alone; Karau & Williams, 1993). Gollwitzer and Bayer (2000) observed that even participants who had strong intentions to perform well nonetheless showed reduced performance in a group task when each person's contribution supposedly could not be identified. Similarly, being mimicked by another person caused participants to comply with a request for funds even though participants had strong intentions to save money (Wieber, Gollwitzer, & Sheeran, 2014). And stereotypes concerning the typical binge drinker also influenced participants' drinking behavior, without participants being aware of, or intending, this influence (Rivis & Sheeran, 2013).

Low willpower has trait and state dimensions, and evidence suggests that both can increase the intention–behavior gap. At the trait level, several studies have shown that participants with low executive function (assessed by Go/No-Go or Stroop task performance) are less successful at translating their intentions into action than those with better executive functions (Allan, Johnston, & Campbell, 2011; Hall, Fong, Epp, & Elias, 2008; Wong & Mullan, 2009). Equivalent findings were observed for personality factors relevant to willpower, including low levels of conscientiousness (Conner, Rodgers, & Murray, 2007), future time orientation (Kovač & Rise, 2007), volitional control (Orbell & Hagger, 2006), mindfulness (Chatzisarantis & Hagger, 2007), and locomotion concerns (Mannetti, Pierro, Higgins, & Kruglanski, 2012). The intentions of adolescents and young adults are also less predictive of action than the intentions of mature adults (Pomery, Gibbons, Reis-Bergan, & Gerrard, 2009). For young people, ratings of behavioral willingness (i.e., the inclination to engage in risk behavior given conducive circumstances) better predicted substance use and unsafe sex compared with intentions to avoid risk (see Gerrard, Gibbons, Houlihan, Stock, & Pomery, 2008; Gibbons, Kingsbury, & Gerrard, 2012, for reviews).

Low willpower is also a state, termed *ego depletion* (Baumeister, Bratslavsky, Muraven, & Tice, 1998), and is apparent in poorer performance on a second self-control task following the exertion of self-control on an initial task. Although there is much debate about the magnitude of the ego-depletion effect and its interpretation (e.g., Carter, Kofler, Forster, & McCullough, 2015; Hagger & Chatzisarantis, 2014; Inzlicht, Schmeichel, & Macrae, 2014), ego depletion appears to moderate the intention–behavior relation. For example, intentions to curb food (Hofmann, Rauch, & Gawronski, 2007) and alcohol intake (Friese, Hofmann, & Wänke, 2008) did not predict subsequent consumption when participants were depleted by an initial self-control task. Among depleted participants, automatic attitudes toward the specified food and drink—indexed by responses to implicit association tests (Greenwald, McGhee, & Schwartz, 1998)—predicted behavior.

The third major self-regulatory problem is continuing to engage in a futile course of action (Gollwitzer & Sheeran, 2006). Disengagement from goals becomes necessary when it becomes clear that the desired outcome is unattainable, or that the costs of continued striving outweigh the benefits. The difficulty lies in recognizing that these circumstances have arisen, overcoming self-defensiveness, concerns about accountability, or sunk costs (Arkes & Blumer, 1985), and effectively calling a halt. Research on escalation of commitment makes it clear, however, that merely intending to disengage is not sufficient to bring goal striving to a halt (Henderson, Gollwitzer, & Oettingen, 2007).

The final problem has to do with failing to conserve capacity for future goal striving. People typically have multiple goals that they wish to pursue (e.g., Fitzsimons & Shah, 2012). As the phenomenon of ego depletion makes clear, however, enacting intentions on an initial task can compromise performance on a second task that also requires self-control (Baumeister et al., 1998). Action control by goal intentions can lead people to overextend themselves. For instance, Martijn et al. (2008) observed that rates of goal attainment and quality of performance both diminished sharply when participants encountered a minor blockage (e.g., a website that they had been asked to visit was temporarily unavailable and had to be visited later)—even though participants held strong intentions to complete the task. In sum, the road to hell presents manifold problems that can prevent the translation of intention into action.

WHAT INTERVENTIONS AID THE REALIZATION OF INTENTIONS?: TOOLS OF THE *GOOD INTENTIONS PAVING COMPANY*

Key approaches to promoting intention realization are mental contrasting, if–then planning, mental contrasting with implementation intentions (MCII), and interventions designed to prompt progress monitoring. We also consider other approaches that have been studied less intensively but may also hold promise in closing the intention–behavior gap.

Mental Contrasting

Fantasizing about (or "indulging" in) a desired future does not make that future more likely, and it may even be counterproductive, as it reduces efforts to achieve the goal (for reviews, see Oettingen, 2012; Oettingen & Sevincer, Chapter 7, this volume). For example, Oettingen and Wadden (1991) found that people who were trying to lose weight who imagined successfully resisting a tempting box of doughnuts lost less weight than those who imagined having a hard time resisting the same temptation (see Kappes, Oettingen, & Mayer, 2012; Oettingen & Mayer, 2002; Sevincer, Wagner, Kalvelage, & Oettingen, 2014, for similar findings). However, evidence also suggests that mentally contrasting a desired future with obstacles in the current reality that stand in the way of achieving that desired future can help people both to identify and abandon goals that are unlikely to be achieved (e.g., learning Mandarin before dinner time) and promote the effective pursuit of feasible goals. Oettingen et al. (2001, Study 3) prompted students to mentally elaborate on a positive outcome of resolving an interpersonal concern (e.g., feeling loved if they improved their relationship with their partner) and then an aspect of the present reality that currently stands in the way of achieving that outcome (e.g., being too emotional). Oettingen et al. (2001) observed that students who mentally contrasted in this manner were more likely to behave in line with their expectations (e.g., to achieve their goals if so doing was possible, and to abandon them if it was futile to try) compared with those in several control conditions. Subsequent research has demonstrated that mental contrasting promotes the effective pursuit of a wide variety of goals, including integrative bargaining in the lab, time management and decision making among health care professionals, school performance among disadvantaged children, and physical activity among sedentary, overweight men (see Oettingen, 2012, for a review). Mental contrasting aids the realization of intentions because this tool helps people to connect future and reality (Kappes & Oettingen, 2014) and realize that they need to take action (and thus forges strong goal commitments; e.g., Oettingen et al., 2001); mental contrasting also energizes goal pursuit (Oettingen et al., 2009) and promotes adaptive handling of negative feedback on goal progress (Kappes, Oettingen, & Pak, 2012).

If–Then Plans

Perhaps the most widely researched and best-validated tool for improving the translation of intentions into action is prompting people to form if–then plans, or *implementation intentions* (see Gollwitzer, 1999, 2014; Gollwitzer & Sheeran, 2006, 2009; Wieber, Thürmer, & Gollwitzer, 2015, for reviews). As Gollwitzer and Crosby (Chapter 17, this volume) present a comprehensive account of research on implementation intentions, here we merely point out that if–then plans have proven highly effective in accomplishing the self-regulatory tasks outlined above and have thereby aided the execution of intended actions (see Gollwitzer & Sheeran, 2006; Adriaanse, Vinkers, de Ridder, Hox, & de Wit, 2011; Bélanger-Gravel, Godin, & Amireault, 2013, for meta-analyses). If–then plans have been shown to help people to get started, stay on track, halt futile goal striving, and conserve self-regulatory capacity (Gollwitzer & Sheeran, 2006). Evidence suggests that people who furnished their intentions with if–then plans better remembered to take their prescribed medications (Brown, Sheeran, & Reuber, 2009; O'Carroll, Chambers, Dennis, Sudlow, & Johnston, 2013), were more likely to seize opportunities to act toward their goals (e.g., Webb, Sheeran, & Pepper, 2012), overcome procrastination (Wieber & Gollwitzer, 2010), and engage in preparatory behaviors (Arden & Armitage, 2008). Forming implementation intentions has been shown to help to overcome a variety of unwanted influences, including distractions (Wieber, von Suchodoletz, Heikamp, Trommsdorff, & Gollwitzer, 2015), temptations (e.g., Armitage & Arden, 2012), and unwelcome social influences (e.g., Rivis & Sheeran, 2013; Wieber et al., 2014). If–then plans lead to considerably better emotion control compared with merely intending to use the respective emotion regulation strategy (d_+ = 0.54; Webb, Schweiger Gallo, Miles, Gollwitzer, & Sheeran, 2012), and have been shown to reduce the impact of anxiety (Webb et al., 2010), worry (Sheeran et al., 2007), unhelpful moods (Bayer et al., 2010; Webb, Sheeran, Totterdell, et al., 2012) and arousal (Webb, Sheeran, Totterdell, et al., 2012) on the performance of intended behaviors. People who formed if–then plans were also better able to disengage from futile goal striving (Henderson et al., 2007) and showed more frequent, higher quality, and more strenuous efforts to realize subsequent intentions (Martijn et al., 2008). Importantly, these effects are observed not only with college students in the lab, but also in the field, over extended periods, using objective measures, among vulnerable groups (e.g., Toli, Webb, & Hardy, 2016), and with consequential issues such as the prevention of teen pregnancy (Martin, Sheeran, Slade, Wright, & Dibble, 2009, 2011) and uptake of smoking among adolescents (Conner & Higgins, 2010), as well as cancer screening (Neter, Stein, Barnett-Griness, Rennert, & Hagoel, 2014).

Mental Contrasting with Implementation Intentions

Recently, researchers have started to investigate the efficacy of combining mental contrasting with implementation intentions to promote the realization of intentions. This combination of self-regulation tools is synergistic, as mental contrasting (1) forges strong goal intentions, and implementation intention effects depend upon strong goal intentions (Sheeran, Webb, & Gollwitzer, 2005), and (2) increases the inclination to plan feasible goals (Oettingen et al., 2001). Whereas most if–then plan inductions are paternalistic in the sense that the self-regulatory problem to be tackled and the components of the if–then plan are specified by the researcher, mental contrasting enables participants themselves to identify their idiosyncratic problems with intention realization and to specify the plan components in a nonpaternalistic and autonomous fashion. Evidence indicates that MCII leads to improved rates of behavioral performance and goal attainment compared with either mental contrasting or forming implementation intentions on its own (Adriaanse et al., 2010; Kirk, Oettingen, & Gollwitzer, 2013). MCII helped students to engage in preparatory activities for an exam (Duckworth, Grant, Loew, Oettingen, & Gollwitzer, 2011) and adults to manage their time (Oettingen, Kappes, Guttenberg, & Gollwitzer, 2015), achieve their intentions to eat less meat (Loy, Wieber, Gollwitzer, & Oettingen, 2016), and reduce behaviors indicative of insecurity in relationships (e.g., looking at a partner's phone log; Houssais, Oettingen, & Mayer, 2013). MCII has proven effective with clinical samples and helped people with depression to engage in physical and social activities (Fritzsche, Schlier, Oettingen, & Lincoln, 2016) and people with schizophrenia to act on their intentions to go jogging (Sailer et al., 2015).

Progress-Monitoring Interventions

Control theory (Powers, 1973) suggests that goals serve as reference values and that perceiving a discrepancy between one's current standing and the standard specified in one's goal serves to motivate goal striving. According to this analysis, monitoring goal progress (i.e., comparing one's current standing relative to the goal) is thus a key step between intention formation and goal attainment (e.g., de Bruin et al., 2012). Research on the ostrich problem shows, however, that people do not always monitor their progress as frequently as is needed to optimize goal striving (Webb et al., 2013).

Accordingly, interventions that promote progress monitoring (e.g., by making it easier for people to identify their current standing or by increasing the frequency of comparing current vs. set standards) should improve the translation of intentions into action. Harkin et al. (2016) meta-analyzed 138 interventions that used a wide variety of techniques to promote progress monitoring (e.g., via food or activity diaries, self-weighing). Findings showed that a large-sized increase in the frequency of progress monitoring ($d_+ = 1.98$) led to a small-to-medium-sized change in behavior ($d_+ = 0.40$). Harkin et al. (2016) also identified several features of progress monitoring that led to greater impact on intended behaviors. For instance, interventions had larger effects when the focus of monitoring (behavior or outcomes) matched the desired outcome (e.g., a change in behavior or outcomes). Thus self-weighing promoted weight loss but not snack consumption, whereas monitoring snack consumption promoted healthy eating behavior but not weight loss. Interventions designed to prompt progress monitoring also proved more effective when progress was physically recorded (e.g., in a diary) or made public (e.g., group weighing sessions).

Other Approaches

These are exciting times for the development of interventions to help people to translate their intentions into action. Interventions based on the strength model of self-control, such as self-control training (Muraven, 2010), have shown promise, although recent research offers more cautious assessments (Inzlicht & Berman, 2015; Miles et al., 2016). Two kinds of training inspired by dual-process theories (e.g., Strack & Deutsch, 2004) that target impulsive responding or intentional control over impulsive responses also show promise. For instance, stop-signal or Go/NoGo training has been found to improve diet and weight control (van Koningsbruggen, Veling, Stroebe, & Aarts, 2014; Veling, van Koningsbruggen, Aarts, & Stroebe, 2014) and approach–avoidance training has been found to have a dramatic effect on relapse rates among patients with alcoholism (Eberl et al., 2013). Working memory training also reduced alcohol consumption (Houben, Wiers, & Jansen, 2011), though there is much debate about the magnitude and mechanisms of training effects (e.g., Shipstead, Redick, & Engle, 2012; von Bastian & Oberauer, 2014). Embodiment simulations (e.g., practicing dental flossing prior to performance of the behavior) have also strengthened intention–behavior consistency (Sherman, Gangi, & White, 2010). It is important to note, however, that not all of these approaches have formally tested whether the treatment moderates the relationship between intentions and behavior; so doing, therefore, constitutes an important avenue for future interventions in this area.

CONCLUSION

This overview indicates that the intention–behavior gap is substantial—intentions get translated into action approximately one-half of the time. Numerous moderators of the intention–behavior relation have been identified. Intention stability appears to promote intention realization, whereas counterintentional habits make it much harder to enact intentions. There has been considerable progress in identifying the problems that thwart the fulfillment of intention, and techniques such as mental contrasting, implementation intentions, and MCII have proven a boon to interventionists and provided effective tools for helping people to do the things they intend to do. Much remains to be done, of course. There is a need for an overarching theoretical perspective on intention–behavior relations that unites the disparate work in this area. Work on interventions is also needed as practitioners and policymakers concerned with promoting public health, energy conservation, and educational and organizational outcomes look for effective, scalable tools to increase intention–behavior consistency (Sheeran, Klein, & Rothman, 2017). In short, we should intend to undertake more research on intention–behavior relations.

ACKNOWLEDGMENTS

This research was supported by grants from the John Templeton Foundation (to Paschal Sheeran and Thomas L. Webb; No. 23145) and the European Research Council (to Thomas L. Webb; ERC-2011-StG-280515). The views expressed are the authors' and do not necessarily reflect the views of the funding bodies. We thank Katelyn Jones for help in preparing the manuscript.

REFERENCES

Abraham, C., & Sheeran, P. (2004). Deciding to exercise: The role of anticipated regret. *British Journal of Health Psychology, 9,* 269–278.

Adriaanse, M. A., Oettingen, G., Gollwitzer, P. M., Hennes, E. P., de Ridder, D. T. D., & de Wit, J. B. F. (2010). When planning is not enough: Fighting unhealthy snacking habits by mental contrasting with implementation intentions (MCII). *European Journal of Social Psychology, 40,* 1277–1293.

Adriaanse, M. A., Vinkers, C. D., De Ridder, D. T., Hox, J. J., & De Wit, J. B. (2011). Do implementation intentions help to eat a healthy diet?: A systematic review and meta-analysis of the empirical evidence. *Appetite, 56,* 183–193.

Ajzen, I. (1991). The theory of planned behaviour. *Organizational Behaviour and Human Decision Processes, 50,* 179–211.

Allan, J. L., Johnston, M., & Campbell, N. (2011). Missed by an inch or a mile?: Predicting the size of intention–behaviour gap from measures of executive control. *Psychology and Health, 26,* 635–650.

Arden, M. A., & Armitage, C. J. (2008). Predicting and explaining transtheoretical model stage transitions in relation to condom-carrying behaviour. *British Journal of Health Psychology, 13,* 719–735.

Arkes, H. R., & Blumer, C. (1985). The psychology of sunk cost. *Organizational Behavior and Human Decision Processes, 35,* 124–140.

Armitage, C. J., & Arden, M. A. (2012). A volitional help sheet to reduce alcohol consumption in the general population: A field experiment. *Prevention Science, 13,* 635–643.

Armitage, C. J., & Conner, M. (2001). Efficacy of the theory of planned behaviour: A meta-analytic review. *British Journal of Social Psychology, 40,* 471–499.

Austin, J. T., & Vancouver, J. B. (1996). Goal constructs in psychology: Structure, process, and content. *Psychological Bulletin, 120,* 338–375.

Bandura, A. (1996). Failures in self-regulation: Energy depletion or selective disengagement? *Psychological Inquiry, 7,* 20–24.

Bandura, A. (1998). Health promotion from the perspective of social cognitive theory. *Psychology and Health, 13*(4), 623–649.

Bargh, J. A. (2006). What have we been priming all these years?: On the development, mechanisms, and ecology of nonconscious social behavior. *European Journal of Social Psychology, 36,* 147–168.

Baumeister, R. F., & Bargh, J. A. (2014). Conscious and unconscious: Toward an integrative understanding of human mental life and action. In J. W. Sherman, B. Gawronski, Y. Trope, J. W. Sherman, B. Gawronski, & Y. Trope (Eds.), *Dual-process theories of the social mind* (pp. 35–49). New York: Guilford Press.

Baumeister, R. F., Bratslavsky, E., Muraven, M., & Tice, D. M. (1998). Ego-depletion: Is the active self a limited resource? *Journal of Personality and Social Psychology, 74,* 1252–1265.

Bayer, U. C., Gollwitzer, P. M., & Achtziger, A. (2010). Staying on track: Planned goal striving is protected from disruptive internal states. *Journal of Experimental Social Psychology, 46,* 505–514.

Bélanger, J. J., Lafrenière, M. K., Vallerand, R. J., & Kruglanski, A. W. (2013). When passion makes the heart grow colder: The role of passion in alternative goal suppression. *Journal of Personality and Social Psychology, 104,* 126–147.

Bélanger-Gravel, A., Godin, G., & Amireault, S. (2013). A meta-analytic review of the effect of implementation intentions on physical activity. *Health Psychology Review, 7,* 23–54.

Brown, I., Sheeran, P., & Reuber, M. (2009). Enhancing antiepileptic drug adherence: A randomized controlled trial. *Epilepsy and Behavior, 16,* 634–639.

Buehler, R., Griffin, D., & Ross, M. (1994). Exploring the "planning fallacy": Why people underestimate their task completion times. *Journal of Personality and Social Psychology, 67*, 366–381.

Carter, E. C., Kofler, L. M., Forster, D. E., & McCullough, M. E. (2015). A series of meta-analytic tests of the depletion effect: Self-control does not seem to rely on a limited resource. *Journal of Experimental Psychology: General, 144*, 796–815.

Carvalho, T., Alvarez, M. J., Barz, M., & Schwarzer, R. (2015). Preparatory behavior for condom use among heterosexual young men: A longitudinal mediation model. *Health Education and Behavior, 42*, 92–99.

Chatzisarantis, N. L., & Hagger, M. S. (2007). Mindfulness and the intention–behavior relationship within the theory of planned behavior. *Personality and Social Psychology Bulletin, 3*, 663–676.

Chiaburu, D. S., Oh, I. S., Berry, C. M., Li, N., & Gardner, R. G. (2011). The five-factor model of personality traits and organizational citizenship behaviors: A meta-analysis. *Journal of Applied Psychology, 96*, 1140–1166.

Conner, M., & Godin, G. (2007). Temporal stability of behavioural intention as a moderator of intention-health behaviour relationships. *Psychology and Health, 22*, 875–897.

Conner, M., & Higgins, A. R. (2010). Long-term effects of implementation intentions on prevention of smoking uptake among adolescents: A cluster randomized controlled trial. *Health Psychology, 29*, 529–538.

Conner, M., McEachan, R., Jackson, C., McMillan, B., Woolridge, M., & Lawton, R. (2013). Moderating effect of socioeconomic status on the relationship between health cognitions and behaviors. *Annals of Behavioral Medicine, 46*, 19–30.

Conner, M., Norman, P., & Bell, R. (2002). The theory of planned behavior and healthy eating. *Health Psychology, 21*, 194–201.

Conner, M., Rodgers, W., & Murray, T. (2007). Conscientiousness and the intention–behavior relationship: Predicting exercise behavior. *Journal of Sport and Exercise Psychology, 29*, 518–533.

Conner, M., Sandberg, T., McMillan, B., & Higgins, A. (2006). Role of anticipated regret, intentions and intention stability in adolescent smoking initiation. *British Journal of Health Psychology, 11*, 85–101.

Cooke, R., & Sheeran, P. (2004) Moderation of cognition–intention and cognition–behaviour relations: A meta-analysis of properties of variables from the theory of planned behaviour. *British Journal of Social Psychology, 43*, 159–186.

Cooke, R., & Sheeran, P. (2013). Properties of intention: Component structure and consequences for behavior, information processing, and resistance. *Journal of Applied Social Psychology, 43*, 749–760.

Corradi, N., Priftis, K., Jacucci, G., & Gamberini, L. (2013). Oops, I forgot the light on!: The cognitive mechanisms supporting the execution of energy saving behaviors. *Journal of Economic Psychology, 34*, 88–96.

de Bruin, M., Sheeran, P., Kok, G., Hiemstra, A., Prins, J. M., Hospers, H. J., . . . van Breukelen, G. J. (2012). Self-regulatory processes mediate the intention–behavior relation for adherence and exercise behaviors. *Health Psychology, 31*, 695–703.

de Witt Huberts, J. C., Evers, C., & de Ridder, D. T. D. (2012). License to sin: Self-licensing as underlying mechanism of hedonic consumption. *European Journal of Social Psychology, 42*, 490–496.

Deci, E. L., & Ryan, R. M. (2000). The "what" and "why" of goal pursuits: Human needs and the self-determination of behavior. *Psychological Inquiry, 11*, 227–268.

Dholakia, U. M., & Bagozzi, R. (2006). As time goes by: How goal and implementation intentions influence enactment of short-fuse behaviors. *Journal of Applied Social Psychology, 33*, 889–922.

DiBonaventura, M., & Chapman, G. B. (2008). The effect of barrier underestimation on weight management and exercise change. *Psychology, Health and Medicine, 13*, 111–122.

Doll, J., & Ajzen, I. (1992). Accessibility and stability of predictors in the theory of planned behavior. *Journal of Personality and Social Psychology, 63*, 754–765.

Duckworth, A. L., Grant, H., Loew, B., Oettingen, G., & Gollwitzer, P. M. (2011) Self-regulation strategies improve self-discipline in adolescents: Benefits of mental contrasting and implementation intentions. *Educational Psychology, 31*, 17–26.

Eberl, C., Wiers, R. W., Pawelczack, S., Rinck, M., Becker, E. S., & Lindenmeyer, J. (2013). Approach bias modification in alcohol dependence: Do clinical effects replicate and for whom does it work best? *Developmental Cognitive Neuroscience, 4*, 38–51.

Einstein, G. O., McDaniel, M. A., Williford, C. L., Pagan, J. L., & Dismukes, R. (2003). Forgetting of intentions in demanding situations is rapid. *Journal of Experimental Psychology: Applied, 9*, 147–162.

Fife-Schaw, C., Sheeran, P., & Norman, P. (2007). Simulating behaviour change interventions based on the theory of planned behaviour: Impacts on intention and action. *British Journal of Social Psychology, 46*, 43–68.

Fishbach, A., Friedman, R. S., & Kruglanski, A. W. (2003). Leading us not into temptation: Momentary allurements elicit overriding goal activation. *Journal of Personality and Social Psychology, 84*, 269–309.

Fitzsimons, G. M., & Shah, J. Y. (2012). Confusing one instrumental other for another: Goal effects on social categorization. *Psychological Science, 20*, 1468–1472.

Friese, M., Hofmann, W., & Wänke, M. (2008). When impulses take over: Moderated predictive validity of explicit and implicit attitude measures in predicting food choice and consumption behaviour. *British Journal of Social Psychology, 47*, 397–419.

Fritzsche, A., Schlier, B., Oettingen, G., & Lincoln, T. M. (2016). Mental contrasting with implementation intentions increases goal-attainment in individuals with mild to moderate depression. *Cognitive Therapy and Research, 40*, 557–564.

Gerrard, M., Gibbons, F. X., Houlihan, A. E., Stock, M. L., & Pomery, E. A. (2008). A dual-process approach to health risk decision making: The prototype willingness model. *Developmental Review, 28*, 29–61.

Gibbons, F. X., Kingsbury, J. H., & Gerrard, M. (2012). Social-psychological theories and adolescent health risk behavior. *Social and Personality Psychology Compass, 6*, 170–183.

Godin, G., & Conner, M. (2008). Intention–behavior relationship based on epidemiologic indices: An application to physical activity. *American Journal of Health Promotion, 22*, 180–182.

Godin, G., Conner, M., & Sheeran, P. (2005). Bridging the intention–behaviour "gap": The role of moral norm. *British Journal of Social Psychology, 44*, 497–512.

Godin, G., Germain, M., Conner, M., Delage, G., & Sheeran, P. (2014). Promoting the return of lapsed blood donors: A seven-arm randomized controlled trial of the question–behavior effect. *Health Psychology, 33*, 646–655.

Gollwitzer, P. M. (1999). Implementation intentions: Strong effects of simple plans. *American Psychologist, 54*, 493–503.

Gollwitzer, P. M. (2014). Weakness of the will: Is a quick fix possible? *Motivation and Emotion, 38*, 305–322.

Gollwitzer, P. M., & Bayer, U. C. (2000, October). *Becoming a better person without changing the self.* Paper presented at the Self and Identity Preconference of the annual meeting of the Society of Experimental Social Psychology, Atlanta, Georgia.

Gollwitzer, P. M., & Sheeran, P. (2006). Implementation intentions and goal achievement: A meta-analysis of effects and processes. *Advances in Experimental Social Psychology, 38*, 69–120.

Gollwitzer, P. M., & Sheeran, P. (2009). Self-regulation of consumer decision making and behavior: The role of implementation intentions. *Journal of Consumer Psychology, 19,* 593–607.

Gollwitzer, P. M., Sheeran, P., Michalski, V., & Seifert, A. E. (2009). When intentions go public: Does social reality widen the intention–behavior gap? *Psychological Science, 20,* 612–618.

Gollwitzer, P. M., Sheeran, P., Trötschel, R., & Webb, T. L. (2011). Self-regulation of priming effects on behavior. *Psychological Science, 22,* 901–907.

Goschke, T., & Kuhl, J. (1993). Representation of intentions: Persisting activation in memory. *Journal of Experimental Psychology: Learning, Memory, and Cognition, 19,* 1211–1226.

Greenwald, A. G., McGhee, D. E., & Schwartz, J. K. (1998). Measuring individual differences in implicit cognition: The Implicit Association Test. In R. H. Fazio, R. E. Petty, R. H. Fazio, & R. E. Petty (Eds.), *Attitudes: Their structure, function, and consequences* (pp. 109–131). New York: Psychology Press.

Hagger, M. S., & Chatzisarantis, N. L. D. (2014). It is premature to regard the ego-depletion effect as "too incredible." *Frontiers in Psychology, 5,* 298.

Hall, P. A., Fong, G. T., Epp, L. J., & Elias, L. J. (2008). Executive function moderates the intention–behavior link for physical activity and dietary behavior. *Psychology and Health, 23,* 309–326.

Harkin, B., Webb, T. L., Chang, B. P., Prestwich, A., Conner, M., Kellar, I., & Sheeran, P. (2016). Does monitoring goal progress promote goal attainment?: A meta-analysis of the experimental evidence. *Psychological Bulletin, 142,* 198–229.

Henderson, M. D., Gollwitzer, P. M., & Oettingen, G. (2007). Implementation intentions and disengagement from a failing course of action. *Journal of Behavioral Decision Making, 20,* 81–102.

Hofmann, W., Baumeister, R. F., Förster, G., & Vohs, K. D. (2012). Everyday temptations: An experience sampling study of desire, conflict, and self-control. *Journal of Personality and Social Psychology, 102,* 1318–1335.

Hofmann, W., Rauch, W., & Gawronski, B. (2007). And deplete us not into temptation: Automatic attitudes, dietary restraint, and self-regulatory resources as determinants of eating behavior. *Journal of Experimental Social Psychology, 43,* 497–504.

Houben, K., Wiers, R. W., & Jansen, A. (2011). Getting a grip on drinking behavior: Training working memory to reduce alcohol abuse. *Psychological Science, 22,* 968–975.

Houssais, S., Oettingen, G., & Mayer, D. (2013). Using mental contrasting with implementation intentions to self-regulate insecurity-based behaviors in relationships. *Motivation and Emotion, 37,* 224–233.

Inzlicht, M., & Berkman, E. (2015). Six questions for the resource model of control (and some answers). *Social and Personality Psychology Compass, 9*(10), 511–524.

Inzlicht, M., Schmeichel, B. J., & Macrae, C. N. (2014). Why self-control seems (but may not be) limited. *Trends in Cognitive Sciences, 18,* 127–133.

Johnson, R. E., Chang, C. H., & Lord, R. G. (2006). Moving from cognition to behavior: What the research says. *Psychological Bulletin, 132,* 381–415.

Kappes, A., & Oettingen, G. (2014). The emergence of goal pursuit: Mental contrasting connects future and reality. *Journal of Experimental Social Psychology, 54,* 25–39.

Kappes, A., Oettingen, G., & Pak, H. (2012). Mental contrasting and the self-regulation of responding to negative feedback. *Personality and Social Psychology Bulletin, 38,* 845–857.

Kappes, H. B., Oettingen, G., & Mayer, D. (2012). Positive fantasies predict low academic achievement in disadvantaged students. *European Journal of Social Psychology, 42,* 53–64.

Kappes, H. B., Singmann, H., & Oettingen, G. (2012). Mental contrasting instigates goal pursuit by linking obstacles of reality with instrumental behavior. *Journal of Experimental Social Psychology, 48,* 811–818.

Karau, S. J., & Williams, K. D. (1993). Social loafing: A meta-analytic review and theoretical integration. *Journal of Personality and Social Psychology, 65,* 681–706.

Kashima, Y., Gallois, C., & McCamish, M. (1993). The theory of reasoned action and cooperative behaviour: It takes two to use a condom. *British Journal of Social Psychology, 32,* 227–239.

Keer, M., Conner, M., Putte, B., & Neijens, P. (2014). The temporal stability and predictive validity of affect-based and cognition-based intentions. *British Journal of Social Psychology, 53,* 315–327.

Kendzierski, D. (1990). Exercise self-schemata: Cognitive and behavioral correlates. *Health Psychology, 9,* 69–82.

Kirk, D., Oettingen, G., & Gollwitzer, P. M. (2013). Promoting integrative bargaining: Mental contrasting with implementation intentions. *International Journal of Conflict Management, 24,* 148–165.

Klinger, E. (1971). *Structure and functions of fantasy.* New York: Wiley.

Klinger, E. (1975). Consequences of commitment to and disengagement from incentives. *Psychological Review, 82,* 1–25.

Klinger, E. (1977). *Meaning and void: Inner experience and the incentives in people's lives.* Minneapolis: University of Minnesota Press.

Kovać, V. B., & Rise, J. (2007). The relation between past behavior, intention, planning, and quitting smoking: The moderating effect of future orientation. *Journal of Applied Biobehavioral Research, 12,* 82–100.

Kuhl, J., & Quirin, M. (2011). Seven steps toward freedom and two ways to lose it: Overcoming limitations of intentionality through self-confrontational coping with stress. *Social Psychology, 42,* 74–84.

Liberman, N., & Dar, R. (2009). Normal and pathological consequences of encountering difficulties in monitoring progress towards goals. In G. B. Moskowitz & H. Grant (Eds.), *The psychology of goals* (pp. 277–303). New York: Guilford Press.

Locke, E. A., & Latham, G. P. (1992). "Process feedback in task groups: An application of goal setting": Comments. *Journal of Applied Behavioral Science, 28,* 42–45.

Loy, L. S., Wieber, F., Gollwitzer, P. M., & Oettingen, G. (2016). Supporting sustainable food consumption: Mental contrasting with implementation intentions (MCII) aligns intentions and behavior. *Frontiers in Psychology, 7,* 607.

Mannetti, L., Pierro, A., Higgins, E. T., & Kruglanski, A. W. (2012). Maintaining physical exercise: How locomotion mode moderates the full attitude–intention–behavior relation. *Basic and Applied Social Psychology, 34,* 295–303.

Martijn, C., Alberts, H., Sheeran, P., Peters, G. J. Y., Mikolajczak, J., & De Vries, N. K. (2008). Blocked goals, persistent action: Implementation intentions engender tenacious goal striving. *Journal of Experimental Social Psychology, 44,* 1137–1143.

Martin, J., Sheeran, P., Slade, P., Wright, A., & Dibble, T. (2009). Implementation intention formation reduces consultations for emergency contraception and pregnancy testing among teenage women. *Health Psychology, 28,* 762–769.

Martin, J., Sheeran, P., Slade, P., Wright, A., & Dibble, T. (2011). Durable effects of implementation intentions: Reduced rates of confirmed pregnancy at 2 years. *Health Psychology, 30,* 368–373.

McEachan, R. R. C., Conner, M., Taylor, N. J., & Lawton, R. J. (2011). Prospective prediction of health-related behaviours with the theory of planned behaviour: A meta-analysis. *Health Psychology Review, 5,* 97–144.

Michie, S., Whittington, C., Abraham, C., McAteer, J., & Gupta, S. (2009). Effective techniques in healthy eating and physical activity interventions: A meta-regression. *Health Psychology, 28,* 690–701.

Miles, E., Sheeran, P., Baird, H. M., Macdonald, I., Webb, T. L., & Harris, P. R. (2016). Does self-control improve with practice?: Evidence from a 6-week training program. *Journal of Experimental Psychology: General, 145*(8), 1075–1091.

Milkman, K. L., Rogers, T., & Bazerman, M. H. (2008). Harnessing our inner angels and demons: What we have learned about want/should conflicts and how that knowledge can help us reduce short-sighted decision making. *Perspectives on Psychological Science, 3*, 324–338.

Muraven, M. (2010). Building self-control strength: Practicing self-control leads to improved self-control performance. *Journal of Experimental Social Psychology, 46*, 465–468.

Myrseth, K. O. R., & Fishbach, A. (2009). Self-control: A function of knowing when and how to exercise restraint. *Current Directions in Psychological Science, 18*, 247–252.

Neter, E., Stein, N., Barnett-Griness, O., Rennert, G., & Hagoel, L. (2014). From the bench to public health: Population-level implementation intentions in colorectal cancer screening. *American Journal of Preventive Medicine, 46*, 273–280.

Nordgren, L. F., van der Pligt, J., & van Harreveld, F. (2008). The instability of health cognitions: Visceral states influence self-efficacy and related health beliefs. *Health Psychology, 27*, 722–727.

O'Carroll, R. E., Chambers, J. A., Dennis, M., Sudlow, C., & Johnston, M. (2013). Improving adherence to medication in stroke survivors: A pilot randomised controlled trial. *Annals of Behavioral Medicine, 46*, 358–368.

O'Carroll, R. E., Chambers, J. A., Dennis, M., Sudlow, C., & Johnston, M. (2014). Improving medication adherence in stroke survivors: Mediators and moderators of treatment effects. *Health Psychology, 33*, 1241–1250.

Oettingen, G. (2012). Future thought and behavior change. *European Review of Social Psychology, 23*, 1–63.

Oettingen, G., Kappes, H. B., Guttenberg, K. B., & Gollwitzer, P. M. (2015). Self-regulation of time management: Mental contrasting with implementation intentions. *European Journal of Social Psychology, 45*, 218–229.

Oettingen, G., & Mayer, D. (2002). The motivating function of thinking about the future: Expectations versus fantasies. *Journal of Personality and Social Psychology, 83*, 1198–1212.

Oettingen, G., Mayer, D., Sevincer, A. T., Stephens, E. J., Pak, H., & Hagenah, M. (2009). Mental contrasting and goal commitment: The mediating role of energisation. *Personality and Social Psychology Bulletin, 35*, 608–622.

Oettingen, G., Pak, H., & Schnetter, K. (2001). Self-regulation of goal setting: Turning free fantasies about the future into binding goals. *Journal of Personality and Social Psychology, 80*, 736–753.

Oettingen, G., & Wadden, T. A. (1991). Expectation, fantasy, and weight loss: Is the impact of positive thinking always positive? *Cognitive Therapy and Research, 15*, 167–175.

Orbell, S., & Hagger, M. (2006). "When no means no": Can reactance augment the theory of planned behavior? *Health Psychology, 25*, 586–594.

Orbell, S., & Sheeran, P. (1998). "Inclined abstainers": A problem for predicting health-related behaviour. *British Journal of Social Psychology, 37*, 151–165.

Ouellette, J. A., & Wood, W. (1998). Habit and intention in everyday life: The multiple processes by which past behavior predicts future behavior. *Psychological Bulletin, 124*, 54–74.

Parks-Stamm, E. J., Gollwitzer, P. M., & Oettingen, G. (2010). Implementation intentions and test anxiety: Shielding academic performance from distraction. *Learning and Individual Differences, 20*, 30–33.

Pomery, E. A., Gibbons, F. X., Reis-Bergan, M., & Gerrard, M. (2009). From willingness to intention: Experience moderates the shift from reactive to reasoned behavior. *Personality and Social Psychology Bulletin, 35*, 894–908.

Poropat, A. E. (2009). A meta-analysis of the five-factor model of personality and academic performance. *Psychological Bulletin, 135,* 322–338.

Powers, W. T. (1973). *Behavior: The control of perception.* New York: Aldine de Gruyter.

Prinsen, S., Evers, C., & De Ridder, D. T. D. (2016). Oops I did it again: Examining self-licensing effects in a subsequent self-regulation dilemma. *Applied Psychology: Health and Well-Being, 8,* 104–126.

Rhodes, R. E., & de Bruijn, G. (2013). How big is the physical activity intention–behaviour gap?: A meta-analysis using the action control framework. *British Journal of Health Psychology, 18,* 296–309.

Rhodes, R. E., & Dickau, L. (2012). Experimental evidence for the intention–behavior relationship in the physical activity domain: A meta-analysis. *Health Psychology, 31,* 724–727.

Rhodes, R. E., & Smith, N. E. I. (2006). Personality correlates of physical activity: A review and meta-analysis. *British Journal of Sports Medicine, 40,* 958–965.

Rivis, A., & Sheeran, P. (2013). Automatic risk behavior: Direct effects of binge drinker stereotypes on drinking behavior. *Health Psychology, 32,* 571–580.

Rogers, R. W. (1983). Preventive health psychology: An interface of social and clinical psychology. *Journal of Social and Clinical Psychology, 1,* 120–127.

Sailer, P., Wieber, F., Pröpster, K., Stoewer, S., Nischk, D., Volk, F., . . . Odenwald, M. (2015). A brief intervention to improve exercising in patients with schizophrenia: A controlled pilot study with mental contrasting and implementation intentions (MCII). *BMC Psychiatry, 15,* 211.

Sevincer, A. T., Wagner, G., Kalvelage, J., & Oettingen, G. (2014). Positive thinking about the future in newspaper reports and presidential addresses predicts economic downturn. *Psychological Science, 25,* 1010–1017.

Shah, J. Y., Friedman, R., & Kruglanski, A. W. (2002). Forgetting all else: On the antecedents and consequences of goal shielding. *Journal of Personality and Social Psychology, 83,* 1261–1280.

Sheeran, P. (2002). Intention–behaviour relations: A conceptual and empirical review. *European Review of Social Psychology, 12,* 1–36.

Sheeran, P., & Abraham, C. (2003). Mediator of moderators: Temporal stability of intention and the intention–behavior relationship. *Personality and Social Psychology Bulletin, 29,* 205–215.

Sheeran, P., Abraham, C., & Orbell, S. (1999). Psychosocial correlates of heterosexual condom use: A meta-analysis. *Psychological Bulletin, 125,* 90–132.

Sheeran, P., Aubrey, R., & Kellett, S. (2007). Increasing attendance for psychotherapy: Implementation intentions and the self-regulation of attendance-related negative affect. *Journal of Consulting and Clinical Psychology, 75,* 853–863.

Sheeran, P., Godin, G., Conner, M., & Germain, M. (2017). Paradoxical effects of experience: Past behavior both strengthens and weakens the intention-behavior relationship. *Journal of the Association for Consumer Research.* Available at *www.researchgate.net/publication/314350932_Paradoxical_Effects_of_Experience_Past_Behavior_Both_Strengthens_and_Weakens_the_Intention-_Behavior_Relationship.*

Sheeran, P., Gollwitzer, P. M., & Bargh, J. A. (2013). Nonconscious processes and health. *Health Psychology, 32,* 460–473.

Sheeran, P., Harris, P. R., & Epton, T. (2014). Does heightening risk appraisals change people's intentions and behavior?: A meta-analysis of experimental studies. *Psychological Bulletin, 140,* 511–544.

Sheeran, P., Klein, W. M. P., & Rothman, A. J. (2017). Health behavior change: Moving from observation to intervention. *Annual Review of Psychology, 68,* 573–600.

Sheeran, P., & Orbell, S. (1998). Do intentions predict condom use?: A meta-analysis and examination of six moderator variables. *British Journal of Social Psychology, 37,* 231–250.

Sheeran, P., & Orbell, S. (1999). Implementation intentions and repeated behaviour: Augmenting the predictive validity of the theory of planned behaviour. *European Journal of Social Psychology, 29,* 349–369.

Sheeran, P., & Orbell, S. (2000). Using implementation intentions to increase attendance for cervical cancer screening. *Health Psychology, 19,* 283–289.

Sheeran, P., Orbell, S., & Trafimow, D. (1999). Does the temporal stability of behavioral intentions moderate intention–behavior and past behavior–future behavior relations? *Personality and Social Psychology Bulletin, 25,* 721–730.

Sheeran, P., Trafimow, D., & Armitage, C. J. (2003). Predicting behavior from perceived behavioural control: Tests of the accuracy assumption of the theory of planned behaviour. *British Journal of Social Psychology, 42,* 393–410.

Sheeran, P., Webb, T. L., & Gollwitzer, P. M. (2005). The interplay between goals and implementation intentions. *Personality and Social Psychology Bulletin, 31,* 87–98.

Sherman, D. K., Gangi, C., & White, M. L. (2010). Embodied cognition and health persuasion: Facilitating intention–behavior consistency via motor manipulations. *Journal of Experimental Social Psychology, 46,* 461–464.

Shipstead, Z., Redick, T. S., & Engle, R. W. (2012). Is working memory training effective? *Psychological Bulletin, 138,* 628–654.

Steel, P. (2007). The nature of procrastination: A meta-analytic and theoretical review of quintessential self-regulatory failure. *Psychological Bulletin, 133,* 65–94.

Strack, F., & Deutsch, R. (2004). Reflective and impulsive determinants of social behavior. *Personality and Social Psychology Review, 8,* 220–247.

Stroebe, W., van Koningsbruggen, G. M., Papies, E. K., & Aarts, H. (2013). Why most dieters fail but some succeed: A goal conflict model of eating behavior. *Psychological Review, 120,* 110–138.

Taylor, C., Webb, T. L., & Sheeran, P. (2014). "I deserve a treat!": Justifications for indulgence undermine the translation of intentions into action. *British Journal of Social Psychology, 53,* 501–520.

Thomas, G. O., Poortinga, W., & Sautkina, E. (2016). Habit discontinuity, self-activation, and the diminishing influence of context change: Evidence from the UK Understanding Society survey. *PLOS ONE, 11.* Available at *https://doi.org/10.1371/journal.pone.0153490.*

Toli, A., Webb, T. L., & Hardy, G. E. (2016). Does forming implementation intentions help people with mental health problems to achieve goals?: A meta-analysis of experimental studies with clinical and analogue samples. *British Journal of Clinical Psychology, 55,* 69–90.

Triandis, H. C. (1980). Values, attitudes, and interpersonal behavior. In H. E. Howe, Jr., & M. Page (Eds.), *Nebraska Symposium on Motivation: Vol. 27. Attitudes, values, and beliefs* (pp. 195–259). Lincoln: University of Nebraska Press.

Turchik, J. A., & Gidycz, C. A. (2012). Exploring the intention–behavior relationship in the prediction of sexual risk behaviors: Can it be strengthened? *Journal of Sex Research, 49,* 50–60.

van Empelen, P., & Kok, G. (2008). Action-specific cognitions of planned and preparatory behaviors of condom use among Dutch adolescents. *Archives of Sexual Behavior, 37,* 626–640.

van Koningsbruggen, G. M., Veling, H., Stroebe, W., & Aarts, H. (2014). Comparing two psychological interventions in reducing impulsive processes of eating behaviour: Effects on self-selected portion size. *British Journal of Health Psychology, 19,* 767–782.

Veling, H., van Koningsbruggen, G. M., Aarts, H., & Stroebe, W. (2014). Targeting impulsive processes of eating behavior via the Internet: Effects on body weight. *Appetite, 78,* 102–109.

Verplanken, B., & Roy, D. (2016). Empowering interventions to promote sustainable lifestyles: Testing the habit discontinuity hypothesis in a field experiment. *Journal of Environmental Psychology, 45,* 127–134.

von Bastian, C. C., & Oberauer, K. (2014). Effects and mechanisms of working memory training: A review. *Psychological Research, 78,* 803–820.

Wagner, D. D., & Heatherton, T. F. (2014) Emotion and self-regulation failure. In J. J. Gross (Ed.), *Handbook of emotion regulation* (2nd ed., pp. 613–628). New York: Guilford Press.

Webb, T. L., Chang, B. P. I., & Benn, Y. (2013). "The ostrich problem": Motivated avoidance or rejection of information about goal progress. *Social and Personality Psychology Compass, 7,* 794–807.

Webb, T. L., Ononaiye, M. S. P., Sheeran, P., Reidy, J. G., & Lavda, A. (2010). Using implementation intentions to overcome the effects of social anxiety on attention and appraisals of performance. *Personality and Social Psychology Bulletin, 36,* 612–627.

Webb, T. L., Schweiger Gallo, I., Miles, E., Gollwitzer, P. M., & Sheeran, P. (2012). Effective regulation of affect: An action control perspective on emotion regulation. *European Review of Social Psychology, 23,* 143–186.

Webb, T. L., & Sheeran, P. (2006). Does changing behavioral intentions engender behavior change?: A meta-analysis of the experimental evidence. *Psychological Bulletin, 132,* 249–268.

Webb, T. L., Sheeran, P., & Pepper, J. (2012). Gaining control over responses to implicit attitude tests: Implementation intentions engender fast responses on attitude-incongruent trials. *British Journal of Social Psychology, 51,* 13–32.

Webb, T. L., Sheeran, P., Totterdell, P., Miles, E., Mansell, W., & Baker, S. (2012). Using implementation intentions to overcome the effect of mood on risky behaviour. *British Journal of Social Psychology, 51,* 330–345.

Wicklund, R. A., & Gollwitzer, P. M. (1982). *Symbolic self-completion.* Hillsdale, NJ: Erlbaum.

Wieber, F., & Gollwitzer, P. M. (2010). Overcoming procrastination through planning. In C. Andreou & M. D. White (Eds.), *The thief of time: Philosophical essays on procrastination* (pp. 185–205). New York: Oxford University Press.

Wieber, F., Gollwitzer, P. M., & Sheeran, P. (2014). Strategic regulation of mimicry effects by implementation intentions. *Journal of Experimental Social Psychology, 5,* 31–39.

Wieber, F., Thürmer, J. L., & Gollwitzer, P. M. (2015). Promoting the translation of intentions into action by implementation intentions: Behavioral effects and physiological correlates. *Frontiers in Human Neuroscience, 9,* 395.

Wieber, F., von Suchodoletz, A., Heikamp, T., Trommsdorff, G., & Gollwitzer, P. M. (2015). If–then planning helps school-aged children to ignore attractive distractions. *Social Psychology, 42,* 39–47.

Wong, C. L., & Mullan, B. A. (2009). Predicting breakfast consumption: An application of the theory of planned behaviour and the investigation of past behaviour and executive function. *British Journal of Health Psychology, 14,* 489–504.

Wood, W., & Neal, D. T. (2007). A new look at habits and the habit–goal interface. *Psychological Review, 114,* 843–863.

Zogg, J. B., Woods, S. P., Sauceda, J. A., Wiebe, J. S., & Simoni, J. M. (2012). The role of prospective memory in medication adherence: A review of an emerging literature. *Journal of Behavioral Medicine, 35,* 47–62.

CHAPTER 26

Multiple Processes in Prospective Memory

Exploring the Nature of Spontaneous Retrieval

Gilles O. Einstein
Mark A. McDaniel
Francis T. Anderson

As is clear from many of the chapters in this volume, a core function of our episodic memory system and our neural architecture is envisioning the future and planning for it (Schacter, Addis, & Buckner, 2007). Survival and success favor individuals who can anticipate future needs, develop appropriate plans for meeting those needs, and then remember to carry out the planned actions at appropriate times. Consistent with this perspective, and despite the fact that research on episodic memory has focused almost exclusively on understanding how we remember past events (retrospective memory), recent findings suggest that much of our mental life is devoted to thinking about the future.

Using an experience sampling procedure, Gardner and Ascoli (2015) telephoned adults ranging in age from 18 to 75 at randomly determined times over several weeks. In response to the calls, participants indicated whether at the moment of the call they happened to be thinking about an event from the personal past (e.g., savoring last night's dinner), thinking about some event in the personal future (e.g., buying groceries for dinner later that day), or not thinking about either type of event (e.g., focused on the task at hand, such as writing a paper). Based on participants' descriptions of the duration of the thoughts, as well as their probability of having a thought of one type or the other, Gardner and Ascoli estimated that people have about 13 autobiographical memories per hour and at least as many thoughts about personal future events. On average, young adults were estimated to have about 17 future-related thoughts per hour, and this estimate jumped to 31 thoughts per hour for older adults! Thus it appears that young adults, and especially older adults, spend a great deal of their mental lives thinking about the future.

Much of our future-thinking involves prospective memory or memory for actions to be performed in the future. From remembering to initiate basic activities such as shopping for groceries or paying bills to fulfilling social obligations such as meeting a friend for lunch to remembering to take care of health-related needs such as taking medication, good prospective memory is important for smooth, efficient, and normal living. Prospective memory research has focused on understanding how we retrieve intentions at appropriate times, and this is the topic of this chapter. This is an interesting issue because, as pointed out by early researchers and theorists (e.g., Craik, 1986), a typical characteristic of prospective memory tasks is that they do not include a specific request to search memory at the moment of retrieval. In remembering to give a friend a message when you see him or her or in remembering to buy groceries on the way home, for example, there is usually no one there to remind you to interrogate memory for the relevant action upon seeing your friend or upon passing the grocery store (i.e., no one is there to put you in a retrieval mode; Tulving, 1983).

This characteristic of prospective memory retrieval can be appreciated by comparing a typical retrospective memory task such as cued recall with a typical event-based prospective memory task. As shown in Table 26.1, in a cued-recall task, the experimenter first asks participants to study a list of cue-target pairs. Next, after a delay, the experimenter tests participants by presenting them with cues and asking them to search memory for the associated items. In doing so, the experimenter explicitly asks participants to search memory for the items associated to the cues (i.e., the experimenter puts participants in a retrieval mode). By contrast, in a typical event-based prospective memory task, participants may be asked to remember to make a designated response (e.g., press the *Q* key) when they later see the word *rake* in the context of performing an ongoing task (e.g., a lexical decision task). As shown in Table 26.1, during Phase 2 testing, the target word *rake* occurs without a prompt to search memory for the significance of the item. Without the benefit of being in an externally prompted retrieval mode, participants have to go beyond seeing the item *rake* as an item to be rated for the lexical decision task and to retrieve the intention to press the designated key.

It is important to note that in most experiments the prospective memory task is relatively simple (as in the example above), and participants are required to verify that they fully understand the instructions (and often tested at the end of the experiment for their retrospective memory of the instructions). Thus the attempt in most experiments is to isolate the prospective memory component as the source of forgetting. That is, the interest is in understanding the conditions under which we forget to perform an intended action (the prospective memory intention) despite having complete retrospective memory for what we intended to do (e.g., we forget to give a friend a message when we see her or him even though we can, when prompted, remember the intention and the message).

One major theoretical approach to understanding how the prospective memory retrieval challenge is accomplished (McDaniel & Einstein, 2000, 2007) is to assume that intentions can be remembered using top-down attentional control processes (or monitoring) as well as bottom-up spontaneous retrieval processes that are initiated by the processing of a relevant cue (see Heathcote, Loft, & Remington, 2015, and Smith, 2003, for alternative views). In this chapter, we first provide behavioral

TABLE 26.1. Comparison of Typical Retrospective and Prospective Memory Tasks

Retrospective memory (cued recall) task	Prospective memory task
Phase 1: Presentation of Word Pairs Participants study pairs of items . . . rake–table . . .	Phase 1: Instructions for the Prospective Memory Task Participants receive instructions and practice with the ongoing lexical decision task. In a lexical decision task, participants press the *yes* key when a string of letters forms a word (*bicycle*) and the *no* key when the string of letters does not form a word (*aczmed*). Next, they receive the prospective memory instruction to press the *Q* key whenever they see the word *rake* in the context of the ongoing lexical decision task.
Delay of 20 minutes or so	Delay of 20 minutes or so filled with activities
Phase 2: Retrieval Phase Participants are presented with cues and explicitly asked to search memory for the associated items . . . rake– . . .	Phase 2: Retrieval Phase The ongoing lexical task is reintroduced without reminding participants of the prospective memory task. They are presented several hundred lexical decision trials, and the target word *rake* is presented three to four times. . . . . rake . .
Successful retrospective memory occurs when participants recall the word *table* in response to the cue *rake*	Successful prospective memory occurs when participants remember to press the Q key when the target word *rake* occurs. Note that participants are not prompted by the experimenter to search memory when *rake* occurs.

evidence for the existence of these two types of processes and then discuss the conditions that encourage reliance on one process or another. We then present theory and evidence regarding the neural pathways that underlie these processes. Next, we focus on one process—spontaneous retrieval—and discuss two characteristics of this process (automaticity and persistence after intention completion) that have important implications for prospective remembering in the real world.

MULTIPLE PROCESSES CAN SUPPORT PROSPECTIVE MEMORY RETRIEVAL

On the basis of noticing that performing a prospective memory task often leads to slowing or costs on an ongoing task (relative to control participants who perform only the ongoing task), researchers (Burgess, Quayle, & Frith, 2001; Marsh, Hicks, Cook, Hansen, & Pallos, 2003; Smith, 2003; Smith, Hunt, McVay, & McConnell, 2007) proposed that people use attentional control processes to maintain activation of the prospective memory intention and/or to search the environment for relevant cues. These attentional control processes are assumed to compete for limited resources with the processes used to perform the ongoing task and thus slow down performance on the ongoing task. In Smith's (2003) research, for example, participants were about 400 milliseconds slower in their lexical decision response times when simultaneously performing a prospective memory task (press a designated key whenever you see one of six prospective memory target words) relative to control group participants who performed only the lexical decision task. Indeed, there is good evidence that people who engage in more monitoring (i.e., show more costs) have higher prospective memory performance in many situations (e.g., Smith, 2003). Thus, when people are relying on a monitoring process, they are in essence endogenously maintaining their system in a retrieval mode.

Although the typical interpretation of costs is that they reflect attentional control processes needed to maintain sufficient activation of the intention (so that later processing of relevant cues triggers retrieval) and/or to actively monitor the environment for prospective memory cues that signal that it is appropriate to perform the prospective memory intention, it should be noted that Heathcote et al. (2015) have recently presented a different view. Their interpretation focuses on participants adopting a more conservative response threshold for the ongoing task when they have a prospective memory demand, so as to allow more accumulation of evidence for the prospective memory task before making a decision.

Prospective memory retrieval can also occur in the absence of monitoring processes or through what we have called spontaneous retrieval processes (Einstein & McDaniel, 2005; McDaniel & Einstein, 2007). Spontaneous retrieval, which we believe is often experienced as a thought "popping into mind," is revealed when the occurrence of a relevant cue triggers retrieval of an intention under conditions of no monitoring. Although participants are often inclined to monitor in experimental tests of prospective memory (McDaniel, Umanath, Einstein, & Waldum, 2015), conditions can be created that eliminate monitoring. For example, Scullin, McDaniel, Shelton, and Lee (2010) varied whether participants were asked to perform a prospective memory task whenever they saw a single target item (i.e., to press a designated key when they saw the target word *crossbar*). To discourage monitoring, participants were told that their primary task was performing the ongoing lexical decision task quickly and accurately, and the experimenters did not present the one target event until trial number 501. As might be expected from the perspective that it is difficult to sustain a controlled monitoring process (cf. Bargh & Chartrand, 1999), there was no evidence of slowing on the lexical decision task (i.e., no evidence of monitoring) in the prospective memory condition (relative to the control condition) by the 500th trial, and yet participants remembered to perform the prospective memory task 73% of the time (see also Harrison & Einstein, 2010, Harrison, Mullet, Whiffen, Ousterhout, & Einstein, 2014, and Mullet et al., 2013, for additional evidence of prospective memory retrieval in the absence of monitoring).

Further evidence for spontaneous retrieval comes from research using an intention interference or suspended intention paradigm (Cohen, Dixon, & Lindsay, 2005; Einstein et al., 2005; Mullet et al., 2013; Scullin, Bugg, McDaniel, & Einstein, 2011). In this paradigm (shown in Figure 26.1), participants are first given instructions for an ongoing task (e.g., a lexical decision task) and then instructions for an embedded prospective memory task (e.g., press a designated key when you see the words *corn* and *dancer*). They then perform a block of lexical decision trials with the embedded

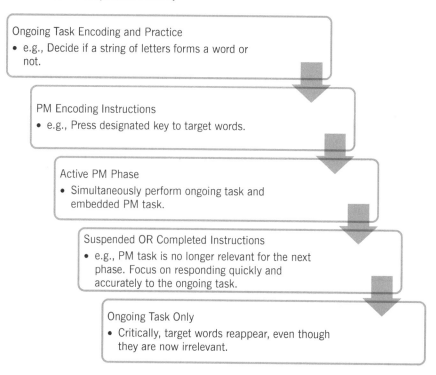

FIGURE 26.1. Basic paradigm for studying the effects of suspended or completed intentions in prospective memory (PM).

prospective memory task. Next, participants are told that the prospective memory task is suspended and should not be performed during the next phase. Participants are told that their sole demand during the next phase is to perform the ongoing task (often a lexical decision task and often called a "speed task") as accurately and quickly as possible. Because the intention has been suspended, participants do not monitor while performing this intervening task (Knight et al., 2011), and the interesting question is how they will respond to the target cues that are presented during this phase. The research consistently shows that lexical decision response times to prospective memory target cues are slower than to matched-control items, and this suggests that the processing of prospective memory target cues (in the absence of monitoring) causes spontaneous retrieval of intention-related information and often full conscious retrieval of the intention (Anderson & Einstein, 2017).

CONDITIONS THAT ENCOURAGE RELIANCE ON MONITORING VERSUS SPONTANEOUS RETRIEVAL PROCESSES

In line with a number of previous researchers (Loft, Kearney, & Remington, 2008; Marsh, Hicks, & Cook, 2005; McDaniel & Einstein, 2007; Rummel & Meiser, 2013), we assume that when people are confronted with a prospective memory demand, they decide how to allocate their attentional resources between the prospective memory and ongoing tasks based on metacognitive expectations. Then, they adjust their allocation policy in response to their experiences and any changes in ongoing task demands. There are also likely to be individual-difference factors (e.g., compulsiveness, working memory capacity) that affect the allocation policy and the willingness and ability to engage in and sustain monitoring processes. Generally, the allocation of resources to the prospective memory task has been shown to depend on the perceived difficulty of noticing the prospective memory target (Rummel & Meiser, 2013), the importance of the prospective memory task, the number of different prospective memory targets, the density of occurrence of the prospective memory targets, the anticipated delay between the prospective memory instructions and the occurrence of the prospective memory cue, momentary lapses in attention, as well as other factors (McDaniel & Einstein, 2007). More specifically, research has shown that participants rely more heavily on monitoring processes early in an ongoing task and less so on later trials (Loft et al., 2008; Einstein et al., 2005), when there are multiple prospective memory targets (six vs. one; Einstein et al., 2005), when performance on the prospective memory task is emphasized (Einstein et al., 2005; Kliegel, Martin, McDaniel, & Einstein, 2004), and when the prospective memory target is presented often (e.g., every 10th trial; Smith et al., 2007, Experiments 3 and 4).

Focal and Nonfocal Processing

An additional important variable that affects the extent to which participants adopt a monitoring or spontaneous retrieval approach to the prospective memory task (as well as the success of that approach) is whether the ongoing task encourages focal or nonfocal processing of the target event. The distinction between focal and non-focal processing is based on the encoding specificity principle that retrieval is facilitated when the cue at retrieval is processed in the same way that it was processed at encoding (Tulving & Thomson, 1973). More specifically, by focal processing, we mean that the ongoing task directs attention to the target item and especially those features of the target that were thought about at encoding. An example of a focal prospective memory task is the one that was used in the Scullin et al. (2010) experiment described earlier in which participants were asked to press a designated key when they saw the word *crossbar* in the context of performing a lexical decision ongoing task. In this case, participants likely thought about the meaning of the word *crossbar* when they encoded the prospective memory intention, and the ongoing lexical decision task required them to decide whether the letter strings formed a meaningful word. Given the match at encoding and retrieval, encountering the word *crossbar* is likely to lead to spontaneous retrieval of the intention—even when participants are not monitoring. As described earlier, Scullin et al. (2010) found no evidence of monitoring by the 501st trial of their experiment, and yet high retrieval (73%) was seen when the prospective memory target occurred.

   By contrast, nonfocal processing occurs when the ongoing task does not direct attention to the target word or directs attention to features other than those that were thought about at encoding. An example of a nonfocal prospective memory task is asking participants to press a designated key when they see a word that begins with the letter *c* in the context of performing a lexical decision task. Because the lexical decision task does not direct participants to evaluate the first letter in a string, processing of the word *crossbar* is less likely to lead to spontaneous retrieval. Scullin et al. (2010) included this condition in their experiment, and, consistent with expectations, retrieval was low (18%) when the nonfocal prospective memory cue occurred on the 501st trial.

In sum, there is clear evidence that people use both monitoring processes and spontaneous retrieval processes to support prospective memory retrieval. There is also evidence that variables differentially affect these processes. For example, aging has a greater negative effect on prospective memory tasks that depend on monitoring processes and less of an effect on tasks in which participants rely on spontaneous retrieval (Kliegel, Jäger, & Phillips, 2008; Mullet et al., 2013). Also, working memory capacity is more highly related to performance on tasks that require monitoring for successful retrieval (i.e., nonfocal prospective memory tasks; Brewer, Knight, Marsh, & Unsworth, 2010). Thus a more complete understanding of prospective memory requires that we examine how different variables affect these processes. An important step on the path to this goal involves using conditions in prospective memory experiments that clearly isolate one process or the other. Our general impression is that it is difficult to eliminate monitoring in laboratory experiments of prospective memory, however, and researchers often use conditions that encourage monitoring when trying to investigate spontaneous retrieval (see McDaniel et al., 2015, for further discussion of this issue and examples). In Table 26.2, we summarize task conditions that encourage reliance on monitoring or spontaneous

TABLE 26.2. Event-Based Prospective Memory Task Conditions That Affect Whether Participants Rely on Monitoring versus Spontaneous Retrieval

Task conditions that encourage monitoring

1. Using multiple different prospective memory target events.
2. Using a nonfocal prospective memory task.
3. Emphasizing the importance of performance on the prospective memory task.
4. Presenting participants with a small number of trials on the ongoing task.
5. Presenting the target event often.
6. Asking participants to perform the prospective memory task response prior to or instead of the ongoing task response.

Task conditions that discourage monitoring and help isolate spontaneous retrieval

1. Using a single focal target event.
2. Minimizing cues or demand characteristics (such as the title of the experiment) that suggest to participants that you are interested in their prospective memory.
3. Emphasizing the importance of the ongoing task, deemphasizing the importance of the prospective memory task, and reminding participants of those priorities from time to time.
4. Presenting participants with a large number of trials on the ongoing task and delaying the onset of the first target.
5. Limiting the number of occurrences of the target event.
6. Making it clear to participants that they can perform the prospective memory task at any point after seeing the target (including several trials later).
7. In some of our experiments (e.g., Harrison, Mullet, Whiffen, Ousterhout, & Einstein, 2015), we have told participants that only 5% of the participants will receive a prospective memory target event and thus not to worry about that task—but to respond should it happen to occur.

retrieval in an effort to facilitate the design of experiments that can isolate these processes.

Neural Mechanisms Underlying Monitoring and Spontaneous Retrieval

To illuminate the neural mechanisms of monitoring and spontaneous retrieval, we believe that it is especially informative to use prospective memory paradigms that encourage participants to rely on either monitoring or spontaneous retrieval processes (cf. Cona, Scarpazza, Sartori, Moscovitch, & Bisiacchi, 2015). As discussed above, participants facing prospective memory tasks with nonfocal cues tend to monitor, whereas participants given prospective memory tasks with focal cues (and appropriate instructions) tend to dispense with monitoring and rely on spontaneous retrieval. We emphasize here that to a large extent neuroimaging studies have not been sensitive to this distinction, either in terms of methodology or theoretical assertions. As it turns out, most studies have used nonfocal tasks. For these nonfocal tasks, the functional neuroimaging research has converged on two main findings. First, there is sustained neural activation unique to the prospective memory trial blocks (relative to the activation present in the control blocks; see, e.g., Gilbert, Gollwitzer, Cohen, Oettingen, & Burgess, 2009), consistent with the assumption that a monitoring process is involved in nonfocal prospective memory. Second, the sustained neural activation patterns are located in regions associated with sustained attentional control. The primary system involved is the anterior prefrontal cortex (aPFC), with the rostrolateral PFC (BA10) being especially indicated (Burgess, Gonen-Yaacovi, & Volle, 2011; Beck, Ruge, Walser, & Goschke, 2014), as well as other regions of the frontoparietal control network, including the dorsolateral–prefrontal cortex (DLPFC; BA46), parietal lobule (BA7), and precuneous (for reviews, see Cona et al., 2015; McDaniel et al., 2015). This pattern is entirely sensible and not unexpected, as monitoring processes are considered to rely on attentional control (Smith, 2003; note also that these patterns seemingly disfavor the Heathcote et al., 2015, model of costs that excludes the idea of an attentional-demanding monitoring process for nonfocal prospective memory).

Converging with the functional neuroimaging patterns is a structural imaging study conducted with older adults, some of whom who had a history of hypertension, and control participants who had no reported history of hypertension (Scullin et al., 2013). Structural magnetic resonance imaging (MRI) on aPFC, DLPFC, and medial temporal structures indicated as expected that the hypertension group had significantly diminished aPFC white matter, but no significant volumetric differences in other regions (or in gray matter). Moreover, the hypertension group showed significant impairment in a nonfocal prospective memory task (but not a focal prospective memory task), and associated with this impairment was an absence of cost on the prospective memory block relative to the control block of trials (for hypertension history but not control group). This pattern is consistent with the idea that monitoring processes assumed to underlie nonfocal prospective memory are related to aPFC structures. Finally, when all participants were considered together, aPFC white matter volume correlated with nonfocal prospective memory performance.

Spontaneous Retrieval

The neural mechanisms underlying spontaneous retrieval are less clear-cut, both because only a couple of functional magnetic resonance imaging (fMRI) studies have used focal prospective memory tasks under conditions that discourage monitoring (with monitoring present, spontaneous retrieval processes may or may not be present and are difficult to isolate) and because the available results diverge somewhat from prevailing theory. Theoretical work in neuroscience suggests that the hippocampus is involved in reflexive (spontaneous) retrieval of information when a cue is encountered (and fully processed) that was previously associated with that information (Eichenbaum & Cohen, 2001; Konkel & Cohen, 2009; Moscovitch, 1994). Upon successful retrieval, that information is then delivered to awareness in an obligatory fashion. Extending this notion to prospective memory retrieval is straightforward: During a focal prospective memory task, upon full processing of the focal cue, the hippocampus would possibly (in probabilistic fashion) spontaneously retrieve the associated intention, and that intention would be delivered to awareness (presumably to aPFC, via parietal pathways) so that control processes could act on the intention (see McDaniel & Einstein, 2011, for development of this view).

Initial support for the role of hippocampal structures in spontaneous retrieval comes from structural MRI results. Gordon, Shelton, Bugg, McDaniel, and Head (2011) examined associations between prospective memory performance in older adults with gray matter volume in frontal and medial temporal regions. There was a significant correlation between hippocampal volume (but not regions of interest in the frontal area) and focal prospective memory but not nonfocal prospective memory performance. These results strongly suggest that hippocampal structures are prominently involved in the spontaneous retrieval specifically associated with focal prospective memory. Further, Kalpouzos, Eriksson, Sjolie, Molin, and Nyberg (2010) have found evidence for hippocampal involvement in a naturalistic focal prospective memory task.

The limited fMRI research on focal prospective memory, however, has not provided direct evidence for transient activation (on successful prospective memory target trials) in the hippocampus (again, limited to paradigms in which monitoring would presumably not have been encouraged; see McDaniel et al., 2015, for details). For instance, McDaniel, LaMontagne, Beck, Scullin, and Braver (2013) reported no sustained activation in the trial blocks with focal prospective memory cues (e.g., in aPFC or the frontoparietal control network), implying an absence of sustained monitoring, as expected, but there was also no evidence for hippocampal activation on successful prospective memory target trials relative to nontarget trials (either in the prospective memory blocks or control blocks). Instead, transient activation associated with prospective memory retrieval to focal cues was especially pronounced in the precuneus and right middle temporal gyrus. Interestingly, these and other areas for which transient activation was evident (e.g., cingulate), align well with a parietal memory network (PMN) that is prominent in retrospective memory (Gilmore, Nelson, & McDermott, 2015). More specifically, the PMN appears to activate strongly when familiar stimuli that are relevant to current tasks are encountered (Gilmore et al., 2015). This function appears to dovetail with at least one theoretical account of spontaneous retrieval, which suggests that items encoded as PM targets gain increased familiarity. The increased familiarity then subsequently supports spontaneous noticing of the items during the PM task, leading to target detection and stimulating retrieval of the intended action (Guynn & McDaniel, 2007; McDaniel, 1995). Thus, finding that the PMN transiently activates during the PMN may help inform potential cognitive underpinnings of spontaneous retrieval.

Yet several other fMRI studies tentatively suggest that Broadman Area 9 is activated in retrieval for focal prospective memory tasks (see McDaniel et al., 2015), and this finding has interesting parallels with activation in BA 9 reported for spontaneous retrieval of autobiographical memory (with positron emission tomography [PET] imaging; Hall, Gjedde, & Kupers, 2008). At this stage there are too few studies to draw strong conclusions. The only certain conclusions are that the theoretical role of the hippocampus in spontaneous retrieval (in prospective and retrospective memory) awaits supporting evidence and that other possible neural candidates for supporting spontaneous retrieval, such as the parietal memory network, are emerging in the early fMRI work with focal prospective memory tasks (tasks supported by spontaneous retrieval, as developed earlier in the chapter).

CHARACTERISTICS OF SPONTANEOUS RETRIEVAL

In the remaining sections of this chapter, we flesh out two characteristics of spontaneous retrieval that have important implications for prospective memory in everyday situations. As noted earlier, research on retrospective memory tends to assume that people start off with a controlled search of memory when retrieving information (McDaniel, Guynn, Einstein, & Breneiser, 2004). We know much less about how the processing of cues triggers the spontaneous retrieval of memories in the absence of a controlled retrieval search (although see Gollwitzer & Crosby, Chapter 17, this volume; see also Berntsen, Staugaard, & Sorensen, 2013; Schlagman & Kvavilashvili, 2008). In this section, we consider whether spontaneous retrieval is fully automatic and whether cues continue to elicit retrieval of intentions after they have been completed.

How Automatic Is Spontaneous Retrieval?

Spontaneous retrieval may be a completely automatic process. As described earlier, within Moscovitch's (1994) view of the hippocampal system, if a good association has been formed between the cue and the intended action, full processing of the cue should produce reflexive retrieval of the intended action—and the thought to perform the intended action should be automatically delivered to conscious awareness. Within this view, full processing of focal cues should obligatorily lead to conscious retrieval of intentions (i.e., the intentions should "pop into mind"), regardless of current attentional demands.

On the other hand, demanding attentional conditions (e.g., dividing attention, high concentration, multitasking) may compromise spontaneous retrieval. From Moscovitch's (1994) view of the hippocampus, full processing of the cue is needed to trigger a spontaneous retrieval process, and dividing attention may compromise processing of the cue. Another possibility is that under demanding attentional conditions, we may set a higher threshold for allowing cue-driven thoughts into conscious awareness (Conway & Pleydell-Pearce, 2000). The idea here is that processing of the cue under divided attention conditions could stimulate the hippocampus to initiate retrieval of the intention, but the thought may be blocked from reaching conscious awareness. This kind of blocking mechanism would be adaptive in the sense of helping people maintain attention on the task at hand and preventing stimuli in the environment from usurping control of limited attentional resources.

The foregoing idea is consistent with research showing that people are more likely to report spontaneous autobiographical memories when they are in a diffuse, as opposed to a focused, attentional state (Kvavilashvili & Mandler, 2004). It is also consistent with research showing that external signals are muted or lessened in intensity when people are performing tasks that demand extensive attentional resources. For example, van der Wal and van Dillen (2013) found that participants rated a sweet solution as less sweet when it was consumed under a high task load. Similarly, Sörqvist and Marsh (2015) reviewed research showing that there is less brain responsiveness to external sounds (sounds that participants were told to ignore while performing an n-back task) when participants were performing a more difficult n-back task. Interestingly, they found that concentrating attention on a difficult task reduced activation from auditory stimuli in the brainstem area, and this was taken as evidence of the attenuation of the sound signals early in their processing (prior to reaching conscious awareness).

A recent psychophysiological experiment using skin conductance measures (Rothen, Nagai, & Rusted, 2015) provides some additional evidence consistent with the dynamics of spontaneous retrieval sketched above. All participants performed a focal and nonfocal prospective memory task. An absence of costs for the focal task (in terms of behavioral response latency to ongoing trials) and significant costs for the nonfocal task (slower response times relative to a no-prospective-memory control block) support the assumption that the focal task (but not the nonfocal task) was accomplished by spontaneous retrieval. Importantly, phasic skin conductance activity was recorded during the prospective memory target trials, as well as during nontarget trials. Phasic skin conductance activity significantly increased for correct target trials (i.e., the trials on which the prospective memory response was executed) relative to nontarget trials for both focal and nonfocal tasks. Critically, increased phasic skin conductance activity was also observed (relative to nontarget trials) for *incorrect* focal target trials (but not incorrect nonfocal trials)—that is, target trials for which no prospective memory response was elicited. Thus, when prospective memory retrieval was supported by spontaneous processes, there were psychophysiological reactions to the target regardless of successful prospective memory performance. This pattern would fit with the above theoretical notion that hippocampal processes could activate the intention in the presence of the target, and thus at some level in the system the significance of the target cue is appreciated. However, this spontaneous activation would not necessarily be conveyed to awareness (e.g., perhaps through parietal pathways to aPFC) and, therefore, not lead to successful prospective remembering.

In behavioral work, Harrison et al. (2014) conducted several experiments to test whether heavy attentional demands affect the spontaneous retrieval of prospective memory intentions. The general procedure involved asking participants to perform an ongoing lexical decision task and to also press a designated key if they saw a particular prospective memory target word. Critically, participants were also required to perform a divided-attention task (either digit detection or random number generation) during alternating segments of the ongoing task. Across the experiment, the prospective memory target occurred twice when attention was divided and twice when it was not divided. As described earlier, it is difficult to isolate spontaneous retrieval in the laboratory, but Harrison et al. (2014) were able to do so by following the recommendations in Table 26.2. Specifically, they presented participants with a single focal target cue, they emphasized the importance of performing the ongoing task, and they deemphasized the importance of performing the prospective memory task. Further, they told participants that they were unlikely to see the prospective memory target (only a 5% chance) and to focus on the ongoing task, but to perform the prospective memory action if they happened to see the target.

The results showed that a less demanding divided-attention task (digit detection) had no effect on prospective memory retrieval but that a more demanding divided-attention task (random number generation) lowered prospective memory performance (on average from 53% to 38%). Thus, under conditions that isolated reliance on spontaneous retrieval processes, the results showed that spontaneous retrieval is not completely automatic. In terms of real-world implications, it appears that stimuli that trigger spontaneous retrieval under less demanding attentional states may not do so when attention is highly focused or divided. At this point, further research is needed to determine whether the reduced spontaneous retrieval when attentional resources are occupied is the result of diminished processing of cues, the inability of activated intentions to reach conscious awareness, or both.

Another technique to promote spontaneous retrieval is to instruct participants to use implementation intentions to accomplish the prospective memory task. (There is also an extensive literature using implementation intentions to help people improve prospective memory and fulfill intentions; see Gollwitzer& Crosby, Chapter 17, this volume; Gollwitzer, 1999, 2014; Oettingen, Kappes, Guttenberg, & Gollwitzer, 2015; Parks-Stamm, Gollwitzer, & Oettingen, 2007.) Implementation intentions involve associating an intended action with a specific stimulus or target event and take the form of "When situation X occurs, I will perform response Y" (Gollwitzer, 1999, p. 494), where X refers to the target event and Y refers to the intended action. The idea is that implementation intentions strengthen the cue–action association such that processing the cue leads to automatic retrieval of the action (Rummel, Einstein, & Rampey, 2012). With implementation encoding, although prospective memory was not reduced under a less demanding divided-attention task (McDaniel, Howard, & Butler, 2008), prospective memory performance was significantly compromised under a demanding divided-attention task (McDaniel & Scullin, 2010). Converging with Harrison et al. (2014), these results suggest that prospective memory retrieval may not be completely automatic, even under ideal encoding conditions (but see Brandstätter, Lengfelder, & Gollwitzer, 2001).

Does Spontaneous Retrieval Persist after Intention Completion?

Whereas much of the research on prospective memory has focused on retrieval processes used to support prospective remembering, in light of the evidence for relatively automatic spontaneous retrieval processes, some researchers have begun to inquire whether our intentions continue to be spontaneously retrieved after completion. Specifically, if some intentions can be retrieved in the absence of monitoring, is it possible that no-longer-relevant cues will continue to drive retrieval after tasks have been completed? This potentially problematic characteristic of spontaneous retrieval could interfere with current goals and task demands and under certain conditions could even lead to commission errors, or the erroneous repetition of a completed prospective memory task (e.g., accidentally taking a double dose of medication). More specifically, strong focal cues for previously completed intentions could trigger spontaneous retrieval, and if there is no physical marker indicating the task's completion, commission errors are possible. If there is evidence of task completion (e.g., if you use a daily pill planner for medication, and the current day's dose is empty), however, then making a commission error is unlikely.

Theoretically, there are at least two possibilities regarding the fate of completed intentions. The first possibility is that representations of completed intentions are deactivated. Some evidence exists to support this possibility: After completing an intention, processing a previously relevant target word does not lead to retrieval of the intention and does not interfere with current tasks (Marsh, Hicks, & Bink, 1998; Scullin et al., 2011; Scullin, Einstein, & McDaniel, 2009). Most of the research, however, seems to support the alternative possibility that activation for the intention persists even after the intention has been completed (the "persisting activation view"; e.g., Walser, Fischer, & Goschke, 2012). This possibility is supported by findings showing that previously associated target words continue to be retrieved, interfere with task demands, and occasionally cause commission errors (Anderson & Einstein, 2015; Bugg & Scullin, 2013; Bugg, Scullin, & McDaniel, 2013; Scullin & Bugg, 2013; Scullin, Bugg, & McDaniel, 2012). Much of this research uses a modified version of the intention interference or suspended intention paradigm (Cohen et al., 2005; Einstein et al., 2005), in which researchers tell participants that the prospective memory task has been completed rather than simply suspended until later. In this completed-intention paradigm (see Figure 26.1), persisting activation is typically measured by examining either response times to old target words when compared with matched-control words, commission errors (pressing the previously designated key to old target words), or both. Next, we summarize the major findings that compel the idea that intentions are not quickly deactivated after execution and continue to influence cognitive processes and behavior.

Using a completed-intention paradigm, Scullin et al. (2012) had participants simultaneously engage in an ongoing task (to decide whether a string of letters forms a word or not) and perform an embedded prospective memory task (press the Q key if the target words *corn* or *dancer* appear). After completing this task, participants were told that they no longer had to press the Q key to target words and that in the next phase of the experiment their only goal was to perform the ongoing task as quickly and accurately as possible. Crucially, the target words (*corn* and *dancer*) appeared during the second phase, and the number of commission errors was recorded as a measure of persisting activation. Overall, this study showed evidence for residual activation, but particularly when the targets were salient, when the ongoing tasks were the same in both phases, and with older adults (see Figure 26.2). Similar research has shown (1) that persisting activation is still obtained when participants are given a *new* prospective memory task to perform in the second phase (Anderson & Einstein, 2017; Walser et al., 2012; Walser, Plessow, Goschke, & Fischer, 2014), (2) that a context shift between the first and second phases can reduce or possibly eliminate persisting activation (Scullin et al., 2009; 2011), and (3) that older adults may have particular difficulty deactivating intentions (McDaniel, Bugg, Ramuschkat, Kliegel, & Einstein 2009; Scullin et al., 2009, 2011).

Further evidence that completed intentions are often spontaneously retrieved comes from research using implementation intentions (Gollwitzer, 1999) at prospective memory encoding. It has been shown that implementation intentions increase the likelihood of spontaneous retrieval, presumably because they strengthen the association between target and intended action (Cohen & Gollwitzer, 2008; McDaniel et al., 2008; McDaniel & Scullin, 2010). If so, implementation intentions should more reliably produce persisting activation in a completed intention paradigm. Bugg et al. (2013) confirmed this hypothesis, finding increased commission errors in an implementation intention condition (relative to a standard prospective memory encoding condition) for both older and younger adults.

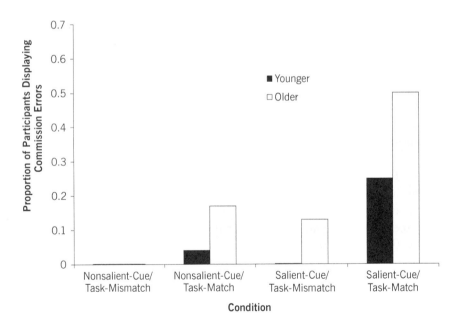

FIGURE 26.2. The proportion of participants who made a commission error in each condition during the post-prospective memory phase. This pattern implies that persisting activation was more pronounced when target items were salient (salient-cue), when the ongoing tasks were the same in both phases (task-match), and for older adults. Copyright © 2011 American Psychological Association. Reprinted by permission from Scullin, M. K., Bugg, J. M., & McDaniel, M. A. (2012). Whoops, I did it again: Commission errors in prospective memory. *Psychology and Aging, 27,* 46–53.

Although there appears to be strong evidence that cues continue to elicit the spontaneous retrieval of an intention after a prospective memory task has been completed, the exact qualitative nature of this retrieval is not clear. For example, slowing to target words could reflect a discrepancy or noticing response (McDaniel et al., 2004; Rummel & Meiser, 2016) rather than full conscious retrieval of the intention. Additionally, *not* obtaining commission errors does not necessarily indicate deactivation. Instead, it could simply reflect good cognitive control (Scullin & Bugg, 2013), in which participants retrieve the intention but successfully suppress the response.

In an attempt to better understand the qualitative nature of persisting activation, Anderson and Einstein (2017) used a novel thought-probe procedure (adapted from Plimpton, Patel, & Kvavilashvili, 2015) during the second phase of their experiment. Specifically, participants were prompted to report their thoughts *after trials following* target or matched-control words (these items were randomly determined in order to reduce the likelihood of participants learning the association between target words and thought probes). They found that participants were much more likely to report thinking about the previous prospective memory task following target words than their matched controls. They also found support for persisting activation on measures of response times and commission errors. Although not conclusive, these results lend support to the claim that residual activation can lead to full, conscious, spontaneous retrieval of the previous intention when presented with unexpected and now irrelevant targets.

Thus it seems that spontaneous retrieval tends to persist even after intentions have been completed. This is particularly likely when highly salient focal cues appear in the same context, with strengthened encoding (e.g., implementation intentions), and for older adults. Because spontaneous retrieval is relatively automatic, persisting activation of completed tasks could be particularly problematic for those with controlled retrieval deficits (e.g., older adults) or for habitual prospective tasks such as taking medication (Einstein, McDaniel, Smith, & Shaw, 1998). In these conditions, for example, retrieval of the intention to take one's medication with breakfast is relatively automatic and likely to "pop into mind." Remembering whether or not you have completed the intention that morning could prove more difficult, however, and if no task completion cue is present it could lead to a commission error, or accidently taking a double dose of medication.

SUMMARY

In summary, the evidence is compelling that people rely on multiple processes for prospective memory retrieval (McDaniel & Einstein, 2000, 2007). There appears to be good behavioral and neuroscience support that prospective memory retrieval can be accomplished through sustained monitoring processes and through transient spontaneous retrieval processes that are initiated by the processing of cues that have been associated with the intention. We probably use both types of processes in real-world settings, and which process we rely on likely depends on the circumstances. For example, in remembering to give a message to a friend whom you do not expect to see for several hours or several days, most people probably depend on spontaneous retrieval and let the appearance of the friend trigger retrieval of the intention (cf. Kvavilashvili & Fisher, 2007). By contrast, in a demanding air traffic control setting, where one has multiple intentions to keep in mind and the consequences of memory failure can be disastrous, operators are likely to rely extensively on monitoring processes (Loft, Smith, & Remington, 2013).

We believe that researchers have tended to use laboratory paradigms that encourage monitoring processes, and, accordingly, we believe that more research needs to be directed toward exploring the nature of spontaneous retrieval processes. In this chapter, we examined two characteristics of spontaneous retrieval. Thus far, the evidence indicates that spontaneous retrieval is spontaneous in the sense that it occurs without the intention to retrieve at the moment that a relevant cue is processed (i.e., when we are not in a retrieval mode), but that retrieval into conscious awareness is not fully automatic. It also appears that the associative link between the cue and the action is not quickly deactivated after the intention has been completed.

Research indicates that we spend a good deal of our mental lives thinking about the future (Gardner & Ascoli, 2015). Much of this thinking involves planning future actions that we intend to perform when the appropriate circumstances arise. The evidence indicates that we use both monitoring and spontaneous retrieval processes to remember to perform these intended actions, and we believe that fuller understanding of these processes and their vulnerabilities to forgetting can only be accomplished by using laboratory paradigms that isolate these processes.

REFERENCES

Anderson, F. T., & Einstein, G. O. (2017). The fate of completed intentions. *Memory, 25*(4), 467–480.

Bargh, J. A., & Chartrand, T. L. (1999). The unbearable automaticity of being. *American Psychologist, 54,* 462–479.

Beck, S. M., Ruge, H., Walser, M., & Goschke, T. (2014). The functional neuroanatomy of spontaneous retrieval and strategic monitoring of delayed intentions. *Neuropsychologia, 52,* 37–50.

Berntsen, D., Staugaard, S. R., & Sørensen, L. M. T. (2013). Why am I remembering this now?: Predicting the occurrence of involuntary (spontaneous) episodic memories. *Journal of Experimental Psychology: General, 142,* 426–444.

Brandstätter, V., Lengfelder, A., & Gollwitzer, P. M. (2001). Implementation intentions and efficient action initiation. *Journal of Personality and Social Psychology, 81,* 946–960.

Brewer, G. A., Knight, J. B., Marsh, R. L., & Unsworth, N. (2010). Individual differences in event-based prospective memory: Evidence for multiple processes supporting cue detection. *Memory and Cognition, 38,* 304–311.

Bugg, J. M., & Scullin, M. K. (2013). Controlling intentions: The surprising ease of stopping after going relative to stopping after never having gone. *Psychological Science, 24,* 2463–2471.

Bugg, J. M., Scullin, M. K., & McDaniel, M. A. (2013). Strengthening encoding via implementation intention formation increases prospective memory commission errors. *Psychonomic Bulletin and Review, 20,* 522–527.

Burgess, P. W., Gonen-Yaacovi, G., & Volle, E. (2011). Functional neuroimaging studies of prospective memory: What have we learnt so far? *Neuropsychologia, 49,* 2246–2257.

Burgess, P. W., Quayle, A., & Frith, C. D. (2001). Brain regions involved in prospective memory as determined by positron emission tomography. *Neuropsychologia, 39,* 545–555.

Cohen, A.-L., Dixon, R. A., & Lindsay, D. S. (2005). The intention interference effect and aging: Similar magnitude of effects for young and old adults. *Applied Cognitive Psychology, 19,* 1177–1197.

Cohen, A.-L., & Gollwitzer, P. M. (2008). The cost of remembering to remember: Cognitive load and implementation intentions influence ongoing task performance. In M. Kliegel, M. A. McDaniel, & G. O. Einstein (Eds.), *Prospective memory: Cognitive, neuroscience, developmental, and applied perspectives* (pp. 367–390). Mahwah, NJ: Erlbaum.

Cona, G., Scarpazza, C., Sartori, G., Moscovitch, M., & Bisiacchi, P. S. (2015). Neural bases of prospective memory: A meta-analysis and the "attention to delayed intention" (AtoDI) model. *Neuroscience and Biobehavioral Reviews, 52,* 21–37.

Conway, M. A., & Pleydell-Pearce, C. W. (2000). The construction of autobiographical memories in the self-memory system. *Psychological Review, 107,* 261–288.

Craik, F. I. M. (1986). A functional account of age differences in memory. In F. Klix & H. Hagendorf (Eds.), *Human memory and cognitive capabilities: Mechanisms and performances* (pp. 409–422). Amsterdam, The Netherlands: North-Holland.

Eichenbaum, H., & Cohen, N. J. (2001). *From conditioning to conscious recollection: Memory systems of the brain.* New York: Oxford University Press.

Einstein, G. O., & McDaniel, M. A. (2005). Prospective memory: Multiple retrieval processes. *Current Directions in Psychological Science, 14,* 286–290.

Einstein, G. O., McDaniel, M. A., Smith, R., & Shaw, P. (1998). Habitual prospective memory and aging: Remembering instructions and forgetting actions. *Psychological Science, 9,* 284–288.

Einstein, G. O., McDaniel, M. A., Thomas, R., Mayfield, S., Shank, H., Morrisette, N., & Breneiser, J. (2005). Multiple processes in prospective memory retrieval: Factors determining monitoring versus spontaneous retrieval. *Journal of Experimental Psychology: General, 134,* 327–342.

Gardner, R. S., & Ascoli, G. A. (2015). The natural frequency of human prospective memory increases with age. *Psychology and Aging, 30,* 209–219.

Gilbert, S. J., Gollwitzer, P. M., Cohen, A. L., Oettingen, G., & Burgess, P. W. (2009). Separable brain systems supporting cued versus self-initiated realization of delayed intentions. *Journal of Experimental Psychology: Learning, Memory, and Cognition, 35,* 905–915.

Gilmore, A. W., Nelson, S. M., & McDermott, K. B. (2015). A parietal memory network revealed by multiple MRI methods. *Trends in Cognitive Sciences, 19,* 534–543.

Gollwitzer, P. M. (1999). Implementation intentions: Strong effects of simple plans. *American Psychologist, 54,* 493–503.

Gollwitzer, P. M. (2014). Weakness of the will: Is a quick fix possible? *Motivation and Emotion, 38,* 305–322.

Gordon, B. A., Shelton, J. T., Bugg, J. M., McDaniel, M. A., & Head, D. (2011). Structural correlates of prospective memory. *Neuropsychologia, 49,* 3795–3800.

Guynn, M. J., & McDaniel, M. A. (2007). Target preexposure eliminates the effect of distraction on event-based prospective memory. *Psychonomic Bulletin and Review, 14*(3), 484–488.

Hall, N. M., Gjedde, A., & Kupers, R. (2008). Neural mechanisms of voluntary and involuntary recall: A PET study. *Behavioural Brain Research, 186,* 261–272.

Harrison, T. L., & Einstein, G. O. (2010). Prospective memory: Are preparatory attentional processes necessary for a single focal cue? *Memory and Cognition, 38,* 860–867.

Harrison, T. L., Mullet, H. G., Whiffen, K. N., Ousterhout, H., & Einstein, G. O. (2014). Prospective memory: Effects of divided attention on spontaneous retrieval. *Memory and Cognition, 42,* 212–224.

Heathcote, A., Loft, S., & Remington, R. (2015). Slow down and remember to remember!: A delay theory of prospective memory costs. *Psychological Review, 122,* 376–410.

Kalpouzos, G., Eriksson, J., Sjolie, D., Molin, J., & Nyberg, L. (2010). Neurocognitive systems related to real-world prospective memory. *PLOS ONE, 5,* e13304.

Kliegel, M., Jäger, T., & Phillips, L. H. (2008). Adult age differences in event-based prospective memory: A meta-analysis on the role of focal versus nonfocal cues. *Psychology and Aging, 23,* 203–208.

Kliegel, M., Martin, M., McDaniel, M. A., & Einstein, G. O. (2004). Importance effects in event-based prospective memory tasks. *Memory, 12,* 553–561

Knight, J. B., Meeks, J. T., Marsh, R. L., Cook, G. I., Brewer, G. A., & Hicks, J. L. (2011). An observation on the spontaneous noticing of prospective memory event-based cues. *Journal of Experimental Psychology: Learning, Memory, and Cognition, 37,* 298–307.

Konkel, A., & Cohen, N. J. (2009). Relational memory and the hippocampus: Representations and methods. *Frontiers in Neuroscience, 3,* 166–174.

Kvavilashvili, L., & Fisher, L. (2007). Is time-based prospective remembering mediated by self-initiated rehearsals?: Role of incidental cues, ongoing activity, age, and motivation. *Journal of Experimental Psychology: General, 136,* 112–132.

Kvavilashvili, L., & Mandler, G. (2004). Out of one's mind: A study of involuntary semantic memories. *Cognitive Psychology, 48,* 47–94.

Loft, S., Kearney, R., & Remington, R. (2008). Is task interference in event-based prospective memory dependent on cue presentation? *Memory and Cognition, 36,* 139–148.

Loft, S., Smith, R., & Remington, R. (2013). Minimizing the disruptive effects of prospective memory in simulated air traffic control. *Journal of Experimental Psychology: Applied, 19,* 254–265.

Marsh, R. L., Hicks, J. L., & Bink, M. L. (1998). Activation of completed, uncompleted, and partially completed intentions. *Journal of Experimental Psychology: Learning, Memory, and Cognition, 24,* 350–361.

Marsh, R. L., Hicks, J. L., & Cook, G. I. (2005). On the relationship between effort toward an ongoing task and cue detection in event-based prospective memory. *Journal of Experimental Psychology: Learning, Memory, and Cognition, 29,* 68–75.

Marsh, R. L., Hicks, J. L., Cook, G. I., Hansen, J. S., & Pallos, A. L. (2003). Interference to ongoing activities covaries with the characteristics of an event-based intention. *Journal of Experimental Psychology: Learning, Memory, and Cognition, 29,* 861–870.

McDaniel, M. A. (1995). Prospective memory: Progress and processes. In D. L. Medin (Ed.), *The psychology of learning and motivation: Advances in research and theory* (Vol. 33, pp. 191–221). San Diego, CA: Academic Press.

McDaniel, M. A., Bugg, J. M., Ramuschkat, G. M., Kliegel, M., & Einstein, G. O. (2009). Repetition errors in habitual prospective memory: Elimination of age differences via complex actions or appropriate resource allocation. *Aging, Neuropsychology, and Cognition, 16,* 563–588.

McDaniel, M. A., & Einstein, G. O. (2000). Strategic and automatic processes in prospective memory retrieval: A multiprocess framework. *Applied Cognitive Psychology, 14,* S127–S144.

McDaniel, M. A., & Einstein, G. O. (2007). *Prospective memory: An overview and synthesis of an emerging field.* Thousand Oaks, CA: SAGE.

McDaniel, M. A., & Einstein, G. O. (2011). The neuropsychology of prospective memory in normal aging: A componential approach. *Neuropsychologia, 49,* 2147–2155.

McDaniel, M. A., Guynn, M. J., Einstein, G. O., & Breneiser, J. (2004). Cue-focused and reflexive-associative processes in prospective memory retrieval. *Journal of Experimental Psychology: Learning, Memory, and Cognition, 30,* 605–614.

McDaniel, M. A., Howard, D. C., & Butler, K. M. (2008). Implementation intentions facilitate prospective memory under high attention demands. *Memory and Cognition, 36,* 716–724.

McDaniel, M. A., LaMontagne, P., Beck, S. M., Scullin, M. K., & Braver, T. S. (2013). Dissociable neural routes to successful prospective memory. *Psychological Science, 24,* 1791–1800.

McDaniel, M. A., & Scullin, M. K. (2010). Implementation intention encoding does not automatize prospective memory responding. *Memory and Cognition, 38,* 221–232.

McDaniel, M. A., Umanath, S., Einstein, G. O., & Waldum, E. R. (2015). Dual pathways to prospective remembering. *Frontiers in Human Neuroscience, 9.* Available at *http://journal.frontiersin.org/article/10.3389/fnhum.2015.00392/full.*

Moscovitch, M. (1994). Memory and working with memory: Evaluation of a component process model and comparisons with other models. In D. L. Schacter & E. Tulving (Eds.), *Memory systems* (pp. 269–310). Cambridge, MA: MIT Press.

Mullet, H. G., Scullin, M. K., Hess, T. J., Scullin, R. B., Arnold, K. M., & Einstein, G. O. (2013) Prospective memory and aging: Evidence for preserved spontaneous retrieval with exact but not related cues. *Psychology and Aging, 28,* 910–922.

Oettingen, G., Kappes, H. B., Guttenberg, K. B., & Gollwitzer, P. M. (2015). Self-regulation of time management: Mental contrasting with implementation intentions. *European Journal of Social Psychology, 45,* 218–229.

Parks-Stamm, E. J., Gollwitzer, P. M., & Oettingen, G. (2007). Action control by implementation intentions: Effective cue detection and efficient response initiation. *Social Cognition, 25,* 248–266.

Plimpton, B., Patel, P., & Kvavilashvili, L. (2015). Role of triggers and dysphoria in mind-wandering about past, present and future: A laboratory study. *Consciousness and Cognition: An International Journal, 33,* 261–276.

Rothen, N., Nagai, Y., & Rusted, J. (2015, September). *Psychophysiology of prospective memory: The effects of autonomic arousal and cue-focality on prospective memory retrieval.* Paper presented at the Society for Swiss Psychology conference, Geneva, Switzerland.

Rummel, J., Einstein, G. O., & Rampey, H. (2012). Implementation-intention encoding in a prospective memory task enhances spontaneous retrieval of intentions. *Memory, 20,* 803–817.

Rummel, J., & Meiser, T. (2013). The role of metacognition in prospective memory: Anticipated task demands influence attention allocation strategies. *Consciousness and Cognition: An International Journal, 22,* 931–943.

Rummel, J., & Meiser, T. (2016). Spontaneous prospective-memory processing: Unexpected fluency experiences trigger erroneous intention executions. *Memory and Cognition, 44,* 89–103.

Schacter, D. L., Addis, D. R., & Buckner, R. L. (2007). Remembering the past to imagine the future: The prospective brain. *Nature Reviews Neuroscience, 8,* 657–661.

Schlagman, S., & Kvavilashvili, L. (2008). Involuntary autobiographical memories in and outside the laboratory: How different are they from voluntary autobiographical memories? *Memory and Cognition, 36,* 920–932.

Scullin, M. K., & Bugg, J. M. (2013). Failing to forget: Prospective memory commission errors can result from spontaneous retrieval and impaired executive control. *Journal of Experimental Psychology: Learning, Memory, and Cognition, 39,* 965–971.

Scullin, M. K., Bugg, J. M., & McDaniel, M. A. (2012). Whoops, I did it again: Commission errors in prospective memory. *Psychology and Aging, 27,* 46–53.

Scullin, M. K., Bugg, J. M., McDaniel, M. A., & Einstein, G. O. (2011). Prospective memory and aging: Preserved spontaneous retrieval, but impaired deactivation, in older adults. *Memory and Cognition, 39,* 1232–1240.

Scullin, M. K., Einstein, G. O., & McDaniel, M. A. (2009). Evidence for spontaneous retrieval of suspended but not finished prospective memories. *Memory and Cognition, 37,* 425–433.

Scullin, M. K., Gordon, B. A., Shelton, J. T., Lee, J. H., Head, D., & McDaniel, M. A. (2013). Evidence for a detrimental relationship between hypertension history, prospective memory, and prefrontal cortex white matter in cognitively-normal older adults. *Cognitive, Affective, and Behavioral Neuroscience, 13,* 405–416.

Scullin, M. K., McDaniel, M. A., Shelton, J. T., & Lee, J. H. (2010). Focal/nonfocal cue effects in prospective memory: Monitoring difficulty or different retrieval processes? *Journal of Experimental Psychology: Learning, Memory, and Cognition, 36,* 736–749.

Smith, R. E. (2003). The cost of remembering to remember in event-based prospective memory: Investigating the capacity demands of delayed intention performance. *Journal of Experimental Psychology: Learning, Memory, and Cognition, 29,* 347–361.

Smith, R. E., Hunt, R. R., McVay, J. C., & McConnell, M. D. (2007). The cost of event-based prospective memory: Salient target events. *Journal of Experimental Psychology: Learning, Memory, and Cognition, 33,* 734–746.

Sörqvist, P., & Marsh, J. E. (2015). How concentration shields against distraction. *Current Directions in Psychological Science, 24,* 267–272.

Tulving, E. (1983). *Elements of episodic memory.* New York: Oxford University Press.

Tulving, E., & Thomson, D. M. (1973). Encoding specificity and retrieval processes in episodic memory. *Psychological Review, 80,* 352–373.

van der Wal, R. C., & van Dillen, L. F. (2013). Leaving a flat taste in your mouth: Task load reduces taste perception. *Psychological Science, 24,* 1277–1284.

Walser, M., Fischer, R., & Goschke, T. (2012). The failure of deactivating intentions: After-effects of completed intentions in the repeated prospective memory cue paradigm. *Journal of Experimental Psychology: Learning, Memory, and Cognition, 38,* 1030–1044.

Walser, M., Plessow, F., Goschke, T., & Fischer, R. (2014). The role of temporal delay and repeated prospective memory cue exposure on the deactivation of completed intentions. *Psychological Research, 78,* 584–596.

CHAPTER 27

The Planning Fallacy

Roger Buehler
Dale Griffin

For over 20 years, we have studied how and how well people predict their task completion times. When we started (Buehler, Griffin, & Ross, 1994), we were motivated by a specific theoretical account of planning biases, the inside–outside model of the "planning fallacy" presented by Kahneman and Tversky 15 years earlier (Kahneman & Tversky, 1979). We first set about testing the model and examining specific underlying processes. Since then, we (and many others) have expanded and broadened the original theoretical account and have explored a variety of theoretically derived methods for reducing the bias. In addition, we have expanded the scope of the planning fallacy to other domains beyond time prediction. In this chapter, we provide an overview of this research stream and outline progress made over the last two decades.

DEFINING AND DOCUMENTING THE PLANNING FALLACY

The planning fallacy refers to a prediction bias wherein people underestimate the time it will take to complete a future task, despite knowing that similar tasks have typically taken longer in the past. The term was first introduced to the literature by Kahneman and Tversky (1979, 1982, p. 415) in noting people's tendency "to underestimate the time required to complete a project, even when they have considerable experience of past failures to live up to planned schedules" and was intended, more generally, "to describe plans and forecasts that are unrealistically close to best-case scenarios" and "could be improved by consulting the statistics of similar cases" (Kahneman, 2011, p. 250). According to founding definitions, then, the signature of the planning fallacy is that people make plans and forecasts that are not only more optimistic than actual outcomes but also more optimistic than a known (or readily knowable) distribution of completion times for similar projects.

Several studies of the planning fallacy have revealed this dual pattern. For example, in one of the first empirical tests of the planning fallacy, we obtained student predictions for completion of a computer-based tutorial session (Buehler et al., 1994). Although students reported that they usually completed similar academic tasks about a day before deadline, they expected to complete the tutorial session, on average, about 6 days in advance of the deadline. In fact, only about 30% completed by their predicted date, and most students finished much closer to the deadline than they predicted. Similarly, moving outside the academic domain, Canadian taxpayers predicted that they would file their tax returns about a week earlier than they had typically done in the past (3 weeks before deadline rather than their usual 2 weeks), but they ended up completing the forms at their typical times (Buehler, Griffin, & MacDonald, 1997). Such findings are consistent with classic definitions of the planning fallacy, revealing a paradoxical combination of optimism about the future with realism about the past.

The term *planning fallacy* is sometimes used in a broader sense to describe the tendency to underestimate the time it will take to complete tasks, without regard to whether predictions depart from a distribution of relevant experience. Although we contend that such definitions miss much of the richness of the planning fallacy as a psychological phenomenon, clearly there is value in understanding causes and consequences of a basic "optimistic bias" or "underestimation bias." The basic tendency to underestimate task completion times has been documented by dozens of studies for a wide range of personal, academic, and work-related tasks (e.g., Buehler & Griffin, 2003; Byram, 1997; Griffin & Buehler, 1999; Kruger & Evans, 2004; Min & Arkes, 2012; Roy, Christenfeld, & McKenzie, 2005; Taylor, Pham, Rivkin, & Armor, 1998).

To further characterize the planning fallacy, we consider two noteworthy distinctions. First, many optimistic forecasts may represent duplicitous attempts to manipulate an audience rather than honest predictions about the future. For example, Flyvbjerg and colleagues (e.g., Flyvbjerg, Bruzelius, & Rothengatter, 2003; Flyvbjerg, Holm, & Buhl, 2004) have demonstrated that estimates of time and cost for large infrastructure projects are plagued by deception and "strategic misrepresentation" in order to gain project approval. These authors acknowledge, however, that time and cost overruns do not always stem from strategic misrepresentation; even when planners attempt to predict as accurately as possible, there are a number of psychological mechanisms that leave them prone to optimistic "delusions" (Flyvbjerg, 2008; Flyvbjerg, Garbuio, & Lovallo, 2009). Psychological research on the planning fallacy is focused on the "honest" forms of prediction bias and explores processes that leave even honest, well-intentioned planners prone to optimistic bias.

Second, the planning fallacy has traditionally focused on task completion times, and over time it has become apparent that there is a need to differentiate two types of time predictions. To do so, we adopt terminology recommended by Halkjelsvik and Jørgensen (2012) for consistency across disciplines. Predictions of *task performance time* refer to the amount of actual working time required to carry out a task, such as the number of hours spent working at the task itself. In contrast, predictions of *task completion time* refer to the point at which the task is finished, such as an estimated delivery date. For example, a scientist asked to review a journal article may estimate that this task will demand about 6 hours of actual working time (performance time prediction) and that the review will be submitted in 3 weeks (completion time prediction). Obviously, task completion times can diverge markedly from task performance times. This is because task completion times include time taken by factors external to the task, such as time spent on competing activities, interruptions, delays, and procrastination.

Although some theorists propose that the same processes and outcomes characterize both types of predictions (Roy et al., 2005; Roy & Christenfeld, 2007) and that underestimation of performance time is the root cause of the planning fallacy, we have argued that optimistic predictions of task completion time reflect processes that differ from those underlying predictions of performance time (Buehler, Griffin, & Ross, 2002; Buehler, Griffin, & Peetz, 2010; Griffin & Buehler, 2005; see also Halkjelsvik & Jørgensen, 2012). In particular, predictions of performance time, where uncertainty is solely about the nature and difficulty of the target task, should be less prone to bias than are predictions of task completion time, where uncertainty is greater and comes not only from the nature of the task but also from a host of other complicating factors (e.g., competing tasks, difficulties in coordinating with others, unexpected interruptions, a lack of necessary materials, challenges in scheduling resources, and self-control failure).

Consistent with this reasoning, literature reviews reveal a clearer and more robust tendency to underestimate task completion times than performance times (Buehler, Griffin, & Peetz, 2010; Halkjelsvik & Jørgensen, 2012). Studies reveal a consistent tendency to underestimate task completion times regardless of task type or length, whereas results for task performance time are mixed, with about as many studies showing overestimation as underestimation. Furthermore, for predictions of task performance time, the degree and direction of bias are highly dependent on the magnitude of the task: For very short laboratory tasks, overestimation is typical, whereas for longer tasks, underestimation is more common (Halkjelsvik & Jørgensen, 2012; Roy & Christenfeld, 2008; Roy et al., 2005). This magnitude-dependent pattern of bias, with short tasks overestimated and long tasks underestimated, is consistent with the effect of random error on task performance time predictions: a "regression to the mean" effect. For short tasks, both floor effects and regression to the mean lead to overestimation of performance time, whereas for long tasks, regression to the mean leads to underestimation of performance time. In contrast, the robust tendency to underestimate task completion times regardless of the length of the task is consistent with a systematic error or bias.

Few studies have compared the two types of predictions for the same target task. However, in one early study (Buehler et al., 1994, Study 2; results reported in Buehler, 1991) and one recent study (Wiese, Buehler, & Griffin, 2016), we collected both performance time and completion time estimates for an upcoming project. In each case, the completion time estimates were optimistically biased, even though estimates of performance time were not, and the two predictions were uncorrelated. In another relevant study, participants asked to perform a standard take-home task were informed either that they could complete the work in a single session or that they were required to spread it out across multiple sessions (Deslauriers, 2002). Even though task requirements were identical, there was greater bias in completion time estimates when the task was spread out over multiple sessions (and thus more prone to delays from factors external to the task). The findings suggest that task completion times are influenced greatly by factors other than the performance time of the target task itself and that the underestimation bias for completion times is not driven by a tendency to underestimate performance times.

Psychological Mechanisms

The Inside View and the Outside View

Psychological explanations for the planning fallacy have been guided by the seminal theorizing of Kahneman and Tversky (1979), who distinguished between two approaches to prediction, the "inside" and "outside" views (Kahneman & Lovallo, 1993). People who adopt an inside view of a prediction problem are looking forward and focusing on "singular" information relevant to only that one task: specific aspects of the target task that might lead to longer or shorter completion times. People who adopt an outside view of the prediction problem are looking across other projects in the past and present and focusing on distributional information: the outcomes of a set of relevant tasks. This approach requires identifying a set of related task outcomes to use as a basis for prediction. Thus the two approaches differ primarily in whether individuals base their predictions on knowledge of the specific case at hand or on knowledge of a relevant set of previous or parallel experiences.

According to the inside–outside account, people typically adopt the inside view when developing plans and predictions, and this leaves them prone to bias (Kahneman & Lovallo, 1993; Kahneman & Tversky, 1979). That is, people are inclined to generate predictions by looking ahead and trying to envision how the project will unfold. For example, when estimating the time needed for a home repair project, people might imagine when they will start the project, the resources that are required, and the specific steps they will take to carry it out. They are likely to consider their goals for the project, including when they hope to be done. They may consider other activities and events that will compete for their time and try to schedule the work accordingly. They may even try to foresee potential obstacles and how these obstacles could be overcome. Essentially, then, the inside view involves sketching out a specific plan or scenario that leads from the beginning to the successful conclusion of the project.

People are less inclined to adopt an outside view and base predictions on historical outcomes or the outcomes of others. This may be partly because prediction, by its very nature, evokes a focus on the future rather than the past. However, a failure to use historical information does not always result from inattention to the past. People may consider the past but fail to incorporate the information into their predictions because it does not seem applicable. People have difficulty extracting an appropriate set of past experiences; the various instances seem so different from each other on a surface level that individuals cannot compare them meaningfully (Kahneman & Lovallo, 1993; Kahneman & Tversky, 1979). People may also make attributions that diminish the relevance of past experiences to the current prediction. To the extent that a previous outcome is attributed to external, unstable, and specific factors—factors unlikely to generalize to other projects—it will not seem relevant to prediction (Buehler et al., 1994).

The problem with basing predictions on a plan-based, future scenario is that such scenarios typically do not provide a comprehensive representation of future events. Mental scenarios tend to be idealized, schematic, and oversimplified (Dunning, 2007). When individuals imagine the future, they often fail to entertain alternatives to their favored scenario and do not appreciate the uncertainty inherent in every detail of a constructed scenario (Griffin, Dunning, & Ross, 1990; Hoch, 1985). Furthermore, given that people plan for success rather than failure, the scenarios tend to focus on positive rather than negative information. When individuals are asked to predict based on "best-guess" scenarios, their forecasts are generally indistinguishable from those generated by "best-case" scenarios (Griffin et al., 1990; Newby-Clark, Ross, Buehler, Koehler, & Griffin, 2000). Finally, the very act of generating a scenario can cause people to inflate the likelihood of that scenario unfolding (for a review, see Koehler, 1991). Focusing on a plan-based scenario, then, may lead predictors to ignore or underweight the chances that different events will occur. This is a formula for overoptimism, because even when a particular success scenario is relatively probable, a priori, chance will still usually favor the whole set of possible alternative events because there are so many (Kahneman & Lovallo, 1993).

Empirical studies provide convergent support for the inside–outside analysis of the planning fallacy. Studies that include "think-aloud" procedures and written "thought listing" measures have shown that a focus on plan-based future scenarios—and a consequent neglect of past experience—is indeed characteristic of the prediction process. For example, in a typical study of academic and home projects (Buehler et al., 1994, Study 3), more than 70% of thoughts reported by participants referred to their plans for the current project, for the most part describing scenarios in which they finished the task without problems arising; the verbal protocols revealed an almost total neglect of other kinds of information, including their own past experiences or others' experiences with similar projects.

Another early experiment (Buehler et al., 1994, Study 4) tested whether the relative neglect of past experience was due to a lack of attention or the perceived irrelevance of the past. Participants predicted when they would finish a standard, 1-hour computer assignment due in a week. Those in the recall condition reported on their previous experiences with similar assignments (and recalled finishing very close to deadline) just before making their predictions. Nonetheless, they underestimated actual completion times to the same degree as participants in a control condition, suggesting that attention to the past is not enough to make it seem relevant to prediction. Participants in a recall-relevance condition were required, before generating predictions, to actively link their past experiences with the upcoming computer assignment by first determining when they would finish the assignment (if they finished as far before deadline as usual) and describing a plausible scenario that would result in this outcome. The manipulation was designed to prevent participants from discounting the relevance of past experiences with similar tasks, and for this task, at least, it eliminated prediction bias.

To test the role of attribution processes in the planning fallacy, we have asked participants to recall and explain occasions when they failed to complete a task by the predicted time and a similar failure experienced by a close acquaintance (Buehler et al., 1994, Study 3). We coded the reasons on dimensions of the

Attributional Style Questionnaire (Peterson et al., 1982). The reasons participants reported for their own lateness were more external, transitory, and specific than the reasons for others' lateness. In a related study (Buehler et al., 1994, Study 4), participants explained why they had either succeeded or failed in meeting a completion time prediction. Those who finished late offered reasons that were more transitory and specific than those who finished on time. These findings suggest that people explain their own past lateness in a manner that diminishes its relevance to prediction (see also Helzer & Dunning, 2012).

Following Kahneman and Tversky (1979), we distinguish between forecasts that are generated through the process of planning and imagining future outcomes (the inside view) and those that are generated through the process of drawing on past experiences and other general "distributional" knowledge (the outside view). Oettingen and Mayer (2002) discuss two modes of thought about the future that may be related to this distinction between views. That is, some thoughts about the future are pure fantasies, unlimited by reality constraints. This type of thought should always fall into the inside thinking category. Other thoughts about the future give rise to expectations, which may be derived from thinking about past experiences, and as such may be linked to the outside mode of thinking. Furthermore, when future fantasies are compared with reality constraints in the form of "mental contrasting" (Oettingen, 2012; Oettingen & Schwörer, 2013), planners are more likely to be aware of obstacles to plan completion, as we discuss further in the later section on debiasing.

Additional Psychological Mechanisms

Motivated Reasoning

In addition to the cognitive processes described in the inside–outside account, motivational forces may contribute to prediction bias. Theories of motivated reasoning (Kunda, 1990) and desirability bias (Krizan & Windschitl, 2007) suggest that predictions in many domains are colored by people's hopes, wishes, and desires. When considering an upcoming task, one pervasive motivation that could bias people's predictions is the desire to finish as soon as possible. Consistent with this account, research on task completion predictions has shown that motivation to finish tasks early, such as that produced by monetary incentives (Buehler et al., 1997; Buehler, Griffin, Lam, & Deslauriers, 2012) or a desire to please others (Pezzo, Pezzo, & Stone, 2006) increases optimistic bias. Furthermore, mediational analyses suggest that the desire to finish tasks promptly elicits optimistic predictions because it heightens people's tendency to adopt an inside view and focus narrowly on a plan for task completion (Buehler et al., 1997; Buehler et al., 2012).

Anchoring

Theorists have also proposed that the planning fallacy may be supported by processes of anchoring and adjustment (Jørgensen & Sjøberg, 2004; König, 2005; LeBoeuf & Shafir, 2009; Thomas & Handley, 2008; Thomas, Newstead, & Handley, 2003). In many domains, people arrive at judgments by first contemplating a salient value that serves as the starting point or anchor and then adjusting (insufficiently) from that value (Strack & Mussweiler, 1997; Tversky & Kahneman, 1974). LeBoeuf and Shafir (2009) proposed that a salient anchor for task completion predictions is the present. In particular, respondents asked to estimate completion times as a number of days might begin at the present (a natural, self-generated anchor) and then adjust incrementally in a forward direction. However, as with other anchoring effects, their adjustments from the anchor are likely to be insufficient. Respondents asked to predict in terms of a calendar date should be less inclined to engage in this process. Supporting this anchoring account, participants predicted they would finish various tasks (e.g., reading a book, going shopping at the mall) sooner when asked to estimate in days rather than in dates.

In many planning contexts, there could be other salient anchors, besides the present, that could systematically influence prediction. Research has shown that performance time predictions can be influenced by an ostensibly arbitrary starting point suggested by the researcher. König (2005) asked participants to first consider whether they would need more or less than 30 minutes (short anchor) or 90 minutes (long anchor) before estimating the time needed for a catalogue search task. Participants made shorter and more biased time estimates after exposure to the short anchor than the long anchor. Related studies demonstrated that performance time predictions can be biased in the direction of anchors emanating from various other sources including the time it took a randomly selected person to carry out the task (Thomas & Handley, 2008) and clients' initial expectations about how long a software project should take (Aranda & Easterbrook, 2005; Jørgensen & Grimstad, 2008; Jørgensen & Sjøberg, 2004).

Memory Bias

Another explanation proposed for the planning fallacy is the "memory bias account" (Roy & Christenfeld, 2007, 2008; Roy et al., 2005). According to this account, people underestimate completion times because they misremember how long similar tasks have taken in the past and then use the faulty estimates of performance time as input for predicting completion time. The problem, then, is not that people disregard historical information but, rather, that people's memories of previous performance times are systematically biased, resulting in a corresponding bias in prediction. In support of this account, researchers have documented that people tend to underestimate in retrospect how long tasks have taken and that the same factors that influence the retrospective biases are also related to prediction biases. Related research has shown that people were able to make more accurate predictions of task performance time when they were provided with accurate records of previous performance times rather than relying on their memories (Roy, Mitten, & Christenfeld, 2008).

As we have previously noted (Buehler, Griffin, & Peetz, 2010; Griffin & Buehler, 2005), the memory bias account may be limited in its ability to explain the planning fallacy. In particular, a hallmark of the planning fallacy is that predictions diverge markedly from reported memories and beliefs about previous completion times. Moreover, as noted earlier, the general tendency to underestimate task completion times does not appear to be driven primarily by performance time estimates. Thus, although it has been argued that the memory bias account explains bias in both types of prediction (Roy et al., 2005), we suggest that this account may be most germane to performance time predictions and that further research is needed to test its applicability to completion time predictions.

Do Plans and Predictions Influence Completion Times?

The degree of optimistic bias is determined not only by processes occurring at prediction but also by what transpires after an optimistic prediction has been generated. There would be no planning fallacy if people acted to bring their actual completion times in line with their optimistic forecasts. Notably, then, whereas self-predictions can sometimes have self-fulfilling effects on subsequent behavior (Morwitz & Fitzsimons, 2004; Sherman, 1980), evidence of the planning fallacy suggests that predicted task completion times may have little impact on actual completion times.

We have proposed that the impact of optimistic completion time predictions on subsequent behavior may vary depending on the nature of the task, and particularly the extent to which the task is prone to unexpected interruptions, problems, and delays. In particular, we tested whether generating an optimistic completion time prediction would help people finish tasks earlier than they would otherwise (Buehler, Peetz, & Griffin, 2010). We proposed that task completion predictions are more "translatable" (Koehler & Poon, 2006) into the one-time action of starting a project than into the continuing actions necessary to complete a project. Accordingly, for tasks that can be completed in a single, continuous session ("closed tasks"), and thus are not usually prone to interruptions and delays once they have been started, we would expect an effect of predictions on actual completion times. In contrast, for tasks that require multiple steps to be completed at different times or locations ("open tasks"), and thus are relatively prone to interruptions and delays even after they have been started, we would expect that differential plans and predictions may not influence the ultimate completion times. Consequently, optimistic predictions will have a greater impact on completion times for closed tasks than for open tasks.

As one test of this logic, we performed a quantitative review of studies with manipulations that affected predicted completion times (Buehler, Peetz, & Griffin, 2010) and classified the target tasks as being either closed (e.g., a 1-hour computer tutorial, a short writing assignment) or open (e.g., major school projects, income tax returns). As hypothesized, effects on prediction were more likely to carry through to behavior for closed tasks than for open tasks. In addition, a set of experiments examined the impact of predictions more directly by using anchoring procedures to manipulate the optimism of participants' task completion predictions. The specific anchoring manipulations varied across studies, from drawing a card to sliding a pointer along a numbered timeline, but in each case they yielded a strong effect on prediction, allowing us to investigate whether completion times would be influenced by these predictions. The type of task (open vs. closed) was varied across studies, as well as experimentally manipulated within a study. Results indicated that for closed tasks, the manipulated differences in prediction carried on to affect actual completion times. For open tasks, predictions influenced the time at which the tasks were started but did not affect final completion times. The findings support the idea that optimistic predictions have their greatest impact on the beginning phases of a project, particularly the initiation time, but this effect diminishes over the course of an extensive, multistage project.

To fully understand the behavioral effects, we believe it is also necessary to consider the role of deadlines in guiding task completion behavior. The target tasks we studied had a firm deadline for completion, and previous research has shown that such deadlines exert a powerful impact on when people actually finish their tasks—even when people hope to finish well in advance of a deadline, their actual time ends up being driven largely by deadlines (Ariely & Wertenbroch, 2002; Buehler et al., 1994; Tversky & Shafir, 1992). We suspect that for open tasks, the salience of an early prediction (and perhaps the task itself) may fade until a looming deadline pulls it back into focus. That is, people's final task completion times may be a function of two psychological forces—people's plans to finish early and their deadlines. Optimistic plans to finish early may get tasks started, but then the effects of external factors take over, and it is the force of deadlines that controls actual completion times.

DEBIASING INTERVENTIONS

Distributional Information

A central implication of the inside–outside model of the planning fallacy is that people can reduce optimistic bias by adopting an outside view wherein they use distributions of similar project outcomes as the basis for prediction rather than relying on goal-based plans and scenarios. Accordingly, some debiasing strategies avoid or diminish the problems associated with overly optimistic plans by prompting predictors to base predictions on "outside" or "distributional" information. For instance, the strategy of reference class forecasting requires forecasters to base predictions on a distribution of outcomes from comparable previous projects (Flyvbjerg, 2008; Lovallo & Kahneman, 2003), and empirical tests support the effectiveness of this strategy in reducing time and cost overruns in large-scale construction projects (Ansar, Flyvbjerg, Budzier, & Lunn, 2014; Flyvbjerg et al., 2009) and software development projects (Shmueli, Pliskin, & Fink, 2015). Our research on smaller, individual projects also found that prompting people to base predictions on past experience (by highlighting the relevance of previous completion times) resulted in unbiased predictions (Buehler et al., 1994).

Note, however, that such strategies are most applicable in those prediction contexts in which a class of comparable projects can be readily identified. In what follows we consider strategies that may minimize bias among forecasters who adopt an inside approach to prediction of a subjectively "unique" project.

Potential Obstacles versus Plans for Success

According to Kahneman and Tversky's (1979) original theory, the inside view includes all case-specific content, including possible problems or obstacles to completion, as well as plans for how to overcome them. Thus an inside view can, at least in theory, vary in the balance of its content between plans for success and possible obstacles or interruptions. However, our research suggests that people naturally focus on positive plans for success, with relatively little attention to obstacles, and that the balance of content (between plans and obstacles) influences their predictions, even though both types of content fit into the inside view. Newby-Clark et al. (2000) found that people generate remarkably similar scenarios about future projects, whether they are instructed to develop a "realistic" or a "best case" scenario, suggesting that planning a task and estimating its completion may often be similar to "assuming the best and working from there." Furthermore, recent studies have found that people asked to elaborate on an important goal spontaneously generated far more thoughts about the desired future than about present reality or obstacles to attaining the desired future (Sevincer & Oettingen, 2013).

What happens if predictors are directly instructed to focus on potential obstacles as they generate predictions? Relevant research findings are mixed. Some studies have found that people predict longer completion times when they are prompted to focus on potential obstacles (Peetz, Buehler, & Wilson, 2010). In other studies, however, people's predictions were not influenced by instructions to consider potential problems or surprises (Byram, 1997; Hinds, 1999) or to generate worst-case scenarios of task completion (Newby-Clark et al., 2000). When people are confronted directly with potential obstacles, they may be reluctant to incorporate this information into their predictions. Furthermore, in some contexts, inducing a focus on obstacles may result in "counteractive optimism," wherein people generate optimistic predictions in order to overcome anticipated obstacles in goal pursuit (Zhang & Fishbach, 2010).

The effectiveness of focusing on obstacles versus plans for success can further depend on the ease of generating these cognitions (Min & Arkes, 2012; Sanna & Schwarz, 2004). Sanna and Schwarz (2004) manipulated the number and type of thoughts (plans for success vs. obstacles) that forecasters were required to list and found that forecasters made more optimistic predictions when success thoughts were experienced as easy to bring to mind (because participants were asked to list only a few) and potential problems were perceived as difficult to bring to mind (because participants were asked to list many). Conversely, forecasters made less optimistic predictions when success thoughts were difficult to bring to mind and potential obstacles were easy to bring to mind. This implies that drawing attention to obstacles may curb optimism only in contexts in which obstacles can be readily identified and that otherwise this strategy could backfire.

Another method to draw attention to future obstacles is mental contrasting, in which a planner is guided to consider a favored outcome through a guided fantasy goal and (only then) to identify specific barriers that stand in the way of achieving the desired outcome (Oettingen, 2012; Oettingen & Schwörer, 2013). That is, "thinking about the future should involve both the desired future and the resisting reality" (Oettingen, 2012, p. 55), and these two contrasting foci give rise to more calibrated behavior because, with mental contrasting, highly likely goals receive greater commitment and less likely goals receive lower commitment. Furthermore, mental contrasting can be combined with implementation intentions (MCII), a combination that has been shown to have a variety of positive effects on future goal attainment (see Oettingen, 2012 for a summary, and the website www.woopmylife. org for practical applications).

Decomposition

Another strategy that varies the content of the "inside view" is to unpack or decompose the target task into smaller segments (Byram, 1997; Connolly & Dean, 1997; Forsyth & Burt, 2008; Kruger & Evans, 2004). Given that plans generated holistically tend to be incomplete and oversimplified, breaking down a larger task into smaller subtasks may highlight steps that need to be completed but that would otherwise be overlooked. Kruger and Evans (2004) found that asking people to unpack a task (i.e., identify all the necessary subtasks) reduced the underestimation bias in performance time predictions for several lab tasks and had a parallel effect on completion time predictions for holiday shopping. Similarly, Forsyth and Burt (2008) reported a "segmentation effect" on performance time predictions: Participants in the segmentation condition provided time estimates separately for each task subcomponent, and these were aggregated to produce an estimate for the task as a whole. The aggregated total of the decomposed estimates was longer than overall estimates, which reduced the underestimation bias for relatively "long" tasks lasting 20–40 minutes and actually produced an overestimation bias for shorter tasks.

However, studies have not always found an effect of unpacking (Byram, 1997; Connolly & Dean, 1997), and a number of moderators have been identified. Unpacking appears to be less effective if there are few task components (Kruger & Evans, 2004), if the unpacked components will be easy to carry out (Hadjichristidis, Summers, & Thomas, 2014), or if the tasks are in the distant future (Moher, 2012). Also, notably, studies of unpacking have focused almost exclusively on predictions of performance time rather than completion time; more research is needed to examine unpacking for extensive tasks that are prone to external interruptions and delays. One intriguing possibility is that unpacking may help planners to identify more of the necessary steps in a task (thereby increasing performance time predictions) but as a result distract attention from complicating factors external to the task (thereby decreasing completion time predictions).

Neutral Observers

Theorists have long noted that people appear to make more realistic estimates about completion times for others than for themselves, and that this actor–observer difference in prediction may reflect differences in the underlying cognitive and motivational processes. Observers typically do not have access to the detailed information that actors possess about their plans and life circumstances, making it less likely that they will focus narrowly on a plan for completing the task by a desired time. In addition, neutral observers do not generally share the same motivations as actors (e.g., a desire to finish promptly), and thus observers' predictions are less likely to be colored by these motives.

Consistent with this theorizing, an early study (Buehler et al., 1994, Study 5) found that observers are generally less attentive than actors to the actors' reported plans and more attentive to potential obstacles, past experiences, and task deadlines—in other words, observers were more likely to adopt the outside view *and* to construct a more problem-focused inside view. Another study found that observers gave little weight to an actor's motivation for early completion. Actors predicted they would finish a school project much earlier in a scenario in which they were offered incentive grades for early completion; however, knowing that the student had been offered this incentive did not affect predictions generated by observer participants (Mulhern, 2006). It appears that observers are more skeptical than actors about whether incentives that operate on the actor are enough to overcome past behavioral tendencies. Along similar lines, prompting actors to contemplate worst-case scenarios of task completion (which included myriad obstacles, interruptions, and delays) had no impact on the actors' own predictions but led observers to predict later completion times (Newby-Clark et al., 2000). Again, this finding suggests that observers are guided less by the actors' desires and are more receptive to potential obstacles than are actors.

Notably, studies examining predictions of task performance time, rather than completion time, have not found a general actor–observer difference in prediction (Byram, 1997; Hinds, 1999; Jørgensen, 2004; Roy, Christenfeld, & Jones, 2013). Byram (1997) asked participants to build a computer stand in the lab and found that participants underestimated the time it would take to an equal degree, whether their predictions concerned themselves or the average person. Roy et al. (2013) found very similar patterns of bias (either underestimation or overestimation, depending on task characteristics) in actor and observer predictions for brief laboratory tasks, suggesting that prediction bias was not driven by the predictors' level of involvement with the task. The divergent results for studies of completion time and performance time is striking and again suggests that bias in these two types of predictions stems from different sources.

The Observer Perspective

We have extended the work on observer prediction by testing whether people can be induced to take on an observer-like perspective for their own tasks and whether this perspective curbs prediction bias for task completion times (Buehler et al., 2012). This approach was motivated by evidence that people can choose strategically to imagine future events from differing visual perspectives (Libby & Eibach, 2011; Pronin & Ross, 2006). People who adopt a *first-person* perspective see a future project unfolding as if they were actually carrying it out, whereas those who adopt a *third-person* perspective see events from an observer's vantage point. The third-person perspective may help to minimize optimistic bias because it elicits cognitive processes similar to those in neutral observers (e.g., Frank & Gilovich, 1989; Pronin & Ross, 2006) and reduces the salience and intensity of emotional engagement with imagined events (e.g., Kross, Ayduk, & Mischel, 2005; McIsaac & Eich, 2002). Thus third-person imagery may attenuate cognitive and motivational processes that contribute to optimistic forecasts.

To test this theorizing, a series of experiments varied the imagery perspective that people adopted as they contemplated an upcoming task (Buehler et al., 2012). Student participants identified a specific upcoming task, and we manipulated the perspective they adopted as they imagined themselves carrying out the task. As hypothesized, the students predicted longer task completion times—and thus were less prone to bias—when they imagined the task from a third-person rather than a first-person perspective. This effect of perspective was mediated partially by people's cognitive focus on plans versus obstacles at the time of prediction: Third-person imagery reduced people's inclination to focus narrowly on optimistic plans and increased their focus on potential obstacles. Taking a third-person perspective also altered the role of task-relevant motivation in prediction. The desire to finish a task promptly was reduced and weighted less heavily when individuals adopted a third-person perspective. In essence, then, the third-person perspective elicited predictions and underlying psychological processes that mimic those found in neutral observers (Buehler et al., 1994; Newby-Clark et al., 2000), suggesting that planners could gain benefits of observer-based prediction without the need to consult with others.

Backward Planning

In a recent program of research, we have examined another prediction strategy—known as backward planning—that alters the perspective people adopt when developing plans (Wiese et al., 2016). Backward planning involves starting a plan at the point of task completion and working back through the required steps in reverse-chronological order. Our research was inspired by ideas gaining currency in applied fields of project management, where practitioners commonly advocate the use of backward planning (also referred to as back-planning or back-casting; Lewis, 2002; Verzuh, 2005) to generate realistic plans and projections. We hypothesized, consistent with anecdotal reports, that backward planning may lead people to predict longer task completion times and thus attenuate the planning fallacy.

In four experiments, we asked participants to develop a plan for completing a target task (e.g., preparing for a date, completing a major school assignment) and manipulated the temporal direction of their planning to create three conditions. In the backward-planning condition, participants were instructed:

> "We want you to develop your plan in a particular way called backward planning. Backward planning involves starting with the very last step that needs to be taken and then moving back from there in reverse chronological order. That is, you should try to picture in your mind the steps you will work through in order to reach your goal in a backward direction."

In the forward-planning condition, participants received parallel instructions to plan in a forward direction, and in the unspecified condition, the instructions did not specify a temporal direction. After planning for the task, participants predicted how far before the deadline it would be finished. In the final study, participants also reported actual completion times in a follow-up session, allowing us to examine the degree of bias in their predictions. As hypothesized, in each study, people predicted the target task would take longer to complete in the backward-planning condition than in the forward and unspecified conditions. Moreover, the final study, which tracked actual task completion times, found that backward planning eliminated the typical optimistic bias. Participants generally predicted they would finish their projects earlier than they actually did; however, the magnitude of this bias was much smaller in the backward-planning condition ($M = 0.18$ days) than in the forward ($M = 1.93$ days) and unspecified conditions ($M = 1.21$ days). The bias was reduced in the backward-planning condition because participants predicted later completion times in this condition than in the other two conditions, and there was no difference across conditions in the times at which the projects were actually completed.

We included measures to assess cognitive processes underlying the effects. In particular, we reasoned that backward planning may counter people's natural inclination to focus on an idealized and hence highly fluent scenario of task completion. Backward planning prompts people to adopt a temporal outlook that may disrupt the chronological, narrative structure of plan-based scenarios, and consequently backward planners may focus less on central, schematic information (e.g., a plan for successful task completion) and focus more on information that is typically neglected (e.g., additional steps, potential obstacles, and competing demands on their time). Consistent with this reasoning, process measures revealed that backward planning led participants to include more steps in their plans, to focus more on potential obstacles, and to report that the planning exercise had elicited more novel planning insights (e.g., helped them to clarify the steps they would need to take, led them to think of steps they would not have considered otherwise). In some studies, though not all, these cognitions were correlated with task completion predictions and mediated the effects of backward planning.

We included an additional exploratory measure to test the possibility that backward planning may also alter the planner's perception of the flow of time. People can view the passing of time either as the individual moving through time (ego-motion perspective) or as time moving toward the individual (time-motion perspective; Boroditsky, 2000). Moreover, previous research has found that adopting the time-motion perspective can result in less optimistic time predictions (Boltz & Yum, 2010). We reasoned that backward planning, which involves moving cognitively from the future toward the present, may emphasize the directional flow of time and induce a time-motion perspective. Consistent with this reasoning, in three of four experiments, participants were more likely to adopt a time-motion perspective (vs. an ego-motion perspective) in the backward-planning condition than in the forward and unspecified conditions. Although this perspective did not mediate the effects of planning direction, these findings suggest that another cognitive consequence of backward planning—and one that may sometimes attenuate bias (Boltz & Yum, 2010)—is that it alters perceptions of the flow of time.

Making Plans and Predictions That Influence Behavior

Whereas the preceding strategies focus on altering predictions, an alternative way to increase the accuracy of prediction is to generate plans and predictions in a manner that increases their impact on subsequent behavior. In this regard, Koole and van't Spijker (2000) tested whether prediction bias is reduced through the formation of implementation intentions at the time of prediction. This research drew on the distinction developed by Gollwitzer between goal intentions (i.e., a commitment to a particular goal) and implementation intentions (i.e., a concrete action plan that specifies when, where, and how to act; Gollwitzer, 1999; Gollwitzer & Crosby, Chapter 17, this volume). Student participants were asked to complete a written report within the coming week and to predict when they would start and finish the report.

Participants assigned to the goal-intention condition simply predicted the day they would finish the report, whereas those in the implementation intention condition were asked, in addition, to specify the specific point in time and the location where they would complete it and to commit themselves to their chosen situation by silently saying "I intend to write the report in situation X." Forming these concrete implementation intentions helped to bring behavior in line with predictions. In the goal-intention condition, participants predicted they would start and finish the task earlier than they actually did, but in the implementation-intention condition there was not a significant difference between predicted and actual times. Forming implementation intentions led participants to predict earlier completion times, relative to the goal-intention condition, but had an even greater impact on actual completion times, and thereby reduced the degree of optimistic bias in prediction.

Another related study examined the effect of inducing differing mindsets on both predicted and actual task completion times (Brandstätter, Giesinger, Job, & Frank, 2015, Study 2). This research drew upon the model of action phases (Gollwitzer, 1990, 2012), which postulates that individuals adopt different mindsets during different phases of goal pursuit. Before committing to a goal, people adopt a deliberative mindset focused on appraising pros and cons regarding whether to pursue the goal; after committing to a goal, people adopt an implemental mindset focused on how to implement the goal. Previous research indicates that the implemental mindset enhances people's evaluations of goal desirability and feasibility and thus heightens their motivation to act (for a review, see Gollwitzer, 2012). Accordingly, Brandstätter et al. (2015) proposed that inducing an implemental mindset (vs. deliberative mindset) at the time of prediction would result in earlier predicted and actual task completion times. To induce these mindsets, independently of the target task, participants were asked to identify with a hypothetical individual who was either pondering a decision on a goal (deliberative mindset) or planning the implementation of the goal (implemental mindset). Participants were then assigned the target task—a written report to complete in the next 2 weeks—and asked to predict when it would be submitted. Consistent with hypotheses, participants in an implemental mindset not only predicted that they would finish the report earlier than those in deliberative mindset, but they actually did submit it earlier. Moreover, because the effects of the mindset on prediction and behavior were equivalent, there was no greater tendency to underestimate completion times in the implemental than in the deliberative condition (for a similar pattern of effects, see Armor & Taylor, 2003). The findings suggest that interventions that induce an implemental mindset can heighten people's motivation to act and thereby help to bring behavior in line with ambitious forecasts.

BEYOND TIME: THE PLANNING FALLACY ACROSS DOMAINS

Although this chapter is focused on the planning fallacy in the domain of task completion predictions, we have documented similar processes underlying people's tendency to overestimate the longevity of their romantic relationships (Buehler, Griffin, & Ross, 1995; see also Lavner, Karney, & Bradbury, 2013; MacDonald & Ross, 1999) and the intensity of their emotional reactions to future events (Buehler

& McFarland, 2001). In each case, we find that people's natural inclination to take an inside approach to prediction and to neglect or dismiss the outside approach leaves them prone to bias.

More recently, a program of research has extended the planning fallacy into the realm of personal finance predictions. This work focused in particular on people's predictions of how much money they would spend in the future. In everyday life, people frequently try to estimate future spending—when withdrawing money from the automatic teller machine, when contemplating a vacation, or when planning next month's budget (Peetz, Simmons, Chen, & Buehler, 2016). Research on spending predictions reveals many parallels with time predictions. Just as people underestimate the time they will spend on future tasks, they commonly underestimate how much money they will spend in the future (Peetz & Buehler, 2009, 2012, 2013; Sussman & Alter, 2012; Ülkümen, Thomas, & Morwitz, 2008). Moreover, consistent with classic definitions of the planning fallacy, this bias coexists with the sobering knowledge of past experiences. For example, Peetz and Buehler (2009, Study 1) asked university students to recall how much money they had spent in a previous week, to predict their spending for the upcoming target week, and later to report their actual spending during the target week. Participants predicted that they would spend significantly less in the target week (M = $94) than they remembered spending the previous week (M = $126); however, the amount they ended up spending in the target week (M = $122) was very similar to that of the previous week. As a result, participants underestimated their actual spending for the target week by about 23%. Clearly, these students could have generated more realistic predictions by utilizing their knowledge of previous spending as a basis for prediction.

As with task completion predictions, the tendency to underestimate future spending may be exacerbated when people are motivated to downplay the relevance of past experience. Within the realm of personal finance, a salient directional goal, shared by many, is to minimize expenses, save money, and keep expenditures under control. We hypothesized that such "savings goals" are pervasive and could often bias spending predictions. As it is relatively easy to generate a prediction that corresponds with current goals and intentions but much more difficult to translate these goals into actual spending behavior, reliance on savings goals to generate predictions could contribute to bias. Consistent with this theorizing, we found that participants with stronger savings goals at the time of prediction generated lower—and more biased—predictions of future spending (Peetz & Buehler, 2009).

The preceding findings suggest that the tendency to underestimate future spending may reflect an inside approach to prediction. To predict their spending for the upcoming week, for instance, people may mentally simulate the upcoming week, imagining the expenses they will encounter as the week unfolds. As discussed previously, however, such scenarios tend to be schematic and oversimplified; predictors may focus on a limited set of salient or representative expenses but fail to anticipate many peripheral events that cost money. Accordingly, there may again be potential for unpacking interventions to improve prediction by prompting predictors to break down the target event (e.g., the upcoming week) into its smaller constituent parts before generating an overall prediction. To test this possibility, in four studies we examined the effects of an unpacking manipulation on predicted spending for various upcoming time periods and events (Peetz, Buehler, Koehler,

& Moher, 2015). In each case, prompting participants to unpack the details of expected expenses resulted in increased spending predictions. This helped to curb underestimation bias but sometimes introduced a new bias. In contexts in which predictions were generally too low (e.g., weekly spending), unpacking eliminated the underestimation bias; however, in contexts in which predictions were unbiased to begin with (e.g., spending for a smaller, discrete event), unpacking created an overestimation bias. It appears that unpacking makes predictions bigger, but not necessarily better, and thus its value as a debiasing tool may depend greatly on the context in which it is applied.

Finally, another set of studies (Peetz & Buehler, 2012) identified cognitive processes that may facilitate an outside approach to prediction. Drawing on construal level theory (CLT; Trope & Liberman, 2003), we reasoned that one way to facilitate the outside approach is to induce a high-level construal of the prediction target. Given that high-level construals emphasize the central or invariant features of the target event—features that should be found in any specific instantiation—this should help people to see beyond unique contextual details and locate the event within a broader class of experiences (Ledgerwood, Wakslak, & Wang, 2010). Accordingly, we proposed that high-level construal would facilitate the outside approach to prediction and thereby attenuate optimistic bias. This proposal was tested in two studies that examined people's predicted spending for the upcoming week. As hypothesized, participants induced to adopt a higher level of construal at the time of prediction generated more accurate predictions of their weekly spending, and this effect on prediction was mediated by a greater reliance on past experience (Peetz & Buehler, 2012).

BUT WAIT—IS THERE MORE?

More than 37 years after the publication of the seminal Kahneman and Tversky (1979) paper on the planning fallacy, we and many others continue to discover sources of insight and improvement in the rich and important psychological processes associated with the planning fallacy and the inside–outside approach to prediction. The richness comes partly from the fact that planning and prediction—whether for time or for money—is such an important and defining part of being human and partly from the fact that the associated cognitive biases are so recognizable (and amusing) to many of us. In this spirit, the future has been defined as "that period of time in which our affairs prosper, our friends are true, and our happiness is assured" (Bierce, 1914, p. 12). Despite all the jewels that have already been extracted from the planning fallacy mine, we are sure that there are plenty more still left down there.

REFERENCES

Ansar, A., Flyvbjerg, B., Budzier, A., & Lunn, D. (2014). Should we build more large dams?: The actual costs of hydropower megaproject development. *Energy Policy, 69,* 43–56.

Aranda, J., & Easterbrook, S. (2005). Anchoring and adjustment in software estimation. *Software Engineering Notes, 30,* 346–355.

Ariely, D., & Wertenbroch, K. (2002). Procrastination, deadlines, and performance: Self-control by precommitment. *Psychological Science, 13,* 219–224.

Armor, D. A., & Taylor, S. E. (2003). The effects of mindset on behavior: Self-regulation in deliberative and implemental frames of mind. *Personality and Social Psychology Bulletin, 29,* 86–95.

Bierce, A. (1914). *The devil's dictionary.* New York: World Publishing.

Boltz, M. G., & Yum, Y. N. (2010). Temporal concepts and predicted duration judgments. *Journal of Experimental Social Psychology, 46,* 895–904.

Boroditsky, L. (2000). Metaphoric structuring: Understanding time through spatial metaphors. *Cognition, 75,* 1–28.

Brandstätter, V., Giesinger, L., Job, V., & Frank, E. (2015). The role of deliberative and implemental mindsets in time prediction and task accomplishment. *Social Psychology, 46,* 104–115.

Buehler, R., (1991). *Why individuals underestimate their own task completion times.* Unpublished doctoral dissertation, University of Waterloo, Waterloo, ON, Canada.

Buehler, R., & Griffin, D. (2003). Planning, personality, and prediction: The role of future focus in optimistic time predictions. *Organizational Behavior and Human Decision Processes, 92,* 80–90.

Buehler, R., Griffin, D., Lam, K. C. H., & Deslauriers, J. (2012). Perspectives on prediction: Does third-person imagery improve task completion estimates? *Organizational Behavior and Human Decision Processes, 117,* 138–149.

Buehler, R., Griffin, D., & MacDonald, H. (1997). The role of motivated reasoning in optimistic time predictions. *Personality and Social Psychology Bulletin, 23,* 238–247.

Buehler, R., Griffin, D., & Peetz, J. (2010). The planning fallacy: Cognitive, motivational, and social origins. In M. P. Zanna & J. M. Olson (Eds.), *Advances in experimental social psychology* (Vol. 43, pp. 1–62). San Diego, CA: Academic Press.

Buehler, R., Griffin, D., & Ross, M. (1994). Exploring the "planning fallacy": Why people underestimate their task completion times. *Journal of Personality and Social Psychology, 67,* 366–381.

Buehler, R., Griffin, D., & Ross, M. (1995). It's about time: Optimistic predictions in work and love. In W. Stroebe & M. Hewstone (Eds.), *European review of social psychology* (Volume 6, pp. 1–32). Chichester, UK: Wiley.

Buehler, R., Griffin, D., & Ross, M. (2002). Inside the planning fallacy: The causes and consequences of optimistic time predictions. In T. Gilovich, D. Griffin, & D. Kahneman (Eds.), *Heuristics and biases: The psychology of intuitive judgment* (pp. 250–270). Cambridge, UK: Cambridge University Press.

Buehler, R., & McFarland, C. (2001). Intensity bias in affective forecasting: The role of temporal focus. *Personality and Social Psychology Bulletin, 27,* 1480–1493.

Buehler, R., Peetz, J., & Griffin, D. (2010). Finishing on time: When do predictions influence actual completion times? *Organizational Behaviour and Human Decision Processes, 111,* 23–32.

Byram, S. J. (1997). Cognitive and motivational factors influencing time predictions. *Journal of Experimental Psychology: Applied, 3,* 216–239.

Connolly, T., & Dean, D. (1997). Decomposed versus holistic estimates of effort required for software writing tasks. *Management Science, 43,* 1029–1045.

Deslauriers, J. (2002). *Should we plan for upcoming tasks?: Effects of planning on prediction accuracy for simple and difficult assignments.* Unpublished honors thesis, Wilfrid Laurier University, Waterloo, ON, Canada.

Dunning, D. (2007). Prediction: The inside view. In A. W. Kruglanski & E. T. Higgins (Eds.), *Social psychology: Handbook of basic principles* (2nd ed., pp. 69–90). New York: Guilford Press.

Flyvbjerg, B. (2008). Curbing optimism bias and strategic misrepresentation in planning: Reference class forecasting in practice. *European Planning Studies, 16,* 3–21.

Flyvbjerg, B., Bruzelius, N., & Rothengatter, W. (2003). *Megaprojects and risk: An anatomy of ambition.* Cambridge, UK: Cambridge University Press.

Flyvbjerg, B., Garbuio, M., & Lovallo, D. (2009). Delusion and deception in large infrastructure projects: Two models for explaining and preventing executive disaster. *California Management Review, 51,* 170–193.

Flyvbjerg, B., Holm, M. K. S., & Buhl, S. L. (2004). What causes cost overrun in transport infrastructure projects? *Transport Reviews, 24,* 3–18.

Forsyth, D. K., & Burt, C. D. B. (2008). Allocating time to future tasks: The effect of task segmentation on planning fallacy bias. *Memory and Cognition, 36,* 791–798.

Frank, M. G., & Gilovich, T. (1989). The effect of memory perspective on retrospective causal attributions. *Journal of Personality and Social Personality, 57,* 399–403.

Gollwitzer, P. M. (1990). Action phases and mindsets. In E. T. Higgins & R. M. Sorrentino (Eds.), *Handbook of motivation and cognition* (Vol. 2, pp. 53–92). New York: Guilford Press.

Gollwitzer, P. M. (1999). Implementation intentions: Strong effects of simple plans. *American Psychologist, 54,* 493–503.

Gollwitzer, P. M. (2012). Mindset theory of action phases. In P. Van Lange, A. W. Kruglanski, & E. T. Higgins (Eds.), *Handbook of theories of social psychology* (pp. 526–545). London: SAGE.

Griffin, D., & Buehler, R. (1999). Frequency, probability, and prediction: Easy solutions to cognitive illusions? *Cognitive Psychology, 38,* 48–78.

Griffin, D., & Buehler, R. (2005). Biases and fallacies, memories and predictions: Comment on Roy, Christenfeld, and McKenzie (2005). *Psychological Bulletin, 131,* 757–760.

Griffin, D., Dunning, D., & Ross, L. (1990). The role of construal processes in overconfident predictions about the self and others. *Journal of Personality and Social Psychology, 59,* 1128–1139.

Hadjichristidis, C., Summers, B., & Thomas, K. (2014). Unpacking estimates of task duration: The role of typicality. *Journal of Experimental Social Psychology, 51,* 45–50.

Halkjelsvik, T., & Jørgensen, M. (2012). From origami to software development: A review of studies on judgment-based predictions of performance time. *Psychological Bulletin, 138,* 238–271.

Helzer, E. G., & Dunning, D. (2012). Why and when peer prediction is superior to self-prediction: The weight given to future aspiration versus past achievement. *Journal of Personality and Social Psychology, 103,* 38–53.

Hinds, P. J. (1999). The curse of expertise: The effects of expertise and debiasing methods on predictions of novice performance. *Journal of Experimental Psychology: Applied, 5,* 205–221.

Hoch, S. J. (1985). Counterfactual reasoning and accuracy in predicting personal events. *Journal of Experimental Psychology: Learning, Memory, and Cognition, 11,* 719–731.

Jørgensen, M. (2004). A review of studies on expert estimation of software development effort. *Journal of Systems and Software, 70,* 37–60.

Jørgensen, M., & Grimstad, S. (2008). Avoiding irrelevant and misleading information when estimating development effort. *IEEE Software, 25,* 78–83.

Jørgensen, M., & Sjøberg, D. I. (2004). The impact of customer expectation on software development effort estimates. *International Journal of Project Management, 22,* 317–325.

Kahneman, D. (2011). *Thinking, fast and slow.* New York: Farrar, Straus, & Giroux.

Kahneman, D., & Lovallo, D. (1993). Timid choices and bold forecasts: A cognitive perspective on risk taking. *Management Science, 39,* 17–31.

Kahneman, D., & Tversky, A. (1979). Intuitive prediction: Biases and corrective procedures. *TIMS Studies in Management Science, 12,* 313–327.

Kahneman, D., & Tversky, A. (1982). Intuitive prediction: Biases and corrective procedures. In D. Kahneman, P. Slovic, & A. Tversky (Eds.), *Judgment under uncertainty: Heuristics and biases* (pp. 414–421). Cambridge, UK: Cambridge University Press.

Koehler, D. (1991). Explanation, imagination, and confidence in judgment. *Psychological Bulletin, 110,* 499–519.

Koehler, D., & Poon, C. S. K. (2006). Self-predictions overweight strength of current intentions. *Journal of Experimental Social Psychology, 42,* 517–524.

König, C. J. (2005). Anchors distort estimates of expected duration. *Psychological Reports, 96,* 253–256.

Koole, S., & van't Spijker, M. (2000). Overcoming the planning fallacy through willpower: Effects of implementation intentions on actual and predicted task-completion times. *European Journal of Social Psychology, 30,* 873–888.

Krizan, Z., & Windschitl, P. D. (2007). The influence of outcome desirability on optimism. *Psychological Bulletin, 133,* 95–121.

Kross, E., Ayduk, O., & Mischel, W. (2005). When asking "why" doesn't hurt: Distinguishing rumination from reflective processing of negative emotions. *Psychological Science, 16,* 709–715.

Kruger, J., & Evans, M. (2004). If you don't want to be late, enumerate: Unpacking reduces the planning fallacy. *Journal of Experimental Social Psychology, 40,* 586–598.

Kunda, Z. (1990). The case for motivated reasoning. *Psychological Bulletin, 108,* 480–498.

Lavner, J. A., Karney, B. R., & Bradbury, T. N. (2013). Newlyweds' optimistic forecasts of their marriage: For better or worse? *Journal of Family Psychology, 27,* 531–540.

LeBoeuf, R. A., & Shafir, E. (2009). Anchoring on the "here" and "now" in time and distance judgments. *Journal of Experimental Psychology: Learning, Memory, and Cognition, 35,* 81–93.

Ledgerwood, A., Wakslak, C. J., & Wang, M. A. (2010). Differential information use for near and distant decisions. *Journal of Experimental Social Psychology, 46,* 538–642.

Lewis, J. (2002). *Fundamentals of project management.* New York: Amacom.

Libby, L. K. & Eibach, R. P. (2011). Visual perspective in mental imagery: A representational tool that functions in judgment, emotion, and self-insight. *Advances in Experimental Social Psychology, 44,* 185–245.

Lovallo, D., & Kahneman, D. (2003). Delusions of success: How optimism undermines executives' decisions. *Harvard Business Review, 81,* 56–63.

MacDonald, T. K., & Ross, M. (1999). Assessing the accuracy of predictions about dating relationships: How and why do lovers' predictions differ from those made by observers? *Personality and Social Psychology Bulletin, 25,* 1417–1429.

McIsaac, H. K., & Eich, E. (2002). Vantage point in episodic memory. *Psychonomic Bulletin and Review, 9,* 409–420.

Min, K. S., & Arkes, H. R. (2012). When is difficult planning good planning?: The effects of scenario-based planning on optimistic prediction bias. *Journal of Applied Social Psychology, 42,* 2701–2729.

Moher, E. (2012). *Tempering optimistic bias in temporal prediction: The role of psychological distance in the unpacking effect.* Unpublished doctoral dissertation, University of Waterloo, Waterloo, ON, Canada.

Morwitz, V. G., & Fitzsimons, G. J. (2004). The mere-measurement effect: Why does measuring intentions change behavior? *Journal of Consumer Psychology, 14,* 64–74.

Mulhern, K. (2006). *Self–other differences in task completion predictions: The impact of motivation.* Unpublished honors thesis, Wilfrid Laurier University, Waterloo, ON, Canada.

Newby-Clark, I. R., Ross, M., Buehler, R., Koehler, D., & Griffin, D (2000). People focus on optimistic and disregard pessimistic scenarios while predicting task completion times. *Journal of Experimental Psychology: Applied, 6,* 171–182.

Oettingen, G. (2012). Future thought and behaviour change. *European Review of Social Psychology, 23,* 1–63.

Oettingen, G., & Mayer, D. (2002). The motivating function of thinking about the future: Expectations versus fantasies. *Journal of Personality and Social Psychology, 83,* 1198–1212.

Oettingen, G., & Schwörer, B. (2013). Mind wandering via mental contrasting as a tool for behavior change. *Frontiers in Psychology, 4,* 562.

Peetz, J., & Buehler, R. (2009). Is there a budget fallacy?: The role of savings goals in the prediction of personal spending. *Personality and Social Psychology Bulletin, 35,* 230–242.

Peetz, J., & Buehler, R. (2012). When distance pays off: The role of construal level in spending predictions. *Journal of Experimental Social Psychology, 48,* 395–398.

Peetz, J., & Buehler, R. (2013). Different goals, different predictions: Accuracy and bias in financial planning for events and time periods. *Journal of Applied Social Psychology, 43,* 1079–1088.

Peetz, J., Buehler, R., Koehler, D., & Moher, E. (2015). Bigger not better: Unpacking future expenses inflates spending predictions. *Basic and Applied Social Psychology, 37,* 19–30.

Peetz, J., Buehler, R., & Wilson, A. (2010). Planning for the near and distant future: How does temporal distance affect task completion predictions? *Journal of Experimental Social Psychology, 46,* 709–720.

Peetz, J., Simmons, M., Chen, J., & Buehler, R. (2016). Predictions on the go: Prevalence of spontaneous spending predictions. *Judgment and Decision Making, 11,* 48–61.

Peterson, C., Semmel, A., von Baeyer, C., Abramson, L. Y., Metalski, G. I., & Seligman, M. E. P. (1982). The Attributional Style Questionnaire. *Cognitive Therapy and Research, 6,* 287–299.

Pezzo, S. P., Pezzo, M. V., & Stone, E. R. (2006). The social implications of planning: How public predictions bias future plans. *Journal of Experimental Social Psychology, 42,* 221–227.

Pronin, E., & Ross, L. (2006). Temporal differences in trait self-ascription: When the self is seen as another. *Journal of Personality and Social Psychology, 90,* 197–209.

Roy, M. M., & Christenfeld, N. J. S. (2007). Bias in memory predicts bias in estimation of future task duration. *Memory and Cognition, 35,* 557–564.

Roy, M. M., & Christenfeld, N. J. S. (2008). Effect of task length on remembered and predicted duration. *Psychonomic Bulletin and Review, 15,* 202–207.

Roy, M. M., Christenfeld, N. J., & Jones, M. (2013). Actors, observers, and the estimation of task duration. *Quarterly Journal of Experimental Psychology, 66,* 121–137.

Roy, M. M., Christenfeld, N. J. S., & McKenzie, C. R. M. (2005). Underestimating the duration of future events: Memory incorrectly used or memory bias? *Psychological Bulletin, 131,* 738–756.

Roy, M. M., Mitten, S. T., & Christenfeld, N. J. S (2008). Correcting memory improves accuracy of predicted task duration. *Journal of Experimental Social Psychology: Applied, 14,* 266–275.

Sanna, L. J., & Schwarz, N. (2004). Integrating temporal biases: The interplay of focal thoughts and accessibility experiences. *Psychological Science, 15,* 474–481.

Sevincer, A. T., & Oettingen, G. (2013). Spontaneous mental contrasting and selective goal pursuit. *Personality and Social Psychology Bulletin, 39,* 1240–1254.

Sherman, S. J. (1980). On the self-erasing nature of errors of prediction. *Journal of Personality and Social Psychology, 39,* 211–221.

Shmueli, O., Pliskin, N., & Fink, L. (2015). Can the outside-view approach improve planning decisions in software development projects? *Information Systems Journal, 26,* 395–418.

Strack, F., & Mussweiler, T. (1997). Explaining the enigmatic anchoring effect: Mechanisms of selective accessibility. *Journal of Personality and Social Psychology, 73,* 437–446.

Sussman, A. B., & Alter, A. L. (2012). The exception is the rule: Underestimating and over-spending on exceptional expenses. *Journal of Consumer Research, 39,* 800–814.

Taylor, S. E., Pham, L. B., Rivkin, I. D., & Armor, D. A. (1998). Harnessing the imagination: Mental simulation, self-regulation, and coping. *American Psychologist, 53,* 429–439.

Thomas, K. E., & Handley, S. J. (2008). Anchoring in time estimation. *Acta Psychologica, 127,* 24–29.

Thomas, K. E., Newstead, S. E., & Handley, S. J. (2003). Exploring the time prediction process: The effects of task experience and complexity on prediction accuracy. *Applied Cognitive Psychology, 17,* 655–673.

Trope, Y., & Liberman, N. (2003). Temporal construal. *Psychological Review, 110,* 403–421.

Tversky, A., & Kahneman, D. (1974). Judgment under uncertainty: Heuristics and biases. *Science, 185,* 1124–1131.

Tversky, A., & Shafir, E. (1992). Choice under conflict: The dynamics of deferred decision. *Psychological Science, 3,* 358–361.

Ülkümen, G., Thomas, M., & Morwitz, V. G. (2008). Will I spend more in 12 months or a year?: The effect of ease of estimation and confidence on budget estimates. *Journal of Consumer Research, 35,* 245–256.

Verzuh, E. (2005). *The fast forward MBA in project management: Quick tips, speedy solutions, and cutting-edge ideas.* Hoboken, NJ: Wiley.

Wiese, J., Buehler, R., & Griffin, D. (2016). Backward planning: Effects of planning direction on predictions of task completion time. *Judgment and Decision Making, 11,* 147–167.

Zhang, Y., & Fishbach, A. (2010). Counteracting obstacles with optimistic predictions. *Journal of Experimental Psychology: General, 139,* 16–31.

Index

Note. *f* or *t* following a page number indicates a figure or a table.